THE PEOPLE'S NUTRITION ENCYCLOPEDIA

THE
PEOPLE'S
NUTRITION
ENCYCLOPEDIA

Lynne S. Hill, M.S., R.D.

A PERIGEE BOOK

Perigee Books
are published by
The Putnam Publishing Group
200 Madison Avenue
New York, NY 10016

Typeset by Fisher Composition, Inc.

Library of Congress Cataloging-in-Publication Data

Hill, Lynne S.
   The people's nutrition encyclopedia.

   1. Food—Composition—Popular works.
2. Food—Composition—Tables. I. Title.
[DNLM: 1. Nutritive Value—popular works.   QU 145 H646p]
TX533.H55   1986   641.1   86-12342
ISBN 0-399-51289-6

Printed in the United States of America

        4   5   6   7   8   9   10

Acknowledgments

Compiling this type of book cannot be successfully accomplished without the support of a team of enthusiastic and hardworking individuals. If the contributions of any of the following individuals were absent, the task would have been much more difficult.

Much appreciation goes to the team at Hill Nutrition Associates who were so generous with their caring, time and help.

Beverly Bumbaugh and Marie Mahar have been invaluable aides in keeping the normal flow of work under control and providing extra efforts on the book, as needed. Nancy Frent and Nancy Sleezer, R.D., provided extra help with the typing and proofing of the manuscript at the same time they maintained their normal work. Julia Bumbaugh's accurate data input during her college vacations was much appreciated.

Invaluable resources outside of the company included Lida Dawson Price, who spent hours with me proofing the final manuscript, and Jodi Kearns, R.D., who reviewed the nutritional information content of the introduction.

A special thanks goes to Judy Linden of Putnam Publishing who conceived of this encyclopedia and put the idea and the author together.

As any author knows, the whole family gets involved with a book in one way or another. Much appreciation goes to each one of them for their contributions: Bill who combined the reassurance of a husband and the advice of a fellow dietitian; Douglas, our son, who got us into, and out of, computer difficulties with the book at any time of the day or night; Suzanne, our daughter, who, although too young to help with the book, undertook many household responsibilities to free me to write.

Last but certainly not least is appreciation for the love and encouragement from other family members and a special group of friends, whose unfailing support enabled me to complete this publication.

To Bill, Douglas and Suzanne, with love

CONTENTS

Introduction

The People's Nutrition Encyclopedia provides information on the nutritional composition of over 9,000 commonly eaten foods, including fresh, processed, kosher and fast foods. The ten nutrients listed for each food commonly concern people on special diets or those who want to be informed about what they are eating. Calories and values for protein, fat and carbohydrate are presented for dieters and diabetics. The sodium, fat and cholesterol values usually interest individuals with cardiac or circulation problems. Calcium and iron information is especially helpful to women who are trying to maintain adequate levels of intake. Information on fiber is supplied because of its probable role in preventing cancer and other intestinal diseases.

A Note on the Data

The more than 9,000 foods listed in this book include representative foods from the United States Department of Agriculture data and from manufacturers. Many food manufacturers were contacted and most cooperated by sending analyses of their products. Other companies, however, refused to provide data. Either they lacked analyses of their products or were unwilling to have their data published.

Some products do not provide data on all ten nutrients. Missing information is marked by a dash (—) in the column for that nutrient. Don't assume that a dash is a zero.

All product information is correct as of publication, but please realize that manufacturers may change their product formulas at any time, thereby affecting nutritional content.

How to Use This Book

1. Foods are arranged in chapters of general food groups such as Baked Goods; Beans and Legumes; Breakfast Items. Each food group or

chapter is broken down alphabetically into its specific types (for example, Chapter 1, Baked Goods, includes bagels, biscuits, etc.), then further subdivided alphabetically by manufacturer. Nutritional values accompany different product varieties sold by the manufacturers.

2. When there is no manufacturer, as in the case of unprocessed and generic foods, items are listed under USDA (United States Department of Agriculture) as the source of the data.

3. All food values except those for fiber and iron are rounded to the nearest whole number.

4. Missing data is marked with a dash (—).

5. An asterisk (*) means there is less than 2 percent of the U.S. Recommended Dietary Allowance for the nutrient.

6. Cholesterol is present only in foods from animal sources. If a food is entirely from non-animal sources, it can be assumed that the cholesterol value is zero. There may be cholesterol in foods containing dairy products or other animal fats.

7. Portions are listed both by weight and by common household measures whenever both are available.

8. All meat, poultry and seafood values refer to only the edible portion; the weight of bones and shells are not included.

9. All foods prepared from mixes are made according to the manufacturer's directions.

10. The use of a straightedge makes reading across lines of numbers easier.

Dietary Guidelines

The dietary guidelines listed below are from a booklet published in 1985 by the federal government titled *Nutrition and Your Health: Dietary Guidelines for Americans.* Based on the best medical research, they offer general suggestions for maximizing nutritional health. Nevertheless, they are subject to change as more information becomes available. The guidelines are suggested for healthy individuals. Persons with diseases or conditions that affect normal nutrient requirements are advised to check with a physician or registered dietitian.

Even though nutritional guidelines do not guarantee good health, they provide a sensible eating plan. Other factors that affect a person's health are heredity, environment, life-style and mental attitude.

"Eat a Variety of Foods"

Although *The People's Nutrition Encyclopedia* lists the nutrient values for ten nutrients, over forty nutrients are known to be essential to good health. Different combinations of vitamins and minerals are found in each food group: grains and enriched breads; fruits and vegetables; meats, poultry and fish; fats; and dairy products. Eating a wide variety of foods within each group assures that you'll get the nutrients you need.

"Maintain Desirable Weight"

Since obesity is linked to diseases such as adult onset diabetes, cardiovascular disease and others, it is important to maintain a desirable weight level. When attempting to lose weight, the loss should be kept to a steady one to two pounds a week. Fad diets should be avoided. Excess weight is generally put on over a period of time, and is most successfully lost slowly. Rapid weight loss is usually followed by an equally rapid return of the weight.

The fuel the body uses is measured in calories. Calories are provided by carbohydrates, fats, protein and alcohol. There are approximately 3,500 calories in a pound of body fat. It follows that a person must eat 3,500 calories less than needed to lose a pound. An alternative is increasing activity in order to burn off 3,500 additional calories to lose a pound.

"Avoid Too Much Fat, Saturated Fat and Cholesterol"

Diets high in saturated fats or cholesterol and those which provide excess calories increase blood cholesterol levels. Avoid this by limiting the use of fats. Lean meats, fish, poultry, peas and beans are low-fat protein sources. Skim and low-fat cheeses and milks provide the benefits of dairy products without the high fat level of their creamier counterparts. Only moderate amounts of egg yolk, organ meats, butter, lard, heavily hydrogenated oils, palm or coconut oils should be consumed; fried foods should be avoided.

"Eat Foods with Adequate Starch and Fiber"

An adequate diet contains complex carbohydrates, grains and whole-grain breads, fruits, vegetables, dry peas and beans, and potatoes instead of simple sugars such as refined sugar, candy or syrups. Foods high in complex carbohydrates offer more vitamins, minerals and fiber per calorie than do refined foods.

Fiber, the undigestible part of plant foods, is thought to play a role in reducing the risk of several diseases such as chronic constipation, some types of "irritable bowel syndrome," diverticular disease and possibly some forms of cancer. It is thought that the risk of developing such diseases can be lowered by increasing the fiber in the diet.

"Avoid Too Much Sugar"

The risk of tooth decay is lowered by limiting high-sugar foods in the diet. When eaten between meals, sugary foods stick to the teeth, increasing the risk of tooth decay. Cakes, candies, dried fruits, sugary snacks and sugar-sweetened soft drinks all contain simple sugars.

"Avoid Too Much Sodium"

Sodium in small quantities is an essential nutrient, but excess sodium in the diet is hazardous to the one in four adults with elevated blood pressure. Sodium is most commonly found in table salt, but is also present in processed foods, condiments, most cheeses, cured meats, pickled foods, salty snacks, baking powders, baking soda, MSG (monosodium glutamate), other additives and some medications such as antacids.

To lower sodium intake, it is necessary to avoid salty foods and highly processed foods such as cured meats and processed cheeses, to cook without salt, and to use products canned without salt. To make a low-sodium diet appealing, herbs, spices, lemon juice, vinegar and other low-sodium flavorings should be used to add flavor to food.

"If You Drink Alcoholic Beverages, Do So in Moderation"

Alcoholic beverages are high in calories and low in nutrients. Heavy drinkers can develop nutrient deficiencies as well as diseases such as cirrhosis of the liver and some forms of cancer. (Cigarette smoking also increases these risks.) Pregnant women should avoid alcoholic beverages. About equal amounts of alcohol are contained in 12 ounces of beer, 5 ounces of wine and 1½ ounces of distilled spirits.

Recommended Dietary Allowances

The Recommended Dietary Allowances (RDAs) are determined by the Committee on Dietary Allowances of the Food and Nutrition Board of the National Academy of Sciences. They are established to set a standard level of intake to meet the needs of groups of persons, not individuals. They are intended to be met by diets containing a variety of foods and not by supplements. Levels are set by age and sex. The requirements quoted in this book are from the most recent revision (1980).

The RDAs are combined to form the U.S. RDAs which are used for food labeling. To allow for individual differences, they represent amounts in excess of the minimum amount of a nutrient required to assure good health, and represents the highest RDA for children age four and older through adult. It allows shoppers to easily gauge the quality of their food choices, permitting easy comparisons between foods.

The Nutrients in this Book

Calories

Calories are a measure of the energy in a food. Energy is needed for all body functions. When the number of calories eaten equals the calories used by the body, weight stays constant. When activity requirements exceed caloric intake, weight loss results. Weight gain occurs when extra calories are stored in the form of body fat. Since there are approximately 3,500 calories in one pound of fat, lowering the normal caloric intake by 500 calories per day should result in a weight loss of one pound per week. Increasing caloric requirements through exercise while eating the same number of calories will also result in weight loss. To gain weight, more calories than the body needs must be eaten.

Recommended levels. The recommended levels for calories are based on the "reference man" (5′ 10″ tall and 154 pounds) and the "reference woman" (5′ 4″ tall and 120 pounds). Recommended allowances change with age. For men the average levels vary from 2,900 calories daily for a 19- to 22-year-old to 2,050 calories for a man of 76 years or older. A 19- to 22-year-old "reference woman" should consume about 2,100 calories daily. By age 76 the level is reduced to 1,600 calories. Body size and activity levels, in addition to age and sex, affect caloric requirements.

Protein

Protein is made up of amino acids, the "building blocks" of the body. Proteins from animal sources are usually "complete," having all the amino acids needed by humans, while plants contain "incomplete" proteins. Plant proteins should be combined in the diet with other, complementary plant proteins. Two such proteins will each supply the amino acids missing in the other.

Functions. Protein is
   a. A component of all body cells, antibodies and enzymes
   b. Essential for growth
   c. Necessary for repair and maintenance of cells
   d. A source of energy when too few calories are available from carbohydrate or fat

Sources. Complete protein is found in meat, fish, eggs, poultry and dairy products. Incomplete protein occurs in dried peas and beans, nuts, cereals and breads.

Recommended levels. The recommended protein level is based on body weight and whether the proteins in the diet are complete. The recommendation for a diet which combines both complete and incomplete proteins is .8 gram of protein per kilogram (2.2 pounds) of body weight.

Fat

Fat is the most concentrated form of energy. Fats are made up of saturated, monounsaturated, and polyunsaturated fatty acids and cholesterol. Saturated fats usually come from animal sources or coconut or palm oil. Polyunsaturated and monounsaturated fats come from the other vegetable oils.

Functions. Fat
  a. Maintains body heat
  b. Provides padding for body organs
  c. Aids in the absorption of fat soluble vitamins
  d. Provides a feeling of satiety after eating

Sources. Animal fats from meats, fish, poultry, butter and lard; vegetable oils and margarines; whole milk, cream and whole-milk cheeses; and fried foods.

Recommended levels. Although there is no specifically recommended level, the government's dietary goals recommend that fat consumption be reduced to a reasonable level and that consumption of saturated fats and cholesterol be limited.

Carbohydrates

Carbohydrates are found in foods in the form of simple sugars, complex carbohydrates and fiber. Carbohydrates are broken down into simple sugars during digestion so they can be absorbed. The remaining undigested material from plants is fiber.

Functions. Carbohydrates
  a. Are a source of energy for the body
  b. Spare protein from being used as an energy source
  c. Are a source of fiber

Sources. Grains, flours, cereals, baked goods, sugars, pastas, vegetables, fruits, dried peas and beans.

Recommended levels. There are no specific recommended levels, although it is suggested that the intake of complex carbohydrates be increased and simple sugars decreased.

Fiber

Fiber is non-digestible carbohydrate. There are five types of fiber: cellulose, hemicellulose, pectin, lignin and gums. Fiber absorbs water and adds bulk, making waste matter pass more quickly through the intestines. Interest in fiber has increased because of the apparent link between low-fiber diets and diseases of the digestive tract. Recent studies also have shown possible relationships between low-fiber diets and cardiovascular diseases, certain cancers and diabetes.

Fiber values are reported in different ways. *Crude fiber* is the fiber remaining after a food is dissolved, first in a strong acid, and then in a strong base. Crude fiber is primarily lignin and cellulose. *Dietary fiber* refers to that fiber not digested by the enzymes in the gastrointestinal tract. The latter category includes more types of fiber than that of crude, and it is thought to be a more helpful indication of fiber for use in nutrition. Most fiber analyses in the past have centered on crude fiber, although more work now is being done on dietary fiber. The letter *d* following a value for fiber in this book indicates that the value is for dietary fiber. Otherwise the value listed is for crude fiber.

Functions. Fiber provides bulk in the intestines, and helps prevent constipation.

Sources. Fruits, vegetables and whole-grain products.

Recommended levels. There is no specific recommendation; however, it is recommended that fiber in the average American diet be increased.

Calcium

Calcium recently has received increased attention because of the discovery of its relationship to osteoporosis and a possible link with high blood pressure.

Functions. Calcium is necessary to
  a. The structure of teeth and bones
  b. Muscle activity
  c. Nervous system activity
  d. Blood clotting
  e. Enzyme activity
  f. Lactation

Sources. Dairy foods, green leafy vegetables, canned salmon and sardines with bones, and raw oysters.

Requirements.

Infants	0–.5 year	360 mg
	.5–1 year	540 mg
Children	1–10 years	800 mg
Males	11–18 years	1,200 mg
	19+ years	800 mg
Females	11–18 years	1,200 mg
	19+ years	800 mg
(Pregnant or lactating, add 400 mg)		
USRDA		1,000 mg

Iron

Iron is found in foods in two forms, heme and non-heme iron. Heme iron is found only in meat and is absorbed better by the body than non-heme iron. Intake of vitamin C improves the body's ability to absorb iron.

Functions. Iron is needed for hemoglobin, the oxygen-carrying component of the blood, and for proper functioning of respiratory enzymes. A deficiency leads to iron-deficiency anemia.

Sources. Variety meats, lean meats, egg yolks, green leafy vegetables, whole-grain and enriched cereals and baked goods.

Requirements.

Infants	0–.5 year	10 mg
	.5–1 year	15 mg
Children	1–3 years	15 mg
	4–10 years	10 mg
Males	11–18 years	18 mg
	19+ years	10 mg
Females	11–50 years	18 mg
	51+ years	10 mg
(Supplementation is recommended for pregnant and lactating women)		
USRDA		18 mg

Sodium

Sodium is found in the fluids surrounding each body cell (extracellular fluids). Since the volume of extracellular fluids is determined largely by the amount of sodium in the body, sodium is frequently restricted in the case of high blood pressure and cardiac conditions. High blood pressure is a risk factor in strokes, coronary heart disease and kidney failure. Normally the kidneys remove excess sodium from the body. When the kidneys do not function properly, sodium in the diet must be restricted.

Functions. Sodium is necessary for
   a. Maintenance of fluid and acid-base balances
   b. Conduction of nerve impulses
   c. Carbohydrate and protein metabolism

Sources. Table salt, pickles, cured meats, processed foods, cheeses and condiments.

Requirements. Although there are no Recommended Dietary Allowances for sodium, there are Recommended Safe and Adequate Daily Dietary Intake levels.

Infants	0–.5 year	115–350 mg
	.5–1 year	250–750 mg
Children and Adolescents	1–3 years	325–975 mg
	4–6 years	450–1,350 mg
	7–10 years	600–1,800 mg
	11+ years	900–2,700 mg
Adults		1,100–3,300 mg

Potassium

Potassium is found in the fluids within body cells (intracellular fluids). The body must maintain a balance between sodium and potassium in order to maintain normal blood pressure.

Functions. Potassium is needed for
   a. Fluid balance and volume
   b. Carbohydrate metabolism
   c. Muscle contractions
   d. Protein synthesis
   e. Nerve impulse conduction

Sources. Fruits, especially bananas, apricots, prunes and cantaloupe; vegetables, especially potatoes, tomatoes, sweet potatoes, and dark green, leafy vegetables; and meats, fish and cereals.

Requirements. Estimated Safe and Adequate Levels

Infants	0–.5 year	350–925 mg
	.5–1 year	425–1,275 mg
Children and Adolescents	1–3 years	550–1,650 mg
	4–6 years	775–2,325 mg
	7–10 years	1,000–3,000 mg
	11+ years	1,525–4,575 mg
Adults		1,875–5,625 mg

Cholesterol

Cholesterol is synthesized in the body as well as obtained through the diet. It is an essential part of the body but excess intake is harmful. The only foods containing cholesterol come from animal sources.

Cholesterol in the diet is one of the factors found to affect the blood cholesterol level. High serum cholesterol is a risk factor in atherosclerosis and coronary heart disease.

Functions. Cholesterol is a part of all cell membranes, and is a precursor for hormones, including the sex hormones, estrogen and testosterone, as well as a precursor for vitamin D.

Sources. Egg yolks, organ meats, cream, whole milk and animal fats such as butter and lard.

Requirements. There is no minimum amount needed since the body will make cholesterol when it is absent from the diet.

Abbreviations

bkd	baked
c	cup
ckd	cooked
cnd	canned
cond	condensed
d	dietary (fiber)
dehyd	dehydrated
dr	drained
env	envelope
ep	edible portion
fr	fresh
fz	frozen
gm	gram
imit	imitation
ls	low sodium
pkg	package
pkt	packet
prep	prepared according to manufacturer's directions
rts	ready to serve
sc	sauce
sl	slice
s&l	solids & liquids
tbsp	tablespoon
tsp	teaspoon
tr	trace
unsw	unsweetened
<	less than

Conversions

Fluid

```
3 tsp  = 1 tablespoon (tbsp)
2 tbsp = 1 fluid ounce (oz)
8 oz   = 1 cup (c)
4 c    = 1 quart (qt)
4 qt   = 1 gallon
```

Weight

```
1 weighed ounce (oz) = 28.35 grams (gm)
16 weighed ounces = 1 pound (lb)
1 pound = 454 grams
```

THE
PEOPLE'S
NUTRITION
ENCYCLOPEDIA

1

BAKED GOODS

FOOD & DESCRIPTION MEASURE OR QUANTITY	CALORIES	PROTEIN (GM)	FAT (GM)	CARBO-HYDRATE (GM)	FIBER (GM)	CALCIUM (MG)	IRON (MG)	SODIUM (MG)	POTASSIUM (MG)	CHO-LESTEROL (MG)
Bagels										
Lender's										
EGG BAGELS, 2 oz	150	7	1	29	—	20	1.08	360	—	5
GARLIC BAGELS, 2 oz	160	6	1	32	—	*	2.70	340	—	0
ONION BAGELETTES, .9 oz	70	3	<1	14	—	*	.36	135	—	0
ONION BAGELS, 2 oz	160	7	1	31	—	40	1.08	290	—	0
PLAIN BAGELETTES .9 oz	70	3	<1	13	—	*	.36	170	—	0
PLAIN BAGELS, 2 oz	150	6	1	30	—	20	1.08	320	—	0
POPPY SEED BAGELS, 2 oz	150	7	1	29	—	20	1.44	370	—	0
PUMPERNICKEL BAGELS, 2 oz	160	6	1	31	—	20	1.44	330	—	0
RAISIN 'N HONEY BAGELS, 2½ oz	200	8	1	40	—	20	1.44	310	—	0
RAISIN 'N WHEAT BAGELS, 2½ oz	190	6	1	39	—	20	1.44	310	—	0
RYE BAGELS, 2 oz	150	6	1	30	—	40	1.44	310	—	0
SESAME SEED BAGELS, 2 oz	160	7	1	31	—	40	1.08	320	—	0
Sara Lee										
CINNAMON & RAISIN, 1 bagel	240	8	2	47	—	*	2.70	260	—	—
EGG BAGEL, 1 bagel	240	9	2	46	—	*	3.60	390	—	—
ONION BAGEL, 1 bagel	220	9	1	44	—	*	3.60	560	—	—
PLAIN BAGEL, 1 bagel	230	9	1	45	—	*	2.70	500	—	—
POPPY SEED BAGEL, 1 bagel	230	9	1	45	—	20	3.60	560	—	—
Biscuits										
Arrowhead Mills										
BISCUIT MIX, prep, 2 oz	100	4	1	19	—	—	—	170	—	—
Jiffy										
BAKING MIX, prep, 1 biscuit	110	3	3	18	—	*	1.08	335	—	—
BUTTERMILK BISCUIT MIX, prep, 1 biscuit	180	4	5	30	—	*	1.62	655	—	—
Pillsbury										
BALLARD OVENREADY, 2 biscuits	100	3	1	20	—	0	1.08	360	210	—
BUTTERMILK, 2 biscuits	100	3	1	20	—	0	1.08	360	210	—
BIG COUNTRY										
BUTTERMILK, 2 biscuits	200	4	8	29	—	0	1.08	650	180	—
SOUTHERN STYLE, 2 biscuits	200	4	8	29	—	0	1.08	650	180	—

FOOD & DESCRIPTION MEASURE OR QUANTITY	CALORIES	PROTEIN (GM)	FAT (GM)	CARBO-HYDRATE (GM)	FIBER (GM)	CALCIUM (MG)	IRON (MG)	SODIUM (MG)	POTASSIUM (MG)	CHOLES-TEROL (MG)
BIG PREMIUM										
HEAT 'N EAT BUTTERMILK, 2 biscuits	280	5	15	32	—	20	1.44	610	75	—
BUTTER, 2 biscuits	100	3	1	20	—	0	1.08	360	210	—
BUTTERMILK, 2 biscuits	100	3	1	20	—	0	1.08	360	210	—
COUNTRY, 2 biscuits	100	3	1	20	—	0	1.08	360	210	—
1869 Brand										
BAKING POWDER, 2 biscuits	200	4	8	27	—	20	1.08	590	60	—
BUTTERMILK, 2 biscuits	200	4	8	27	—	20	1.08	590	60	—
BUTTER TASTIN', 2 biscuits	200	4	8	27	—	20	1.08	590	55	—
EXTRA LIGHTS FLAKY BUTTERMILK, 2 biscuits	110	2	4	18	—	0	.72	340	200	—
GOOD 'N BUTTERY BIG COUNTRY, 2 biscuits	190	4	8	27	—	0	1.08	650	180	—
HEAT 'N EAT BUTTERMILK, 2 biscuits	170	4	5	27	—	20	1.08	530	55	—
HUNGRY JACK										
BUTTER TASTIN' FLAKY, 2 biscuits	180	3	9	23	—	0	1.08	550	30	—
BUTTERMILK FLAKY, 2 biscuits	170	3	7	25	—	0	1.08	590	40	—
BUTTERMILK FLUFFY, 2 biscuits	180	3	8	24	—	0	1.44	560	35	—
EXTRA RICH BUTTERMILK, 2 biscuits	110	2	3	19	—	0	.72	350	200	—
FLAKY, 2 biscuits	170	3	7	24	—	0	1.44	590	35	—
TENDERFLAKE										
BAKING POWDER, 2 biscuits	110	2	5	14	—	0	.72	360	20	—
BUTTERMILK, 2 biscuits	110	2	5	14	—	0	.72	340	20	—
USDA										
BISCUIT, 2″ diam, 1¼″ high, 1 biscuit										
made with enriched flour, 1 oz, 28 gm	103	2	5	13	—	34	.40	175	33	—
made with self-rising enriched flour, 1 oz, 28 gm	104	2	5	13	—	59	.50	185	18	—
BISCUIT MIX with enriched flour, dry, 1 c, 120 gm	509	9	15	82	—	32	3.70	1560	96	—
1 biscuit, made with milk, 2″ diam, 1¼″ high, 1 oz, 28 gm	91	2	3	15	—	19	.60	272	32	—
Weight Watchers										
BUTTERMILK BISCUITS, 2 biscuits, 37 gm	80	2	1	16	—	9	.60	346	87	—
WHEAT BISCUITS, 2 biscuits, 37 gm	80	2	1	16	—	9	.80	379	56	—

Breads & Rolls

Arrowhead Mills

CORN BREAD MIX, prep, 1 oz	100	4	1	19	—	—	—	220	—	—
MULTIGRAIN MIX, prep, 2 oz	150	6	2	29	—	—	—	225	—	—
WHOLE WHEAT MIX, prep, 2 oz	150	6	2	27	—	—	—	225	—	—

Aunt Jemima–Quaker

CORN BREAD, ⅙ bread	205	4	6	34	.10	15	1.48	519	55	—

FOOD & DESCRIPTION MEASURE OR QUANTITY	CALORIES	PROTEIN (GM)	FAT (GM)	CARBO-HYDRATE (GM)	FIBER (GM)	CALCIUM (MG)	IRON (MG)	SODIUM (MG)	POTASSIUM (MG)	CHOLES-TEROL (MG)
Ballard–Pillsbury										
CORN BREAD, prep, ⅛ recipe	140	3	3	25	—	0	.36	570	75	—
Chico-San										
RICE CAKES, sodium free, 1 cake, 9.3 gm	35	1	0	8	—	*	*	0	25	—
RICE CAKES, very low sodium, 1 cake, 9.3 gm	35	1	0	8	—	*	*	10	25	—
Continental Baking										
CINNAMON RAISIN, 1 sl, 1 oz	80	2	1	15	.10	20	.72	140	—	<5
DICARLO										
PARISIAN FRENCH, 1 sl, 1 oz	70	3	1	13	.10	40	.72	180	—	<5
SOUR DOUGH, 1 sl, 1 oz	70	3	1	12	.10	20	.72	140	—	0
FRESH & NATURAL WHEAT, 1 sl, 1 oz	70	3	1	13	.40	0	.72	140	—	0
FRESH HORIZONS										
WHEAT, 1 sl, 1 oz	50	3	1	10	2.10	40	1.08	140	—	0
WHITE, 1 sl, 1 oz	50	3	1	10	2.10	40	1.08	140	—	0
HEARTY/MILD RYE, 1 sl, 1 oz	70	3	1	13	.10	40	1.08	180	—	<5
HILLBILLY, 1 sl, 1 oz	70	3	1	14	.10	40	1.08	140	—	<5
HOLLYWOOD										
DARK, 1 sl, 1 oz	70	3	1	13	.30	40	1.08	160	—	<5
LIGHT, 1 sl, 1 oz	70	3	1	13	.10	40	1.08	150	—	<5
HOME PRIDE										
DINNER ROLLS, 1 roll, 1 oz	80	2	2	14	.10	40	.72	170	—	<5
7 GRAIN, 1 sl, 1 oz	70	3	1	13	.10	20	1.08	140	—	<5
WHEATBERRY, 1 sl, 1 oz	70	3	1	12	.40	40	1.08	160	—	<5
HOME PRIDE BUTTERTOP										
WHEAT, 1 sl, 1 oz	70	3	1	13	.20	40	.72	140	—	<5
WHITE, 1 sl, 1 oz	70	3	1	13	.10	40	.72	160	—	<5
ROMAN MEAL, 1 sl, 1 oz	70	3	1	13	.40	40	1.08	140	—	<5
WONDER										
BROWN 'N SERVE ROLLS										
GEM STYLE, 1 roll, 1 oz	80	2	2	13	.10	40	.72	140	—	<5
HALF & HALF, 1 roll, 1 oz	80	2	2	13	.10	40	.72	140	—	<5
HOME BAKE, 1 roll, 1 oz	80	2	2	13	.10	40	.72	130	—	<5
WITH BUTTERMILK, 1 roll, 1 oz	80	2	2	13	.10	40	.72	140	—	<5
CRACKED WHEAT, 1 sl, 1 oz	70	3	1	13	.20	40	.72	180	—	<5
FAMILY ITALIAN, 1 sl, 1 oz	70	2	1	13	.10	40	1.08	160	—	<5
FAMILY WHEAT, 1 sl, 1 oz	70	3	1	13	.20	40	1.08	140	—	<5
FRENCH, 1 sl, 1 oz	70	3	1	13	.10	40	1.08	180	—	0
HAMBURGER BUNS, 1 bun, 1 oz	80	2	1	14	.10	40	.72	150	—	<5
HOT DOG ROLLS, 1 roll, 1 oz	80	2	1	14	.10	40	.72	150	—	<5
HOAGIE ROLLS, 1 roll, 5 oz	400	13	7	73	.50	200	5.40	840	—	<5
100% WHOLE WHEAT, 1 sl, 1 oz	70	3	1	12	.40	20	1.08	160	—	<5
PAN, DINNER or BISCUITS, 1 oz	80	2	1	14	.10	40	.72	140	—	<5
SOFT 100% WHOLE WHEAT, 1 sl, 1 oz	70	4	1	10	.40	20	1.08	140	—	0
WHITE, 1 sl, 1 oz	70	3	1	13	.10	40	.72	140	—	<5
WHITE WITH BUTTERMILK, 1 sl, 1 oz	70	2	1	13	.10	40	1.08	160	—	<5
Dromedary–Nabisco										
CORN BREAD MIX, prep, 2 × 2″	130	3	3	20	—	60	1.08	480	65	—
DATE NUT ROLL, ½″ sl	80	1	2	13	—	20	.36	160	60	—

FOOD & DESCRIPTION MEASURE OR QUANTITY	CALORIES	PROTEIN (GM)	FAT (GM)	CARBO- HYDRATE (GM)	FIBER (GM)	CALCIUM (MG)	IRON (MG)	SODIUM (MG)	POTASSIUM (MG)	CHOLES- TEROL (MG)
El Saha Pocket Bread										
CINNAMON RAISIN, 5″ diam, 2 oz	174	5	<1	37	—	17	1.62	331	—	—
ONION, 6″ diam, 2 oz	178	6	<1	37	—	12	1.58	364	—	—
WHITE, 6″ diam, 2 oz	174	5	<1	37	—	10	1.55	363	—	—
WHOLE WHEAT, 6″ diam, 2 oz	167	6	<1	35	—	16	1.66	364	—	—
Finn Crisp—Wasa										
DARK, 22 gm, 4 pieces	80	2	0	17	3.60d	7	.92	238	15	—
WITH CARAWAY SEEDS, 22 gm, 4 pieces	80	2	0	17	3.60d	7	.92	238	15	—
LIGHT, 20.3 gm, 4 pieces	70	5	1	14	1.60d	5	1.05	186	10	—
Home Hearth—Nabisco										
FRENCH BREAD MIX, prep, 2⅜″ sl	170	6	3	29	—	*	.36	320	70	—
OLD FASHIONED WHITE BREAD MIX, prep, 2⅜″ sl	150	6	1	29	—	*	.36	260	70	—
RYE BREAD MIX, prep, 2⅜″ sl	150	6	1	28	—	20	.72	360	90	—
Ideal—Wasa										
EXTRA-THIN, 9.4 gm, 3 pieces	36	1	0	8	.35d	—	.19	52	47	—
FIBER, 8.8 gm, 2 pieces	34	1	0	8	1.40d	—	.27	78	44	—
WHOLE GRAIN NO SALT, 9.3 gm, 2 pieces	36	1	0	8	.87d	—	.29	<1	—	—
Mrs. Dash—Alberto Culver										
COATING MIX, ¼ env, .6 oz	63	5	<1	10	—	—	—	3	229	0
Old London—Borden										
BACON ROUNDS, 5 rounds, ½ oz	60	2	2	9	—	*	.36	130	35	—
CHEESE ROUNDS, 5 rounds, ½ oz	60	2	2	9	—	*	.36			—
GARLIC ROUNDS, 5 rounds, ½ oz	50	2	1	9	—	*	.36	130	25	—
ONION ROUNDS, 5 rounds, ½ oz	50	2	1	9	—	*	.36	160	25	—
PUMPERNICKEL MELBA TOAST, 3 sl, ½ oz	50	2	0	10	—	*	.36	—	—	—
RYE MELBA TOAST, 3 sl, ½ oz	50	2	0	10	—	*	.36	—	—	—
SALTY RYE, 5 rounds, ½ oz	50	2	1	9	—	*	.36	—	—	—
SESAME ROUNDS, 5 rounds, ½ oz	60	2	2	8	—	20	.72	160	25	—
TOASTED BREAD CRUMBS, reg style, 2 oz	210	7	2	40	—	60	1.44	—	—	—
WHITE MELBA TOAST, 3 sl, ½ oz	50	2	0	10	—	*	.36	—	—	—
UNSALTED, 3 sl, ½ oz	50	2	0	10	—	*	.36	5	—	—
WHOLE GRAIN MELBA TOAST, 3 sl, ½ oz	60	2	1	10	—	*	.36	130	30	—
Pepperidge Farm—Campbell										
BUTTER CRESCENT ROLLS, 1 roll	110	2	6	13	—	20	.72	160	—	—
CINNAMON, 2 sl	170	4	4	27	—	20	1.44	200	—	—

FOOD & DESCRIPTION MEASURE OR QUANTITY	CALORIES	PROTEIN (GM)	FAT (GM)	CARBO-HYDRATE (GM)	FIBER (GM)	CALCIUM (MG)	IRON (MG)	SODIUM (MG)	POTASSIUM (MG)	CHOLES-TEROL (MG)
CLUB BROWN 'N SERVE										
ROLLS, 1 roll	100	3	1	20	—	40	1.08	220	—	—
CRACKED WHEAT, 2 sl	140	4	2	26	—	20	1.44	290	—	—
DIJON RYE, 2 sl	110	4	2	18	—	40	1.80	340	—	—
FAMILY PUMPERNICKEL, 2 sl	160	6	2	30	—	40	1.80	610	—	—
FAMILY RYE, 2 sl	170	6	2	31	—	40	1.80	490	—	—
FRENCH STYLE ROLLS, 1 roll	110	4	1	19	—	40	.72	250	—	—
GOLDEN TWIST ROLLS, 1 roll	110	2	6	14	—	20	.72	160	—	—
HAMBURGER ROLLS, 1 roll	130	4	3	21	—	40	1.08	260	—	—
HONEY BRAN, 2 sl	190	5	2	36	—	20	1.80	350	—	—
MULTI-GRAIN, very thin, 2 sl	80	3	1	14	—	*	.72	150	—	—
OATMEAL, 2 sl	140	4	3	25	—	40	1.44	370	—	—
ONION SANDWICH BUNS with										
poppy seeds, 1 roll	150	5	3	26	—	40	1.80	240	—	—
PARKER HOUSE ROLLS, 1 roll	50	2	1	9	—	20	.36	90	—	—
PARTY ROLLS, 1 roll	30	1	1	5	—	*	.36	50	—	—
RAISIN WITH CINNAMON, 2 sl	150	4	3	28	—	20	1.08	190	—	—
SANDWICH ROLLS with										
sesame seeds, 1 roll	130	5	3	23	—	40	1.80	210	—	—
SANDWICH WHITE, 2 sl	130	4	2	23	—	40	1.08	270	—	—
SEEDLESS RYE, 2 sl	160	6	2	31	—	40	1.80	500	—	—
SOURDOUGH STYLE FRENCH										
ROLLS, 1 roll	100	4	1	19	—	20	1.08	240	—	—
TOASTING WHITE, 2 sl	170	6	2	32	—	60	1.80	460	—	—
WHEAT, 2 sl	190	6	3	35	—	20	1.80	390	—	—
WHITE, 2 sl	150	4	3	25	—	40	1.08	270	—	—
VERY THIN, 2 sl	80	3	1	16	—	40	.72	170	—	—
WHOLE WHEAT, 2 sl	130	5	3	24	—	40	1.80	250	—	—
VERY THIN, 2 sl	80	3	2	15	—	20	1.08	160	—	—
Pillsbury										
APPLESAUCE SPICE MIX,										
prep, 1/12 loaf	150	2	3	28	—	0	.72	150	30	—
APRICOT NUT MIX, prep, 1/12										
loaf	160	2	4	27	—	0	1.08	150	65	—
BAKERY STYLE COUNTRY										
WHITE ROLLS, 1 roll	100	3	1	20	—	0	1.08	350	20	—
BANANA MIX, prep, 1/12 loaf	150	2	4	27	—	0	.72	150	30	—
BLUEBERRY NUT MIX, prep,										
1/12 loaf	150	2	4	26	—	20	.72	150	25	—
BUTTERFLAKE ROLLS, 1 roll	110	2	4	16	—	0	.72	410	20	—
CARROT NUT MIX, prep, 1/12										
loaf	150	2	4	27	—	20	.72	180	60	—
CHERRY NUT MIX, prep, 1/12										
loaf	180	2	5	29	—	0	.72	150	30	—
CINNAMON ROLL WITH										
ICING, 2 rolls	230	3	9	34	—	0	1.08	520	40	—
CRANBERRY MIX, prep, 1/12										
loaf	160	2	3	30	—	0	.36	150	60	—
CRESCENT ROLLS, 2 rolls	200	3	11	22	—	0	1.08	460	125	—
DATE MIX, prep, 1/12 loaf	160	2	3	31	—	0	.72	150	55	—
HOT ROLL MIX, prep, 2 rolls	240	7	4	42	—	0	1.80	430	90	—
HUNGRY JACK BUTTER										
TASTIN' CINNAMON										
ROLL WITH ICING, 2										
rolls	290	3	14	37	—	0	.72	570	30	—
NUT MIX, prep, 1/12 loaf	160	2	3	31	—	0	.36	180	60	—
PARKERHOUSE ROLLS, 2 rolls	150	3	3	27	—	0	1.08	600	35	—
PIPIN' HOT										
HOT CINNAMON ROLLS, 1										
roll	210	2	9	29	—	0	1.08	260	25	—
SOFT BREAD STICKS, 1 stick	100	3	2	17	—	0	1.08	230	20	—
WHITE LOAF, 1" sl	80	2	2	13	—	0	.36	170	15	—

35

FOOD & DESCRIPTION MEASURE OR QUANTITY	CALORIES	PROTEIN (GM)	FAT (GM)	CARBO-HYDRATE (GM)	FIBER (GM)	CALCIUM (MG)	IRON (MG)	SODIUM (MG)	POTASSIUM (MG)	CHOLES-TEROL (MG)
WHEAT LOAF, 1″ sl	80	3	2	12	—	0	.36	170	30	—
PLAIN WEINER WRAP, 1 wrap	60	1	2	10	—	0	.36	430	25	—
RYE BREAD MIX, prep, ½″ sl	110	3	2	21	—	0	1.08	200	45	—
WHITE BREAD MIX, prep, ½″ sl	110	3	2	21	—	0	.72	200	40	—

Rich's

BREAD DOUGH, white, prep, 2 sl	116	4	1	23	—	110	2.10	300	51	0
ROLL DOUGH, HOME STYLE, prep, 2 rolls	152	5	2	28	—	27	2.04	335	68	0

Thomas

PROTEIN BREAD, 2 sl, 39 gm	93	7	<1	15	.20	44	1.50	180	—	0
SAHARA BREAD 100% WHOLE WHEAT, 1 loaf, 28 gm	75	4	<1	14	.30	30	1.10	170	—	0
REGULAR, 1 loaf, 28 gm	80	3	1	16	.40	*	1.10	190	—	0

USDA

BOSTON BROWN BREAD, 1/10 can, 45 gm	95	3	<1	21	—	41	.90	113	131	—
BREAD CRUMBS, dry, 1 c, 100 gm	392	13	5	73	—	122	3.60	736	152	—
CHEESE STRAWS, 5 × ¾ × ⅜″, 10 straws, 60 gm	272	7	18	21	—	155	.40	433	38	—
CLOVERLEAF ROLLS BROWN AND SERVE, 2½″ diam, 1 oz, 28 gm	84	2	2	14	—	20	.50	136	25	—
FROM MIX, 2½″ diam, 35 gm	105	3	2	19	—	20	.70	110	43	—
CORN BREAD MIX, prep, 2½ × 2½ × 1⅜″ piece, 55 gm	178	4	6	28	—	133	.80	263	61	—
SOUTHERN STYLE, 2½ × 2½ × 1½″ piece, 78 gm	161	6	6	23	—	94	.90	490	122	—
1″ cube, 8.3 gm	17	<1	<1	2	—	10	.10	52	13	—
CORN PONE, 9″ diam pone, 485 gm	989	22	26	176	—	301	5.80	1921	296	—
⅛ pone, 3½″ arc, 60 gm	122	3	3	22	—	37	.70	238	37	—
CRACKED WHEAT, commercial, 1 sl, 25 gm	66	2	<1	13	.10	16	.67	108	33	—
FRENCH BREAD, 5 × 2½ × 1″ sl, 35 gm	102	3	1	19	—	15	.80	203	32	—
2½ × 2 × ½″ sl, 15 gm	44	1	<1	8	—	6	.30	87	14	—
FRENCH/VIENNA, commerical, 1 sl, 28 gm	79	3	1	14	.05	31	.87	156	24	—
HAMBURGER/HOTDOG ROLL, 1 bun, 40 gm	119	3	2	21	—	30	.80	202	38	—
HARD ROLL, 3¾″ diam, 50 gm	156	5	2	30	—	24	1.20	313	49	—
ITALIAN BREAD, 4½ × 3¼ × ¾″ sl, 30 gm	83	3	<1	17	—	5	.70	176	22	—
3¼ × 2½ × ½″ sl, 10 gm	28	1	<1	6	—	2	.20	59	7	—
MIXED GRAIN, commercial, 1 oz, 28 gm	73	3	1	13	.20	29	.92	117	62	—
PARKERHOUSE ROLL, from fz dough, 2⅜ × 2 × 1⅜″ roll, 28 gm	75	2	1	13	—	9	.50	127	23	—
PUMPERNICKEL, 2½ × 2 × ¼″ sl, 7 gm	17	<1	<1	4	—	6	.20	40	32	—
commercial, 1 sl, 32 gm	82	3	1	15	.34	23	.88	173	43	—
RAISIN BREAD, commercial, 1 sl, 25 gm	70	2	<1	13	.23	26	.78	94	60	—

FOOD & DESCRIPTION MEASURE OR QUANTITY	CALORIES	PROTEIN (GM)	FAT (GM)	CARBO- HYDRATE (GM)	FIBER (GM)	CALCIUM (MG)	IRON (MG)	SODIUM (MG)	POTASSIUM (MG)	CHOLES- TEROL (MG)
RUSK, 3⅜″ diam × ½″, 9 gm	38	1	<1	6	—	2	.10	22	14	—
RYE BREAD, commercial, 1 sl, 25 gm	66	2	<1	12	.1	20	.68	174	51	—
SPOON BREAD, white cornmeal, 1 c, 240 gm	468	16	27	41	—	230	2.40	1157	317	—
VIENNA BREAD, 4¾ × 4 × ½″, 1 sl, 25 gm	73	2	<1	14	—	11	.60	145	23	—
WHEAT BREAD, commercial, 1 sl, 1 oz	72	3	1	13	.18	36	.99	153	39	—
WHITE BREAD, commercial										
4⅜ × 4 × 9/16″ sl, 28 gm	76	2	1	14	.08	36	.81	146	32	—
3¾ × 4 × 7/16″ sl, 24 gm	64	2	<1	12	.07	30	.68	123	27	—
bread cubes, 1 c, 30 gm	80	2	1	15	.09	38	.85	154	34	—
bread crumbs, 1 c, 45 gm	120	4	2	22	.13	57	1.28	231	50	—
WHOLE WHEAT, commercial, 1 sl, 25 gm	61	2	1	11	.38	18	.86	159	44	—
sandwich style, 3⅛ × 3⅝ × 7/16″, 1 sl, 23 gm	56	2	1	10	.35	17	.79	146	40	—
ZWIEBACK, 3½ × 1½ × ½″ piece, 7 gm	30	<1	<1	5	—	1	tr	18	11	—

Wasa Crispbreads

BREAKFAST, 1 sl, 13.3 gm	54	2	2	9	.7 d	17	1.30	75	39	—
EXTRA CRISP CRACKERBREAD, 1 sl, 6.1 gm	22	1	<1	5	—	—	—	40	—	—
FIBER PLUS, 1 sl, 10.4 gm	35	1	1	4	2.7 d	7	.98	46	98	—
GOLDEN RYE, 1 sl, 10.4 gm	39	1	0	8	1.3 d	6	.30	43	57	—
HEARTY RYE, 1 sl, 15.6 gm	52	1	1	11	2.2 d	9	.45	38	93	—
LITE RYE, 1 sl, 8.3 gm	30	2	0	7	1.2 d	7	.34	20	40	—
SESAME, 1 sl, 13.3 gm	54	2	2	8	.6 d	21	.69	63	47	—
SPORT, 1 sl, 12.5 gm	44	1	0	9	1.8 d	11	.36	66	71	—

Weight Watchers

THICK SLICED COUNTRY WHITE, enriched, 1 sl, 21 gm	40	2	0	9	—	20	.72	95	—	—
MULTI-GRAIN, 1 sl, 21 gm	40	2	0	9	—	20	.72	95	—	—
RYE, 1 sl, 21 gm	40	2	0	9	—	20	.72	95	—	—
WHEAT, 1 sl, 21 gm	40	2	0	9	—	20	.72	95	—	—

Cakes, Brownies & Bars

Arrowhead Mills

CAROB CAKE MIX, prep, 2 oz	150	6	2	27	—	—	—	225	—	—
CHOICE CAKE MIX, prep, 1 oz	100	3	1	21	—	—	—	170	—	—
MULTI-CAKE MIX, prep, 1 oz	100	3	1	21	—	—	—	170	—	—

Aunt Jemima–Quaker

EASY MIX COFFEE CAKE, prep, ⅛ cake, 1.3 oz	162	2	4	29	.10	58	.73	225	32	—

Betty Crocker– General Mills

APPLE CINNAMON SUPERMOIST CAKE, prep, 1/12 cake	250	3	10	36	—	80	.72	280	45	—
APPLESAUCE RAISIN SNACKIN' CAKE, prep, 1/9 cake	190	2	6	33	—	40	.72	260	85	—

FOOD & DESCRIPTION MEASURE OR QUANTITY	CALORIES	PROTEIN (GM)	FAT (GM)	CARBO-HYDRATE (GM)	FIBER (GM)	CALCIUM (MG)	IRON (MG)	SODIUM (MG)	POTASSIUM (MG)	CHOLES-TEROL (MG)
BANANA WALNUT SNACKIN' CAKE, prep, ⅑ cake	200	2	7	31	—	40	.72	260	80	—
BOSTON CREAM PIE, CLASSIC DESSERT, prep, ⅛ cake	270	4	6	50	—	150	.72	390	110	—
BUTTER BRICKLE SUPERMOIST CAKE, prep, 1/12 cake	260	3	11	38	—	60	1.08	280	40	—
BUTTER PECAN SUPERMOIST CAKE, prep, 1/12 cake	250	3	11	35	—	80	.72	320	45	—
BUTTER RECIPE YELLOW SUPERMOIST CAKE, prep, 1/12 cake	260	3	11	37	—	60	1.08	350	40	—
CARROT CAKE LOVERS, prep, 1/12 cake	330	4	17	40	—	80	1.44	310	—	—
CARROT SUPERMOIST CAKE, prep, 1/12 cake	260	3	12	34	—	40	.72	260	65	—
CARROT CAKE/CREAM CHEESE FROSTING, STIR 'N FROST, prep, ⅙ cake	230	2	6	43	—	60	.72	210	85	—
CHERRY CHIP SUPERMOIST CAKE, prep, 1/12 cake	190	3	3	37	—	*	.72	270	35	—
CHOCOLATE ALMOND CAKE LOVERS, prep, 1/12 cake	360	5	20	41	—	60	1.80	280	—	—
CHOCOLATE ANGEL FOOD CAKE, prep, 1/12 cake	150	3	0	34	—	*	.36	300	80	0
CHOCOLATE CHIP SUPERMOIST CAKE, prep, 1/12 cake	280	3	14	36	—	80	.72	300	60	—
CHOCOLATE CHIP CAKE/CHOCOLATE FROSTING, STIR 'N FROST, prep, ⅙ cake	230	2	6	41	—	40	.72	200	125	—
CHOCOLATE CHOCOLATE CHIP SUPERMOIST CAKE, 1/12 cake	250	3	12	34	—	60	1.08	430	115	—
CHOCOLATE CHOCOLATE CHIP CAKE/CHOCOLATE CHOCOLATE CHIP FROSTING, STIR 'N FROST, prep, ⅙ cake	230	2	6	41	—	20	1.08	260	120	—
CHOCOLATE DEVIL'S FOOD CAKE/CHOCOLATE FROSTING, STIR 'N FROST, prep, ⅙ cake	230	2	6	41	—	20	1.44	260	180	—
CHOCOLATE FUDGE SUPERMOIST CAKE, prep, 1/12 cake	250	3	11	35	—	60	1.08	450	100	—
CHOCOLATE FUDGE CAKE/VANILLA FROSTING, STIR 'N FROST, prep, ⅙ cake	230	2	5	43	—	20	1.80	270	120	—
CHOCOLATE FUDGE CHIP SNACKIN' CAKE, prep, ⅑ cake	190	2	6	33	—	60	1.08	210	110	—
CHOCOLATE PUDDING CAKE, prep, ⅙ cake	230	3	5	44	—	40	.72	250	170	—
COCONUT MACAROON, prep, 1/24 pkg	80	1	4	10	—	20	*	15	80	—
CONFETTI ANGEL FOOD CAKE, prep, 1/12 cake	160	3	0	36	—	60	*	310	45	0
DATE BAR, prep, 1/32 pkg	60	<1	2	9	—	*	*	40	35	—
DEVIL' S FOOD SUPERMOIST CAKE, prep, 1/12 cake	270	3	13	35	—	20	1.80	430	160	—

FOOD & DESCRIPTION MEASURE OR QUANTITY	CALORIES	PROTEIN (GM)	FAT (GM)	CARBO-HYDRATE (GM)	FIBER (GM)	CALCIUM (MG)	IRON (MG)	SODIUM (MG)	POTASSIUM (MG)	CHOLES-TEROL (MG)
DOUBLE CHOCOLATE CAKE LOVERS, prep, 1/12 cake	340	4	17	43	—	40	1.80	270	—	—
DUTCH APPLE CAKE LOVERS, prep, 1/12 cake	290	3	12	42	—	60	1.08	310	—	—
FUDGE PEANUT BUTTER CHIP SNACKIN' CAKE, prep, 1/9 cake	200	3	7	32	—	60	1.08	250	50	—
GERMAN CHOCOLATE SUPERMOIST CAKE, prep, 1/12 cake	260	3	11	37	—	60	1.08	430	65	—
GERMAN CHOCOLATE COCONUT PECAN SNACKIN' CAKE, prep, 1/9 cake	190	2	5	33	—	60	.72	270	90	—
GINGERBREAD, prep, 1/9 cake	210	3	6	35	—	20	1.80	330	150	—
GOLDEN CHOCOLATE CHIP SNACKIN' CAKE, prep, 1/9 cake	190	2	5	34	—	60	.72	260	80	—
GOLDEN POUND CAKE, prep, 1/12 cake	200	2	9	28	—	20	.72	170	25	—
LEMON CHIFFON CAKE, prep, 1/12 cake	190	4	4	35	—	20	.72	190	60	—
LEMON CUSTARD ANGEL FOOD CAKE, prep, 1/12 cake	150	3	0	35	—	60	*	260	45	0
LEMON PUDDING CAKE, prep, 1/6 cake	230	2	5	45	—	40	.36	270	35	—
LEMON SUPERMOIST CAKE, prep, 1/12 cake	260	3	11	37	—	*	1.08	280	30	—
MARBLE SUPERMOIST CAKE, prep, 1/12 cake	260	3	11	36	—	80	.72	300	60	—
MILK CHOCOLATE SUPERMOIST CAKE, prep, 1/12 cake	250	3	11	35	—	40	1.08	290	120	—
PINEAPPLE UPSIDE DOWN CAKE, 1/9 cake	260	2	9	43	—	60	.72	230	70	—
SOUR CREAM CHOCOLATE SUPERMOIST CAKE, prep, 1/12 cake	250	3	10	36	—	60	1.08	450	115	—
SOUR CREAM WHITE SUPERMOIST CAKE, prep, 1/12 cake	180	3	3	36	—	*	1.08	300	40	—
SPICE SUPERMOIST CAKE, prep, 1/12 cake	250	2	11	36	—	100	1.08	320	50	—
SPICE CAKE/VANILLA FROSTING, STIR 'N FROST, prep, 1/6 cake	280	2	9	48	—	20	.72	310	30	—
STRAWBERRY ANGEL FOOD CAKE, prep, 1/12 cake	150	3	0	35	—	60	*	260	45	0
TRADITIONAL WHITE ANGEL FOOD CAKE, prep, 1/12 cake	140	3	0	31	—	40	*	160	60	0
VIENNA DREAM BAR, prep, 1/24 pkg	90	1	5	10	—	*	*	65	30	—
WHITE ANGEL FOOD CAKE, prep, 1/12 cake	150	3	0	34	—	60	*	300	60	0
WHITE SUPERMOIST CAKE, prep, 1/12 cake	250	3	10	37	—	60	1.08	250	35	—
YELLOW CAKE/CHOCOLATE FROSTING, STIR 'N FROST, prep, 1/6 cake	230	2	8	37	—	20	.72	210	60	—
YELLOW SUPERMOIST CAKE, prep, 1/12 cake	250	2	11	36	—	80	.72	300	35	—

FOOD & DESCRIPTION MEASURE OR QUANTITY	CALORIES	PROTEIN (GM)	FAT (GM)	CARBO-HYDRATE (GM)	FIBER (GM)	CALCIUM (MG)	IRON (MG)	SODIUM (MG)	POTASSIUM (MG)	CHOLES-TEROL (MG)
Borden										
DEVIL DOGS, 1 piece	170	2	8	22	—	*	.72	165	80	—
FUNNY BONES, 1 piece	160	2	9	18	—	20	.72	130	95	—
RING DING, JR, 1 piece	160	1	9	20	—	*	.72	120	65	—
YANKEE DOODLES, 1 piece	110	1	5	15	—	*	.36	130	45	—
Dromedary–Nabisco										
GINGERBREAD MIX, prep, 2 × 2″ piece	100	1	2	19	—	20	.72	190	90	—
POUND CAKE MIX, prep, ½″ slice	150	2	6	21	—	20	.36	340	65	—
Duncan Hines– Procter & Gamble										
ANGEL FOOD CAKE, prep, 1/12 cake	140	3	0	30	—	20	*	130	—	—
APPLE CAKE, prep, 1/12 cake	260	3	12	34	—	60	1.08	265	—	—
BANANA SUPREME CAKE, prep, 1/12 cake	260	3	11	36	—	60	1.08	285	—	—
BROWNIE										
family size, prep, 1/24 batch	120	1	3	22	—	<20	.36	100	—	—
regular size, prep, 1/16 batch	120	1	3	23	—	<20	.36	105	—	—
BROWNIE, CHEWY										
family size, prep, 1/24 batch	160	2	7	22	—	<20	.36	105	—	—
regular size, prep, 1/16 batch	160	2	7	23	—	<20	.36	110	—	—
BUTTER RECIPE FUDGE CAKE, prep, 1/12 cake	270	4	13	34	—	20	1.08	350	—	—
BUTTER RECIPE GOLDEN CAKE, prep, 1/12 cake	270	3	13	36	—	40	.72	270	—	—
CARROT CAKE, prep, 1/12 cake	250	3	11	34	—	60	1.08	265	—	—
CHERRY SUPREME CAKE, prep, 1/12 cake	260	3	11	36	—	60	1.08	285	—	—
CHOCOLATE CHIP CAKE, prep, 1/12 cake	260	3	12	34	—	60	1.08	265	—	—
DEEP CHOCOLATE CAKE, prep, 1/12 cake	280	4	15	33	—	61	1.08	375	—	—
DEVIL'S FOOD CAKE, prep, 1/12 cake	280	4	15	33	—	60	1.08	375	—	—
FUDGE MARBLE CAKE, prep, 1/12 cake	260	3	11	36	—	60	1.08	285	—	—
GOLDEN VANILLA CAKE, prep, 1/12 cake	260	3	11	36	—	60	1.08	285	—	—
LEMON SUPREME CAKE, prep, 1/12 cake	260	3	11	36	—	60	1.08	285	—	—
ORANGE SUPREME CAKE, prep, 1/12 cake	260	3	11	36	—	60	1.08	285	—	—
PINEAPPLE SUPREME CAKE, prep, 1/12 cake	260	3	11	36	—	60	1.08	285	—	—
SOUR CREAM CHOCOLATE CAKE, prep, 1/12 cake	280	4	15	33	—	60	1.08	375	—	—
SPICE CAKE, prep, 1/12 cake	260	3	11	36	—	60	1.08	285	—	—
STRAWBERRY SUPREME CAKE, prep, 1/12 cake	260	3	11	36	—	60	1.08	285	—	—
SWISS CHOCOLATE CAKE, prep, 1/12 cake	280	4	15	33	—	100	1.08	375	—	—
YELLOW CAKE, prep, 1/12 cake	260	3	11	36	—	60	1.08	285	—	—
WHITE CAKE, prep, 1/12 cake	250	3	10	36	—	60	.72	260	—	—
Estee										
BROWNIE, prep, 2″ square	45	1	2	8	—	—	—	15	—	30
CAKE MIX, CHOCOLATE, prep, 1/10 cake	100	2	2	17	—	—	—	110	—	0

FOOD & DESCRIPTION MEASURE OR QUANTITY	CALORIES	PROTEIN (GM)	FAT (GM)	CARBO-HYDRATE (GM)	FIBER (GM)	CALCIUM (MG)	IRON (MG)	SODIUM (MG)	POTASSIUM (MG)	CHOLES-TEROL (MG)
CAKE MIX (all others), prep, 1/10 cake	100	2	2	18	—	—	—	60–75	—	0

Hostess

CHIP FLIPS, 1 piece, 2.75 oz	330	2	16	47	—	20	1.08	165	—	25
CHOCO-DILES, 1 piece, 2 oz	240	2	11	35	—	20	.72	280	—	22
CHOCOLATE CUP CAKES, 1 cupcake, 1.75 oz	170	2	6	29	—	20	.72	250	—	3
CRUMB CAKES, 1 cake, 1.25 oz	130	1	4	22	—	20	.72	95	—	10
DESSERT CUPS, 1 cup, .75 oz	60	1	0	14	—	20	.36	120	—	9
DING DONGS/BIG WHEELS, 1 piece, 1.33 oz	170	1	9	21	—	20	.36	130	—	6
FRUIT LOAF, 1 loaf, 5 oz	400	4	9	77	—	40	1.80	520	—	7
HO HOs, 1 piece, 1 oz	120	1	6	17	—	20	.36	90	—	13
HONEY BUNS, glazed, 1 bun, 3.75 oz	450	5	27	49	—	20	1.44	650	—	24
HOSTESS O's, 1 piece, 2.25 oz	240	3	11	33	—	40	.36	265	—	14
LIL' ANGELS, 1 piece, 1 oz	90	1	2	14	—	20	.36	95	—	2
ORANGE CUP CAKES, 1 cupcake, 1.5 oz	150	1	5	28	—	20	.36	175	—	13
PEANUT PUTTERS, filled, 1 piece, 3 oz	360	5	15	46	—	40	1.44	240	—	4
PEANUT PUTTERS, unfilled, 1 piece, 3 oz	410	7	21	43	—	40	1.08	240	—	4
SNO BALLS, 1 piece, 1.5 oz	150	1	4	28	—	20	.36	170	—	2
SUZY Q's, BANANA, 1 piece, 2.25 oz	240	2	9	38	—	40	.72	195	—	21
SUZY Q's, CHOCOLATE, 1 piece, 2.25 oz	240	2	10	37	—	20	.72	300	—	16
TIGER TAIL, 1 piece, 2.25 oz	210	2	6	38	—	20	.72	240	—	25
TWINKIES, 1 piece, 1.5 oz	160	1	5	26	—	20	.36	150	—	20

Jiffy

DARK FUDGE CAKE, prep, 4 × 2" piece	140	2	3	25	—	*	1.62	285	—	—
DEVIL'S FOOD CAKE, prep, 4 × 2" piece	140	3	4	25	—	*	2.16	315	—	—
GOLDEN YELLOW CAKE, prep, 4 × 2" piece	140	3	3	26	—	*	1.08	240	—	—
SPICE CAKE, prep, 4 × 2" piece	150	3	6	22	—	*	1.08	265	—	—
WHITE CAKE, prep, 4 × 2" piece	140	2	3	25	—	*	1.08	235	—	—

Pepperidge Farm–Campbell

BOSTON CREAM SUPREME CAKE, 2.88 oz	290	3	14	39	—	20	.72	190	—	—
BUTTER POUND CAKE, 1 oz	130	1	7	16	—	*	*	150	—	—
BUTTERSCOTCH PECAN LAYER CAKE, 1.63 oz	160	1	7	23	—	20	.36	110	—	—
CARROT CAKE/CREAM CHEESE ICING, 1.38 oz	140	1	8	17	—	*	.36	150	—	—
CHOCOLATE FUDGE LAYER CAKE, 1.63 oz	180	1	10	23	—	*	.72	140	—	—
CHOCOLATE MINT LAYER CAKE, 1.63 oz	170	1	9	22	—	20	1.08	140	—	—
CHOCOLATE SUPREME CAKE, 2.88 oz	310	3	17	37	—	20	1.08	140	—	—
COCONUT LAYER CAKE, 1.63 oz	180	1	9	25	—	*	.36	120	—	—

FOOD & DESCRIPTION MEASURE OR QUANTITY	CALORIES	PROTEIN (GM)	FAT (GM)	CARBO-HYDRATE (GM)	FIBER (GM)	CALCIUM (MG)	IRON (MG)	SODIUM (MG)	POTASSIUM (MG)	CHOLES-TEROL (MG)
DEVIL'S FOOD LAYER CAKE, 1.63 oz	180	1	9	24	—	*	.36	135	—	—
DUTCH CHOCOLATE SUPREME CAKE, 1.75 oz	190	1	10	25	—	20	1.08	115	—	—
GERMAN CHOCOLATE LAYER CAKE, 1.63 oz	180	1	10	23	—	20	.36	170	—	—
GOLDEN LAYER CAKE, 1.63 oz	180	1	9	24	—	*	.36	115	—	—
GRAND MARNIER SUPREME CAKE, 1.5 oz	160	1	18	22	—	20	.72	85	—	—
LEMON COCONUT SUPREME CAKE, 3 oz	280	2	13	38	—	*	.36	220	—	—
PEACH MELBA SUPREME, 3.13 oz	270	2	7	50	—	20	1.44	135	—	—
PINEAPPLE CREAM SUPREME CAKE, 2 oz	190	2	7	28	—	20	.72	130	—	—
RASPBERRY MOCHA SUPREME CAKE, 3.13 oz	310	3	14	43	—	20	1.80	170	—	—
STRAWBERRY CREAM SUPREME, 2 oz	190	1	7	30	—	20	.72	120	—	—
VANILLA LAYER CAKE, 1.63 oz	190	1	8	25	—	*	*	120	—	—

Pillsbury

APPLE CINNAMON COFFEE CAKE, prep, ⅛ cake	240	3	7	40	—	60	1.08	160	90	—
APPLESAUCE SPICE CAKE, prep, ¹⁄₁₂ cake	250	3	11	36	—	40	.72	300	80	—
BANANA CAKE, prep, ¹⁄₁₂ cake	250	3	11	36	—	40	.72	290	80	—
BOSTON CREAM BUNDT CAKE, prep, ¹⁄₁₆ cake	270	3	10	43	—	40	.72	310	55	—
BROWN SUGAR & OATMEAL FUDGE JUMBLES, prep, ¹⁄₃₆ pkg	100	1	4	15	—	0	.36	60	45	—
BUTTER CAKE, prep, ¹⁄₁₂ cake	240	3	9	36	—	40	.72	350	85	—
CARROT 'N SPICE, prep, ¹⁄₁₂ cake	260	3	11	36	—	40	.72	330	85	—
CHOCOLATE CHIP OATMEAL FUDGE JUMBLES, prep, ¹⁄₃₆ pkg	100	1	4	14	—	0	0	60	30	—
CHOCOLATE MACAROON BUNDT CAKE, prep, ¹⁄₁₆ cake	250	3	11	37	—	0	.72	300	55	—
CHOCOLATE MINT CAKE, prep, ¹⁄₁₂ cake	260	3	12	35	—	100	1.08	340	80	—
CHOCOLATE MOUSSE BUNDT CAKE, prep, ¹⁄₁₆ cake	230	3	9	35	—	40	1.08	310	100	—
CINNAMON STREUSEL SWIRL, prep, ¹⁄₁₆ cake	260	3	11	38	—	40	1.08	200	40	—
COCONUT OATMEAL FUDGE JUMBLES, prep, ¹⁄₃₆ pkg	100	1	5	14	—	0	.36	60	50	—
DARK CHOCOLATE CAKE, prep, ¹⁄₁₂ cake	260	3	12	35	—	100	1.44	440	95	—
DEVIL'S FOOD CAKE, prep, ¹⁄₁₂ cake	250	3	11	35	—	100	1.08	400	80	—
DEVIL'S FOOD CHOCOLATE FILLING/CHOCOLATE FROSTING, prep, 1 cupcake	210	2	8	34	—	20	.72	240	95	—
DEVIL'S FOOD/VANILLA FILLING/CHOCOLATE FROSTING, prep, 1 cupcake	210	2	8	34	—	20	.36	250	80	—

FOOD & DESCRIPTION MEASURE OR QUANTITY	CALORIES	PROTEIN (GM)	FAT (GM)	CARBO-HYDRATE (GM)	FIBER (GM)	CALCIUM (MG)	IRON (MG)	SODIUM (MG)	POTASSIUM (MG)	CHOLES-TEROL (MG)
DUTCH APPLE STREUSEL SWIRL, prep, 1/16 cake	260	3	11	38	—	20	1.08	200	45	—
FUDGE BROWNIE family size pkg, prep, 2" square	150	1	7	20	—	0	.36	95	30	—
regular size pkg, prep, 2" square	150	2	6	21	—	0	.36	100	35	—
FUDGE MARBLE CAKE, prep, 1/12 cake	270	4	12	36	—	40	1.08	300	55	—
FUDGE MARBLE STREUSEL SWIRL, prep, 1/16 cake	260	3	11	38	—	20	1.08	200	35	—
GERMAN CHOCOLATE CAKE, prep, 1/12 cake	250	3	11	36	—	40	.36	340	80	—
GINGERBREAD, prep, 3" square	190	2	4	36	—	40	1.80	310	160	—
LEMON BLUEBERRY BUNDT CAKE, prep, 1/16 cake	200	3	8	28	—	40	1.08	270	40	—
LEMON CAKE, prep, 1/12 cake	260	3	11	36	—	40	.72	310	30	—
LEMON STREUSEL SWIRL, prep, 1/16 cake	270	3	11	39	—	60	.72	340	45	—
MOCHA CAKE, prep, 1/12 cake	260	3	12	35	—	100	1.44	440	95	—
OATS 'N BROWN SUGAR CAKE, prep, 1/12 cake	260	3	12	35	—	40	1.08	310	80	—
PEANUT BUTTER OATMEAL FUDGE JUMBLES, prep, 1/36 pkg	100	1	4	14	—	0	.36	55	55	—
PECAN BROWN SUGAR STREUSEL SWIRL, prep, 1/16 cake	260	3	11	37	—	20	1.08	200	45	—
POUND BUNDT CAKE, prep, 1/16 cake	230	3	9	33	—	20	.72	260	30	—
STRAWBERRY CAKE, prep, 1/12 cake	260	3	11	37	—	40	.72	300	85	—
TUNNEL OF FUDGE BUNDT CAKE, prep, 1/16 cake	270	3	12	37	—	20	.72	310	115	—
TUNNEL OF LEMON BUNDT CAKE, prep, 1/16 cake	270	2	9	45	—	40	.72	300	90	—
WALNUT BROWNIE, family size, prep, 2" square	150	2	8	19	—	0	.36	90	40	—
WHITE CAKE, prep, 1/12 cake	240	3	10	35	—	20	0	290	75	—
YELLOW CAKE, prep, 1/12 cake	260	3	12	36	—	40	.72	300	80	—
YELLOW CAKE/VANILLA FILLING/CHOCOLATE FROSTING, prep, 1 cupcake	210	2	7	35	—	40	.72	230	75	—

Sara Lee

ALL BUTTER POUND CAKE, 1/10 cake	130	2	7	14	—	*	.72	85	—	—
BLACK FOREST CAKE, 1/8 cake	190	2	8	28	—	20	1.44	100	—	—
CLASSIC ELEGANT ENDINGS CHEESECAKE, 1/6 cake	350	10	22	29	—	60	1.08	250	—	—
CHOCOLATE CHIP ELEGANT ENDINGS CHEESECAKE, 1/6 cake	420	7	27	38	—	60	1.44	390	—	—
CHOCOLATE CHIP POUND CAKE, 1/10 cake	130	2	5	19	—	*	1.08	150	—	—
CHOCOLATE MOUSSE BAVARIAN CAKE, 1/8 cake	250	3	16	23	—	20	1.44	140	—	—
FRENCH CREAM COFFEECAKE, 1/8 cake	260	4	17	23	—	40	.72	150	—	—
PECAN COFFEE CAKE, 1/8 cake	160	3	8	19	—	*	1.08	240	—	—

FOOD & DESCRIPTION MEASURE OR QUANTITY	CALORIES	PROTEIN (GM)	FAT (GM)	CARBO-HYDRATE (GM)	FIBER (GM)	CALCIUM (MG)	IRON (MG)	SODIUM (MG)	POTASSIUM (MG)	CHOLES-TEROL (MG)
PECAN PRALINE ELEGANT ENDINGS CHEESECAKE, ⅙ cake	430	7	30	32	—	60	1.08	410	—	—
STRAWBERRY FRENCH CREAM CHEESECAKE, ⅛ cake	250	3	13	29	—	20	.72	170	—	—
STRAWBERRY SHORTCAKE, ⅙ cake	190	2	8	26	—	20	.72	90	—	—
WALNUT COFFEE CAKE, ⅛ cake	170	3	9	18	—	*	1.08	160	—	—
WALNUT RAISIN POUND CAKE, 1/10 cake	140	3	5	20	—	20	.72	170	—	—

Sweet 'N Low

FOOD & DESCRIPTION MEASURE OR QUANTITY	CALORIES	PROTEIN (GM)	FAT (GM)	CARBO-HYDRATE (GM)	FIBER (GM)	CALCIUM (MG)	IRON (MG)	SODIUM (MG)	POTASSIUM (MG)	CHOLES-TEROL (MG)
BANANA CAKE, prep, 1/10 cake	90	2	2	16	—	150	*	40	—	<5
CHOCOLATE CAKE, prep, 1/10 cake	90	2	2	16	—	150	*	40	—	<5
GINGERBREAD, prep, 1/10 cake	90	2	2	16	—	150	*	20	18	<5
LEMON CAKE, prep, 1/10 cake	90	2	2	16	—	150	*	40	—	<5
MINT CHOCOLATE CAKE, 1/10 cake	90	2	2	16	—	150	*	40	—	<5
WHITE CAKE, 1/10 cake	90	2	2	16	—	150	*	40	—	<5
YELLOW CAKE, 1/10 cake	90	2	2	16	—	150	*	40	—	<5

Tastykake

FOOD & DESCRIPTION MEASURE OR QUANTITY	CALORIES	PROTEIN (GM)	FAT (GM)	CARBO-HYDRATE (GM)	FIBER (GM)	CALCIUM (MG)	IRON (MG)	SODIUM (MG)	POTASSIUM (MG)	CHOLES-TEROL (MG)
BANANA TREATS, 1 piece	147	1	4	26	—	—	—	99	—	—
BUTTERSCOTCH KRIMPET, 1 piece	129	1	5	20	—	—	—	94	—	—
CHOCOLATE CREAMIE, 1 piece	195	2	9	25	—	—	—	114	—	—
CHOCOLATE CUP CAKE, 1 cupcake	113	1	4	19	—	—	—	111	—	—
CHOCOLATE JUNIOR, 1 piece	354	4	12	56	—	—	—	292	—	—
CHOCOLATE KANDY KAKE, 1 piece	95	1	4	12	—	—	—	64	—	—
CHOCOLATE TEMPTY, 1 piece	97	1	4	15	—	—	—	76	—	—
COCONUT JUNIOR, 1 piece	330	4	7	60	—	—	—	327	—	—
COCONUT KANDY KAKE, 1 piece	106	1	5	14	—	—	—	44	—	—
CREME FILLED BUTTERCREAM CUP, 1 cup	129	1	5	20	—	—	—	121	—	—
CREME FILLED CHOCOLATE CUP, 1 cup	137	2	6	20	—	—	—	131	—	—
CREME FILLED CHOCOLATE KRIMPET, 1 piece	148	1	7	21	—	—	—	122	—	—
CREME FILLED KOFFEE KAKE, 1 piece	147	2	6	21	—	—	—	135	—	—
CREME FILLED VANILLA KRIMPET, 1 piece	149	1	7	21	—	—	—	83	—	—
FUDGE BAR, 1 bar	266	3	11	38	—	—	—	144	—	—
JELLY KRIMPET, 1 piece	112	1	2	22	—	—	—	85	—	—
KOFFEE KAKE, 1 piece	329	4	12	49	—	—	—	314	—	—
KREME KUPS, 1 piece	115	1	5	15	—	—	—	134	—	—
OATMEAL RAISIN BAR, 1 bar	239	4	8	37	—	—	—	269	—	—
ORANGE JUNIOR, 1 piece	347	4	11	58	—	—	—	258	—	—
PEANUT BUTTER KANDY KAKE, 1 piece	105	2	6	11	—	—	—	48	—	—
VANILLA CREAMIE, 1 piece	209	1	10	28	—	—	—	126	—	—
VANILLA CUP CAKES, 1 cupcake	116	2	5	17	—	—	—	129	—	—

FOOD & DESCRIPTION MEASURE OR QUANTITY	CALORIES	PROTEIN (GM)	FAT (GM)	CARBO- HYDRATE (GM)	FIBER (GM)	CALCIUM (MG)	IRON (MG)	SODIUM (MG)	POTASSIUM (MG)	CHOLES- TEROL (MG)
USDA										
ANGELFOOD CAKE, from mix, 9¾" diam, ¹⁄₁₂ cake, 53 gm	137	3	<1	32	—	50	.20	77	32	—
ANGELFOOD CAKE, home recipe										
9¾" diam, ¹⁄₁₂ cake, 60 gm	161	4	<1	36	—	5	.10	170	53	—
8½" diam, ¹⁄₁₂ cake, 39 gm	105	3	<1	24	—	4	.10	110	34	—
BOSTON CREAM PIE, home recipe, 8" diam, ¹⁄₁₂ cake, 69 gm	208	4	7	34	—	46	.30	128	61	—
CARAMEL CAKE/CARAMEL ICING, home recipe										
9" diam, ¹⁄₁₂ cake, 105 gm	398	4	16	62	—	88	1.60	265	67	—
8" diam, ¹⁄₁₂ cake, 83 gm	315	3	12	49	—	70	1.20	209	53	—
CHOCOLATE MALT CAKE/WHITE ICING, from mix, ¹⁄₁₂ cake, 89 gm	308	3	8	59	—	56	.60	283	71	—
COFFEE CAKE, from mix 2⅝ × 2¾ × 1¼" piece, 72 gm	232	5	7	38	—	44	1.20	310	78	—
COTTAGE PUDDING CAKE, home recipe, 2 × 4 × 1½" piece										
plain, 54 gm	186	4	6	29	—	49	.80	161	48	—
with chocolate sauce, 74 gm	235	4	7	42	—	53	1.00	172	104	—
with strawberry sauce, 70 gm	204	4	6	34	—	51	.80	163	65	—
CUPCAKES, from mix, 2½" diam, 25 gm	88	1	3	14	—	40	.10	113	21	—
with chocolate icing, 36 gm	129	2	5	21	—	47	.30	121	42	—
DEVIL'S FOOD CAKE										
from mix, ¹⁄₁₂ cake, 92 gm	312	4	11	54	—	54	.70	241	120	—
fz, 7½" diam, with chocolate icing, ⅙ cake, 85 gm	323	4	15	47	—	46	.70	357	101	—
layer cake with chocolate icing/cream filling, 7¼" diam, ⅙ cake, 85 gm	315	3	19	37	—	68	.50	162	96	—
DEVIL'S FOOD CUPCAKE, from mix, 2½" cupcake, 35 gm	119	2	4	20	—	21	.30	92	46	—
FRUITCAKE, dark										
tube style, ¹⁄₃₂ cake, 43 gm	163	2	7	26	—	31	1.10	68	213	—
loaf style, 2 × 1½ × ¼" sl, 15 gm	57	<1	2	9	—	11	.40	24	74	—
FRUITCAKE, light										
tube style, ¹⁄₃₂ cake, 43 gm	167	3	7	25	—	29	.70	83	100	—
loaf style, 2 × 1½ × ¼" sl, 15 gm	58	<1	3	9	—	10	.20	29	35	—
GINGERBREAD, from mix, ⅑ cake, 63 gm	174	2	4	32	—	57	1.00	192	173	—
HONEY SPICE CAKE/CARAMEL ICING, from mix, ¹⁄₁₂ cake, 103 gm	363	4	11	63	—	73	.80	252	84	—
MARBLE CAKE/BOILED ICING, from mix, ¹⁄₁₂ cake, 87 gm	288	4	8	54	—	68	.70	225	106	—
PLAIN CAKE, 3 × 3 × 2" piece, 86 gm	313	4	12	48	—	55	.30	258	68	—
with boiled icing, 3 × 3 × 2" piece, 114 gm	401	4	12	71	—	56	.30	299	73	—
with chocolate icing, 3 × 3 × 2" piece, 123 gm	453	5	17	73	—	77	.70	282	140	—

FOOD & DESCRIPTION MEASURE OR QUANTITY	CALORIES	PROTEIN (GM)	FAT (GM)	CARBO-HYDRATE (GM)	FIBER (GM)	CALCIUM (MG)	IRON (MG)	SODIUM (MG)	POTASSIUM (MG)	CHOLES-TEROL (MG)
with white icing, home recipe, 3 × 3 × 2", 121 gm	444	4	14	77	—	61	.40	275	74	—
PLAIN CUPCAKE, 2½" diam, 25 gm	91	1	4	14	—	16	.10	75	20	—
with boiled icing, 2½" diam, 33 gm	116	1	4	20	—	16	.10	86	21	—
POUND CAKE										
home recipe, old fashioned loaf, 3½ × 3 × ½" sl, 30 gm	142	2	9	14	—	6	.20	33	18	—
modified home recipe, 3½ × 3 × ½" sl, 29 gm	119	2	5	16	—	12	.20	52	23	—
WHITE CAKE										
with chocolate icing, from mix, 1/12 cake, 95 gm	333	4	10	60	—	94	.50	216	110	—
with coconut icing, home recipe										
9" diam, 1/12 cake, 104 gm	386	4	14	63	—	47	.30	267	110	—
8" diam, 1/12 cake, 81 gm	301	3	11	49	—	36	.20	208	86	—
with white icing, home recipe										
9" diam, 1/12 cake, 104 gm	390	3	13	65	—	50	.10	243	60	—
8" diam, 1/12 cake, 82 gm	308	3	11	52	—	39	.10	192	48	—
YELLOW CAKE										
with caramel icing, home recipe, 9" diam, 1/12 cake, 108 gm	391	4	13	66	—	83	.80	244	79	—
with chocolate icing, home recipe, 9" diam, 1/12 cake, 100 gm	365	4	13	60	—	68	.60	208	108	—

Cookies

Drake–Borden

OATMEAL, 3 cookies	190	3	7	29	—	*	.72	200	60	—

Duncan Hines– Procter & Gamble

ALMOND FUDGE CHOCOLATE CHIP, 1 cookie	55	<1	3	7	—	*	*	45	—	—
BUTTERSCOTCH CHOCOLATE CHIP, 1 cookie	55	<1	3	7	—	*	*	35	—	—
CHOCOLATE CHIP, 1 cookie	55	<1	3	7	—	*	*	35	—	—
CHOCOLATE CHIP MIX, 2 cookies	150	1	8	19	—	*	.36	95	—	—
DOUBLE CHOCOLATE CHIP MIX, 2 cookies	140	1	7	19	—	*	.72	80	—	—
GOLDEN SUGAR MIX, 2 cookies	130	1	6	17	—	*	.36	70	—	—
MINT CHOCOLATE CHIP, 1 cookie	55	<1	3	7	—	*	*	35	—	—
OATMEAL RAISIN MIX, 2 cookies	130	2	6	18	—	20	.72	70	—	—
PEANUT BUTTER MIX, 2 cookies	140	3	7	15	—	*	.36	120	—	—
PEANUT BUTTER 'N FUDGE CHOCOLATE CHIP, 1 cookie	55	<1	3	7	—	*	*	45	—	—

Estee

COOKIES, ASSORTED, 1 cookie	25	<1	1-2	3	—	—	—	<5	—	0-5

FOOD & DESCRIPTION MEASURE OR QUANTITY	CALORIES	PROTEIN (GM)	FAT (GM)	CARBO-HYDRATE (GM)	FIBER (GM)	CALCIUM (MG)	IRON (MG)	SODIUM (MG)	POTASSIUM (MG)	CHOLES-TEROL (MG)
CREME FILLED COOKIES, CHOCOLATE/VANILLA FILLING, 1 cookie	20	<1	1	3	—	—	—	<5	—	0
WAFERS, ASSORTED, 1 cookie	30	<1	2	4	—	—	—	5	—	0
DUPLEX SANDWICH, 1 cookie	40	<1	2	5	—	—	—	5	—	0
SNACK WAFERS, all flavors, 1 cookie	80	<1	4	11	—	—	—	<5	—	0
SNACK WAFERS, CHOCOLATE COATED, 1 cookie	120	2	7	14	—	—	—	10	—	<5

Featherweight

FOOD & DESCRIPTION	CALORIES	PROTEIN	FAT	CARBO	FIBER	CALCIUM	IRON	SODIUM	POTASSIUM	CHOL
CHOCOLATE CHIP, 1 cookie	40	1	2	4	—	—	—	6	30	—
CHOCOLATE WAFER, 1 wafer	30	0	2	3	—	—	—	12	60	—
LEMON, 1 cookie	40	1	2	4	—	—	—	3	25	—
PEANUT BUTTER WAFERS, 1 wafer	30	0	2	3	—	—	—	12	64	—
VANILLA, 1 cookie	40	1	2	4	—	—	—	6	31	—
VANILLA WAFER, 1 wafer	30	0	2	3	—	—	—	12	57	—

General Mills

FOOD & DESCRIPTION	CALORIES	PROTEIN	FAT	CARBO	FIBER	CALCIUM	IRON	SODIUM	POTASSIUM	CHOL
CHOCOLATE CHIP, BIG BATCH, 2 cookies	120	1	6	16	—	*	.36	100	75	—
CHOCOLATE CHIP BROWNIE, 1/24 batch	130	1	5	20	—	*	.72	75	85	—
FUDGE BROWNIE family size, 1/24 batch	130	1	5	21	—	*	.72	95	90	—
regular size, 1/16 batch	150	1	6	23	—	*	.72	100	95	—
FROSTED FAMILY FUDGE BROWNIE, 1/24 batch	160	1	5	27	—	*	.72	105	105	—
SUPREME FUDGE BROWNIE, 1/24 batch	120	1	3	21	—	*	.36	85	65	—
SUPREME GOLDEN BROWNIE, 1/24 batch	130	1	5	19	—	*	*	30	30	—
SUGAR, BIG BATCH, 2 cookies	120	1	5	18	—	*	.36	95	25	—
WALNUT BROWNIE family size, 1/24 batch	130	1	6	19	—	*	.72	85	90	—
regular size, 1/16 batch	160	1	7	22	—	*	.72	105	105	—

Jiffy

FOOD & DESCRIPTION	CALORIES	PROTEIN	FAT	CARBO	FIBER	CALCIUM	IRON	SODIUM	POTASSIUM	CHOL
FUDGE BROWNIE, 2 × 2½" piece, 31 gm	130	2	5	18	—	20	1.08	135		

Keebler

FOOD & DESCRIPTION	CALORIES	PROTEIN	FAT	CARBO	FIBER	CALCIUM	IRON	SODIUM	POTASSIUM	CHOL
CHIPS DELUXE, 1 cookie	90	<1	4	10	—	*	.36	75	—	—
DELUXE GRAHAMS, 2 cookies	80	<1	4	11	—	*	.36	50	—	—
FUDGE CREMES, 1 cookie	60	<1	3	8	—	*	*	30	—	—
FUDGE STRIPES, 1 cookie	50	<1	3	7	—	*	*	50	—	—
OATMEAL CREMES, 1 cookie	80	<1	3	11	—	*	*	60	—	—
OLD FASHIONED OATMEAL, 1 cookie	80	1	3	12	—	*	.36	115	—	—
PECAN SANDIES, 1 cookie	80	<1	5	9	—	*	.36	75	—	—
PITTER PATTER, 1 cookie	90	1	4	11	—	*	.36	120	—	—
RICH 'N CHIPS, 1 cookie	80	1	4	10	—	*	*	70	—	—
VANILLA WAFERS, 3 cookies	60	<1	3	8	—	*	*	50	—	—

Nabisco

FOOD & DESCRIPTION	CALORIES	PROTEIN	FAT	CARBO	FIBER	CALCIUM	IRON	SODIUM	POTASSIUM	CHOL
ALMOST HOME APPLE FRUIT STICKS, 1 piece, .67 oz	70	0	2	14	—	*	.36	30	30	—

FOOD & DESCRIPTION MEASURE OR QUANTITY	CALORIES	PROTEIN (GM)	FAT (GM)	CARBO-HYDRATE (GM)	FIBER (GM)	CALCIUM (MG)	IRON (MG)	SODIUM (MG)	POTASSIUM (MG)	CHOLES-TEROL (MG)
BLUEBERRY FRUIT STICKS, 1 piece, .67 oz	70	0	2	14	—	*	.36	90	20	—
CHERRY FRUIT STICKS, 1 piece, .67 oz	70	0	2	14	—	*	.36	100	20	—
FUDGE CHOCOLATE CHIP, 2 cookies, 1 oz	130	1	5	20	—	*	.72	130	60	—
RAISIN, 2 cookies, 1 oz	130	1	5	18	—	20	.36	85	60	—
FUDGE 'N CHOCOLATE CREME SANDWICHES, 1 cookie, 1.13 oz	140	2	6	20	—	20	.72	120	40	—
FUDGE 'N NUT BROWNIE, 1 piece, 1.25 oz	160	1	7	23	—	*	.36	75	50	—
FUDGE 'N VANILLA CREME SANDWICHES, 1 cookie, 1.13 oz	140	1	6	20	—	20	.36	110	35	—
ICED APPLESAUCE RAISIN, 2 cookies, 1 oz	140	2	8	17	—	20	.72	70	60	—
ICED DUTCH APPLE FRUIT STICKS, 1 piece, .67 oz	70	0	1	14	—	*	.36	40	40	—
ICED OATMEAL RAISIN, 2 cookies, 1 oz	130	2	5	19	—	*	.72	80	55	—
OATMEAL CREME SANDWICH, 1 piece, 1.13 oz	140	2	5	21	—	20	.72	150	60	—
OATMEAL RAISIN, 2 cookies, 1 oz	130	2	5	20	—	*	.72	100	55	—
OLD FASHIONED CINNAMON RAISIN, 2 cookies, 1 oz	140	3	7	16	—	*	.72	95	85	—
PEANUT BUTTER, 2 cookies, 1 oz	140	3	7	16	—	20	.36	95	85	—
CREME SANDWICH, 1 piece, 1.13 oz	140	2	6	20	—	20	.36	120	60	—
FUDGE, 2 cookies, 1 oz	140	3	7	16	—	20	.36	90	85	—
REAL CHOCOLATE CHIP COOKIES, 2 cookies, 1 oz	130	1	5	20	—	*	.36	100	35	—
APPLE NEWTON, 1½ cookies, 1 oz	110	1	2	21	—	*	.36	45	35	—
BAKERS BONUS OATMEAL, 2 cookies, 1 oz	130	2	5	20	—	*	.72	90	35	—
SUGAR RING, 2 cookies, 1 oz	130	2	5	20	—	*	.36	100	25	—
BARNUM'S ANIMAL CRACKERS, 11 cookies, 1 oz	130	2	4	21	—	*	.36	120	30	—
BARONET CREME SANDWICH, 3 cookies, 1 oz	140	1	6	20	—	*	.36	75	30	—
BISCOS SUGAR WAFERS, 8 wafers, 1 oz	150	1	7	20	—	*	.36	35	15	—
WAFFLE CREMES, 3 cookies, 1 oz	150	1	7	20	—	*	.36	30	5	—
BLUEBERRY NEWTON, 1½ cookies, 1 oz	110	1	2	21	—	*	.36	80	25	—
BROWN EDGE WAFERS, 5 wafers, 1 oz	140	1	6	20	—	*	.36	80	30	—
BUGS BUNNY GRAHAM, 9 cookies, 1 oz	120	2	4	20	—	20	.36	130	60	—
BUTTER FLAVOR, 6 cookies, 1 oz	130	2	5	20	—	*	.36	140	35	—
CAMEO CREME SANDWICH, 3 cookies, 1 oz	140	1	5	21	—	*	.36	85	40	—
CHERRY NEWTON, 1½ cookies, 1 oz	110	1	2	20	—	*	.36	80	30	—

FOOD & DESCRIPTION MEASURE OR QUANTITY	CALORIES	PROTEIN (GM)	FAT (GM)	CARBO-HYDRATE (GM)	FIBER (GM)	CALCIUM (MG)	IRON (MG)	SODIUM (MG)	POTASSIUM (MG)	CHOLES-TEROL (MG)
CHEWY CHIPS AHOY, 2 cookies, 1 oz	130	1	6	18	—	*	.36	110	25	—
CHIPS AHOY, 3 cookies, 1 oz	140	2	7	18	—	*	.72	95	35	—
CHIPS 'N MORE CHOCOLATE CHIP COOKIES										
COCONUT, 2 cookies, 1 oz	150	1	8	18	—	*	.72	95	45	—
FUDGE, 3 cookies, 1 oz	140	2	6	19	—	*	.36	90	45	—
ORIGINAL, 2 cookies, 1 oz	150	2	7	18	—	*	.36	70	35	—
CHOCOLATE CHIP SNAP, 6 cookies, 1 oz	130	2	4	21	—	*	.36	100	30	—
CHOCOLATE GRAHAM, 3 cookies, 1 oz	150	2	7	19	—	*	1.08	70	80	—
CHOCOLATE SNAP, 7 cookies, 1 oz	130	2	4	21	—	*	.72	140	50	—
COCONUT MACAROON SOFT CAKES, 1 cookie, 1.33 oz	190	1	9	23	—	*	1.08	65	95	—
COOKIE BREAK VANILLA CREME, 3 cookies, 1 oz	140	1	6	20	—	*	.36	95	20	—
DEVIL'S FOOD CAKES, 1 cookie, 1.33 oz	140	1	1	30	—	*	.72	90	50	—
FAMOUS CHOCOLATE WAFERS, 5 cookies, 1 oz	130	2	4	21	—	*	1.08	200	75	—
FIG NEWTON, 2 cookies, 1 oz	100	1	2	20	—	20	.72	100	60	—
FUDGE STRIPED SHORTBREAD, 3 cookies, 1 oz	150	1	7	19	—	*	.36	110	30	—
GAIETY FUDGE CHOCOLATE, 3 cookies, 1 oz	150	2	7	19	—	*	.72	120	50	—
GIGGLES SANDWICH										
CHOCOLATE, 2 cookies, 1 oz	140	1	6	17	—	*	.36	70	20	—
VANILLA, 2 cookies, 1 oz	140	1	6	17	—	*	.36	50	15	—
HEYDAY BARS, 1 bar, 1 oz	140	2	8	15	—	60	.36	45	80	—
IDEAL BARS, 2 bars, 1 oz	150	2	8	17	—	*	.36	130	80	—
IMPORTED DANISH, 5 cookies, 1 oz	150	1	8	18	—	20	.72	70	25	—
I SCREAMS DOUBLE DIP CREME SANDWICH										
CHOCOLATE, 2 cookies, 1 oz	150	1	7	20	—	*	.72	70	55	—
VANILLA, 2 cookies, 1 oz	150	1	7	20	—	*	.36	70	20	—
KETTLE, 4 cookies, 1 oz	130	2	5	20	—	*	.72	115	30	—
LORNA DOONE SHORTBREAD, 4 cookies, 1 oz	140	2	7	18	—	*	.36	135	30	—
MALLOMARS CHOCOLATE CAKES, 2 cakes, 1 oz	130	1	6	18	—	*	.72	35	55	—
MARSHMALLOW PUFF, 1 cookie, 1 oz	120	1	4	20	—	*	*	55	50	—
MARSHMALLOW SANDWICH, 4 cookies, 1 oz	120	1	3	22	—	*	.36	80	20	—
MARSHMALLOW TWIRLS CAKES, 1 cake, 1 oz	130	1	5	19	—	*	.72	55	55	—
MYSTIC MINT SANDWICH, 2 cookies, 1 oz	150	1	8	19	—	*	.72	95	70	—
NATIONAL ARROWROOT BISCUIT, 6 cookies, 1 oz	130	2	4	21	—	20	.36	80	25	—
NILLA WAFER, 7 cookies, 1 oz	130	1	4	21	—	*	.36	95	30	—
NUTTER BUTTER PEANUT BUTTER										
CREME PATTIES, 4 cookies, 1 oz	150	3	8	17	—	*	.36	95	70	—
SANDWICH, 2 cookies, 1 oz	140	3	6	18	—	*	.36	100	55	—
OLD FASHIONED GINGER SNAP, 4 cookies, 1 oz	120	2	3	22	—	20	1.44	200	100	—

FOOD & DESCRIPTION MEASURE OR QUANTITY	CALORIES	PROTEIN (GM)	FAT (GM)	CARBO- HYDRATE (GM)	FIBER (GM)	CALCIUM (MG)	IRON (MG)	SODIUM (MG)	POTASSIUM (MG)	CHOLES- TEROL (MG)
OREO										
CHOCOLATE SANDWICH, 3 cookies, 1 oz	140	1	6	20	—	*	.72	170	50	—
DOUBLE STUFF, 2 cookies, 1 oz	140	1	7	19	—	*	.36	120	35	—
MINT CREME, 2 cookies, 1 oz	140	1	6	20	—	*	.72	160	50	—
PANTRY MOLASSES, 2 cookies, 1 oz	130	2	4	21	—	20	1.44	130	120	—
PARTY GRAHAM, 3 cookies, 1 oz	140	1	7	19	—	*	.36	100	50	—
PECAN SHORTBREAD, 2 cookies, 1 oz	150	2	9	16	—	*	.36	80	20	—
PINWHEEL, 1 cake, 1 oz	130	1	5	20	—	*	.36	35	40	—
PURE CHOCOLATE MIDDLES, 2 cookies, 1 oz	150	2	8	18	—	*	.72	65	50	—
SOCIAL TEA BISCUIT, 6 biscuits, 1 oz	130	2	4	21	—	*	.72	105	30	—
SUPER HEROES, 11 cookies, 1 oz	135	2	5	20	—	*	.36	120	50	—
Pepperidge Farm— Campbell										
ALMOND SUPREME, 2 cookies	140	2	10	13	—	20	.72	45	—	—
APRICOT-RASPBERRY FRUIT, 3 cookies	150	1	6	23	—	*	*	80	—	—
BLUEBERRY FRUIT, 3 cookies	170	2	6	27	—	*	.36	80	—	—
BORDEAUX, 3 cookies	110	1	5	16	—	*	*	70	—	—
BROWNIE CHOCOLATE NUT, 3 cookies	170	1	10	19	—	*	.72	80	—	—
BRUSSELS, 3 cookies	160	1	8	20	—	*	.36	95	—	—
BRUSSELS MINT, 3 cookies	200	1	10	25	—	*	.36	120	—	—
CAPPUCINO, 3 cookies	160	1	9	18	—	*	*	60	—	—
CAPRI, 2 cookies	160	1	9	20	—	*	.36	90	—	—
CHAMPAGNE, 3 cookies	95	1	5	12	—	*	.36	55	—	—
CHESSMEN, 3 cookies	130	1	6	18	—	*	.36	80	—	—
CHOCOLATE CHIP, 3 cookies	150	1	8	20	—	*	.36	90	—	—
CHOCOLATE CHOCOLATE CHIP, 3 cookies	160	1	9	19	—	*	.72	75	—	—
CHOCOLATE CHUNK PECAN, 2 cookies	130	1	7	15	—	*	.36	50	—	—
CHOCOLATE LACED PIROUETTES, 3 cookies	110	0	7	13	—	*	.36	45	—	—
DATE NUT GRANOLA, 3 cookies	160	1	9	20	—	*	.72	95	—	—
DATE PECAN, 3 cookies	160	1	8	22	—	*	.36	60	—	—
GENEVA, 3 cookies	170	2	10	19	—	*	.72	65	—	—
GINGERMAN, 3 cookies	100	1	4	15	—	*	.36	75	—	—
HAZELNUT, 3 cookies	170	1	9	22	—	*	.36	110	—	—
IRISH OATMEAL, 3 cookies	140	1	7	20	—	*	.36	120	—	—
LEMON NUT CRUNCH, 3 cookies	170	1	10	19	—	*	.72	75	—	—
LIDO, 2 cookies	190	1	11	21	—	*	.36	85	—	—
MILANO, 3 cookies	180	1	10	21	—	*	*	80	—	—
MILK CHOCOLATE MACADAMIA, 2 cookies	120	2	7	13	—	20	.36	60	—	—
MINT MILANO, 3 cookies	230	0	13	25	—	*	.36	105	—	—
MOCHA CHOCOLATE CHIP, 3 cookies	120	1	6	16	—	20	.36	65	—	—
MOLASSES CRISPS, 3 cookies	100	1	5	12	—	20	.36	75	—	—
NASSAU, 2 cookies	170	2	10	18	—	*	.36	90	—	—
OATMEAL RAISIN, 3 cookies	170	2	8	23	—	*	.72	170	—	—
ORANGE MILANO, 3 cookies	230	1	13	25	—	*	.36	105	—	—

FOOD & DESCRIPTION MEASURE OR QUANTITY	CALORIES	PROTEIN (GM)	FAT (GM)	CARBO-HYDRATE (GM)	FIBER (GM)	CALCIUM (MG)	IRON (MG)	SODIUM (MG)	POTASSIUM (MG)	CHOLES-TEROL (MG)
ORIGINAL PIROUETTES, 3 cookies	110	0	7	13	—	*	*	55	—	—
ORLEANS, 3 cookies	90	0	6	11	—	*	.36	30	—	—
PEANUT BUTTER CHOCOLATE CHIP, 3 cookies	140	2	8	16	—	80	.36	125	—	—
RAISIN BRAN, 3 cookies	160	1	8	20	—	*	.36	80	—	—
SEVILLE, 2 cookies	110	1	6	14	—	*	.36	50	—	—
SHORTBREAD, 2 cookies	150	1	8	17	—	*	*	85	—	—
SOUTHPORT, 2 cookies	150	1	9	18	—	*	.72	70	—	—
STRAWBERRY FRUIT, 3 cookies	150	1	7	23	—	*	.36	70	—	—
SUGAR, 3 cookies	150	1	8	20	—	*	.36	115	—	—
TAHITI, 2 cookies	170	1	11	17	—	*	.36	50	—	—

Pillsbury

FOOD & DESCRIPTION MEASURE OR QUANTITY	CALORIES	PROTEIN (GM)	FAT (GM)	CARBO-HYDRATE (GM)	FIBER (GM)	CALCIUM (MG)	IRON (MG)	SODIUM (MG)	POTASSIUM (MG)	CHOLES-TEROL (MG)
CHOCOLATE CHIP, 3 cookies	200	2	10	27	—	0	.72	160	55	—
DOUBLE CHOCOLATE, 3 cookies	150	1	6	23	—	0	.36	160	50	—
FUDGE BROWNIES, 1 bar	140	1	5	22	—	0	.36	115	60	—
OATMEAL RAISIN, 3 cookies	190	3	8	27	—	0	.72	190	80	—
PEANUT BUTTER, 3 cookies	200	4	10	24	—	0	.72	220	85	—
SUGAR, 3 cookies	190	2	8	28	—	0	.72	210	25	—

Stella D'Oro

FOOD & DESCRIPTION MEASURE OR QUANTITY	CALORIES	PROTEIN (GM)	FAT (GM)	CARBO-HYDRATE (GM)	FIBER (GM)	CALCIUM (MG)	IRON (MG)	SODIUM (MG)	POTASSIUM (MG)	CHOLES-TEROL (MG)
ALMOND TOAST, 1 toast	56	1	1	10	—	—	—	—	—	—
ANGEL BARS, 1 bar	69	<1	4	7	—	—	—	—	—	—
ANGEL WINGS, 1 cookie	75	<1	5	7	—	—	—	—	—	—
ANGELICA GOODIES, 1 cookie	104	2	4	16	—	—	—	—	—	—
ANGINETTI, 1 cookie	32	<1	1	5	—	—	—	—	—	—
ANISETTE SPONGE, 1 cookie	52	1	<1	10	—	—	—	—	—	—
ANISETTE TOAST, 1 toast	46	<1	<1	10	—	—	—	—	—	—
JUMBO, 1 toast	138	3	1	29	—	—	—	—	—	—
CHINESE DESSERT, 1 cookie	178	3	10	20	—	—	—	—	—	—
COCONUT, dietetic, 1 cookie	50	<1	2	6	—	—	—	<10	—	—
COCONUT MACAROON, 1 cookie	64	<1	4	7	—	—	—	—	—	—
COMO DELIGHT, 1 cookie	138	2	7	17	—	—	—	—	—	—
EGG BISCUIT, 1 biscuit	44	2	1	7	—	—	—	—	—	—
dietetic, 1 biscuit	40	2	1	7	—	—	—	<10	—	—
EGG JUMBO, 1 piece	46	1	<1	9	—	—	—	—	—	—
GOLDEN BARS, 1 bar	109	2	4	16	—	—	—	—	—	—
HOLIDAY TRINKET, 1 cookie	37	<1	2	5	—	—	—	—	—	—
HOSTESS ASSORTMENT, 1 cookie	37	<1	2	5	—	—	—	—	—	—
KICHEL, dietetic, 1 cookie	8	<1	<1	<1	—	—	—	<10	—	—
LADY STELLA ASSORTMENT, 1 cookie	39	<1	2	5	—	—	—	—	—	—
LOVE, dietetic, 1 cookie	110	2	6	14	—	—	—	<10	—	—
MARGHERITE CHOCOLATE, 1 cookie	72	1	3	10	—	—	—	—	—	—
VANILLA, 1 cookie	75	1	3	11	—	—	—	—	—	—
MINIATURE FRUIT CAKES, 1 cake	54	<1	3	7	—	—	—	—	—	—
PEACH APRICOT PASTRY, 1 cookie	97	1	4	14	—	—	—	—	—	—
dietetic, 1 cookie	90	2	4	13	—	—	—	<10	—	—
PFEFFERNUSSE, 1 cookie	37	<1	<1	7	—	—	—	—	—	—
ROMAN EGG BISCUITS, 1 biscuit	125	3	5	18	—	—	—	—	—	—
ROYAL NUGGETS, dietetic, 1 cookie	1	<1	<1	<1	—	—	—	<10	—	—
SESAME/REGINA, 1 cookie	48	<1	2	6	—	—	—	—	—	—
dietetic, 1 cookie	43	<1	2	6	—	—	—	<10	—	—

FOOD & DESCRIPTION MEASURE OR QUANTITY	CALORIES	PROTEIN (GM)	FAT (GM)	CARBO-HYDRATE (GM)	FIBER (GM)	CALCIUM (MG)	IRON (MG)	SODIUM (MG)	POTASSIUM (MG)	CHOLES-TEROL (MG)
SUGARED EGG BISCUIT, 1 biscuit	75	2	1	14	—	—	—	—	—	—
SWISS FUDGE, 1 cookie	67	<1	3	8	—	—	—	—	—	—

Sweet 'N Low

CHOCOLATE CHIP MIX, prep, 1 cookie	25	<1	<1	5	—	20	*	9	37	<5

Tastykake

VANILLA SHORTBREAD, 1 cookie	49	<1	2	6	—	—	—	23	—	—

USDA

BUTTER, 10 cookies, 50 gm	229	3	9	36	—	63	.30	209	30	—
CHOCOLATE CHIP, 2¼″ diam, 10 cookies, 105 gm	495	6	22	73	—	41	1.90	421	141	—
COCONUT BAR, 3 × 1¼ × ¼″, 10 pieces, 90 gm	445	6	22	58	—	65	1.30	133	205	—
GINGERSNAP, 2 × ¼″, 10 cookies, 70 gm	294	4	6	56	—	51	1.60	400	323	—
LADYFINGERS, 3¼ × 1⅜ × 1⅛″, 4 cookies, 44 gm	158	3	3	28	—	18	.70	31	31	—
MACAROONS, 2¾″ diam, 2 cookies, 38 gm	181	2	9	25	—	10	.30	13	176	—
MOLASSES, 3⅝ × ¾″, 1 cookie, 33 gm	137	2	3	25	—	17	.70	125	45	—
OATMEAL WITH RAISINS, 2⅝ × ¼″, 4 cookies, 52 gm	235	3	8	38	—	11	1.50	84	192	—
PEANUT SANDWICH, 1¾ × ½″, 4 cookies, 49 gm	232	5	9	33	—	21	.40	85	86	—
PEANUT SUGAR WAFER, 1¾ × 1⅜ × ⅜″, 10 cookies, 70 gm	331	7	13	47	—	29	.60	121	123	—
RAISIN, buscuit type, 2¼ × 2½ × ¼″, 4 cookies, 71 gm	269	3	4	57	—	50	1.50	37	193	—
SHORTBREAD, 1⅝ × 1⅝ × ¼″, 10 cookies, 75 gm	374	5	17	49	—	53	.40	45	50	—
SUGAR WAFERS, 2½ × ¾ × ¼″, 10 cookies, 35 gm	170	2	7	26	—	13	.10	66	21	—
VANILLA WAFERS, 1¾ × ¼″ 10 cookies, 40 gm	185	2	6	30	—	16	.20	101	29	—
1 cup crumbs, 80 gm	370	4	13	60	—	33	.30	202	58	—

Crackers

Estee

SIX CALORIE WHEAT WAFER, 1 cracker	6	<1	<1	1	—	—	—	<5	—	<5
UNSALTED, 2 crackers	30	<1	1	5	—	—	—	<5	—	<1

Featherweight

BRAN WAFER, 4 wafers	50	1	1	8	—	—	—	2	35	—
CRACKERS, 2 crackers	30	0	1	5	—	—	—	1	67	—
WHEAT WAFERS, 4 wafers	50	1	1	9	—	—	—	2	35	—

Hain

CHEESE, 11 crackers, 1 oz	130	3	6	17	—	20	1.44	180	80	—
ONION SALT FREE, 11 crackers, 1 oz	130	3	6	17	—	20	.72	5	0	—

FOOD & DESCRIPTION MEASURE OR QUANTITY	CALORIES	PROTEIN (GM)	FAT (GM)	CARBO-HYDRATE (GM)	FIBER (GM)	CALCIUM (MG)	IRON (MG)	SODIUM (MG)	POTASSIUM (MG)	CHOLES-TEROL (MG)
SALTED, 11 crackers, 1 oz	130	3	6	17	—	20	.72	160	75	—
PUMPERNICKEL										
SALT FREE, 10 crackers, 1 oz	130	3	6	16	—	*	.72	10	70	—
SALTED, 10 crackers, 1 oz	130	3	6	16	—	*	.72	180	70	—
RICH										
SALT FREE, 8 crackers, 1 oz	130	3	5	18	—	*	.72	15	200	—
SALTED, 8 crackers, 1 oz	130	3	5	18	—	*	.72	160	200	—
RYE										
SALT FREE, 11 crackers, 1 oz	120	3	4	19	—	20	.72	10	80	—
SALTED, 11 crackers, 1 oz	120	3	4	19	—	20	.72	200	80	—
SESAME										
SALT FREE, 11 crackers, 1 oz	140	3	7	16	—	*	.72	5	85	—
SALTED, 11 crackers, 1 oz	140	3	7	16	—	*	.72	210	85	—
SOUR CREAM & CHIVE										
SALT FREE, 11 crackers, 1 oz	130	3	6	15	—	20	.36	25	85	—
SALTED, 11 crackers, 1 oz	130	3	6	15	—	20	.36	150	85	—
SOURDOUGH										
SALT FREE, 11 crackers, 1 oz	130	3	5	18	—	20	.36	10	60	—
SALTED, 11 crackers, 1 oz	130	3	5	18	—	20	.36	200	60	—
TOASTED CHEESE CRACKERS										
BLUE CHEESE & ONION, LOW SALT, 14 crackers, 1 oz	140	3	6	17	—	40	.36	100	160	—
CHEESE STYLE PIZZA, 14 crackers, 1 oz	140	4	7	15	—	20	.36	340	160	—
PARMESAN & GARLIC, 14 crackers, 1 oz	150	3	8	15	—	20	.36	310	65	—
SWISS CHEESE & RYE LOW SALT, 14 crackers, 1 oz	140	3	6	17	—	40	.36	100	110	—
SALTED, 14 crackers, 1 oz	140	3	6	17	—	40	.36	330	110	—
VEGETABLE										
SALT FREE, 11 crackers, 1 oz	130	3	5	10	—	20	1.44	50	60	—
SALTED, 11 crackers, 1 oz	130	3	5	10	—	20	1.44	180	60	—

Keebler

CINNAMON CRISP, 4 graham crackers	70	1	2	11	—	*	.36	85	—	—
CLUB, 4 crackers	60	1	3	8	—	*	.36	155	—	—
HARVEST WHEATS, 3 crackers	70	1	4	8	—	*	.36	115	—	—
HONEY GRAHAM, 4 crackers	70	1	2	12	—	*	.36	85	—	—
TOASTED RYE, 5 crackers	80	1	4	10	—	*	.36	145	—	—
TOASTED SESAME, 5 crackers	80	1	4	10	—	*	.36	140	—	—
TOASTED WHEAT, 5 crackers	80	1	4	10	—	*	.36	150	—	—
TOWN HOUSE, 5 crackers	80	1	5	9	—	*	.36	145	—	—
TUC SNACK, 3 crackers	70	1	4	8	—	*	.36	85	—	—
ZESTA SALTINES, 5 crackers	60	1	2	10	—	*	.36	205	—	—

Manischewitz

AMERICAN MATZO, 1 oz	115	—	1	—	—	—	—	175	—	0
DAILY THIN TEA MATZOS, .91 oz	103	—	<1	—	—	—	—	<5	—	0
DIETETIC MATZO THINS, .83 oz	91	—	<1	—	—	—	—	<5	—	0
EGG MATZO, 10 crackers	108	—	2	—	—	—	—	<10	—	20
EGG N'ONION MATZOS, 1 oz	112	—	<1	—	—	—	—	180	—	0
GARLIC TAMS, 10 crackers	153	—	8	—	—	—	—	165	—	0
MATZO, 1 oz	110	—	<1	—	—	—	—	<5	—	0
MATZO MINIATURES, 1 cracker	9	—	0	—	—	—	—	0	—	0
ONION TAMS, 10 crackers	150	—	8	—	—	—	—	157	—	0
TAM TAM, 10 crackers	147	—	8	—	—	—	—	171	—	0
no salt, 5 crackers	70	—	4	—	—	—	—	<5	—	0

FOOD & DESCRIPTION MEASURE OR QUANTITY	CALORIES	PROTEIN (GM)	FAT (GM)	CARBO-HYDRATE (GM)	FIBER (GM)	CALCIUM (MG)	IRON (MG)	SODIUM (MG)	POTASSIUM (MG)	CHOLES-TEROL (MG)
WHEAT TAMS, 10 crackers	150	—	8	—	—	—	—	180	—	0
WHEAT MATZO, 1 cracker	9	—	0	—	—	—	—	0	—	0

Nabisco

FOOD & DESCRIPTION MEASURE OR QUANTITY	CALORIES	PROTEIN (GM)	FAT (GM)	CARBO-HYDRATE (GM)	FIBER (GM)	CALCIUM (MG)	IRON (MG)	SODIUM (MG)	POTASSIUM (MG)	CHOLES-TEROL (MG)
BACON FLAVORED THINS, 7 crackers, ½ oz	70	1	4	8	—	*	.36	210	20	—
BETTER										
BLUE CHEESE SNACK, 10 crackers, ½ oz	70	1	4	8	—	*	.36	260	15	—
CHEDDAR SNACK THINS, 11 crackers, ½ oz	70	2	4	8	—	*	.36	220	15	—
NACHO SNACK THINS, 9 crackers, ½ oz	70	1	4	8	—	*	.36	220	15	—
SWISS SNACK THINS, 10 crackers, ½ oz	70	1	4	8	—	*	.36	230	15	—
CHEESE NIPS, 13 crackers, ½ oz	70	1	3	9	—	*	.36	130	25	—
CHEESE PEANUT BUTTER SANDWICH, 2 pieces, ½ oz	70	2	3	8	—	20	.36	150	25	—
CHEESE RITZ, 5 crackers, ½ oz	70	1	3	8	—	20	.36	120	15	—
CHEESE SANDWICH, 2 pieces, ½ oz	70	2	3	8	—	20	.36	180	40	—
CHEESE TID-BIT, 16 bits, ½ oz	70	1	4	8	—	20	.36	200	20	—
CHEESE WHEAT THINS, 9 crackers, ½ oz	70	2	3	9	—	20	.36	220	35	—
CHICKEN IN A BISKIT, 7 crackers, ½ oz	70	1	4	8	—	*	.36	115	20	—
CINNAMON TREATS, 2 crackers, ½ oz	60	1	1	11	—	*	.36	80	20	—
COUNTRY, 5 crackers, ½ oz	80	1	4	9	—	*	.36	120	20	—
CRACKER MEAL, 2 tbsp, ½ oz	50	1	0	12	—	*	.36	0	20	—
CROWN PILOT, 1 cracker, ½ oz	60	1	1	11	—	*	.36	65	20	—
DANDY SOUP & OYSTER, 20 crackers, ½ oz	60	1	1	10	—	*	.72	220	20	—
DIP IN A CHIP, CHEESE 'N CHIVE, 8 pieces, ½ oz	70	1	4	8	—	20	.36	130	40	—
ESCORT, 3 crackers, ½ oz	80	1	4	9	—	*	.36	110	20	—
GRAHAM, 2 crackers, ½ oz	60	1	1	11	—	*	.36	115	20	—
crumbs, 2 tbsp, ½ oz	60	1	1	11	—	*	.36	90	15	—
GREAT CRISPS										
CHEESE 'N CHIVE, 9 crackers, ½ oz	70	2	4	8	—	*	.36	170	20	—
FRENCH ONION, 7 crackers, ½ oz	70	1	4	8	—	*	.36	90	20	—
NACHO, 8 crackers, ½ oz	70	1	4	8	—	*	.36	250	30	—
REAL BACON, 9 crackers, ½ oz	70	2	4	8	—	*	.36	230	20	—
SAVORY GARLIC, 8 crackers, ½ oz	70	1	3	9	—	20	.36	190	20	—
SESAME, 9 crackers, ½ oz	70	2	4	8	—	20	.36	190	25	—
TOMATO & CELERY, 9 crackers, ½ oz	70	1	4	8	—	20	.36	160	35	—
HOLLAND RUSK INSTANT TOAST, 1 toast, ½ oz	60	2	1	10	—	*	.36	35	35	—
HONEY MAID GRAHAM, 2 crackers, ½ oz	60	1	1	11	—	*	.36	90	20	—
MALTED MILK PEANUT BUTTER SANDWICH, 2 sandwiches, ½ oz	70	2	3	9	—	*	.36	150	30	—

FOOD & DESCRIPTION MEASURE OR QUANTITY	CALORIES	PROTEIN (GM)	FAT (GM)	CARBO- HYDRATE (GM)	FIBER (GM)	CALCIUM (MG)	IRON (MG)	SODIUM (MG)	POTASSIUM (MG)	CHOLES- TEROL (MG)
MEAL MATES SESAME BREAD WAFERS, 3 wafers, ½ oz	70	1	3	9	—	20	.36	140	30	—
NUTTY WHEAT THINS, 7 crackers, ½ oz	80	1	5	8	—	*	.36	250	35	—
OYSTERETTES, 18 crackers, ½ oz	60	1	1	10	—	*	.36	130	20	—
PREMIUM SALTINES, 5 crackers, ½ oz	60	1	2	10	—	20	.72	180	20	—
UNSALTED TOPS, 5 crackers, ½ oz	60	1	2	10	—	20	.72	115	20	—
RITZ, 4 crackers, ½ oz	70	1	4	9	—	20	.36	120	15	—
LOW SALT, 4 crackers, ½ oz	70	1	4	9	—	20	.36	60	15	—
ROYAL LUNCH MILK, 1 cracker, ½ oz	60	1	2	10	—	20	.36	80	15	—
SEA ROUNDS, 1 cracker, ½ oz	60	1	2	10	—	*	.72	140	20	—
SOCIABLES, 6 crackers, ½ oz	70	1	3	9	—	20	.36	130	30	—
SULTANA SODA, 4 crackers, ½ oz	60	1	1	11	—	*	.36	115	20	—
TOASTED PEANUT BUTTER SANDWICH, 5 crackers, ½ oz	80	1	2	8	—	20	.36	150	30	—
TRISCUIT WAFERS, 3 crackers, ½ oz	60	1	2	10	—	*	.36	90	40	—
LOW SALT, 3 crackers, ½ oz	60	1	2	10	—	*	.36	35	40	—
TWIGS, SESAME & CHEESE, 5 twigs, ½ oz	70	1	4	8	—	40	.36	200	25	—
UNEEDA BISCUIT, unsalted tops, 3 crackers, ½ oz	60	1	2	10	—	*	.72	100	20	—
VEGETABLE THINS, 7 crackers, ½ oz	70	1	4	8	—	40	.36	100	30	—
WAVERLY, 4 crackers, ½ oz	70	1	3	10	—	20	.36	160	15	—
WHEAT THINS, 8 crackers, ½ oz	70	1	3	9	—	*	.36	120	25	—
LOW SALT, 8 crackers, ½ oz	70	1	3	9	—	*	.36	35	25	—
WHEATSWORTH STONE GROUND WHEAT, 5 crackers, ½ oz	70	1	3	9	—	*	.36	135	35	—
ZWIEBACK TOAST, 2 toasts, ½ oz	60	2	1	10	—	*	.36	20	20	—

Pepperidge Farm— Campbell

FOOD & DESCRIPTION MEASURE OR QUANTITY	CALORIES	PROTEIN (GM)	FAT (GM)	CARBO- HYDRATE (GM)	FIBER (GM)	CALCIUM (MG)	IRON (MG)	SODIUM (MG)	POTASSIUM (MG)	CHOLES- TEROL (MG)
BUTTER FLAVORED THIN, 4 crackers	80	1	3	10	—	*	.36	100	—	—
CHEDDAR CHEESE TINY GOLDFISH, 45 pieces	140	3	6	18	—	20	.36	180	—	—
CHEESE SNACK STICKS, 8 sticks	140	3	6	18	—	20	.36	350	—	—
CHEESE THINS, 4 crackers	70	1	3	8	—	20	.36	105	—	—
CRACKED WHEAT, 4 crackers	110	2	4	14	—	*	.36	200	—	—
ENGLISH WATER BISCUIT, 4 crackers	70	1	1	13	—	*	.36	90	—	—
HEARTY WHEAT, 4 crackers	100	2	4	13	—	*	.36	180	—	—
ORIGINAL SNACK STICKS, 8 sticks	130	2	5	20	—	*	.36	320	—	—
ORIGINAL TINY GOLDFISH, 45 pieces	140	2	7	18	—	*	*	180	—	—
PARMESAN CHEESE TINY GOLDFISH, 45 pieces	140	3	6	18	—	20	.36	250	—	—
PIZZA FLAVORED TINY GOLDFISH, 45 pieces	140	2	7	18	—	*	.36	180	—	—
PRETZEL TINY GOLDFISH, 40 pieces	120	2	3	21	—	*	.36	160	—	—

55

FOOD & DESCRIPTION MEASURE OR QUANTITY	CALORIES	PROTEIN (GM)	FAT (GM)	CARBO-HYDRATE (GM)	FIBER (GM)	CALCIUM (MG)	IRON (MG)	SODIUM (MG)	POTASSIUM (MG)	CHOLES-TEROL (MG)
PUMPERNICKEL SNACK STICKS, 8 sticks	130	2	5	20	—	*	.36	380	—	—
RYE SNACK STICKS, 8 sticks	130	2	4	20	—	*	.36	390	—	—
SESAME, 4 crackers	80	2	3	11	—	*	.36	105	—	—
SESAME SNACK STICKS, 8 sticks	130	2	6	18	—	*	.36	350	—	—
TOASTED WHEAT WITH ONION, 4 crackers	80	3	3	12	—	*	.36	110	—	—

Planters—Nabisco

ROUND TOAST, 1 oz	140	4	7	15	—	20	.72	270	85	—
SQUARE CHEESE, 1 oz	140	4	7	15	—	20	.72	270	85	—

Ralston Purina

ANIMAL, 15 crackers	130	2	3	22	.40d	3	.88	113	25	—
CHEDDAR SNACKS, 18 crackers, 1 oz	130	3	5	20	.50d	22	1.22	258	39	—
CHEESE & CHIVE SNACKS, 18 crackers, 1 oz	130	2	5	20	.80d	26	1.17	258	38	—
CHEESE SNACKS, 25 crackers, 1 oz	140	3	7	18	.70d	24	1.25	259	41	—
CRACKERS, UNSALTED TOPS, 10 crackers, 1 oz	120	3	3	21	.50d	5	1.13	212	35	—
GRAHAM, 8 crackers, 1 oz	120	2	3	22	.90d	6	.79	105	38	—
OYSTER, 65 pieces, 1 oz	120	3	3	20	.50d	4	1.20	347	33	—
RICH & CRISP, 9 crackers, 1 oz	140	2	6	19	.80d	18	.80	187	23	—
RY KRISP, 2 triples, .44 oz	45	2	<1	10	1.60d	5	.55	111	61	—
seasoned, 2 triples, .47 oz	50	1	1	10	1.50d	5	.45	160	65	—
sesame, 2 triples, .53 oz	50	2	1	11	1.70d	6	.53	172	69	—
RYE SNACKS, 15 crackers, 1 oz	130	2	5	20	1.70d	5	.97	209	49	—
SALTINES, 10 crackers, 1 oz	120	3	3	21	.60d	4	1.02	320	33	—
SESAME & WHEAT SNACKS, 15 crackers, 1 oz	130	2	6	20	2.00d	20	1.19	258	54	—
SNACKERS, 8 crackers, 1 oz	140	2	6	18	.90d	5	.83	188	32	—
WHEAT SNACKS, 15 crackers, 1 oz	130	2	6	19	1.20d	7	1.10	183	50	—

Rokeach

GRAHAM, 8 crackers	120	2	3	21	—	*	.72	—	—	—
KOSHER SALTINE, 10 crackers	120	2	3	20	—	*	.72	—	—	—
SNACK, 9 crackers	130	2	5	19	—	20	.72	—	—	—

Stella D'Oro

BREADSTICKS										
ONION, 1 piece	40	1	1	6	—	—	—	—	—	—
PLAIN, 1 piece	43	1	1	7	—	—	—	—	—	—
PLAIN, dietetic, 1 piece	43	1	1	7	—	—	—	<10	—	—
SESAME, 1 piece	52	1	2	7	—	—	—	—	—	—
SESAME, dietetic, 1 piece	57	1	2	7	—	—	—	<10	—	—
WHEAT, 1 piece	40	1	1	6	—	—	—	—	—	—
BREAKFAST TREATS, 1 piece	102	2	4	16	—	—	—	—	—	—

USDA

ANIMAL, 10 crackers, 26 gm	112	2	2	21	—	14	.10	79	25	0
BUTTER ROUND, 1⅛ × ³⁄₁₆", 10 pieces, 33 gm	151	2	6	22	—	49	.20	360	37	0
CRUMBS, 1 c, 80 gm	366	6	14	54	—	118	.50	874	90	0
GRAHAM CRACKERS										

FOOD & DESCRIPTION MEASURE OR QUANTITY	CALORIES	PROTEIN (GM)	FAT (GM)	CARBO-HYDRATE (GM)	FIBER (GM)	CALCIUM (MG)	IRON (MG)	SODIUM (MG)	POTASSIUM (MG)	CHOLES-TEROL (MG)
CHOCOLATE COATED, 2½ × ½ × ¼″, 1 square, 13 gm	62	<1	3	9	—	15	.30	53	42	0
PLAIN, 2 squares, 14 gm	55	1	1	10	—	6	.20	95	55	0
CRUMBS, 1 c, 85 gm	326	7	8	62	—	34	1.30	570	326	0
CRUMBS, packed, 1 c, 105 gm	403	8	10	77	—	42	1.60	704	403	0
SUGAR HONEY, 2 squares, 14 gm	58	1	2	11	—	12	.20	72	38	0
CRUMBS, not packed, 1 c, 85 gm	349	6	10	65	—	75	1.40	428	230	0
CRUMBS, packed, 1 c, 105 gm	432	7	12	80	—	92	1.70	529	284	0
SALTINE, 10 crackers, 28.4 gm	123	3	3	20	—	6	.30	312	34	0
CRUMBS, 1c, .70 gm	303	6	8	50	—	15	.80	770	84	0
SANDWICH/CHEESE-PEANUT BUTTER, 4 pieces, 1 oz	139	4	7	16	—	16	.20	281	64	5
SODA, 2⅜ × 2⅛″, 10 crackers, 28 gm	221	5	7	36	—	11	.80	554	60	0
1⅞″, square, 10 crackers, 28 gm	125	3	4	20	—	6	.40	312	34	0
SOUP/OYSTER, 10 crackers, 8 gm	33	1	1	5	—	2	.10	83	9	0

Donuts

Hostess

CHOCOLATE COATED DONETTES, 1 donut, .45 oz	60	1	3	6	—	0	.36	50		4
CHOCOLATE COATED DONUTS, 1 donut, 1 oz	130	1	8	14	—	0	.36	150	—	4
CINNAMON DONUTS, 1 donut, 1 oz	110	1	6	15	—	20	.36	140	—	6
KRUNCH DONUTS, 1 donut, 1 oz	110	1	4	16	—	20	.36	130	—	4
OLD FASHIONED DONUTS, 1 donut, 1.5 oz	180	2	10	22	—	20	.72	220	—	9
OLD FASHIONED GLAZED DONUTS, 1 donut, 2 oz	230	2	12	30	—	20	.72	200	—	11
PLAIN DONUTS, 1 donut, 1 oz	110	1	7	12	—	20	.36	135	—	7
POWDERED SUGAR DONETTES, 1 donut, .33 oz	40	0	2	5	—	0	0	40	—	2
POWDERED SUGAR DONUTS, 1 donut, 1 oz	110	1	5	15	—	0	.36	140	—	6

Tastykake

CINNAMON DONUTS, 1 donut	193	3	10	24	—	—	—	225	—	—
COATED MINI DONUTS, 1 donut	75	<1	5	7	—	—	—	57	—	—
FUDGE ICED DONUTS, 1 donut	339	2	18	40	—	—	—	219	—	—
FUDGE WALNUT BROWNIE DONUTS, 1 donut	394	4	19	53	—	—	—	169	—	—
HONEY WHEAT DONUTS, 1 donut	302	3	14	40	—	—	—	170	—	—
HONEY WHEAT MINI DONUTS, 1 donut	66	<1	3	9	—	—	—	53	—	—
ORANGE GLAZED DONUTS, 1 donut	336	3	16	44	—	—	—	227	—	—
PLAIN DONUTS, 1 donut	197	3	11	22	—	—	—	250	—	—

FOOD & DESCRIPTION MEASURE OR QUANTITY	CALORIES	PROTEIN (GM)	FAT (GM)	CARBO-HYDRATE (GM)	FIBER (GM)	CALCIUM (MG)	IRON (MG)	SODIUM (MG)	POTASSIUM (MG)	CHOLES-TEROL (MG)
POWDERED SUGAR DONUTS, 1 donut	207	3	11	23	—	—	—	233	—	—
POWDERED SUGAR DONUTS, 1 from 12-oz pkg	118	2	6	15	—	—	—	130	—	—
POWDERED SUGAR MINI DONUTS, 1 donut	59	<1	3	8	—	—	—	55	—	—

USDA

CAKE DONUTS, 3⅝" diam, 1 donut, 2 oz	227	3	11	30	—	23	.80	291	52	—
YEAST-RAISED DONUTS, 3¼" diam, 1 donut, 1½ oz	176	3	11	16	—	16	.60	99	34	—

Frostings

Betty Crocker– General Mills

MIXES, 1/12 pkg, prep										
BUTTER BRICKLE	170	0	6	30	—	*	0	115	—	—
BUTTER PECAN	170	0	6	30	—	*	0	100	—	—
CHOCOLATE FUDGE	170	0	6	30	—	*	.36	50	—	—
COCONUT ALMOND	140	0	8	18	—	*	0	90	—	—
COCONUT PECAN	160	0	9	19	—	*	0	45	—	—
CREAM CHEESE & NUTS	160	0	6	26	—	*	0	100	—	—
CREAMY CHERRY	180	0	6	31	—	*	0	100	—	—
CREAMY VANILLA	190	0	6	33	—	*	0	50	—	—
LEMON	180	0	6	31	—	*	0	100	—	—
MILK CHOCOLATE	170	0	5	30	—	*	.36	40	—	—
SOUR CREAM CHOCOLATE FUDGE	180	1	6	30	—	*	.72	80	—	—
SOUR CREAM WHITE	170	0	5	31	—	*	0	100	—	—
WHITE	60	0	0	16	—	*	0	10	—	—
READY-TO-SPREAD-FROSTING, 1/12 tub										
BUTTER PECAN	160	0	7	25	—	*	0	90	20	—
CHERRY	160	0	6	26	—	*	0	100	15	—
CHOCOLATE	170	<1	8	23	—	*	.36	100	110	—
CHOCOLATE CHIP	160	<1	7	25	—	*	0	85	30	—
CHOCOLATE CHOCOLATE CHIP	160	<1	8	23	—	*	.72	85	110	—
CHOCOLATE NUT	160	<1	8	22	—	*	.72	100	100	—
COCONUT PECAN	170	<1	10	19	—	*	0	50	55	—
CREAM CHEESE	160	0	6	26	—	*	0	100	15	—
DARK DUTCH FUDGE	160	<1	7	23	—	*	.36	100	150	—
LEMON	160	0	6	26	—	*	0	100	15	—
MILK CHOCOLATE	160	<1	7	24	—	*	0	100	70	—
ORANGE	160	0	6	26	—	*	0	90	15	—
SOUR CREAM CHOCOLATE	170	<1	8	22	—	*	.72	100	115	—
SOUR CREAM WHITE	160	0	6	26	—	*	0	100	15	—
VANILLA	160	0	6	27	—	*	0	100	15	—

Duncan Hines– Procter & Gamble

CHOCOLATE, 1/12 tub	160	0	7	24	—	*	.36	90	—	—
DARK CHOCOLATE FUDGE, 1/12 tub	160	0	7	24	—	*	.36	95	—	—
MILK CHOCOLATE, 1/12 tub	160	0	7	24	—	*	.36	85	—	—
VANILLA, 1/12 tub	160	0	7	24	—	*	*	80	—	—

Estee

FROSTING MIX, 1.5 tbsp	50-60	1	1-2	10-11	—	—	—	0	—	0

FOOD & DESCRIPTION MEASURE OR QUANTITY	CALORIES	PROTEIN (GM)	FAT (GM)	CARBO-HYDRATE (GM)	FIBER (GM)	CALCIUM (MG)	IRON (MG)	SODIUM (MG)	POTASSIUM (MG)	CHOLES-TEROL (MG)
Jiffy										
JIFFY CARAMEL FROSTING, dry, .94 oz	120	<1	3	22	—	*	<.54	85	—	—
JIFFY FUDGE FROSTING, dry, .94 oz	120	1	3	22	—	*	1.08	155	—	—
JIFFY WHITE FROSTING, dry, .94 oz	120	<1	3	22	—	*	<.54	70	—	—
Pillsbury										
FROSTING SUPREME, READY TO SPREAD, 1/12 tub										
CARAMEL PECAN	160	0	8	21	—	0	0	70	35	—
CHOCOLATE FUDGE	150	<1	6	24	—	0	0	80	95	—
CHOCOLATE MINT	150	<1	6	24	—	0	0	80	95	—
COCONUT ALMOND	150	1	9	17	—	0	0	60	60	—
COCONUT PECAN	160	0	10	17	—	0	0	60	55	—
CREAM CHEESE	160	0	6	26	—	0	0	115	10	—
DOUBLE DUTCH	150	1	7	22	—	0	0	45	135	—
LEMON	160	0	6	26	—	0	0	80	10	—
MILK CHOCOLATE	150	0	6	23	—	0	0	60	80	—
MOCHA	160	<1	6	25	—	0	0	60	60	—
SOUR CREAM VANILLA	160	0	6	27	—	0	0	80	20	—
STRAWBERRY	160	0	6	26	—	0	0	75	10	—
VANILLA	160	0	6	26	—	0	0	75	10	—
RICH 'N EASY, 1/12 pkg, prep										
CHOCOLATE FUDGE	150	<1	4	27	—	0	0	70	65	—
COCONUT ALMOND	160	1	10	16	—	20	0	85	85	—
COCONUT PECAN	150	1	7	20	—	20	0	105	60	—
DOUBLE DUTCH	150	1	4	26	—	0	0	80	95	—
FLUFFY WHITE	60	0	0	15	—	0	0	65	5	—
STRAWBERRY	140	<1	5	25	—	0	0	55	0	—
VANILLA	150	0	5	25	—	0	0	30	0	—
Sweet 'N Low										
CHOCOLATE FROSTING MIX, 1½ tsp.	30	<1	2	3	—	*	*	10	30	<5
FUDGE TOPPING MIX, 1 tsp	30	<1	2	3	—	*	*	10	30	<5
WHITE FROSTING LITE MIX, 1½ tsp	30	<1	2	3	—	*	*	<10	—	<5
Muffins										
Arrowhead Mills										
BRAN MIX, 2 muffins	270	10	7	43	—	—	—	330	—	—
Continental Baking Company										
WONDER										
ENGLISH MUFFIN, 2 oz	130	4	1	26	.20	150	1.80	280	—	0
RAISIN ROUNDS, 2 oz	140	4	2	27	.20	100	1.80	280	—	0
SOUR DOUGH MUFFIN, 2 oz	130	4	1	27	.20	150	1.80	250	—	0
Dromedary–Nabisco										
CORN MUFFIN, prep, 1 muffin	120	3	4	20	—	40	.72	270	50	—
Duncan Hines– Procter & Gamble										
BANANA NUT, 1 muffin	130	2	5	20	—	*	.72	175	—	—
BRAN & HONEY, 1 muffin	120	2	4	18	—	*	.72	170	—	—

FOOD & DESCRIPTION MEASURE OR QUANTITY	CALORIES	PROTEIN (GM)	FAT (GM)	CARBO-HYDRATE (GM)	FIBER (GM)	CALCIUM (MG)	IRON (MG)	SODIUM (MG)	POTASSIUM (MG)	CHOLES-TEROL (MG)
SPICY APPLE, 1 muffin	120	2	4	20	—	*	.72	185	—	—
WILD BLUEBERRY, 1 muffin	110	2	3	17	—	*	.36	155	—	—

Flako–Quaker

CORN, 1 muffin	140	3	4	23	—	20	.36	370	35	—

General Mills

APPLE CINNAMON MIX, prep, 1 muffin	120	2	4	19	—	20	.36	140	40	—
BANANA NUT MIX, prep, 1 muffin	150	2	6	21	—	40	.72	200	65	—
CORN MIX, prep, 1 muffin	160	3	5	25	—	40	.72	310	75	—
TART CHERRY MIX, prep, 1 muffin	120	2	4	18	—	20	.36	140	40	—
WILD BLUEBERRY MIX, prep, 1 muffin	120	2	4	18	—	40	.36	150	40	—

Jiffy

APPLE CINNAMON, 2 muffins	200	3	5	36	—	20	1.62	360	—	—
BLUEBERRY, 2 muffins	220	4	8	32	—	*	2.70	405	—	—
BRAN DATE, 2 muffins	220	5	7	33	—	*	2.70	380	—	—
CORN, 2 muffins	230	5	8	33	—	*	2.16	480	—	—
HONEY DATE, 2 muffins	210	5	6	33	—	20	1.62	275	—	—

Pepperidge Farm–Campbell

APPLE WITH SPICE, 1 muffin	170	3	8	23	—	40	.36	230	—	—
BLUEBERRY, 1 muffin	180	2	7	27	—	20	.36	250	—	—
BRAN WITH RAISIN, 1 muffin	180	2	7	28	—	20	1.44	300	—	—
CARROT WALNUT, 1 muffin	170	6	4	27	—	40	1.80	220	—	—
CHOCOLATE CHIP, 1 muffin	200	3	8	28	—	20	.36	170	—	—
CINNAMON SWIRL, 1 muffin	190	2	6	30	—	20	.36	170	—	—
CORN, 1 muffin	180	3	7	27	—	20	.36	260	—	—
ENGLISH MUFFIN, 1 muffin	140	5	2	26	—	20	1.44	180	—	—
CINNAMON RAISIN, 1 muffin	150	5	2	28	—	40	1.44	180	—	—

Thomas

ENGLISH MUFFIN, 1 muffin	130	4	1	26	.30	91	2	210	—	0
HONEY WHEAT, 1 muffin	129	5	1	24	.40	27	1.10	200	—	0
RAISIN, 1 muffin	153	5	2	30	.15	26	1.71	200	—	0
TOAST-R-CAKE										
BLUEBERRY, 1 cake	100	2	3	16	.19	15	.71	220	—	—
BRAN, 1 cake	100	2	3	16	.34	28	1.33	240	—	—
CORN, 1 cake	110	2	4	17	.10	17	.69	240	—	—

USDA

BLUEBERRY MUFFIN, home recipe, 2⅜″ diam, 1½″ high, 40 gm	112	3	4	17	—	34	.60	253	46	—
BRAN MUFFIN, home recipe, 2⅝″ diam, 1¾″ high, 40 gm	104	3	4	17	—	57	1.50	179	172	—
CORN MUFFIN, home recipe, 2⅜″ diam, 1½″ high, 40 gm	126	3	4	19	—	42	.70	192	54	—
mix, dry, 12 oz pkg, 340 gm	1418	21	39	244	—	1020	6.10	2244	258	—
mix, dry, 1 c packed, 170 gm	709	11	20	122	—	510	3.10	1122	129	—
mix, dry, 1 c not packed, 130 gm	542	8	15	93	—	390	2.30	858	99	—
mix, prep, 1 muffin, 40 gm	130	3	4	20	—	96	.60	192	44	—

FOOD & DESCRIPTION MEASURE OR QUANTITY	CALORIES	PROTEIN (GM)	FAT (GM)	CARBO-HYDRATE (GM)	FIBER (GM)	CALCIUM (MG)	IRON (MG)	SODIUM (MG)	POTASSIUM (MG)	CHOLES-TEROL (MG)
MUFFIN, plain, home recipe, 3″ diam, 1½″ high, 40 gm	118	3	4	17	—	42	.60	176	50	—

Pastries

Flako–Quaker

POPOVER MIX, prep, 1 popover	170	7	5	25	—	60	.72	360	110	—

Hostess

DANISH										
APPLE, 3.5 oz	360	4	20	43	—	60	1.80	410	—	19
BUTTERHORN, 2.85 oz	330	5	18	39	—	20	1.44	520	—	8
RASPBERRY, 2.85 oz	300	4	10	48	—	160	1.80	360	—	20

Pepperidge Farm–Campbell

APPLE CRISS CROSS PASTRY, 2 oz	180	1	9	24	—	*	*	140	—	—
APPLE DUMPLINGS, 3 oz	260	2	14	33	—	*	.36	240	—	—
APPLE STRUDEL, 3 oz	240	1	11	35	—	*	.72	220	—	—
FRUIT SQUARES										
APPLE, 1 square	230	1	12	27	—	*	.36	180	—	—
BLUEBERRY, 1 square	220	1	11	29	—	*	.72	190	—	—
CHERRY, 1 square	230	1	12	29	—	*	.72	190	—	—
PATTY SHELL, 1 shell	210	2	15	17	—	*	.36	180	—	—
PUFF PASTRY SHEETS, ¼ sheet	260	4	17	22	—	*	.72	290	—	—
TURNOVERS										
APPLE, 1 turnover	310	3	17	35	—	*	.72	220	—	—
BLUEBERRY, 1 turnover	320	3	19	32	—	*	.72	240	—	—
CHERRY, 1 turnover	310	3	19	32	—	*	.72	290	—	—
PEACH, 1 turnover	320	3	19	34	—	*	.36	260	—	—
RASPBERRY, 1 turnover	320	3	18	37	—	*	.72	270	—	—

Rich's

BAVARIAN CREAM PUFFS, 1 puff	146	2	8	17	—	9	.62	66	34	35
CHOCOLATE ECLAIRS, 1 eclair	205	2	10	27	—	10	.84	113	47	35

Sara Lee

CROISSANTS										
ALL BUTTER, 1 croissant, 42.5 gm	170	4	9	19	—	20	1.08	240	—	—
APPLE FILLED, 1 croissant, 92.3 gm	260	4	11	36	—	20	1.44	400	—	—
CHEESE, 1 croissant, 42.5 gm	170	4	8	19	—	20	.72	260	—	—
CHOCOLATE FILLED, 1 croissant, 73.4 gm	320	6	18	34	—	40	1.80	310	—	—
CINNAMON-NUT RAISIN FILLED, 1 croissant, 92.3 gm	350	7	17	44	—	40	1.80	420	—	—
STRAWBERRY FILLED, 1 croissant, 80.5 gm	270	5	11	38	—	20	1.80	290	—	—
WHEAT 'N HONEY, 1 croissant, 42.5 gm	170	4	9	18	—	20	1.08	310	—	—
DANISH										
APPLE, 1 roll, 36.5 gm	120	2	6	15	—	*	.72	120	—	—
CHEESE, 1 roll, 36.5 gm	130	2	8	13	—	*	.36	130	—	—

FOOD & DESCRIPTION MEASURE OR QUANTITY	CALORIES	PROTEIN (GM)	FAT (GM)	CARBO-HYDRATE (GM)	FIBER (GM)	CALCIUM (MG)	IRON (MG)	SODIUM (MG)	POTASSIUM (MG)	CHOLES-TEROL (MG)
CINNAMON RAISIN, 1 roll, 36.5 gm	150	2	8	17	—	*	1.08	140	—	—
RASPBERRY, 1 roll, 36.5 gm	130	2	6	18	—	*	.72	120	—	—

Pies

Banquet

APPLE, ⅙ pie, 3.33 oz	253	2	11	37	—	12	1	282	49	—
1 individual size, 8 oz	578	5	24	88	—	29	2	598	119	—
BANANA CREAM, ⅙ pie, 2.33 oz	177	2	10	21	—	32	1	146	94	—
BLACKBERRY, ⅙ pie, 3.38 oz	268	3	11	40	—	23	1	342	65	—
BLUEBERRY, ⅙ pie, 3.33 oz	266	3	11	40	—	17	1	342	45	—
CHERRY, ⅙ pie, 3.33 oz	252	3	11	36	—	13	1	258	72	—
1 individual size, 8 oz	575	6	23	87	—	32	2	534	181	—
CHOCOLATE CREAM, ⅙ pie, 2.33 oz	185	2	10	24	—	38	1	106	86	—
COCONUT CREAM, ⅙ pie, 2.33 oz	187	2	11	22	—	30	1	113	77	—
LEMON CREAM, ⅙ pie, 2.33 oz	173	2	9	23	—	30	1	111	70	—
MINCE MEAT, ⅙ pie, 3.33 oz	258	3	11	38	—	19	1	364	110	—
PEACH, ⅙ pie, 3.33 oz	244	3	11	35	—	11	1	275	69	—
1 individual size, 8 oz	553	5	23	82	—	25	2	579	172	—
PUMPKIN, ⅙ pie, 3.33 oz	197	3	8	29	—	53	1	341	138	—
STRAWBERRY CREAM, ⅙ pie, 2.33 oz	168	2	9	22	—	30	1	112	80	—

Drake—Borden

APPLE, 1 individual size	220	2	10	30	—	*	.72	230	35	—

Flako—Quaker

PIE CRUST MIX, ⅙ pkg, 1.7 oz	244	3	14	25	.10	48	1.12	314	35	—

General Mills

PIE CRUST MIX, ¹⁄₁₆ pkt	120	1	8	10	—	*	*	140	15	—
PIE CRUST STICK, ⅛ stick	120	1	8	10	—	*	*	140	15	—

Hostess

APPLE, 4.5 oz	390	5	20	45	—	20	1.44	540	—	18
BERRY, 4.5 oz	390	3	20	48	—	40	1.80	490	—	18
BLUEBERRY, 4.5 oz	390	3	20	49	—	20	1.44	450	—	18
CHERRY, 4.5 oz	390	5	20	55	—	20	1.44	530	—	18
LEMON, 4.5 oz	400	3	22	53	—	20	1.44	471	—	30
PEACH, 4.5 oz	400	4	20	53	—	40	1.80	445	—	18
STRAWBERRY, 4.5 oz	340	3	14	56	—	20	1.08	400	—	13

Jell-O—General Foods

CHOCOLATE MOUSSE PIE mix only, 1 serving	140	2	5	23	tr	*	.72	310	180	—
prep with whole milk, ⅛ pie	220	3	12	26	tr	80	.72	400	260	—

Jiffy

PIE CRUST MIX, 1 serving, 1.12 oz	160	2	9	17	—	*	1.08	280	—	—

Pillsbury

ALREADY PIECRUST MIX, prep, ⅙ 2-crust pie	240	2	15	23	—	0	0	280	30	—

FOOD & DESCRIPTION MEASURE OR QUANTITY	CALORIES	PROTEIN (GM)	FAT (GM)	CARBO-HYDRATE (GM)	FIBER (GM)	CALCIUM (MG)	IRON (MG)	SODIUM (MG)	POTASSIUM (MG)	CHOLES-TEROL (MG)
PIE CRUST STICKS, ⅙ 2-crust pie	270	4	17	25	—	0	1.08	430	80	—
Royal–Nabisco										
NO BAKE PIE MIXES										
CHOCOLATE MINT, mix only, 1.13 oz	140	3	4	24	—	60	*	140	180	—
prep with whole milk, ⅛ pie	260	5	15	25	—	100	.72	280	260	—
LITE CHEESE CAKE, mix only, 1.13 oz	140	4	4	21	—	150	1.08	260	180	—
prep with whole milk, ⅛ cake	210	5	10	23	—	200	1.08	380	250	—
REAL CHEESE CAKE, mix only, 1⅜ oz	160	4	3	29	—	80	*	250	115	—
prep with whole milk, ⅛ cake	280	5	9	31	—	150	*	370	210	—
Salada–Kellogg										
DANISH DESSERT PIE GLAZE, ½ cup	130	0	0	32	—	*	*	5	3	—
Tastykake										
APPLE	362	4	14	52	—	—	—	458	—	—
BLUEBERRY	376	3	11	62	—	—	—	406	—	—
CHERRY	356	4	10	62	—	—	—	389	—	—
COCONUT CREME	507	7	32	44	—	—	—	285	—	—
FRENCH APPLE	420	4	11	72	—	—	—	442	—	—
LEMON	373	4	15	54	—	—	—	320	—	—
PEACH	333	4	13	48	—	—	—	391	—	—
PINEAPPLE	369	4	12	59	—	—	—	393	—	—
PUMPKIN	358	6	12	55	—	—	—	339	—	—
TASTY KLAIR	446	7	17	64	—	—	—	240	—	—
USDA [All pies are made with nonenriched flour and vegetable shortening]										
APPLE										
9″ pie, ⅙, 158 gm	404	4	18	60	—	13	.50	476	126	—
8″ pie, fz, ⅙, 92 gm	231	2	9	37	—	8	.20	195	66	—
BANANA CUSTARD, 9″ pie, ⅙, 152 gm	336	7	14	47	—	100	.80	295	309	—
BLACKBERRY, 9″ pie, ⅙, 158 gm	384	4	17	54	—	30	.80	423	158	—
BLUEBERRY, 9″ pie, ⅙, 158 gm	382	4	17	55	—	17	.90	423	103	—
BUTTERSCOTCH, 9″ pie, ⅙, 152 gm	406	7	17	58	—	114	1.40	325	144	—
CHERRY										
9″ pie, ⅙, 158 gm	412	4	18	61	—	22	.50	480	166	—
8″ pie, fz, ⅙, 97 gm	282	21	12	43	—	12	.20	222	79	—
CHOCOLATE CHIFFON, 9″ pie, ⅙, 108 gm	354	7	17	47	—	26	1.30	272	119	—
CHOCOLATE MERINGUE, 9″ pie, ⅙, 152 gm	383	7	18	51	—	105	1.10	389	211	—
COCONUT CUSTARD										
9″ pie, ⅙, 152 gm	357	9	19	38	—	143	1.10	375	248	—
8″ pie, fz, ⅙, 100 gm	249	6	12	30	—	95	.60	252	172	—
CUSTARD, 9″ pie, ⅙, 152 gm	331	9	17	36	—	146	.90	436	208	—
LEMON CHIFFON, 9″ pie, ⅙, 108 gm	338	8	14	47	—	25	1.00	282	87	—

FOOD & DESCRIPTION MEASURE OR QUANTITY	CALORIES	PROTEIN (GM)	FAT (GM)	CARBO- HYDRATE (GM)	FIBER (GM)	CALCIUM (MG)	IRON (MG)	SODIUM (MG)	POTASSIUM (MG)	CHOLES- TEROL (MG)
LEMON MERINGUE, 9″ pie, ⅙, 140 gm	357	5	14	53	—	20	.70	395	70	—
MINCE, 9″ pie, ⅙, 158 gm	428	4	18	65	—	44	1.60	708	281	—
PEACH, 9″ pie, ⅙, 158 gm	403	4	17	60	—	16	.80	423	235	—
PECAN, 9″ pie, ⅙, 138 gm	577	7	32	71	—	65	3.90	305	170	—
PIE CRUST, with enriched flour, 1 shell, 194 gm	900	11	60	79	—	25	3.10	1102	89	—
nonenriched flour, 1 shell, 194 gm	900	11	60	79	—	25	.90	1100	89	—
mix, 10 oz pkg	1482	20	93	141	—	131	1.40	1968	179	—
mix, 1 c packed, 195 gm	1018	14	64	97	—	90	1.00	1351	123	—
mix, 1 c not packed, 120 gm	626	9	39	59	—	55	.60	832	76	—
prep from 10 oz pkg, 320 gm	1485	21	93	141	—	131	1.30	2602	179	—
PINEAPPLE, 9″ pie, ⅙, 158 gm	400	4	17	60	—	21	.80	428	114	—
PINEAPPLE CHIFFON, 9″ pie, ⅙, 108 gm	311	7	13	42	—	26	1.00	276	106	—
PINEAPPLE CUSTARD, 9″ pie, ⅙, 152 gm	334	6	13	49	—	76	.60	283	147	—
PUMPKIN, 9″ pie, ⅙, 152 gm	321	6	17	37	—	78	.80	325	243	—
RAISIN, 9″ pie, ⅙, 152 gm	427	4	17	68	—	28	1.40	450	303	—
RHUBARB, 9″ pie, ⅙, 158 gm	400	4	17	60	—	101	1.10	427	251	—
STRAWBERRY, 9″ pie, ⅙, 124 gm	246	2	10	38	—	20	.90	241	149	—
SWEET POTATO, 9″ pie, ⅙, 152 gm	324	7	17	36	—	105	.80	331	248	—

2

BEANS & LEGUMES

FOOD & DESCRIPTION MEASURE OR QUANTITY	CALORIES	PROTEIN (GM)	FAT (GM)	CARBO-HYDRATE (GM)	FIBER (GM)	CALCIUM (MG)	IRON (MG)	SODIUM (MG)	POTASSIUM (MG)	CHO-LESTEROL (MG)
Canned										
Campbell										
BARBEQUE BEANS, 7.88 oz.	250	10	4	43	—	80	2.70	1110	—	—
BEANS & FRANKS IN TOMATO & MOLASSES SAUCE, 7.88 oz	360	14	14	43	—	100	3.60	1140	—	—
HOME STYLE BEANS, 8 oz	270	11	4	48	—	100	3.60	1130	—	—
OLD FASHIONED BEANS IN BROWN SUGAR AND MOLASSES SAUCE, 8 oz	270	11	3	49	—	100	3.60	1160	—	—
PORK & BEANS IN TOMATO SAUCE, 8 oz	240	9	3	42	—	60	2.70	820	—	—
Del Monte										
BEAN BURRITO FILLING MIX, ½ c, 120.5 gm	110	6	1	20	—	40	1.80	900	640	—
BEANS, REFRIED, ½ c, 120.5 gm	130	6	2	20	—	40	1.80	530	660	—
BEANS, SPICY REFRIED, ½ c, 120.5 gm	130	6	2	20	—	40	1.80	480	485	—
Grandma Brown										
HOME-BAKED BEANS, 8 oz	289	14	2	54	—	120	3.60	—	—	—
Heinz										
PORK 'N' BEANS, 8 oz	250	11	4	46	—	150	3.60	745	—	—
VEGETARIAN BEANS, 8 oz	230	11	2	43	—	100	3.60	980	—	—
Libby's—Seneca										
DEEP BROWN BEANS PORK & MOLASSES, ½ c	140	7	2	25	—	150	4.50	320	410	—
PORK & TOMATO SAUCE, ½ c	140	7	2	25	—	100	3.60	320	410	—
VEGETARIAN, ½ c	130	7	1	25	—	100	3.60	300	390	—
Progresso										
BLACK EYE PEAS, 8 oz	165	11	1	29	—	20	2.70	—	—	—
BLACK TURTLE BEANS, 8 oz	205	14	1	37	—	60	4.50	—	—	—
CANNELLINI BEANS (white kidney), 8 oz	180	12	1	30	—	60	3.60	717	—	—
CHICK PEAS, 8 oz	200	10	4	32	—	60	2.70	691	—	—
FAVA BEANS, 8oz	180	14	1	31	—	60	2.70	—	—	—

FOOD & DESCRIPTION MEASURE OR QUANTITY	CALORIES	PROTEIN (GM)	FAT (GM)	CARBO- HYDRATE (GM)	FIBER (GM)	CALCIUM (MG)	IRON (MG)	SODIUM (MG)	POTASSIUM (MG)	CHOLES- TEROL (MG)
PINTO BEANS, 8 oz	165	10	1	31	—	60	3.60	—	—	—
RED KIDNEY BEANS, 8 oz	190	12	1	34	—	60	3.60	1080	—	—
ROMAN BEANS, 8 oz	210	14	1	36	—	100	3.60	—	—	—

USDA

FOOD & DESCRIPTION	CALORIES	PROTEIN	FAT	CARBO-HYDRATE	FIBER	CALCIUM	IRON	SODIUM	POTASSIUM	CHOLESTEROL
BEANS CANNED WITH PORK & SWEET SAUCE,1 c, 255 gm	383	16	12	54	—	161	5.90	969	—	—
BEANS CANNED WITH PORK & TOMATO SAUCE, 1 c, 255 gm	311	16	7	49	—	138	4.60	1181	536	—
BEANS CANNED WITHOUT PORK, 1c, 255 gm	306	16	1	59	—	173	5.10	862	683	—
KIDNEY, RED, with solids & liquid, salt-free, 1 c, 255 gm	230	15	1	42	—	74	4.60	8	673	—

Van Camp–Quaker

FOOD & DESCRIPTION	CALORIES	PROTEIN	FAT	CARBO-HYDRATE	FIBER	CALCIUM	IRON	SODIUM	POTASSIUM	CHOLESTEROL
BEANEE WEENEE, 1c, 7.75 oz	326	15	15	32	2.70	95	4.27	990	565	—
BROWN SUGAR BEANS, 1c 8oz	284	12	5	48	3.20	121	3.83	692	535	—
BUTTER BEANS, 1 c, 8 oz	162	11	<1	28	2.80	41	3.78	752	639	—
CHILEE WEENEE, 1c, 7.75 oz.	309	14	16	28	2.20	68	4.63	1057	527	—
CHILI WITH BEANS, 1 c, 7.75 oz	352	15	23	21	2.30	63	4.83	1215	537	—
KIDNEY BEANS DARK RED, 1 c, 8 oz	182	12	<1	33	2.30	52	3.31	732	549	—
LIGHT RED, 1 c, 8 oz	184	12	<1	33	2.20	55	2.96	688	494	—
NEW ORLEANS STYLE, 1 c, 8 oz	178	12	<1	31	2.40	59	3.10	793	586	—
MEXICAN STYLE CHILI BEANS, 1 c, 8 oz	210	11	2	36	2.60	75	4.42	718	640	—
PORK & BEANS, 1c, 8 oz	216	11	2	39	2.40	97	4.29	1011	563	—
RED BEANS, 1 c, 8 oz	194	12	<1	36	2.40	84	3.65	928	546	—
VEGETARIAN STYLE BEANS, 1 c, 8 oz	206	11	<1	39	2.40	93	4.55	987	602	—
WESTERN STYLE BEANS, 1 c, 8 oz	207	11	4	32	2.40	73	2.71	1006	589	—

Dried

Arrowhead Mills

FOOD & DESCRIPTION	CALORIES	PROTEIN	FAT	CARBO-HYDRATE	FIBER	CALCIUM	IRON	SODIUM	POTASSIUM	CHOLESTEROL
ADZUKI BEANS, 2 oz	190	13	1	35	—	—	—	5	—	—
BLACK TURTLE BEANS, 2 oz	190	13	1	35	—	—	—	15	—	—
BLACKEYE PEAS, 2 oz	70	5	0	12	—	—	—	1	—	—
CHICKPEAS, 2 oz	200	12	3	35	—	—	—	15	—	—
GREAT NORTHERN BEANS, 2 oz	190	13	1	35	—	—	—	10	—	—
KIDNEY BEANS, 2 oz	190	13	1	35	—	—	—	5	—	—
LENTILS, GREEN, 2 oz	190	13	1	35	—	—	—	15	—	—
LENTILS, RED, 2 oz	195	14	1	34	—	—	—	17	—	—
LIMA BEANS, 2 oz	70	5	0	13	—	—	—	1	—	—
NAVY BEANS, 2 oz	190	13	1	35	—	—	—	10	—	—
PINTO BEANS, 2 oz	200	13	1	36	—	—	—	5	—	—
SOYBEANS, 2 oz	230	19	10	19	—	—	—	3	—	—
SPLIT PEAS, GREEN, 2 oz	200	14	1	35	—	—	—	25	—	—
SPLIT PEAS, YELLOW, 2 oz	200	14	1	35	—	—	—	25	—	—

66

FOOD & DESCRIPTION MEASURE OR QUANTITY	CALORIES	PROTEIN (GM)	FAT (GM)	CARBO- HYDRATE (GM)	FIBER (GM)	CALCIUM (MG)	IRON (MG)	SODIUM (MG)	POTASSIUM (MG)	CHOLES- TEROL (MG)
USDA [All beans are cooked without salt]										
BLACK, BROWN, BAYO, 1 c, 200 gm	678	45	3	122	—	270	15.80	50	2076	—
GREAT NORTHERN, 1 c, 180 gm	612	40	3	110	—	259	14.00	34	2153	—
cooked, 1 c, 180 gm	212	14	1	38	—	90	4.90	13	749	—
KIDNEY BEANS, RED, 1 c, 185 gm	635	42	3	115	—	204	12.80	19	1820	—
cooked, 1 c, 185 gm	218	14	<1	40	—	70	4.40	6	629	—
LIMA										
BABY, 1 c, 190 gm	656	39	3	122	—	137	14.80	8	2905	—
FORDHOOK, 1 c, 180 gm	621	37	3	115	—	130	14.00	7	2752	—
cooked, 1 c, 190 gm	262	16	1	49	—	55	5.90	4	1163	—
MUNG BEANS, 1 c, 210 gm	714	51	3	127	—	248	16.20	13	2159	—
PEA BEANS—NAVY, 1 c, 205 gm	697	46	3	126	—	295	16.00	39	2452	—
cooked, 1 c, 190 gm	224	15	1	40	—	95	5.10	13	790	—
PINTO, 1 c, 190 gm	663	44	2	121	—	257	12.20	19	1870	—
SOYBEANS, 1 c, 210 gm	846	72	37	70	—	475	17.60	11	3522	—
cooked, 1 c, 180 gm	234	20	10	19	—	131	4.90	4	972	—

3

BEVERAGES

Note: Sodium from water
source is usually not
included in analysis

FOOD & DESCRIPTION MEASURE OR QUANTITY	CALORIES	PROTEIN (GM)	FAT (GM)	CARBO-HYDRATE (GM)	FIBER (GM)	CALCIUM (MG)	IRON (MG)	SODIUM (MG)	POTASSIUM (MG)	CHOLES-TEROL (MG)
Alcoholic										
Bols										
ADVOCKATT, 34 proof, 1 oz	93	—	—	—	—	—	—	—	—	—
AMARETTO, 91 proof, 1 oz	91	—	—	—	—	—	—	—	—	—
APPLE SCHNAPPS, 48 proof, 1 oz	82	—	—	—	—	—	—	—	—	—
APRICOT FLAVORED BRANDY, 70 proof, 1 oz	94	—	—	—	—	—	—	—	—	—
APRICOT LIQUEUR, 58 proof, 1 oz	90	—	—	—	—	—	—	—	—	—
BLACKBERRY FLAVORED BRANDY, 70 proof, 1 oz	94	—	—	—	—	—	—	—	—	—
BLACKBERRY LIQUEUR, 50 proof, 1 oz	84	—	—	—	—	—	—	—	—	—
BLACKBERRY SCHNAPPS, 48 proof, 1 oz	74	—	—	—	—	—	—	—	—	—
BLUE CURACAO, 60 proof, 1 oz	98	—	—	—	—	—	—	—	—	—
BROWN CREME DE CACAO, 50 proof, 1 oz	96	—	—	—	—	—	—	—	—	—
CHERRY FLAVORED BRANDY, 70 proof, 1 oz	94	—	—	—	—	—	—	—	—	—
CHERRY LIQUEUR, 48 proof, 1 oz	82	—	—	—	—	—	—	—	—	—
CHOCOLATE LIQUEUR, 54 proof, 1 oz	106	—	—	—	—	—	—	—	—	—
CHOCOLATE MINT LIQUEUR, 54 proof, 1 oz	106	—	—	—	—	—	—	—	—	—
COFFEE FLAVORED BRANDY, 70 proof, 1 oz	100	—	—	—	—	—	—	—	—	—
CREME DE BANANA, 50 proof, 1 oz	96	—	—	—	—	—	—	—	—	—
CREME DE CASSIS, 35 proof, 1 oz	90	—	—	—	—	—	—	—	—	—
CREME DE NOYAUX, 50 proof, 1 oz	104	—	—	—	—	—	—	—	—	—
GINGER FLAVORED BRANDY, 70 proof, 1 oz	94	—	—	—	—	—	—	—	—	—
GOLD SCHNAPPS, 48 proof, 1 oz	86	—	—	—	—	—	—	—	—	—
GREEN CREME DE MENTHE, 60 proof, 1 oz	101	—	—	—	—	—	—	—	—	—
MELON LIQUEUR, 46 proof, 1 oz	74	—	—	—	—	—	—	—	—	—

FOOD & DESCRIPTION MEASURE OR QUANTITY	CALORIES	PROTEIN (GM)	FAT (GM)	CARBO- HYDRATE (GM)	FIBER (GM)	CALCIUM (MG)	IRON (MG)	SODIUM (MG)	POTASSIUM (MG)	CHOLES- TEROL (MG)
MOCHA JAVA, 53 proof, 1 oz	116	—	—	—	—	—	—	—	—	—
ORANGE CURACAO, 60 proof, 1 oz	92	—	—	—	—	—	—	—	—	—
PEACH FLAVORED BRANDY, 70 proof, 1 oz	94	—	—	—	—	—	—	—	—	—
PEPPERMINT SCHNAPPS, 48 proof, 1 oz	86	—	—	—	—	—	—	—	—	—
SLOE GIN, 60 proof, 1 oz	74	—	—	—	—	—	—	—	—	—
STRAWBERRY LIQUEUR, 44 proof, 1 oz	81	—	—	—	—	—	—	—	—	—
TRIPLE SEC, 60 proof, 1 oz	92	—	—	—	—	—	—	—	—	—
WHITE ANISETTE, 50 proof, 1 oz	105	—	—	—	—	—	—	—	—	—
WHITE CREME DE CACAO, 50 proof, 1 oz	96	—	—	—	—	—	—	—	—	—
WHITE CREME DE MENTHE, 60 proof, 1 oz	101	—	—	—	—	—	—	—	—	—

Brown–Forman

CANADIAN MIST IMPORTED CANADIAN WHISKEY, 80 proof, 1 oz	65	—	—	—	—	—	—	—	—	—
EARLY TIMES KENTUCKY STRAIGHT BOURBON WHISKEY, 80 proof, 1 oz	65	—	—	—	—	—	—	—	—	—
MARTELL COGNAC, IMPORTED, 80 proof, 1 oz	65	—	—	—	—	—	—	—	—	—
PEPE LOPEZ TEQUILA, IMPORTED, 80 proof, 1 oz	65	—	—	—	—	—	—	—	—	—
OLD BUSHMILLS IMPORTED IRISH WHISKEY, 80 proof, 1 oz	65	—	—	—	—	—	—	—	—	—
OLD FORESTER KENTUCKY STRAIGHT BOURBON WHISKEY, 86 proof, 1 oz	70	—	—	—	—	—	—	—	—	—
SOUTHERN COMFORT, 100 proof, 1 oz	95	—	—	—	—	—	—	—	—	—
USHER'S GREEN STRIPE IMPORTED SCOTCH WHISKEY, 80 proof, 1 oz	65	—	—	—	—	—	—	—	—	—

USDA

BEER, can or bottle, 12 oz	151	1	0	14	—	18	tr	25	90	—
BEER, 8 oz	101	<1	0	9	—	12	tr	17	60	—
BEER, 1 oz	13	<1	0	1	—	2	tr	2	8	—
GIN, RUM, VODKA, WHISKEY										
80 proof, 1 oz	65	—	—	tr	—	—	—	tr	1	—
86 proof, 1 oz	70	—	—	tr	—	—	—	tr	1	—
90 proof, 1 oz	74	—	—	tr	—	—	—	tr	1	—
94 proof, 1 oz	77	—	—	tr	—	—	—	tr	1	—
100 proof, 1 oz	83	—	—	tr	—	—	—	tr	1	—
WINE										
DESSERT, 1 oz	41	tr	0	2	—	2	—	1	23	—
TABLE, 1 oz	25	tr	0	1	—	3	.10	1	27	—

FOOD & DESCRIPTION MEASURE OR QUANTITY	CALORIES	PROTEIN (GM)	FAT (GM)	CARBO-HYDRATE (GM)	FIBER (GM)	CALCIUM (MG)	IRON (MG)	SODIUM (MG)	POTASSIUM (MG)	CHOLES-TEROL (MG)
Carbonated										
Coca-Cola										
COCA-COLA, 6 oz	77	—	—	20	—	—	—	3	tr	—
COCA-COLA, CAFFEINE FREE, 6 oz	77	—	—	20	—	—	—	3	tr	—
COCA-COLA, CHERRY, 6 oz	77	—	—	20	—	—	—	7	tr	—
COCA-COLA, CLASSIC, 6 oz	72	—	—	19	—	—	—	7	tr	—
DIET COKE, 6 oz	<1	—	—	<1	—	—	—	4	19	—
DIET COKE, CAFFEINE FREE, 6 oz	<1	—	—	<1	—	—	—	4	19	—
FRESCA, 6 oz	2	—	—	<1	—	—	—	tr	38	—
MELLO YELLO, 6 oz	86	—	—	22	—	—	—	14	4	—
MR. PIBB, 6 oz	71	—	—	19	—	—	—	11	tr	—
MR. PIBB SUGAR FREE, 6 oz	<1	—	—	<1	—	—	—	19	tr	—
RAMBLIN' ROOT BEER, 6 oz	88	—	—	23	—	—	—	10	tr	—
RAMBLIN' ROOT BEER SUGAR FREE, 6 oz	<1	—	—	<1	—	—	—	29	tr	—
SPRITE, 6 oz	71	—	—	18	—	—	—	23	tr	—
SPRITE, DIET, 6 oz	2	—	—	0	—	—	—	tr	28	—
TAB, 6 oz	<1	—	—	<1	—	—	—	15	tr	—
TAB, CAFFEINE FREE, 6 oz	<1	—	—	<1	—	—	—	15	tr	—
Fanta–Coca-Cola										
GINGER ALE, 6 oz	63	—	—	16	—	—	—	14	tr	—
GRAPE, 6 oz	86	—	—	22	—	—	—	7	tr	—
ORANGE, 6 oz	88	—	—	23	—	—	—	7	tr	—
ROOT BEER, 6 oz	78	—	—	20	—	—	—	10	tr	—
Nehi–Royal Crown										
FRUIT PUNCH, 6 oz	91	—	—	23	—	—	—	8	0	—
GINGERALE, 6 oz	69	—	—	17	—	—	—	0	0	—
GRAPE, bottle, 6 oz	87	—	—	22	—	—	—	8	0	—
GRAPE, can, 6 oz	87	—	—	22	—	—	—	7	0	—
ORANGE, 6 oz	95	—	—	24	—	—	—	11	0	—
PEACH, 6 oz	92	—	—	23	—	—	—	16	0	—
ROOT BEER, 6 oz	87	—	—	22	—	—	—	9	<1	—
STRAWBERRY, bottle, 6 oz	87	—	—	22	—	—	—	0	0	—
STRAWBERRY, can, 6 oz	87	—	—	22	—	—	—	7	0	—
DR NEHI, 6 oz	73	—	—	18	—	—	—	13	<1	—
PepsiCo										
MOUNTAIN DEW, 6 oz	89	—	—	22	—	—	—	16	5	—
PEPSI-COLA, 6 oz	80	—	—	20	—	—	—	1	7	—
PEPSI, DIET, 6 oz	<1	—	—	<1	—	—	—	1	27	—
PEPSI, DIET FREE, 6 oz	<1	—	—	<1	—	—	—	1	50	—
PEPSI FREE, 6 oz	80	—	—	20	—	—	—	1	7	—
PEPSI LIGHT, 6 oz	<1	—	—	<1	—	—	—	1	23	—
SLICE, 6 oz	76	—	—	20	—	—	—	5	50	—
SLICE, DIET, 6 oz	13	—	—	3	—	—	—	5	50	—
Royal Crown										
DIET RC 100, 6 oz	<1	—	—	<1	—	—	—	0	30	—
DIET RITE, SALT FREE, 6 oz	<1	—	—	<1	—	—	—	0	30	—
KICK, 6 oz	89	—	—	22	—	—	—	25	0	—
ROYAL CROWN COLA, 6 oz	78	—	—	20	—	—	—	<1	6	—
RC 100, CAFFEINE FREE, 6 oz	78	—	—	20	—	—	—	<1	6	—
UPPER 10, 6 oz	76	—	—	19	—	—	—	20	0	—
SALT FREE, 6 oz	76	—	—	19	—	—	—	0	13	—
SALT FREE, DIET, 6 oz	2	—	—	<1	—	—	—	0	41	—

FOOD & DESCRIPTION MEASURE OR QUANTITY	CALORIES	PROTEIN (GM)	FAT (GM)	CARBO- HYDRATE (GM)	FIBER (GM)	CALCIUM (MG)	IRON (MG)	SODIUM (MG)	POTASSIUM (MG)	CHOLES- TEROL (MG)
Shasta										
BIRCH BEER, DIET, 6 oz	0	—	—	0	—	—	—	24	3	—
BLACK CHERRY, 6 oz	79	—	—	22	—	—	—	15	3	—
DIET, 6 oz	0	—	—	0	—	—	—	26	4	—
CHERRY COLA, 6 oz	68	—	—	19	—	—	—	12	4	—
DIET, 6 oz	0	—	—	0	—	—	—	23	3	—
CHOCOLATE, DIET, 6 oz	0	—	—	0	—	—	—	14	3	—
CITRUS MIST, 6 oz	83	—	—	23	—	—	—	9	2	—
CLUB SODA, 6 oz	0	—	—	0	—	—	—	23	0	—
COLA, 6 oz	72	—	—	20	—	—	—	2	2	—
DIET, 6 oz	0	—	—	0	—	—	—	25	2	—
SHASTA FREE, 6 oz	74	—	—	20	—	—	—	1	2	—
SHASTA FREE, DIET, 6 oz	0	—	—	0	—	—	—	24	2	—
CREME, 6 oz	75	—	—	21	—	—	—	11	1	—
DIET, 6 oz	0	—	—	0	—	—	—	20	<1	—
DR. DIABLO, 6 oz	68	—	—	19	—	—	—	5	2	—
FROLIC, DIET, 6 oz	0	—	—	0	—	—	—	25	3	—
FRUIT PUNCH, 6 oz	84	—	—	23	—	—	—	16	<1	—
GINGERALE, 6 oz	59	—	—	16	—	—	—	11	1	—
DIET, 6 oz	0	—	—	0	—	—	—	17	1	—
GRAPE, 6 oz	86	—	—	24	—	—	—	14	4	—
DIET, 6 oz	0	—	—	0	—	—	—	25	4	—
GRAPEFRUIT, DIET, 6 oz	2	—	—	<1	—	—	—	21	2	—
LEMONADE, 6 oz	71	—	—	19	—	—	—	53	3	—
LEMON LIME, 6 oz	71	—	—	19	—	—	—	24	2	—
DIET, 6 oz	0	—	—	0	—	—	—	40	4	—
ORANGE, 6 oz	86	—	—	24	—	—	—	14	5	—
DIET, 6 oz	0	—	—	0	—	—	—	25	4	—
RED POP, 6 oz	77	—	—	21	—	—	—	2	16	—
DIET, 6 oz	0	—	—	0	—	—	—	44	2	—
ROOT BEER, 6 oz	75	—	—	21	—	—	—	18	1	—
DIET, 6 oz	0	—	—	0	—	—	—	23	3	—
STRAWBERRY, 6 oz	72	—	—	20	—	—	—	22	3	—
DIET, 6 oz	0	—	—	0	—	—	—	22	4	—
TONIC WATER, 6 oz	59	—	—	16	—	—	—	7	2	—
Spree—Shasta										
COLA, 6 oz	72	—	—	20	—	—	—	<1	<1	—
GINGERALE, 6 oz	59	—	—	16	—	—	—	<1	2	—
GRAPEFRUIT, 6 oz	75	—	—	21	—	—	—	<1	1	—
LEMON LIME, 6 oz	75	—	—	21	—	—	—	<1	2	—
LEMON TANGERINE, 6 oz	81	—	—	22	—	—	—	<1	2	—
MANDARIN LIME, 6 oz	75	—	—	21	—	—	—	<1	2	—
ROOT BEER, 6 oz	75	—	—	21	—	—	—	1	1	—
USDA										
CARBONATED WATERS										
SWEETENED, QUININE, 1 oz	9	0	0	2	—	—	—	—	—	—
UNSWEETENED, CLUB										
SODA, 1 oz	0	0	0	0	—	—	—	—	—	—
COLA TYPE, 1 oz	12	0	0	3	—	—	—	—	—	—
CREAM SODA, 1 oz	13	0	0	3	—	—	—	—	—	—
FRUIT-FLAVORED, 1 oz	14	0	0	4	—	—	—	—	—	—
GINGER ALE, 1 oz	9	0	0	2	—	—	—	—	—	—
ROOT BEER, 1 oz	13	0	0	3	—	—	—	—	—	—
Yoo-Hoo										
CHOCOLATE, 9 oz	140	3	1	27	—	100	.36	130	200	—

FOOD & DESCRIPTION MEASURE OR QUANTITY	CALORIES	PROTEIN (GM)	FAT (GM)	CARBO-HYDRATE (GM)	FIBER (GM)	CALCIUM (MG)	IRON (MG)	SODIUM (MG)	POTASSIUM (MG)	CHOLES-TEROL (MG)
Coffees & Teas										
Borden										
KAVA INSTANT COFFEE, 1 tsp	2	0	0	1	—	*	*	<5	115	—
Crystal Light– General Foods										
ICED TEA, sugar-free, prep, 8 oz	4	0	0	0	0	*	*	0	30	—
General Foods										
INTERNATIONAL COFFEES										
CAFE AMARETTO, 6 oz	50	0	2	7	tr	*	*	25	230	—
SUGAR FREE, 6 oz	35	0	3	3	tr	*	*	20	250	—
CAFE FRANCAIS, 6 oz	50	0	3	6	tr	*	*	25	280	—
CAFE IRISH CREME, 6 oz	60	0	3	8	tr	*	*	20	220	—
SUGAR FREE, 6 oz	30	0	2	3	tr	*	*	15	230	—
CAFE VIENNA, 6 oz	60	0	2	10	tr	*	*	105	110	—
SUGAR FREE, 6 oz	30	0	2	3	tr	*	*	95	120	—
IRISH MOCHA MINT, 6 oz	50	0	2	8	tr	*	*	20	250	—
SUGAR FREE, 6 oz	25	1	2	3	tr	*	*	20	210	—
ORANGE CAPPUCCINO, 6 oz	60	0	2	10	tr	*	*	105	125	—
SUGAR FREE, 6 oz	30	0	2	3	tr	*	*	50	130	—
SUISSE MOCHA, 6 oz	50	0	2	8	tr	*	*	25	150	—
SUGAR FREE, 6 oz	30	0	2	3	tr	*	*	20	150	—
Hills Brothers										
FLAVORED COFFEES										
AMARETTO, 6 oz	57	<1	1	12	—	4	.20	16	—	—
SUGAR FREE, 6 oz	43	<1	2	7	—	14	.29	44	—	—
BAVARIAN MINT, 6 oz	57	<1	1	12	—	5	.22	15	—	—
SUGAR FREE, 6 oz	43	<1	2	7	—	16	.38	58	—	—
CAFE, 6 oz	58	<1	1	12	—	4	.24	59	—	—
CAFE VIENNA, SUGAR FREE, 6 oz	43	<1	2	7	—	14	.28	47	—	—
CINNAMON, 6 oz	59	<1	1	12	—	11	.23	22	—	—
GERMAN CHOCOLATE, 6 oz	64	<1	2	11	—	20	.26	19	—	—
SUGAR FREE, 6 oz	44	<1	2	7	—	14	.33	41	—	—
SWISS MOCHA, SUGAR FREE, 6 oz	44	1	2	6	—	16	.74	130	—	—
Lipton										
DECAFFEINATED, 8 oz	2	0	0	0	—	*	*	0	—	—
CANNED TEA, LEMON FLAVORED										
aseptically packed, 6 oz	70	0	0	18	—	*	*	0	—	—
SUGAR FREE, 8 oz	2	0	0	0	—	*	*	25	—	—
WITH SUGAR, 8 oz	90	0	0	22	—	*	*	20	—	—
CHILLED TEA, LEMON FLAVORED										
SUGAR FREE, 8 oz	2	0	0	0	—	*	*	25	—	—
WITH SUGAR, 8 oz	90	0	0	22	—	*	*	20	—	—
FLAVORED TEA BAGS										
AMARETTO, BLACKBERRY, CHERRY ALMOND, CINNAMON, LEMON AND SPICE, MINT, SPICY APPLE, 1 c	2	0	0	<1	—	*	*	0	—	—
HERBAL TEA										
ALMOND PLEASURE, CHAMOMILE, CITRUS										

FOOD & DESCRIPTION MEASURE OR QUANTITY	CALORIES	PROTEIN (GM)	FAT (GM)	CARBO-HYDRATE (GM)	FIBER (GM)	CALCIUM (MG)	IRON (MG)	SODIUM (MG)	POTASSIUM (MG)	CHOLES-TEROL (MG)
SUNSET, GENTLE ORANGE, LEMON SOOTHER, TANGY ORANGE, 1 c	2	0	0	<1	—	*	*	0	—	—
TOASTY SPICE, 1 c	6	0	0	1	—	*	*	0	—	—
ICED TEA MIX										
SUGAR FREE, LEMON FLAVORED, 8 oz	2	0	0	0	—	*	*	5	—	—
WITH NUTRASWEET, LEMON FLAVORED, 8 oz	4	0	0	1	—	*	*	0	—	—
WITH SUGAR, LEMON FLAVORED, 8 oz	60	0	0	16	—	*	*	0	—	—
INSTANT TEA, 8 oz	2	0	0	0	—	*	*	0	—	—
LEMON FLAVORED, 8 oz	2	0	0	0	—	*	*	0	—	—
TEA BAG, 8 oz	2	0	0	0	—	*	*	0	—	—

Nestle

NESCAFE COFFEE										
INSTANT, 1.8 gm	4	<1	<1	1	—	*	*	0	70	—
DECAFFEINATED, 1.8 gm	4	<1	<1	1	—	*	*	0	70	—
NESTEA										
100% INSTANT TEA										
COLD, .7 gm	0	0	0	0	—	*	*	0	60	—
HOT, .6 gm	0	0	0	0	—	*	*	0	50	—
ICED TEA MIX										
LEMON FLAVOR prep, 8 oz, 1.8 gm	6	0	0	0	—	*	*	0	80	—
WITH ASPARTAME, prep, 8 oz, 1.56 gm	4	0	0	1	—	*	*	0	25	—
WITH SUGAR & LEMON, prep, 6 oz, 19.5 gm	70	0	0	9	—	*	*	0	40	—
SUNRISE, 1.89 gm	6	<1	<1	1	—	*	*	0	64	—
TASTER'S CHOICE FREEZE DRIED COFFEE										
DECAFFEINATED, 1.8 gm	4	<1	<1	1	—	*	*	0	70	—
REGULAR, 1.8 gm	4	<1	<1	1	—	*	*	0	70	—

Postum–General Foods

POSTUM INSTANT HOT BEVERAGE, prep, 6 oz	12	0	0	3	tr	*	*	0	100	—
COFFEE FLAVOR, 6 oz	12	0	0	3	tr	*	*	0	100	—

Shasta

ICED TEA, 6 oz	61	—	—	17	—	—	—	14	3	—

USDA

COFFEE										
INSTANT, 1 tsp, dry	1	tr	tr	<1	—	1	tr	1	26	—
INSTANT, FREEZE-DRIED, 1 tsp dry	1	tr	tr	<1	—	2	.10	1	29	—
PREPARED, 6 oz	2	tr	tr	tr	—	4	.20	2	65	—

Wyler's–Borden

ICED TEA MIX, prep, 8 oz	80	0	0	21	—	*	*	—	—	—

Fruit-Flavored

Bama–Borden

FRUIT PUNCH, 6 oz	90	0	0	22	—	*	*	—	—	—
ORANGE DRINK, 6 oz	90	0	0	22	—	*	*	—	—	—

FOOD & DESCRIPTION MEASURE OR QUANTITY	CALORIES	PROTEIN (GM)	FAT (GM)	CARBO- HYDRATE (GM)	FIBER (GM)	CALCIUM (MG)	IRON (MG)	SODIUM (MG)	POTASSIUM (MG)	CHOLES- TEROL (MG)
Borden										
NATURAL ORANGE FLAVOR INSTANT BREAKFAST DRINK, 4 oz	60	0	0	16	—	40	*	40	0	—
Capri Sun—Shasta										
APPLE, 6.75 oz	90	0	0	23	—	*	*	2	4	—
FRUIT PUNCH, 6.75 oz	102	0	0	26	—	*	*	1	18	—
GRAPE, 6.75 oz	104	0	0	26	—	*	*	19	1	—
LEMONADE, 6.75 oz	92	0	0	23	—	*	*	2	5	—
ORANGE, 6.75 oz	103	0	0	26	—	*	*	2	7	—
RED BERRY, 6.75 oz	110	0	0	28	—	*	*	7	11	—
WATERMELON, 6.75 oz	101	0	0	26	—	*	*	3	1	—
WILD CHERRY, 6.75 oz	118	0	0	30	—	*	*	9	17	—
Country Time— General Foods										
LEMONADE										
SUGAR FREE, prep, 8 oz	4	0	0	0	0	*	*	0	30	—
SUGAR-SWEETENED, prep, 8 oz	90	0	0	22	0	*	*	30	15	—
LEMON-LIME										
SUGAR FREE, prep, 8 oz	4	0	0	0	0	*	*	0	15	—
SUGAR-SWEETENED, prep, 8 oz	90	0	0	22	0	*	*	30	10	—
PINK LEMONADE										
SUGAR FREE, prep, 8 oz	4	0	0	0	0	*	*	0	30	—
SUGAR-SWEETENED, prep, 8 oz	90	0	0	22	0	*	*	30	15	—
Crystal Light— General Foods										
SUGAR FREE DRINK MIX										
CARIBBEAN COOLER, prep, 8 oz	4	0	0	0	0	*	*	0	45	—
CITRUS BLEND, prep, 8 oz	4	0	0	0	0	*	*	0	45	—
FRUIT PUNCH, prep, 8 oz	4	0	0	0	0	*	*	0	45	—
GRAPE, prep, 8 oz	4	0	0	0	0	*	*	0	45	—
LEMONADE, prep, 8 oz	4	0	0	0	0	*	*	0	60	—
LEMON-LIME, prep, 8 oz	4	0	0	0	0	*	*	0	5	—
ORANGE, prep, 8 oz	4	0	0	0	0	*	*	0	45	—
Del Monte										
PINEAPPLE GRAPEFRUIT, 6 oz	90	0	0	24	—	*	.36	50	105	—
PINEAPPLE ORANGE, 6 oz	90	0	0	24	—	*	.36	20	85	—
PINEAPPLE PINK GRAPEFRUIT, 6 oz	90	0	0	24	—	*	.36	50	85	—
Gatorade										
CONSUMER										
LEMON-LIME, prep, 8 oz	60	0	0	15	0	*	*	110	27	—
ORANGE, prep, 8 oz	60	0	0	15	0	*	*	110	27	—
ATHLETIC or INSTITUTIONAL										
LEMON-LIME, 8 oz	50	0	0	14	0	*	*	110	27	—
ORANGE, 8 oz	50	0	0	14	0	*	*	110	27	—
Hi-C—Coca-Cola										
GRAPE, 6 oz	77	—	—	20	—	—	—	6	10	—
LEMON, 6 oz	73	—	—	18	—	—	—	6	10	—
ORANGE, 6 oz	77	—	—	20	—	—	—	7	12	—
PUNCH, 6 oz	77	—	—	20	—	—	—	6	9	—

FOOD & DESCRIPTION MEASURE OR QUANTITY	CALORIES	PROTEIN (GM)	FAT (GM)	CARBO-HYDRATE (GM)	FIBER (GM)	CALCIUM (MG)	IRON (MG)	SODIUM (MG)	POTASSIUM (MG)	CHOLES-TEROL (MG)
Kool-Aid– General Foods										
BLACK CHERRY										
UNSWEETENED, prep, 8 oz	2	0	0	0	tr	*	*	0	0	—
with sugar added, prep, 8 oz	100	0	0	25	tr	*	*	0	0	—
CHERRY										
SUGAR FREE, 8 oz	4	0	0	0	tr	40	*	5	0	—
SUGAR-SWEETENED, 8 oz	90	0	0	23	tr	*	*	5	0	—
UNSWEETENED, prep, 8 oz	2	0	0	0	tr	*	*	0	0	—
with sugar added, prep, 8 oz	100	0	0	25	tr	*	*	0	0	—
GRAPE										
SUGAR FREE, 8 oz	4	0	0	0	tr	40	*	0	0	—
SUGAR SWEETENED, 8 oz	90	0	0	23	0	*	*	0	0	—
UNSWEETENED, prep, 8 oz	2	0	0	0	tr	*	*	0	0	—
with sugar added, prep, 8 oz	100	0	0	25	tr	*	*	0	0	—
LEMONADE										
SUGAR FREE, 8 oz	4	0	0	0	tr	20	*	0	25	—
SUGAR SWEETENED, 8 oz	90	0	0	22	tr	40	*	0	0	—
UNSWEETENED, prep, 8 oz	2	0	0	0	tr	20	*	0	0	—
with sugar added, prep, 8 oz	100	0	0	25	tr	20	*	0	0	—
LEMON-LIME										
UNSWEETENED, prep, 8 oz	2	0	0	0	tr	*	*	0	0	—
with sugar added, prep, 8 oz	100	0	0	25	tr	*	*	0	0	—
MOUNTAIN BERRY PUNCH										
SUGAR FREE, 8 oz	4	0	0	0	tr	20	*	35	0	—
SUGAR-SWEETENED, 8 oz	90	0	0	22	tr	*	*	15	0	—
UNSWEETENED, prep, 8 oz	2	0	0	0	tr	*	*	15	0	—
with sugar added, prep, 8 oz	100	0	0	25	tr	*	*	15	0	—
ORANGE										
SUGAR-SWEETENED, 8 oz	90	0	0	22	0	*	*	0	0	—
UNSWEETENED, prep, 8 oz	2	0	0	0	tr	*	*	0	0	—
with sugar added, prep, 8 oz	100	0	0	25	tr	*	*	0	0	—
PINK LEMONADE										
SUGAR-SWEETENED, 8 oz	90	0	0	22	tr	40	*	0	0	—
UNSWEETENED, prep, 8 oz	2	0	0	0	tr	20	*	0	0	—
with sugar added, prep, 8 oz	100	0	0	25	tr	20	*	0	0	—
RAINBOW PUNCH										
SUGAR FREE, 8 oz	4	0	0	0	tr	20	*	0	0	—
SUGAR-SWEETENED, 8 oz	90	0	0	24	0	*	*	0	0	—
UNSWEETENED, prep, 8 oz	2	0	0	0	tr	*	*	0	0	—
with sugar added, prep, 8 oz	100	0	0	25	tr	*	*	0	0	—
RASPBERRY										
SUGAR-SWEETENED, 8 oz	90	0	0	22	0	*	*	0	0	—
UNSWEETENED, prep, 8 oz	2	0	0	0	0	*	*	0	0	—
with sugar added, prep, 8 oz	100	0	0	25	0	*	*	0	0	—
STRAWBERRY										
SUGAR FREE, 8 oz	4	0	0	0	tr	20	*	0	0	—
SUGAR-SWEETENED, 8 oz	90	0	0	22	0	*	*	0	0	—
UNSWEETENED, prep, 8 oz	2	0	0	0	tr	*	*	35	0	—
with sugar added, prep, 8 oz	100	0	0	25	tr	*	*	35	0	—
SUNSHINE PUNCH										
SUGAR FREE, 8 oz	4	0	0	0	tr	*	*	0	45	—
SUGAR-SWEETENED, 8 oz	90	0	0	23	0	20	*	0	0	—
UNSWEETENED, prep, 8 oz	2	0	0	0	tr	20	*	0	0	—
with sugar added, prep, 8 oz	100	0	0	25	tr	20	*	0	0	—
TROPICAL PUNCH										
SUGAR FREE, 8 oz	4	0	0	0	tr	40	*	0	0	—
SUGAR-SWEETENED, 8 oz	90	0	0	24	0	*	*	0	0	—
UNSWEETENED, prep, 8 oz	2	0	0	0	tr	*	*	0	0	—
with sugar added, prep, 8 oz	100	0	0	25	tr	*	*	0	0	—
Libby										
BANANA FROST MIX, ½ oz	50	0	0	14	—	*	*	—	—	—

FOOD & DESCRIPTION MEASURE OR QUANTITY	CALORIES	PROTEIN (GM)	FAT (GM)	CARBO-HYDRATE (GM)	FIBER (GM)	CALCIUM (MG)	IRON (MG)	SODIUM (MG)	POTASSIUM (MG)	CHOLES-TEROL (MG)
BANANA FROST, RTS, 7 oz	120	2	2	25	—	60	*	—	—	—
ORANGE FROST MIX, ½ oz	60	0	0	14	—	*	*	—	—	—
ORANGE FROST, RTS, 8 oz	120	1	0	29	—	*	*	—	—	—
PINEAPPLE FROST MIX, ½ oz	60	0	0	14	—	*	*	—	—	—
PINEAPPLE FROST, RTS, 6 oz	110	2	2	22	—	60	*	—	—	—
STRAWBERRY FROST MIX, ½ oz	60	0	0	14	—	*	*	—	—	—
STRAWBERRY FROST, rts, 8 oz	120	3	3	21	—	80	.36	—	—	—

Ocean Spray

CRANAPPLE, 6 oz	130	0	0	32	—	*	*	<10	51	—
LOW CALORIE, 6 oz	30	0	0	7	—	*	*	<10	—	—
CRANBERRY JUICE COCKTAIL, 6 oz	110	0	0	26	—	*	*	<10	—	—
LOW CALORIE, 6 oz	35	0	0	9	—	*	*	<10	40	—
CRANGRAPE, 6 oz	110	0	0	26	—	*	*	<10	45	—
CRANICOT, 6 oz	110	0	0	26	—	*	*	<10	115	—
CRANRASPBERRY, 6 oz	110	0	0	27	—	*	*	<10	34	—
CRANTASTIC, 6 oz	110	0	0	27	—	*	*	<10	45	—
PINK GRAPEFRUIT JUICE COCKTAIL, 6 oz	80	0	0	20	—	*	*	15	125	—
PINEAPPLE GRAPEFRUIT JUICE COCKTAIL, 6 oz	110	0	0	26	—	*	*	<10	110	—

Sunkist—Lipton

ASEPTIC

APPLE PUNCH, 8.45 oz	140	0	0	34	—	*	*	0	—	—
FRUIT PUNCH, 8.45 oz	140	0	0	34	—	*	*	0	—	—
GRAPE, 8.45 oz	140	<1	0	33	—	*	*	0	—	—
ORANGE, 8.45 oz	140	<1	0	33	—	*	*	0	—	—

LIGHT, SUGAR-FREE

CITRUS BERRY BLEND FLAVOR, 8 oz	6	0	0	2	—	*	*	20	—	—
NATURAL FRUIT PUNCH FLAVOR, 8 oz	6	0	0	2	—	*	*	20	—	—
NATURAL GRAPE FLAVOR, 8 oz	6	0	0	2	—	*	*	25	—	—
NATURAL LEMONADE FLAVOR, 8 oz	8	0	0	2	—	*	*	35	—	—
NATURAL ORANGE FLAVOR, 8 oz	8	0	0	2	—	*	*	70	—	—

Sweet 'N Low

CHERRY, prep, 8 oz	40	<1	0	9	—	*	*	25	2	—
CRANBERRY-APPLE, prep, 4 oz	40	<1	<1	9	—	20	*	—	—	—
FRUIT PUNCH, prep, 8 oz	40	<1	0	9	—	*	*	25	2	—
GRAPE, prep, 8 oz	40	<1	0	9	—	*	*	25	2	—
LEMONADE, prep, 8 oz	40	<1	0	9	—	*	*	25	2	—
ORANGE, prep, 4 oz	40	<1	<1	9	—	20	*	—	—	—

Tang—General Foods

BREAKFAST BEVERAGE CRYSTALS, prep, 6 oz	90	0	0	22	tr	20	*	0	50	—
SUGAR FREE BREAKFAST BEVERAGE CRYSTALS, prep, 6 oz	6	0	0	1	tr	20	*	0	50	—

Welch

WELCHADE GRAPE DRINK, 6 oz	90	0	0	23	—	*	*	20	15	—

FOOD & DESCRIPTION MEASURE OR QUANTITY	CALORIES	PROTEIN (GM)	FAT (GM)	CARBO-HYDRATE (GM)	FIBER (GM)	CALCIUM (MG)	IRON (MG)	SODIUM (MG)	POTASSIUM (MG)	CHOLES-TEROL (MG)
WELCH'S GRAPE JUICE										
DRINK, 6 oz	110	0	0	27	—	*	*	5	170	—
Wyler's–Borden										
APPLE, prep, 8 oz	90	0	0	22	—	*	*	25	0	—
BLACK CHERRY										
sugar added, prep, 8 oz	100	0	0	26	—	*	*	—	—	—
unsweetened, prep, 8 oz	2	0	0	1	—	*	*	—	—	—
LEMONADE, 8 oz	90	0	0	22	—	*	*	—	—	—
pre-sweetened with										
Nutrasweet, prep, 8 oz	6	0	0	2	—	*	*	35	0	—
ORANGE										
sugar added, 8 oz	100	0	0	26	—	*	*	—	—	—
unsweetened, prep, 8 oz	2	0	0	1	—	*	*	—	—	—
TROPICAL PUNCH, 8 oz	90	0	0	22	—	*	*	—	—	—
pre-sweetened with										
Nutrasweet, 8 oz	4	0	0	1	—	*	*	30	0	—
WILD CHERRY, 8 oz	90	0	0	22	—	*	*	—	—	—
pre-sweetened with										
Nutrasweet, prep, 8 oz	4	0	0	1	—	*	*	20	0	—
WILD GRAPE										
crystals, prep, 8 oz	90	0	0	22	—	*	*	—	—	—
pre-sweetened with										
Nutrasweet, prep, 8 oz	4	0	0	1	—	*	*	20	0	—

Milk-Based

Alba–Heinz

HOT COCOA, 19.14 gm dry	62	5	<1	10	—	323	.07	160	425	4

Alba 77, Fit 'N Frosty

CHOCOLATE, 1 env, 21.26 gm	76	6	<1	12	—	232	1.57	206	477	—
CHOCOLATE MARSHMALLOW,										
1 env, 21.26 gm	76	6	<1	12	—	280	.78	251	439	—
STRAWBERRY, 1 env, 21.26										
gm	73	6	<1	11	—	202	.18	154	474	—
VANILLA, 1 env, 21.26 gm	73	6	<1	12	—	194	.13	152	430	—

Borden

FROSTED [a melloream beverage]										
CHOCOLATE, 8 oz	260	5	11	36	—	250	1.44	205	340	—
STRAWBERRY, 8 oz	270	8	10	36	—	250	*	190	310	—

Catelli

MILK MATE [sweetened milk flavorings]										
BANANA, 1.5 tbsp	55	tr	tr	14	.17	3	.31	12	<1	—
CHOCOLATE, 1.5 tbsp	45	<1	<1	12	.04	7	.54	70	8	—
CHOCOLATE FUDGE, 1.5 tbsp	62	<1	<1	16	.23	3	.2	67	23	—
STRAWBERRY, 1.5 tbsp	62	tr	tr	16	tr	<1	.03	9	<1	—

Diet-Trim 70–Bernard

CHOCOLATE, prep, 12 oz	70	6	<1	11	—	600	9.00	145	310	<5
VANILLA, prep, 12 oz	70	4	<1	12	—	700	9.00	180	290	<5

Estee

COCOA, 6 oz	50	4	<1	9	—	—	—	75	—	2

FOOD & DESCRIPTION MEASURE OR QUANTITY	CALORIES	PROTEIN (GM)	FAT (GM)	CARBO-HYDRATE (GM)	FIBER (GM)	CALCIUM (MG)	IRON (MG)	SODIUM (MG)	POTASSIUM (MG)	CHOLES-TEROL (MG)
Featherweight										
COCOA MIX, prep with water, 6 oz	40	3	0	7	—	—	—	71	254	—
Hills Brothers										
HOT COCOA, prep with water, 6 oz	110	2	2	22	—	223	.65	108	—	—
HOT COCOA, sugar-free, prep with water, 6 oz	57	2	2	9	—	150	.59	136	—	—
Nestle										
RICH 'N CREAMY HOT COCOA MIX										
PLAIN, 1 oz	120	3	3	22	—	80	*	125	—	—
WITH MARSHMALLOWS, 1 oz	120	2	3	22	—	80	*	120	—	—
Ovaltine										
COCOA MIX										
50 CALORIE, .45 oz, prep, 6 oz	50	1	2	8	—	100	1.8	135	135	—
HOT 'N RICH, 5 tsp, prep, 6 oz	120	1	3	22	—	100	1.8	140	368	—
SUGAR FREE, .41 oz, prep, 6 oz	40	2	1	7	—	100	1.80	195	—	—
MILK FLAVORING										
CHOCOLATE, dry mix, ¾ oz	80	<1	<1	18	—	19	3.80	145	145	<1
prep with 2% milk, 8 oz	200	9	5	30	—	310	3.90	270	530	20
SUGAR FREE, 5.7 gm	12	<1	<1	2	—	22	3.90	103	160	<1
prep with 2% milk, 8 oz	140	9	5	14	—	310	4.00	230	540	20
MALT, dry mix, ¾ oz	80	2	<1	18	—	29	3.70	65	124	<1
prep with 2% milk, 8 oz	200	10	5	30	—	320	3.80	190	500	20
STRAWBERRY, SUGAR FREE, dry mix, 5.7 gm	19	<1	<1	4	—	39	3.4	57	116	<1
prep with 2% milk, 8 oz	140	9	5	16	—	330	3.5	180	500	20
PDQ [with 8 oz whole milk and 3–4 tsp powder]										
CHOCOLATE	220	8	26	9	—	290	.12	119	368	—
EGGNOG	270	8	36	8	—	290	.12	119	368	—
STRAWBERRY	215	8	26	8	—	290	.12	119	368	—
Pillsbury										
INSTANT BREAKFAST										
CHOCOLATE MIX, 1 env	130	6	0	26	—	80	4.50	190	270	—
prep with whole milk, 8 oz	290	14	9	38	—	250	4.50	310	620	—
CHOCOLATE MALT MIX, 1 env	130	6*	0	26	—	80	4.50	190	260	—
prep with whole milk, 8 oz	290	14	9	38	—	250	4.50	310	610	—
STRAWBERRY MIX, 1 env	130	5	0	27	—	80	4.50	180	250	—
prep with whole milk, 8 oz	290	14	9	39	—	250	4.50	300	600	—
VANILLA MIX, 1 env	140	6	0	29	—	80	4.50	210	240	—
prep with whole milk, 8 oz	300	14	9	41	—	250	4.50	330	600	—
Quick–Nestle										
CHOCOLATE FLAVOR, dry, 2 tsp, 21.6 gm	90	1	1	19	—	*	.36	35	125	0
STRAWBERRY FLAVOR, dry, 2 tsp, 21.6 gm	90	0	0	22	—	*	*	0	—	—
QUIK CHOCOLATE MILK, 1 c	220	8	8	30	—	250	*	—	—	—

FOOD & DESCRIPTION MEASURE OR QUANTITY	CALORIES	PROTEIN (GM)	FAT (GM)	CARBO- HYDRATE (GM)	FIBER (GM)	CALCIUM (MG)	IRON (MG)	SODIUM (MG)	POTASSIUM (MG)	CHOLES- TEROL (MG)
Rich										
FRESH 'N FROSTY [Mellorine]										
CHOCOLATE, 12 oz	372	9	14	53	—	214	1.44	142	395	6
STRAWBERRY, 12 oz	376	9	13	55	—	247	.41	166	349	6
VANILLA, 12 oz	368	9	13	54	—	247	.31	166	351	6
Shapely Shake– Bernard										
CHOCOLATE, 1 env	60	5	<1	10	—	500	9.00	140	416	<5
VANILLA, 1 env	60	4	<1	12	—	500	9.00	124	273	<5
USDA										
MALTED MILK, powder, 2–3 tsp, 21 gm										
CHOCOLATE FLAVOR	83	1	<1	18	.08	13	.38	49	130	1
with whole milk, 1 c	233	9	9	29	.08	304	.50	168	500	34
NATURAL FLAVOR	86	3	2	15	.13	56	.16	96	159	4
with whole milk, 1 c	236	11	10	27	.13	347	.29	215	529	37

4

BREAKFAST FOODS

FOOD & DESCRIPTION MEASURE OR QUANTITY	CALORIES	PROTEIN (GM)	FAT (GM)	CARBO-HYDRATE (GM)	FIBER (GM)	CALCIUM (MG)	IRON (MG)	SODIUM (MG)	POTASSIUM (MG)	CHOLES-TEROL (MG)
Cereals, Cold										
Arrowhead Mills										
BARLEY FLAKES, 2 oz	200	5	1	45	—	—	—	2	—	—
NATURE O'S, 1 oz	110	5	1	20	—	—	—	14	—	—
OAT FLAKES, 2 oz	220	10	4	39	—	—	—	1	—	—
PUFFED CORN, .5 oz	50	3	0	11	—	—	—	1	—	—
PUFFED MILLET, .5 oz	50	2	0	11	—	—	—	1	—	—
PUFFED RICE, .5 oz	50	1	0	12	—	—	—	1	—	—
PUFFED WHEAT, .5 oz	50	2	0	11	—	—	—	1	—	—
RICE FLAKES, 2 oz	200	4	1	44	—	—	—	5	—	—
RICE & SHINE, ¼ c	160	3	1	35	—	—	—	1	—	—
RYE FLAKES, 2 oz	190	7	1	42	—	—	—	1	—	—
SEVEN GRAIN CEREAL, 1 oz	100	4	1	17	—	—	—	1	—	—
SOY BEAN FLAKES, 2 oz	250	20	11	18	—	—	—	3	—	—
TRITICALE FLAKES, 2 oz	190	7	1	41	—	—	—	1	—	—
WHEAT FLAKES, 2 oz	210	8	1	42	—	—	—	2	—	—
Featherweight										
CORN FLAKES, LOW SODIUM, 1 oz	110	2	0	25	—	—	—	<10	13	—
CRISP RICE, LOW SODIUM, 1 oz	110	2	0	26	—	—	—	<10	26	—
WHEAT FLAKES, LOW SODIUM, 1 oz	100	4	0	23	—	—	—	5	138	—
General Mills										
BODY BUDDIES BROWN SUGAR & HONEY, 1 c, 1 oz	110	2	<1	24	—	100	8.10	290	50	—
NATURAL FRUIT FLAVOR, 1 c, 1 oz	110	2	1	24	—	100	8.10	280	40	—
BOOBERRY, 1 c, 1 oz	110	1	1	24	—	20	4.50	210	45	—
BRAN MUFFIN CRISP, ⅔ c, 1.4 oz	130	3	1	30	4d	60	4.5 0	250	190	—
CHEERIOS, 1¼ c, 1 oz	110	4	2	20	2d	40	4.5 0	290	105	—
CINNAMON TOAST CRUNCH, 1 oz	120	1	3	23	—	40	4.50	220	40	—
COCOA PUFFS, 1 c, 1 oz	110	1	1	25	—	*	4.50	200	45	—
CORN TOTAL, 1 c, 1 oz	110	2	1	24	—	40	18.00	310	30	—
COUNT CHOCULA, 1 c, 1 oz	110	2	1	24	—	20	4.50	210	65	—
COUNTRY CORN FLAKES, 1 c, 1 oz	110	2	<1	25	—	*	8.10	310	30	—

FOOD & DESCRIPTION MEASURE OR QUANTITY	CALORIES	PROTEIN (GM)	FAT (GM)	CARBO-HYDRATE (GM)	FIBER (GM)	CALCIUM (MG)	IRON (MG)	SODIUM (MG)	POTASSIUM (MG)	CHOLES-TEROL (MG)
CRISPY WHEATS 'N RAISINS,										
¾ c, 1 oz	110	2	1	23	—	40	4.50	180	100	—
FIBER ONE, ½ c, 1 oz	60	4	1	21	12d	60	4.50	230	340	—
FRANKENBERRY, 1 c, 1 oz	110	1	1	24	—	20	4.50	210	45	—
GOLDEN GRAHAMS, ¾ c, 1 oz	110	2	1	24	—	*	4.50	280	55	—
HONEY BUC*WHEAT CRISP,										
¾ c, 1 oz	110	2	<1	24	—	60	8.10	250	50	—
HONEY NUT CHEERIOS, ¾ c, 1										
oz	110	3	1	23	—	20	4.50	250	95	—
KABOOM, 1 c, 1 oz	110	2	1	23	—	40	8.10	370	65	—
KIX, 1½ c, 1 oz	110	2	1	24	—	40	8.10	310	45	—
LUCKY CHARMS, 1 c, 1 oz	110	2	1	24	—	20	4.50	180	75	—
PAC-MAN, 1 c, 1 oz	110	1	<1	25	—	20	4.50	200	30	—
RAISIN NUT BRAN, ½ c, 1 oz	110	2	3	21	3d	40	4.50	150	150	—
ROCKY ROAD, ⅔ c, 1 oz	120	1	3	23	—	20	4.50	120	50	—
S'MORES CRUNCH, ¾ c, 1 oz	120	1	2	24	—	*	4.50	250	230	—
TOTAL, 1 c, 1 oz	110	3	1	23	2d	40	18.00	280	110	—
TRIX, 1 c, 1 oz	110	1	<1	25	—	*	4.50	170	25	—
WHEATIES, 1 c, 1 oz	110	3	1	23	2d	40	4.50	370	110	—
Grainfield's										
ALPEN, 1 oz	102	4	1	18	2.21d	61	1.42	51	136	—
no salt/no sugar, 1 oz	98	4	1	17	2.98d	65	1.42	50	152	—
BROWN RICE, 1 oz	111	3	<1	24	.34d	14	.57	4	81	—
CORN FLAKES, 1 oz	109	2	<1	25	.43d	13	.68	2	22	—
CRISPY RICE, 1 oz	112	3	<1	25	.34d	6	.57	3	31	—
RAISIN BRAN, 1 oz	90	2	<1	20	1.87d	16	.85	4	130	—
WEETABIX, 1 oz	102	3	<1	20	2.49d	28	1.53	106	106	—
WHEAT FLAKES, 1 oz	100	3	<1	20	1.98d	28	.28	2	99	—
Kellogg										
ALL-BRAN, ⅓ c, 1 oz	70	4	1	22	9d	22	4.50	260	320	0
ALL-BRAN with extra fiber, ½										
c, 1 oz	60	3	1	22	13d	28	4.50	270	270	0
APPLE-JACKS, 1 c, 1 oz	110	2	0	26	trd	3	4.50	125	30	0
APPLE RAISIN CRISP, ⅔ c,										
1.4 oz	140	2	0	35	2d	6	1.80	220	120	0
BRAN-BUDS, ⅓ c, 1 oz	70	3	1	22	8d	20	4.50	150	310	0
BRAN FLAKES, ⅔ c, 1 oz	90	3	0	23	4d	13	18.00	220	170	0
COCOA KRISPIES, ¾ c, 1 oz	110	1	0	25	trd	6	1.80	190	45	0
CORN FLAKES, 1 c, 1 oz	110	2	0	25	trd	1	1.80	290	35	0
CORN POPS, 1 c, 1 oz	110	1	0	26	trd	2	1.80	90	20	0
CRACKLIN' OAT BRAN, ½ c, 1										
oz	110	3	4	20	4d	15	1.80	150	160	0
CRISPIX, ¾ c, 1 oz	110	2	0	25	trd	4	1.80	220	30	0
FROOT LOOPS, 1 c, 1 oz	110	2	1	25	trd	3	4.50	125	30	0
FROSTED FLAKES, ¾ c, 1 oz	110	1	0	26	trd	1	1.80	200	25	0
FROSTED KRISPIES, ¾ c, 1 oz	110	1	0	25	trd	2	1.80	210	20	0
FROSTED MINI-WHEATS, 4										
biscuits, 1 oz	110	3	0	24	3d	10	1.80	5	80	0
FRUITFUL BRAN, ⅔ c, 1.3 oz	120	3	0	30	4d	12	18.00	230	180	0
HONEY & NUT CORN FLAKES,										
⅔ c, 1 oz	110	2	1	24	trd	4	1.80	200	40	0
HONEY SNACKS, ¾ c, 1 oz	110	2	0	25	trd	3	1.80	70	40	0
JUST RIGHT, ⅔ c, 1 oz	100	3	0	24	2d	7	18.00	190	65	0
JUST RIGHT WITH FRUIT, ¾										
c, 1.3 oz	140	3	1	30	2d	13	18.00	190	110	0
MARSHMALLOW KRISPIES,										
1¼ c, 1.3 oz	140	2	0	33	trd	3	1.80	290	30	0
NUTRI-GRAIN										
ALMOND RAISIN, ⅔ c, 1.4										
oz	150	3	2	32	3d	16	.60	220	130	0
CORN, ½ c, 1 oz	100	2	1	24	2d	1	.60	170	75	0

FOOD & DESCRIPTION MEASURE OR QUANTITY	CALORIES	PROTEIN (GM)	FAT (GM)	CARBO- HYDRATE (GM)	FIBER (GM)	CALCIUM (MG)	IRON (MG)	SODIUM (MG)	POTASSIUM (MG)	CHOLES- TEROL (MG)
WHEAT, ⅔ c, 1 oz	100	3	0	24	2d	9	1.00	170	90	0
WHEAT & RAISINS, ⅔ c, 1.4 oz	130	3	0	32	2d	13	1.10	170	180	0
OJ'S, 1 c, 1 oz	120	2	2	23	—	tr	1.80	135	40	0
PRODUCT 19, 1 c, 1 oz	110	2	0	24	trd	4	18.00	320	45	0
RAISIN BRAN, ¾ c, 1.4 oz	120	3	1	30	4d	19	18.00	220	230	0
RAISIN SQUARES, ½ c, 1 oz	90	2	0	22	3d	14	1.80	0	130	0
RAISINS, RICE & RYE, ¾ c, 1.3 oz	140	2	0	31	2d	9	4.50	235	120	0
RICE KRISPIES, 1 c, 1 oz	110	2	0	25	trd	3	1.80	290	35	0
SPECIAL K, 1 c, 1 oz	110	6	0	20	trd	10	4.50	230	50	0

Nabisco

FOOD & DESCRIPTION MEASURE OR QUANTITY	CALORIES	PROTEIN (GM)	FAT (GM)	CARBO- HYDRATE (GM)	FIBER (GM)	CALCIUM (MG)	IRON (MG)	SODIUM (MG)	POTASSIUM (MG)	CHOLES- TEROL (MG)
100% BRAN, 1 oz	70	3	2	21	10d	20	2.70	190	350	—
SHREDDED WHEAT, 1 biscuit, .83 oz	90	2	1	19	3d	*	.72	0	95	—
SHREDDED WHEAT 'N BRAN, 1 oz	110	3	1	23	4d	*	1.44	0	135	—
SPOON SIZE SHREDDED WHEAT, 1 oz	110	3	0	23	3d	*	.72	0	115	—
TEAM FLAKES, 1 oz	110	2	1	24	0.3d	*	1.44	190	65	—
TOASTED WHEAT AND RAISINS CEREAL, 1 oz	100	2	1	23	3d	*	1.08	0	110	—

Post–General Foods

FOOD & DESCRIPTION MEASURE OR QUANTITY	CALORIES	PROTEIN (GM)	FAT (GM)	CARBO- HYDRATE (GM)	FIBER (GM)	CALCIUM (MG)	IRON (MG)	SODIUM (MG)	POTASSIUM (MG)	CHOLES- TEROL (MG)
ALPHA BITS, 1 oz	110	2	1	24	1d	*	2.70	180	60	—
C.W. POST HEARTY GRANOLA CEREAL, 1 oz	130	2	4	21	1d	*	4.50	85	65	—
C.W. POST HEARTY GRANOLA CEREAL WITH RAISINS, 1 oz	120	2	4	21	1d	*	4.50	80	75	—
COCOA PEBBLES, 1 oz	110	1	1	25	trd	*	1.80	160	40	—
FORTIFIED OAT FLAKES, 1 oz	100	6	1	20	1d	20	8.10	250	150	—
40% BRAN FLAKES, 1 oz	90	3	0	23	4d	*	8.10	230	190	—
FRUIT & FIBRE APPLES & CINNAMON, 1 oz	90	2	0	23	3d	*	4.50	160	150	—
DATES, RAISINS, WALNUTS, 1 oz	90	2	1	22	3d	*	4.50	170	180	—
TROPICAL FRUIT, 1 oz	90	2	1	21	3d	*	4.50	160	190	—
FRUITY PEBBLES, 1 oz	110	1	1	25	trd	*	1.80	150	20	—
GRAPE-NUTS BRAND CEREAL, 1 oz	110	3	0	23	2d	*	1.08	190	85	—
GRAPE-NUTS FLAKES, 1 oz	100	3	1	23	2d	*	4.50	170	95	—
HONEYCOMB, 1 oz	110	1	1	25	trd	*	1.80	195	40	—
HONEY NUT CRUNCH RAISIN BRAN, 1 oz	90	2	1	22	3d	*	3.60	150	160	—
POST TOASTIES CORN FLAKES, 1 oz	110	2	0	24	trd	*	.36	280	30	—
RAISIN BRAN, 1 oz	80	2	0	22	3d	*	4.50	160	170	—
RAISIN GRAPE-NUTS, 1 oz	100	3	0	22	2d	*	.72	140	100	—
SMURF-BERRY CRUNCH, 1 oz	110	1	1	25	trd	*	4.50	75	30	—
SUPER GOLDEN CRISP, 1 oz	110	2	0	26	trd	*	2.70	45	50	—

Quaker

FOOD & DESCRIPTION MEASURE OR QUANTITY	CALORIES	PROTEIN (GM)	FAT (GM)	CARBO- HYDRATE (GM)	FIBER (GM)	CALCIUM (MG)	IRON (MG)	SODIUM (MG)	POTASSIUM (MG)	CHOLES- TEROL (MG)
CAP'N CRUNCH, ¾ c, 1 oz	121	1	3	23	.1	5	4.50	185	37	—
CHOCO CRUNCH, ¾ c, 1 oz	116	2	2	24	.20	5	4.50	172	45	—
CRUNCHBERRIES, ¾ c, 1 oz	120	1	3	23	.1	9	4.50	166	40	—
PEANUT BUTTER CEREAL, ¾ c, 1 oz	127	2	4	21	.2	6	4.50	210	54	—
CORN BRAN, ⅔ c, 1 oz	109	2	<1	23	1.2	23	8.10	244	62	—
HALFSIES, ¾ c, 1 oz	113	2	1	24	.10	12	8.10	243	37	—

FOOD & DESCRIPTION MEASURE OR QUANTITY	CALORIES	PROTEIN (GM)	FAT (GM)	CARBO-HYDRATE (GM)	FIBER (GM)	CALCIUM (MG)	IRON (MG)	SODIUM (MG)	POTASSIUM (MG)	CHOLES-TEROL (MG)
KING VITAMAN, 1¼ c, 1 oz	112	2	1	23	.20	6	8.10	250	49	—
LIFE, .67 c, 1 oz	111	5	2	19	.30	60	8.10	150	172	—
CINNAMON, .67c, 1 oz	110	5	2	19	.30	60	8.10	150	175	—
RAISIN, .67 c, 1⅓ oz	105	6	2	17	.50	60	8.10	161	232	—
MR T., 1 c, 1 oz	121	1	3	23	.10	9	2.70	189	37	—
100% NATURAL CEREAL, ¼ c, 1 oz	136	4	6	18	.3	38	.85	11	150	—
WITH APPLES & CINNAMON, ¼ c, 1 oz	133	3	5	18	.50	40	.89	15	141	—
WITH RAISINS & DATES, ¼ c, 1 oz	132	4	5	18	.3	36	.86	11	156	—
PUFFED RICE, 1 c, ½ oz	55	<1	<1	13	.1	3	.41	1	16	—
PUFFED WHEAT, 1 c, ½ oz	54	2	<1	11	.3	3	.67	1	50	—
QUISP, 1.17 c, 1 oz	121	1	3	23	.1	9	2.70	189	37	—
SHREDDED WHEAT, 2 biscuits, 1.33 oz	104	3	<1	22	.6	11	.86	1	107	—

Ralston Purina

BRAN CHEX, .67 c, 1 oz	90	3	<1	23	4.9d	17	4.50	299	204	—
COOKIE CRISP										
CHOCOLATE CHIP FLAVOR, 1 c, 1 oz	110	2	1	25	.4d	11	4.50	189	32	—
VANILLA WAFER FLAVOR, 1 c, 1 oz	110	2	1	25	.3d	8	4.50	201	28	—
CORN CHEX, 1 c, 1 oz	110	2	<1	25	.6d	2	1.80	328	23	—
CORN FLAKES, 1 c, 1 oz	110	2	<1	25	.7d	1	1.80	277	24	—
CRISPY RICE, 1 c, 1 oz	110	2	<1	25	.3d	4	1.80	204	29	—
DONKEY KONG, 1 c, 1 oz	110	1	1	25	.7d	—	4.50	119	36	—
JUNIOR, 1 c, 1 oz	110	2	1	25	.3d	5	4.50	111	23	—
40% BRAN FLAKES, ¾ c, 1 oz	90	3	<1	20	4.0d	20	4.50	289	184	—
FRUIT RINGS, 1 c, 1 oz	110	2	1	26	.3d	5	4.50	112	—	—
RAISIN BRAN, ¾ c, 1.33 oz	120	3	<1	30	3.6d	19	4.50	299	207	—
RICE CHEX, 1.13 c, 1 oz	110	2	<1	25	.3d	4	1.80	252	36	—
SUGAR FROSTED FLAKES, ¾ c, 1 oz	110	2	<1	26	.6d	3	1.80	176	18	—
SUGAR FROSTED RICE, 1 c, 1 oz	110	2	<1	26	.3d	5	1.80	192	21	—
TASTEEOS, 1¼ c, 1 oz	110	4	<1	22	.8d	13	4.50	209	82	—
WHEAT CHEX, .67 c, 1 oz	100	3	<1	23	2.1d	11	4.50	200	107	—
WHEAT & RAISIN CHEX, ¾ c, 1.33 oz	130	4	<1	31	2.5d	24	5.40	198	125	—

Cereals, Hot

Arrowhead Mills

BEAR MUSH, 1 oz	100	3	0	21	—	—	—	1	—	—
BULGUR-SOY GRITS, 2 oz	200	10	1	40	—	—	—	0	—	—
BULGUR WHEAT, 2 oz	200	6	1	43	—	—	—	0	—	—
CORN GRITS, 2 oz	200	5	1	43	—	—	—	1	—	—
CRACKED WHEAT CEREAL, 2 oz	180	7	1	40	—	—	—	2	—	—
4 GRAIN CEREAL + FLAX, 2 oz	94	4	1	18	—	—	—	1	—	—
STEEL CUT OATS, 2 oz	220	10	4	37	—	—	—	1	—	—

Catelli–Ogilvie

INSTANT QUICK ROLLED SCOTCH OATMEAL, ¾ c, ckd, 25 gm dry	98	4	2	17	.35	16	1.13	<1	45	—
VITA B, ¾ c, ckd, 30 gm dry	108	4	<1	21	.48	12	1.89	<1	111	—
WHEAT HEARTS, ¾ c, ckd, 30 gm dry	107	3	<1	23	.09	8	.39	<1	25	—

FOOD & DESCRIPTION MEASURE OR QUANTITY	CALORIES	PROTEIN (GM)	FAT (GM)	CARBO-HYDRATE (GM)	FIBER (GM)	CALCIUM (MG)	IRON (MG)	SODIUM (MG)	POTASSIUM (MG)	CHOLES-TEROL (MG)
Nabisco										
CREAM OF RICE, 1 oz dry	100	2	0	23	—	*	1.08	0	25	—
INSTANT CREAM OF WHEAT, 1 oz dry	100	3	0	22	—	150	8.10	0	35	—
MIX 'N EAT CREAM OF WHEAT APPLE CINNAMON, 1.25 oz pkt	130	2	0	30	—	40	8.10	240	65	—
BROWN SUGAR CINNAMON, 1.25 oz pkt	130	2	0	30	—	40	8.10	180	65	—
MAPLE BROWN SUGAR, 1.25 oz pkt	130	2	0	30	—	40	8.10	180	40	—
OUR ORIGINAL, 1 oz pkt	100	3	0	21	—	40	8.10	180	30	—
STRAWBERRY, 1.25 oz pkt	140	2	2	29	—	40	8.10	200	50	—
QUICK CREAM OF WHEAT, 1 oz dry	100	3	0	22	—	40	8.10	130	40	—
REGULAR CREAM OF WHEAT, 1 oz dry	100	3	0	22	—	40	8.10	0	35	—
Quaker										
OAT BRAN, .33 c dry	110	6	3	16	.50	20	1.63	1	170	—
OATMEAL, INSTANT REGULAR, 1 pkt, ¾ c ckd	105	5	2	18	.3	100	8.10	281	101	—
WITH APPLES & CINNAMON, 1 pkt, ¾ c ckd	134	4	2	26	.4	100	4.50	181	108	—
WITH BRAN & RAISINS, 1 pkt, ¾ c ckd	153	5	2	29	1	100	4.50	240	227	—
WITH CINNAMON & SPICE, 1 pkt, ¾ c ckd	176	5	2	35	.40	100	8.10	258	106	—
WITH HONEY & GRAHAM, 1 pkt, ¾ c ckd	136	4	2	27	.3	100	4.50	224	87	—
WITH MAPLE & BROWN SUGAR, 1 pkt, ¾ c ckd	163	5	2	32	.3	100	8.10	228	98	—
WITH PEACHES & CREAM, 1 pkt, ¾ c ckd	136	4	2	26	.40	100	4.50	134	130	—
WITH RAISINS & SPICE, 1 pkt, ¾ c ckd	159	5	2	31	.3	100	4.50	217	155	—
WITH RAISINS, DATES & WALNUTS, 1 pkt, ¾ c ckd	150	4	4	25	.40	100	4.50	155	128	—
WITH STRAWBERRIES & CREAM, 1 pkt, ¾ c ckd	136	3	2	26	.40	100	4.50	172	158	—
OATS, QUICK or OLD FASHIONED, .33 c dry, .67 c ckd	109	5	2	18	.3	14	1.08	1	105	—
QUICK CREAMY WHEAT FARINA, 2½ tbsp dry	101	3	<1	22	.10	6	.81	1	31	—
WHOLE WHEAT NATURAL CEREAL, .33 c dry, .67 c ckd	106	3	<1	22	.6	9	.94	1	106	—
Ralston Purina										
INSTANT & REGULAR RALSTON, ¼ c dry, 1 oz	90	4	<1	20	2.7d	10	1.19	2	112	—
REGULAR & QUICK OATS, .33 c dry, 1 oz	110	5	2	18	2.4d	15	1.24	3	103	—
Uhlman Co.										
MALTEX, OLD FASHIONED, ½ c ckd	86	3	<1	15	.38	7	.98	3	78	—
MAYPO, ½ c ckd	109	4	1	17	.24	79	7.15	2	82	—

FOOD & DESCRIPTION MEASURE OR QUANTITY	CALORIES	PROTEIN (GM)	FAT (GM)	CARBO-HYDRATE (GM)	FIBER (GM)	CALCIUM (MG)	IRON (MG)	SODIUM (MG)	POTASSIUM (MG)	CHOLES-TEROL (MG)
MAYPO, VERMONT STYLE, ½ c ckd	90	3	<1	15	.31	59	5.94	3	71	—
WHEATENA, ½ c ckd	79	3	<1	14	.50	7	.93	1	86	—

Entrees: Mixes

Arrowhead Mills

PANCAKE MIX BUCKWHEAT, ½ c	270	17	2	53	—	—	—	500	—	—
PANCAKE MIX GRIDDLE LITE, ½ c	260	8	3	50	—	—	—	417	—	—
PANCAKE MIX MULTIGRAIN, ½ c	350	12	2	70	—	—	—	830	—	—
PANCAKE MIX TRITICALE, ½ c	270	11	2	53	—	—	—	495	—	—

Aunt Jemima–Quaker

BUCKWHEAT PANCAKE & WAFFLE MIX, 3 4" pancakes	200	7	8	25	—	150	1.08	520	200	—
BUTTERMILK COMPLETE PANCAKE & WAFFLE MIX, 3 4" pancakes	260	8	3	57	—	400	1.80	960	85	—
BUTTERMILK PANCAKE & WAFFLE MIX, 3 4" pancakes	300	10	11	40	—	300	1.80	990	220	—
COMPLETE PANCAKE & WAFFLE MIX, 3 4" pancakes	280	8	4	52	—	100	1.80	460	65	—
ORIGINAL PANCAKE & WAFFLE MIX, 3 4" pancakes	220	7	8	26	—	150	1.08	550	170	—
WHOLE WHEAT PANCAKE & WAFFLE MIX, 3 4" pancakes	250	10	9	32	—	200	1.80	730	320	—

Dia Mel

PANCAKE MIX, 3 3" pancakes	100	3	0	21	—	—	—	175	—	0

General Mills
Dry mixes, prepared

BUTTERMILK PANCAKE MIX, 3 4" pancakes	280	8	10	39	—	150	1.44	810		—
COMPLETE BUTTERMILK PANCAKE MIX, 3 4" pancakes	210	5	3	41	—	100	1.44	500	150	—

Hungry Jack–Pillsbury
Dry mixes, prepared

BLUEBERRY, 3 4" pancakes	320	7	15	40	—	100	1.80	820	150	—
BUTTERMILK, 3 4" pancakes	240	7	11	29	—	60	1.08	570	130	—
BUTTERMILK COMPLETE, 3 4" pancakes	180	5	1	38	—	150	2.70	710	75	—
BUTTERMILK COMPLETE PACKETS, 3 4" pancakes	170	4	1	35	—	150	1.80	650	70	—
EXTRA LIGHT, 3 4" pancakes	210	6	7	30	—	150	1.44	490	200	—
EXTRA LIGHT COMPLETE, 3 4" pancakes	180	4	1	39	—	100	2.70	700	45	—

FOOD & DESCRIPTION MEASURE OR QUANTITY	CALORIES	PROTEIN (GM)	FAT (GM)	CARBO-HYDRATE (GM)	FIBER (GM)	CALCIUM (MG)	IRON (MG)	SODIUM (MG)	POTASSIUM (MG)	CHOLES-TEROL (MG)
Pillsbury										
Microwave										
BUTTERMILK PANCAKES, 3 pancakes	220	4	3	43	—	80	1.08	510	70	—
ORIGINAL PANCAKES, 3 pancakes	260	5	6	46	—	80	1.08	540	85	—
Sweet 'N Low										
Dry mixes, prepared										
PANCAKE & CREPE MIX, 4 3″ pancakes	140	4	5	23	—	80	*	40	—	5
1 7″ crepe	70	2	2	12	—	40	*	20	—	<5
POTATO PANCAKES, LOW SODIUM, 2 2¼″ pancakes	76	2	<1	17	—	130	.54	35	21	<1
USDA										
PANCAKE & WAFFLE MIX										
BUCKWHEAT, dry,										
not packed, 1 c, 130 gm	426	14	3	91	—	606	4.00	1734	619	—
packed, 1 c, 135 gm	443	14	3	95	—	629	4.20	1801	643	—
1 6″ pancake, 73 gm	146	5	7	17	—	161	.90	339	179	—
1 4″ pancake, 27 gm	54	2	3	6	—	59	.40	125	66	—
PLAIN & BUTTERMILK, dry										
made with mix, not packed, 1 c, 135 gm	481	12	2	102	—	608	4.20	1935	219	—
eggs and milk, packed, 1 c, 147 gm	523	13	3	111	—	662	4.60	2107	238	—
made with mix, eggs and milk, 1 6″ pancake, 73 gm	164	5	5	24	—	157	.90	412	112	—
1 4″ pancake, 27 gm	61	2	2	9	—	58	.30	152	42	—
WAFFLES, HOME BATTER RECIPE, 1 7″ round waffle, 76 gm	209	7	7	28	—	85	1.30	356	109	—
WAFFLES, HOME RECIPE, 9 × 9″ square, 1.13 c batter, 1 waffle, 200 gm	558	19	20	75	—	226	3.40	950	290	—
Entrees: Frozen										
Aunt Jemima–Quaker										
BLUEBERRY PANCAKES, 3 4″ pancakes	240	7	4	45	.20	76	2.06	778	103	—
BLUEBERRY PANCAKE BATTER, 3 4″ pancakes	205	6	2	42	.20	68	1.44	698	93	—
BUTTERMILK PANCAKES, 3 4″ pancakes	240	7	4	45	.20	76	2.06	778	103	—
BUTTERMILK PANCAKE BATTER, prep, 3 4″ pancakes, 4 oz	212	7	2	43	.10	91	1.70	733	129	—
CINNAMON SWIRL FRENCH TOAST, 2 sl, 3 oz	190	6	6	28	.30	94	1.44	359	126	—
FRENCH TOAST, 2 sl, 3 oz	168	6	4	27	.10	94	1.44	430	97	—
RAISIN, 2 sl, 3 oz	185	7	4	29	.20	96	1.44	423	160	—
PANCAKE BATTER, 3 4″ pancakes, 4 oz	210	7	2	42	.20	68	1.51	857	92	—
WAFFLES										
APPLE & CINNAMON, 2 waffles, 2.5 oz	173	5	4	29	.10	100	3.60	503	87	—
BLUEBERRY, 2 waffles, 2.5 oz	173	5	4	29	.10	100	3.60	503	87	—

FOOD & DESCRIPTION MEASURE OR QUANTITY	CALORIES	PROTEIN (GM)	FAT (GM)	CARBO-HYDRATE (GM)	FIBER (GM)	CALCIUM (MG)	IRON (MG)	SODIUM (MG)	POTASSIUM (MG)	CHOLES-TEROL (MG)
BUTTERMILK, 2 waffles, 2.5 oz	175	5	4	29	.10	100	3.60	550	79	—
ORIGINAL, 2 waffles, 2.5 oz	173	5	4	29	.10	100	3.60	539	86	—
RAISIN, 2 waffles, 2.88 oz	200	5	4	36	.30	100	3.60	526	163	—

Eggo–Kellogg

FOOD & DESCRIPTION	CALORIES	PROTEIN	FAT	CARBO-HYDRATE	FIBER	CALCIUM	IRON	SODIUM	POTASSIUM	CHOLES-TEROL
APPLE CINNAMON WAFFLE, 1 waffle, 1.4 oz	130	3	5	18	—	20	1.80	300	—	—
BLUEBERRY FLAVORED WAFFLE, 1 waffle, 1.4 oz	130	3	5	18	·	20	1.80	300	—	—
BUTTERMILK WAFFLE, 1 waffle, 1.4 oz	120	3	5	16	—	20	1.80	300	—	—
HOMESTYLE WAFFLE, 1 waffle, 1.4 oz	120	3	5	16	—	20	1.80	300	—	—
NUTRI-GRAIN WAFFLE, 1 waffle, 1.4 oz	130	3	5	18	—	20	1.80	300	—	—
STRAWBERRY WAFFLE, 1 waffle, 1.4 oz	130	3	5	18	—	20	1.80	300	—	—

Swanson–Campbell

FOOD & DESCRIPTION	CALORIES	PROTEIN	FAT	CARBO-HYDRATE	FIBER	CALCIUM	IRON	SODIUM	POTASSIUM	CHOLES-TEROL
CINNAMON SWIRL FRENCH TOAST WITH SAUSAGES, 6.5 oz	480	16	29	39	—	100	3.60	710	—	—
FRENCH TOAST WITH SAUSAGES, 6.5 oz	450	17	26	36	—	100	4.50	770	—	—
OMELETS WITH CHEESE SAUCE AND HAM, 7 oz	400	18	31	12	—	250	2.70	1160	—	—
PANCAKES AND BLUEBERRY SAUCE, 7 oz	400	9	9	70	—	60	1.80	800	—	—
PANCAKES AND SAUSAGES, 6 oz	460	14	22	52	—	80	2.70	940	—	—
PANCAKES WITH STRAWBERRIES, 7 oz	430	8	8	82	—	60	2.70	820	—	—
SCRAMBLED EGGS AND SAUSAGE WITH HASHED BROWN POTATOES, 6.25 oz	410	12	33	17	—	60	2.70	790	—	—
SPANISH STYLE OMELET, 7.75 oz	250	9	17	14	—	80	2.70	840	—	—

Toaster Pastries

Pillsbury

FOOD & DESCRIPTION	CALORIES	PROTEIN	FAT	CARBO-HYDRATE	FIBER	CALCIUM	IRON	SODIUM	POTASSIUM	CHOLES-TEROL
TOASTER STRUDEL										
BLUEBERRY, 1 pastry	190	2	8	28	—	0	.72	200	40	—
CINNAMON, 1 pastry	190	2	8	26	—	0	.72	200	35	—
RASPBERRY, 1 pastry	190	2	8	27	—	0	.72	200	40	—
STRAWBERRY, 1 pastry	190	2	8	27	—	0	.72	200	40	—

Kellogg

FOOD & DESCRIPTION	CALORIES	PROTEIN	FAT	CARBO-HYDRATE	FIBER	CALCIUM	IRON	SODIUM	POTASSIUM	CHOLES-TEROL
FROSTED POP-TARTS										
BLUEBERRY, 1 tart	200	3	5	38	—	13	1.80	220	50	—
BROWN SUGAR CINNAMON, 1 tart	210	3	7	34	—	—	1.80	200	70	—
CHERRY, 1 tart	210	3	5	37	—	15	1.80	230	60	—
CHOCOLATE FUDGE, 1 tart	200	3	4	36	—	—	1.80	230	100	—
CHOCOLATE VANILLA CREAM, 1 tart	200	3	4	38	trd	—	1.80	240	70	—
CONCORD GRAPE, 1 tart	210	3	6	36	—	—	1.80	215	70	—
DUTCH APPLE, 1 tart	210	3	6	36	—	—	1.80	210	60	—
RASPBERRY, 1 tart	210	3	6	36	—	14	1.80	220	70	—
STRAWBERRY, 1 tart	200	3	5	38	—	12	1.80	210	50	—

FOOD & DESCRIPTION MEASURE OR QUANTITY	CALORIES	PROTEIN (GM)	FAT (GM)	CARBO-HYDRATE (GM)	FIBER (GM)	CALCIUM (MG)	IRON (MG)	SODIUM (MG)	POTASSIUM (MG)	CHOLES-TEROL (MG)
POP-TARTS										
BLUEBERRY, 1 tart	210	3	5	36	—	14	1.80	220	60	—
BROWN SUGAR CINNAMON, 1 tart	210	3	8	33	—	—	1.80	210	80	—
CHERRY, 1 tart	210	3	5	36	—	15	1.80	230	70	—
STRAWBERRY, 1 tart	200	3	4	37	—	13	1.80	220	60	—

Nabisco

FOOD & DESCRIPTION MEASURE OR QUANTITY	CALORIES	PROTEIN (GM)	FAT (GM)	CARBO-HYDRATE (GM)	FIBER (GM)	CALCIUM (MG)	IRON (MG)	SODIUM (MG)	POTASSIUM (MG)	CHOLES-TEROL (MG)
FROSTED TOASTETTES PASTRIES										
BROWN SUGAR CINNAMON, 1 pastry	200	2	5	36	—	*	2.70	170	45	—
FUDGE, 1 pastry	200	2	6	35	—	*	2.70	210	45	—
STRAWBERRY, 1 pastry	200	2	5	36	—	*	2.70	200	45	—
TOASTETTES PASTRIES										
APPLE, 1 pastry	200	2	5	36	—	*	2.70	170	45	—
BLUEBERRY, 1 pastry	200	2	5	36	—	*	2.70	200	45	—
CHERRY, 1 pastry	200	2	5	36	—	*	2.70	200	45	—
STRAWBERRY, 1 pastry	200	2	5	36	—	*	2.70	200	45	—

5

CANDY & GUM

FOOD & DESCRIPTION MEASURE OR QUANTITY	CALORIES	PROTEIN (GM)	FAT (GM)	CARBO-HYDRATE (GM)	FIBER (GM)	CALCIUM (MG)	IRON (MG)	SODIUM (MG)	POTASSIUM (MG)	CHOLES-TEROL (MG)
Beech-Nut–Nabisco										
BEECHIES CANDY COATED GUM, all flavors, 1 stick	6	0	0	2	—	*	*	0	0	—
COUGH DROPS, 1 piece	10	0	0	3	—	*	*	0	0	—
GUM, all flavors, 1 stick	10	0	0	2	—	*	*	0	0	—
Borden										
CAMPFIRE MARSHMALLOWS, 2 large or 24 mini	40	0	0	10	—	*	*	10	0	—
Boyer Bros.										
PEANUT BUTTER CUP, 2 cups, 1.6 oz	250	5	15	23	—	40	*	—	—	—
MALLO CUP, 2 cups, 1.6 oz	224	1	11	29	—	*	*	—	—	—
SMOOTHIE, 2 cups, 1.6 oz	250	5	15	24	—	60	*	—	—	—
Bubble Yum–Nabisco										
BUBBLE YUM BUBBLE GUM, all flavors, 1 stick	25	0	0	7	—	*	*	0	0	—
SUGARLESS, all flavors, 1 stick	20	0	0	5	—	*	*	0	0	—
Care-free–Nabisco										
CARE-FREE SUGARLESS BUBBLE GUM, all flavors, 1 stick	10	0	0	2	—	*	*	0	0	—
GUM, all flavors, 1 stick	8	0	0	2	—	*	*	0	0	—
Chuckles–Nabisco										
CHERRY JELLIES, 1 oz, 28 gm	100	0	0	23	—	*	*	10	0	—
CINNAMON SOFTEES, 1 oz, 28 gm	110	0	0	26	—	*	*	15	0	—
FAMILY ASSORTMENT, 1 oz, 28 gm	100	0	0	23	—	*	*	10	0	—
FRUIT JELLIES 7 JELLS, 1 oz, 28 gm	100	0	0	23	—	*	*	10	0	—
JELLY BEANS, 1 oz, 28 gm	110	0	0	26	—	*	*	10	0	—
JELLY BUNNY FRUIT SOFTEES, 1 oz, 28 gm	100	0	0	23	—	*	*	10	0	—
JELLY CANDY BAR, 1 oz, 28 gm	100	0	0	25	—	*	*	10	0	—
JELLY EGGS, 1 oz, 28 gm	110	0	0	26	—	*	*	10	0	—

FOOD & DESCRIPTION MEASURE OR QUANTITY	CALORIES	PROTEIN (GM)	FAT (GM)	CARBO-HYDRATE (GM)	FIBER (GM)	CALCIUM (MG)	IRON (MG)	SODIUM (MG)	POTASSIUM (MG)	CHOLES-TEROL (MG)
JELLY MINT SOFTEES, 1 oz, 28 gm	100	0	1	23	—	*	*	10	0	—
JELLY RABBITS, 1 oz, 28 gm	100	0	0	23	—	*	*	10	0	—
JELLY RINGS, 1 oz, 28 gm	100	0	1	22	—	*	*	10	0	—
JU JUBES, 1 oz, 28 gm	110	0	0	25	—	*	*	15	5	—
JU JU RABBITS, 1 oz, 28 gm	110	0	0	25	—	*	*	15	0	—
JU JU SOFTEES, 1 oz, 28 gm	100	0	0	25	—	*	*	15	0	—
LICORICE JELLIES, 1 oz, 28 gm	100	0	0	23	—	*	*	10	0	—
LICORICE JELLY EGGS, 1 oz, 28 gm	110	0	0	26	—	*	*	10	0	—
LICORICE SOFTEES, 1 oz, 28 gm	100	0	0	26	—	*	*	25	0	—
MARSHMALLOW EGGS, PLAIN & SPECKLED, 1 oz, 28 gm	110	0	0	27	—	*	*	0	0	—
NOUGAT CENTERS, 1 oz, 28 gm	110	0	0	26	—	*	*	10	0	—
NOUGAT EGGS, 1 oz, 28 gm	110	0	0	26	—	*	*	10	0	—
ORANGE SLICES, 1 oz, 28 gm	110	0	1	24	—	*	*	10	0	—
SPEARMINT LEAVES, 1 oz, 28 gm	110	0	1	15	—	*	*	15	0	—
SPICE DROPS, 1 oz, 28 gm	110	0	1	24	—	*	*	15	0	—
SPICE STICKS & DROPS, 1 oz, 28 gm	100	0	1	23	—	*	*	10	0	—
SPICE STRINGS, 1 oz, 28 gm	110	0	1	24	—	*	*	10	0	—
WILD FRUIT BERRIES, 1 oz, 28 gm	110	0	0	25	—	*	*	15	0	—
Cortina-Welch—Nabisco										
CHOCOLATE COVERED CHERRIES										
DARK, 2 pieces, 1.5 oz	180	1	5	32	—	*	*	20	40	—
REGULAR, 2 pieces, 1.5 oz	170	1	4	32	—	*	*	20	30	—
THIN MINTS, 3 pieces, 1 oz	120	1	2	23	—	*	.36	10	20	—
Del Monte										
YOGURT COATED RAISINS, 1 oz, 28 gm	120	1	3	22	—	20	*	10	65	—
Durkee—Mower										
MARSHMALLOW FLUFF, 100 gm	325	<1	<1	80	—	—	—	27	—	0
1 serving, 18 gm	59	<1	<1	14	—	—	—	5	—	0
Estee										
CHOCOLATE BARS, 2 squares	60	1	4-6	4-5	—	—	—	10	—	2
CHOCOLATE COATED RAISINS, 6 pieces	30	1	2	4	—	—	—	10	—	<1
CRUNCH CHOCOLATE BAR, 2 squares	45	1	3	4	—	—	—	10	—	2
ESTEE-ETS, 5 pieces	35	1	2	4	—	—	—	10	—	<1
FRUIT AND NUT MIX, 4 pieces	35	1	2	3	—	—	—	10	—	<1
GUM DROPS, 4 pieces	12	0	0	3	—	—	—	5	—	0
HARD CANDY, 2 pieces	25	0	0	6	—	—	—	5	—	0
LOLLIPOPS, 1 lollipop	12	0	0	3	—	—	—	5	—	0
MINTS, 1 mint	4	0	1	1	—	—	—	0	—	0
PEANUT BUTTER CUPS, 1 cup	45	1	3	3	—	—	—	10	—	<1
Featherweight										
CHOCOLATE CRISP BAR, 2 pieces	100	2	6	9	—	—	—	—	66	—

FOOD & DESCRIPTION MEASURE OR QUANTITY	CALORIES	PROTEIN (GM)	FAT (GM)	CARBO- HYDRATE (GM)	FIBER (GM)	CALCIUM (MG)	IRON (MG)	SODIUM (MG)	POTASSIUM (MG)	CHOLES- TEROL (MG)
HARD CANDY, 1 piece	12	0	0	3	—	—	—	—	0	—
MILK CHOCOLATE BAR, 2 pieces	90	2	6	8	—	—	—	—	72	—

Fruit Stripe—Nabisco

BUBBLE GUM, 1 stick	10	0	0	2	—	*	*	0	0	—
GUM, 1 stick	9	0	0	2	—	*	*	0	0	—

M&M—Mars

M&M, PEANUT, 47.3 gm	241	5	12	28	1.35d	59	.67	29	163	6
PLAIN, 48.1 gm	237	3	10	33	.24d	79	.76	41	172	8
MARS BAR, 1 bar, 50 gm	242	4	11	30	.83d	83	.52	75	165	7
MILKY WAY, 1 bar, 59.5 gm	272	3	10	41	.10d	78	.42	113	156	11
ROYALS, 43.1 gm	212	3	9	30	.19d	70	.63	36	157	7
SKITTLES, 1 oz, 28 gm	115	<1	<1	26	—	<1	.03	8	7	0
SNICKERS, 1 bar, 56.7 gm	274	6	13	33	1.39d	64	.44	141	190	9
STARBURST, 1 oz, 28 gm	118	<1	2	24	—	1	.03	13	<1	0
TWIX, CARAMEL, 1 bar, 58.4 gm	290	3	14	38	.12d	68	.38	115	123	5
PEANUT BUTTER, 1 bar, 53.6 gm	286	6	16	30	—	69	1.28	156	173	4
3 MUSKETEERS, 1 bar, 64.6 gm	282	2	8	49	.36d	50	.5	134	116	7

Nabisco

BABY RUTH CANDY BAR, ½ bar, 1 oz, 28 gm	130	2	6	18	—	*	.36	60	60	—
BONKERS FRUIT CANDY, all flavors, 1 piece	20	0	0	5	—	*	*	0	0	—

BREATH SAVERS MINTS,
  SUGAR FREE, all flavors,
  1 piece
	8	0	0	2	—	*	*	0	0	—

BRIDGE MIX, 14 pieces, 1 oz, 28 gm	140	1	6	20	—	*	.36	15	55	—
BUTTERFINGER CANDY BAR, ½ bar, 1 oz, 28 gm	130	2	6	19	—	*	.36	50	60	—

CHARLESTON CHEW
  CHOCOLATE, ½ bar, 1 oz, 28
  gm
	120	1	3	22	—	*	*	40	30	—

STRAWBERRY, ½ bar, 1 oz, 28 gm	120	1	3	22	—	*	*	40	30	—
VANILLA, ½ bar, 1 oz, 28 gm	120	1	3	22	—	*	.36	40	30	—

CHOCOLATE COVERED
  PEANUTS, 14 pieces, 1
  oz, 28 gm
	160	4	9	14	—	20	.36	15	120	—

CHOCOLATE COVERED
  RAISINS, 29 pieces, 1
  oz, 28 gm
	130	1	5	21	—	20	.72	20	150	—

FUDGE BAR, 2 pieces, 1.38 oz	170	1	5	29	—	*	.36	40	50	—
GOODSTUFF BAR, 1 bar, 1.79 oz	250	4	14	29	—	60	.72	90	150	—

LIFESAVERS
  LOLLIPOPS, all flavors, 1
  lollipop
	45	0	0	11	—	*	*	10	0	—

ROLL CANDY
   CIN-O-MON, PEP-O-MINT,
   SPEAR-O-MINT, WINT-
   O-GREEN, 1 piece
	7	0	0	3	—	*	*	0	0	—

OTHER FLAVORS, 1 piece	<10	0	0	3	—	*	*	0	0	—
SOURS, 1 piece	10	0	0	3	—	*	*	0	0	—
JUNIOR MINTS, 12 pieces, 1 oz, 28 gm	120	1	3	24	—	*	*	10	25	—

FOOD & DESCRIPTION MEASURE OR QUANTITY	CALORIES	PROTEIN (GM)	FAT (GM)	CARBO-HYDRATE (GM)	FIBER (GM)	CALCIUM (MG)	IRON (MG)	SODIUM (MG)	POTASSIUM (MG)	CHOLES-TEROL (MG)
MILK CHOCOLATE STARS, 13 pieces, 1 oz, 28 gm	160	2	8	19	—	40	.36	35	85	—
NUT FUDGE SQUARES, 2 pieces, 1 oz, 28 gm	130	1	5	21	—	*	.36	25	30	—
PEPPERMINT PATTIES, 2 pieces, 1 oz, 28 gm	110	1	0	25	—	*	.36	10	25	—
PINE BROS. COUGH DROPS, ASSORTED, HONEY, WILD CHERRY, 13 pieces, 1 oz, 28 gm	130	0	0	31	—	*	*	0	75	—
POM POMS CARAMEL CANDY, ½ box, 1 oz, 28 gm	100	1	3	15	—	20	.36	70	45	—
SUGAR BABIES MILK CARAMEL TIDBITS, 1 pkg, 1.63 oz	180	1	2	40	—	20	.36	85	50	—
SUGAR DADDY MILK CARAMEL POP, 1 pop, 1.38 oz	150	1	1	33	—	20	.36	85	50	—
SUGAR MAMA CARAMEL CANDY, 1 piece, ¾ oz	90	0	3	17	—	20	*	30	30	—

Necco

CANADA MINT & WINTERGREEN LOZENGES, 1 piece, 3.1 gm	12	—	0	3	—	—	—	<1	—	—
NECCO SKY BARS, 1 bar, 39 gm	176	—	8	26	—	—	—	39	—	—
NECCO WAFERS ASSORTED FLAVORS, 1 roll, 57.25 gm	160	—	0	55	—	—	—	5	—	—

Nestle

CRUNCH BAR, 1.06 oz	160	2	8	19	—	60	*	50	110	5
MILK CHOCOLATE BAR, 1 oz, 28 gm	150	2	9	17	—	60	*	20	95	—
WITH ALMONDS, 1 oz, 28 gm	160	3	10	15	—	60	.36	15	125	—
$100,000 BAR, 1.5 oz, 42 gm	200	2	8	31	—	40	*	75	70	—

Pearson—Nabisco

CARAMEL NIP, 4 pieces, 1 oz	120	1	3	23	—	20	*	70	70	—
CHOCOLATE PARFAIT, 4 pieces, 1 oz	120	1	3	23	—	20	*	70	60	—
COFFEE NIP, 4 pieces, 1 oz	120	1	3	23	—	20	*	70	50	—
COFFIOCA PARFAIT, 4 pieces, 1 oz	120	1	3	23	—	20	*	70	85	—
LICORICE NIP, 4 pieces, 1 oz	120	1	3	23	—	20	*	70	50	—
MINT PARFAIT, 4 pieces, 1 oz	120	1	3	23	—	20	*	70	60	—
PEANUT BUTTER PARFAIT, 4 pieces, 1 oz	120	1	3	23	—	20	*	70	70	—

Peter Paul Cadbury, Inc.

ALMOND JOY, I.55 oz	220	2	12	26	—	20	.36	90	—	—
CADBURY ALMOND, 2 oz	310	6	18	31	—	140	.72	80	—	—
CADBURY BRAZIL NUT, 2 oz	310	5	18	32	—	140	.72	80	—	—
CADBURY CARAMELLO, 2 oz	280	4	13	37	—	100	.36	110	—	—
CADBURY CREME EGGS, 1 oz	136	1	6	19	—	7	.40	—	—	—
CADBURY FRUIT AND NUT, 2 oz	300	5	16	33	—	120	1.08	80	—	—
CADBURY DAIRY MILK, 2 oz	300	4	16	34	—	140	1.44	90	—	—

FOOD & DESCRIPTION MEASURE OR QUANTITY	CALORIES	PROTEIN (GM)	FAT (GM)	CARBO-HYDRATE (GM)	FIBER (GM)	CALCIUM (MG)	IRON (MG)	SODIUM (MG)	POTASSIUM (MG)	CHOLES-TEROL (MG)
CADBURY WHOLE HAZELS, 2 oz	310	5	17	32	—	140	.72	90	—	—
MOUNDS, 1.65 oz	230	2	12	28	—	*	.72	90	—	—
POWERHOUSE, 2 oz	260	4	11	38	—	40	.72	195	—	—
WISPA, 1 oz	150	2	8	17	—	60	.72	45	—	—
YORK PEPPERMINT PATTIE, 1.25 oz	160	1	4	28	—	*	.36	15	—	—
Planters–Nabisco										
PEANUT BAR, 4 bars, 1.6 oz	240	8	14	21	—	*	.36	110	130	—
PEANUT CANDY, 4 pieces, 1 oz	140	4	9	13	—	*	*	70	130	—
Sahadi–Lipton										
HALVAH, 1 oz	150	3	10	13	—	20	.72	45	—	—
USDA										
BUTTERSCOTCH, 1 oz, 28 gm	113	tr	1	27	—	5	.40	19	1	—
CANDY CORN, 1 c (approximately 143 pieces)	728	<1	4	179	—	28	2.20	424	10	—
CARAMELS, plain or chocolate, 1 oz, 28 gm	113	1	3	22	—	42	.40	64	54	—
WITH NUTS, 1 oz, 28 gm	121	1	5	20	—	40	.40	58	66	—
CHOCOLATE										
BITTERSWEET, 1 oz, 28 gm	135	2	11	13	—	16	1.40	1	174	—
MILK, PLAIN, 1 oz, 28 gm	147	2	9	16	—	65	.30	27	109	—
WITH ALMONDS, 1 oz, 28 gm	151	3	10	15	—	65	.50	23	125	—
WITH PEANUTS, 1 oz, 28 gm	154	4	11	13	—	49	.40	19	138	—
SEMISWEET, 1 oz, 28 gm	144	1	10	16	—	9	.70	1	92	—
1 c, 170 gm	862	7	61	97	—	51	4.40	3	553	—
SWEET, 1 oz, 28 gm	150	1	10	16	—	27	.40	9	76	—
CHOCOLATE-COATED CANDY										
ALMONDS, 1 oz, 28 gm	161	4	12	11	—	58	.80	17	155	—
CHOCOLATE FUDGE, 1 oz, 28 gm	122	1	5	21	—	29	.40	65	55	—
WITH NUTS, 1 oz, 28 gm	128	1	6	19	—	29	.40	58	62	—
COCONUT CENTER, 1 oz, 28 gm	124	<1	5	20	—	14	.30	56	47	—
FONDANT MINTS, ROUND, 1 oz, 28 gm	116	<1	3	23	—	16	.30	52	26	—
FUDGE CARAMELS & PEANUTS, 1 oz, 28 gm	123	2	5	18	—	51	.40	58	85	—
FUDGE PEANUTS & CARAMEL, 1 oz, 28 gm	130	3	7	17	—	36	.30	36	63	—
HONEYCOMBED HARD CANDY WITH PEANUT BUTTER, 1 oz, 28 gm	131	2	6	20	—	23	.50	46	64	—
NOUGAT AND CARAMEL, 1 oz, 28 gm	118	1	4	21	—	36	.50	49	60	—
PEANUTS, 1 oz, 28 gm	159	5	12	11	—	33	.40	17	143	—
RAISINS, 1 oz, 28 gm	120	2	5	20	—	43	.70	18	171	—
VANILLA CREAMS, 1 oz, 28 gm	123	1	5	20	—	36	.20	52	50	—
CHOCOLATE DISKS, 1 oz, 28 gm	132	2	6	21	—	38	.40	20	71	—
CHOCOLATE-FLAVORED ROLL, 1 oz, 28 gm	112	<1	2	23	—	19	.50	56	35	—
FUDGE										
CHOCOLATE, 1 oz, 28 gm	113	<1	4	21	—	22	.30	54	42	—

FOOD & DESCRIPTION MEASURE OR QUANTITY	CALORIES	PROTEIN (GM)	FAT (GM)	CARBO-HYDRATE (GM)	FIBER (GM)	CALCIUM (MG)	IRON (MG)	SODIUM (MG)	POTASSIUM (MG)	CHOLES-TEROL (MG)
WITH NUTS, 1 oz	121	1	5	20	—	22	.30	48	50	—
VANILLA, 1 oz, 28 gm	113	<1	3	21	—	32	.10	59	36	—
WITH NUTS, 1 oz, 28 gm	120	1	5	20	—	31	.20	53	32	—
GUMDROPS, STARCH JELLY PIECES, 1 oz, 28 gm	98	tr	<1	25	—	2	.10	10	1	—
HARD CANDY, 1 oz, 28 gm	109	0	<1	28	—	6	.50	9	1	—
JELLY BEANS, ¾ × 2", 1 oz, 28 gm	104	tr	<1	26	—	3	.30	3	tr	—
MARSHMALLOWS, PLAIN LARGE, REGULAR TYPE, 1 marshmallow	23	<1	tr	6	—	1	.10	3	tr	—
MINIATURE packed, 1 c, 56 gm	179	1	tr	45	—	10	.90	22	3	—
unpacked, 1 c, 46 gm	147	<1	tr	37	—	8	.70	18	3	—
PEANUT BARS, 1 oz, 28 gm	146	5	9	13	—	12	.50	3	127	—
PEANUT BRITTLE, no added salt or soda, 1 oz, 28 gm	119	2	3	23	—	10	.70	9	43	—
SUGAR-COATED ALMONDS, 1 oz, 28 gm	129	2	5	20	—	28	.50	6	72	—

Wrigley

FOOD & DESCRIPTION MEASURE OR QUANTITY	CALORIES	PROTEIN (GM)	FAT (GM)	CARBO-HYDRATE (GM)	FIBER (GM)	CALCIUM (MG)	IRON (MG)	SODIUM (MG)	POTASSIUM (MG)	CHOLES-TEROL (MG)
EXTRA SUGARFREE GUM, 1 stick	8	—	—	—	—	5	—	—	—	—
HUBBA BUBBA BUBBLE GUM, BLUEBERRY, GRAPE, RASPBERRY, STRAWBERRY, 1 stick	23	—	<1	6	—	<1	—	<1	<1	—
ORIGINAL FLAVOR	23	—	<1	6	—	30	—	<1	<1	—
SPEARMINT, DOUBLEMINT, JUICY FRUIT, BIG RED, FREEDENT, 1 stick	10	—	<1	2	—	3	—	<1	<1	—

6

CONDIMENTS & SEASONINGS

FOOD & DESCRIPTION MEASURE OR QUANTITY	CALORIES	PROTEIN (GM)	FAT (GM)	CARBO- HYDRATE (GM)	FIBER (GM)	CALCIUM (MG)	IRON (MG)	SODIUM (MG)	POTASSIUM (MG)	CHOLES- TEROL (MG)
Bacon Bits, Imitation										
Durkee										
BACON CHIPS, 1 tbsp	44	3	2	4	—	—	—	279	—	—
IMITATION BACON BITS, 1 tsp	8	<1	<1	<1	—	—	—	229	—	—
General Mills										
BAC-OS, 1 tbsp	30	3	1	2	—	*	.36	130	210	—
Hormel										
BACON BITS, 1 tbsp	30	3	2	0	—	—	—	313	—	—
PEPPERONI BITS, 1 tbsp	35	2	3	0	—	—	—	—	—	—
Libby's										
BACON CRUMBLES, 1 tbsp	25	2	1	2	—	*	*	—	—	—
McCormick										
IMITATION BACON CHIPS, 1 tbsp, 7 gm	28	3	1	2	—	—	—	—	—	—
R.T. French										
IMITATION BACON CRUMBLES, 1 tbsp, 1.6 gm	6	1	<1	<1	—	*	*	40	—	—
Condiments										
Arrowhead Mills										
TAMARI SOY SAUCE, 1 tbsp	15	2	0	2	—	—	—	800	—	—
Del Monte										
TOMATO CATSUP, ¼ c, 57 gm	60	1	0	16	—	*	.36	675	310	—
TOMATO CATSUP, NO SALT ADDED, ¼ c, 57 gm	60	1	0	16	—	*	.36	25	310	—
TOMATO CHILI SAUCE, ¼ c, 57 gm	70	1	0	17	—	*	.72	835	400	—
TOMATO SEAFOOD COCKTAIL, ¼ c, 57 gm	70	1	0	17	—	*	.36	765	285	—
Dia-Mel										
BARBECUE SAUCE, 1 tbsp	18	<1	<1	3	—	—	—	0	—	0

FOOD & DESCRIPTION MEASURE OR QUANTITY	CALORIES	PROTEIN (GM)	FAT (GM)	CARBO-HYDRATE (GM)	FIBER (GM)	CALCIUM (MG)	IRON (MG)	SODIUM (MG)	POTASSIUM (MG)	CHOLES-TEROL (MG)
CATSUP, 1 tbsp	6	0	0	1	—	—	—	20	—	0
COCKTAIL SAUCE, 1 tbsp	10	<1	<1	2	—	—	—	35	—	0
PICANTE SAUCE, 2 tbsp	8	<1	0	2	—	—	—	60	—	0
STEAK SAUCE, ½ oz	15	<1	<1	3	—	—	—	10	—	0
TACO SAUCE, 2 tbsp	14	<1	0	3	—	—	—	25	—	0

Durkee

CHRIS & PITT'S BARBECUE SAUCE, 1 tbsp	15	<1	<1	4	—	—	—	141	40	—
FAMOUS SAUCE, 1 tbsp	69	<1	7	2	—	—	—	67	<1	—
FRANK'S HOT SAUCE, ½ tsp	<1	<1	1	<1	—	—	—	131	5	—
MR. MUSTARD, 1 tsp	11	<1	<1	<1	—	—	—	90	<1	—

Featherweight

BARBECUE SAUCE, LOW CALORIE, LOW SODIUM, 2 tbsp	14	0	0	4	—	—	—	38	172	—
CATSUP, LOW SODIUM, 1 tbsp	6	0	0	1	—	—	—	5	111	—
CHILI SAUCE, LOW SODIUM, 1 tbsp	8	0	0	2	—	—	—	10	86	—
MUSTARD, LOW SODIUM, 1 tsp	5	<1	<1	<1	—	—	—	1	24	—

Habitant—Catelli

BARBECUE SAUCE, 2 tbsp	10	<1	<1	<1	.01	1	.03	170	9	—
FRUIT CATSUP, 2 tbsp	27	<1	<1	6	.12	3	.12	90	44	—
HOT CHICKEN SAUCE, 2 tbsp	7	<1	<1	1	tr	<1	.03	171	3	—

Heinz

BARBECUE SAUCE, REGULAR, 1 tbsp	20	0	0	4	—	*	*	140	—	—
HICKORY, 1 tbsp	20	0	0	5	—	*	*	135	—	—
MUSHROOM, 1 tbsp	20	0	0	5	—	*	*	130	—	—
HOT, 1 tbsp	20	0	0	5	—	*	*	120	—	—
ONION, 1 tbsp	20	0	0	5	—	*	*	130	—	—
CHILI SAUCE, 1 tbsp	17	<1	<1	4	—	*	*	191	—	—
KETCHUP, 1 tbsp	18	<1	<1	4	—	7	.10	180	—	—
HOT, 1 tbsp	18	<1	<1	4	—	7	.10	180	—	—
LITE, 1 tbsp	8	<1	<1	2	—	7	.10	110	—	—
LOW SODIUM, LITE, 1 tbsp	8	<1	<1	2	—	7	.10	90	—	—
MUSTARD, BROWN, 1 tsp	8	<1	<1	<1	—	1	.10	58	—	—
MILD, 1 tsp	5	<1	<1	<1	—	4	.10	71	—	—
POURABLE, 1 tsp	5	<1	<1	<1	—	4	.10	71	—	—
57 SAUCE, 1 tbsp	15	<1	<1	3	—	*	*	265	—	—

La Victoria

GREEN TACO SAUCE, 1 tbsp, .5 oz	4	—	—	1	—	—	—	85	—	—
RED TACO SAUCE, 1 tbsp, .5 oz	6	—	—	1	—	—	—	85	—	—
SALSA BRAVA, 1 tbsp, .5 oz	6	—	—	1	—	—	—	100	—	—

Mcilhenny Co.

TABASCO SAUCE, ¼ tsp, 1.3 gm	0	0	0	0	—	*	*	9	2	—

Mrs. Dash—Alberto Culver

STEAK SAUCE, 1 tsp	17	<1	<1	4	—	—	—	8	70	0

FOOD & DESCRIPTION MEASURE OR QUANTITY	CALORIES	PROTEIN (GM)	FAT (GM)	CARBO-HYDRATE (GM)	FIBER (GM)	CALCIUM (MG)	IRON (MG)	SODIUM (MG)	POTASSIUM (MG)	CHOLES-TEROL (MG)
R.T. French										
BARBECUE SAUCE, REGULAR, 1 tbsp, 17 gm	25	0	0	5	—	*	*	250	—	—
SMOKY, 1 tbsp, 17 gm	25	0	0	5	—	*	*	295	—	—
BROWN 'N SPICY MUSTARD, 1 tbsp, 16 gm	15	1	1	1	—	*	*	150	—	—
CREAM SALAD MUSTARD, 1 tbsp, 15 gm	10	1	1	1	—	*	*	180	—	—
MEDFORD MUSTARD, 1 tbsp, 16 gm	16	1	1	1	—	*	*	250	—	—
MUSTARD WITH HORSERADISH, 1 tbsp, 16 gm	15	1	1	1	—	*	*	280	—	—
MUSTARD WITH ONION, 1 tbsp, 17 gm	25	1	1	5	—	*	*	200	—	—
VIVA LA DIJON! MUSTARD, 1 tsp, 5 gm	8	<1	<1	<1	—	—	—	155	—	—
WORCESTERSHIRE SAUCE, REGULAR, 1 tbsp, 16 gm	10	0	0	2	—	*	*	180	—	—
SMOKY, 1 tbsp, 16 gm	10	0	0	2	—	*	*	180	—	—
Smucker's										
KETCHUP, 1 tsp	14	0	0	3	—	*	*	90	—	—
USDA										
GINGER ROOT										
CRYSTALLIZED, 1 oz, 28 gm	96	<1	<1	25	—	—	—	—	—	—
FRESH, ¼ c, sliced, 24 gm	17	<1	<1	4	.25	4	.12	3	100	0
HORSERADISH, prep, 1 tsp, 5 gm	2	<1	<1	<1	—	3	tr	5	15	—
MUSTARD, BROWN, prep, 1 tsp, 5 gm	5	<1	<1	<1	—	6	.10	65	7	—
MUSTARD, YELLOW, prep, 1 tsp, 5 gm	4	<1	<1	<1	—	4	.10	63	7	—
SOY SAUCE, 1 tbsp, 18 gm	12	1	<1	2	—	15	.90	1319	66	—
TARTAR SAUCE, 1 tbsp, 14 gm	74	<1	8	<1	—	3	.10	99	11	—
LOW CALORIE, 1 tbsp, 14 gm	31	<1	3	<1	—	3	.10	99	11	—
VINEGAR, CIDER, 1 tbsp, 15 gm	2	tr	0	<1	—	1	.10	tr	15	—
VINEGAR, DISTILLED, 1 tbsp, 15 gm	2	—	—	<1	—	—	—	tr	2	—
Croutons										
Libby										
SALAD CRUNCHIES, 1 tbsp	35	2	1	4	—	*	*	—	—	—
Pepperidge Farm–Campbell										
CHEESE & GARLIC, ½ oz, 14 gm	70	2	3	9	—	20	.36	180	—	—
ONION & GARLIC, ½ oz, 14 gm	70	2	3	9	—	*	.36	160	—	—
SEASONED, ½ oz, 14 gm	70	2	3	9	—	20	.36	210	—	—

Pickles, Olives & Relishes
(See also *Vegetables*)

Featherweight

DILL, WHOLE, 1 pickle	4	0	0	1	—	—	—	5	473	—
KOSHER, WHOLE, 1 pickle	4	0	0	1	—	—	—	5	473	—
SLICED 3–4 slices	12	0	0	3	—	—	—	5	28	—

Habitant—Catelli

BABY DILLS, 1 pickle	3	<1	<1	<1	.12	6	.21	240	31	—
BEETS, PICKLED, cubed, 3–4 pieces	20	<1	<1	5	.22	10	.19	12	46	—
BEETS, PICKLED, sliced, 4 sl	25	<1	<1	6	.22	5	.19	15	45	—
BEETS, PICKLED, WHOLE BABY, 2 beets	47	<1	<1	11	.50	12	.45	28	106	—
BREAD & BUTTER, 4 sl	35	<1	<1	9	.13	6	.24	163	34	—
CUBED RELISH, 1 tbsp	17	<1	<1	4	.15	6	.27	57	39	—
DILL, 1 pickle	6	<1	<1	1	.23	13	.42	480	62	—
GREEN TOMATO CHOW CHOW, 2 tbsp	37	<1	<1	9	.11	7	.13	117	56	—
HAMBURGER RELISH, 1 tbsp	13	<1	<1	3	.09	4	.17	167	28	—
HOT DOG RELISH, 1 tbsp	14	<1	<1	3	.10	5	.18	182	24	—
OLIVES, 1 queen, 4 cocktail, or 3–4 manzanilla, 10 gm	13	<1	1	<1	.14	9	.16	143	3	—
ONIONS, SOUR PICKLED, 4 onions	7	<1	<1	2	.12	6	.10	155	31	—
ONIONS, SWEET PICKLED, 4 onions	17	<1	<1	4	.10	5	.09	140	27	—
RED TOMATO CHOW CHOW, 2 tbsp	23	<1	<1	5	.12	5	.10	165	51	—
SOUR GHERKINS, 2 pickles	3	<1	<1	<1	.12	7	.22	310	31	—
SOUR MIXED PICKLES, 3–4 pieces	5	<1	<1	1	.18	11	.32	500	49	—
SWEET GHERKINS, 2 pickles	16	<1	<1	4	.10	5	.18	175	26	—
SWEET MIXED PICKLES, 3–4 pieces	27	<1	<1	7	.15	8	.26	279	40	—
SWEET MUSTARD MIXED PICKLES, 2–3 pieces	33	<1	<1	8	.12	10	.25	267	26	—
SWEET RELISH, 1 tbsp	24	<1	<1	6	.21	9	.39	88	56	—

Heinz

BREAD 'N BUTTER CUCUMBER SLICES, 1 oz, 28 gm	25	0	0	6	—	*	*	170	—	—
HAMBURGER RELISH, 1 oz, 28 gm	30	0	0	7	—	*	*	325	—	—
HOT DOG RELISH, 1 oz, 28 gm	35	0	0	8	—	*	*	200	—	—
INDIA RELISH, 1 oz, 28 gm	35	0	0	9	—	*	*	215	—	—
PICALILLI, 1 oz, 28 gm	30	0	0	7	—	*	*	145	—	—
SWEET CUCUMBER SLICES, 1 oz, 28 gm	20	0	0	5	—	*	*	195	—	—
SWEET CUCUMBER STIX, 1 oz, 28 gm	25	0	0	6	—	*	*	145	—	—
SWEET GHERKINS, 1 oz, 28 gm	35	0	0	8	—	*	*	210	—	—
SWEET MIDGET GHERKINS, 1 oz, 28 gm	35	0	0	8	—	*	*	205	—	—
SWEET MIXED PICKLES, 1 oz, 28 gm	40	0	0	9	—	*	*	200	—	—

FOOD & DESCRIPTION MEASURE OR QUANTITY	CALORIES	PROTEIN (GM)	FAT (GM)	CARBO-HYDRATE (GM)	FIBER (GM)	CALCIUM (MG)	IRON (MG)	SODIUM (MG)	POTASSIUM (MG)	CHOLES-TEROL (MG)
SWEET PICKLES, 1 oz, 28 gm	35	0	0	8	—	*	*	210	—	—
SWEET PICKLE SLICES, 1 oz, 28 gm	35	0	0	8	—	*	*	205	—	—
SWEET RELISH, 1 oz, 28 gm	35	0	0	9	—	*	*	205	—	—
SWEET SALAD CUBES, 1 oz, 28 gm	30	0	0	7	—	*	*	270	—	—

USDA

FOOD & DESCRIPTION MEASURE OR QUANTITY	CALORIES	PROTEIN (GM)	FAT (GM)	CARBO-HYDRATE (GM)	FIBER (GM)	CALCIUM (MG)	IRON (MG)	SODIUM (MG)	POTASSIUM (MG)	CHOLES-TEROL (MG)
CHOWCHOW or MUSTARD PICKLES, SOUR, 1 c, 240 gm	70	3	3	10	—	77	6.20	3211	—	—
CHOWCHOW or MUSTARD PICKLES, SWEET, 1 c, 245 gm	284	4	2	66	—	56	3.70	1291	—	—
OLIVES, GREEN										
LARGE, 10, 46 gm	45	<1	5	<1	—	24	.60	926	21	—
GIANT, 10, 78 gm	76	<1	8	<1	—	40	1.00	1572	36	—
SMALL, 10, 34 gm	33	<1	4	<1	—	17	.50	686	16	—
OLIVES, RIPE, ASCOLANO										
EXTRA LARGE, 10, 55 gm	61	<1	7	1	—	40	.80	385	16	—
MAMMOTH, 10, 65 gm	72	<1	8	2	—	47	.90	454	19	—
GIANT, 10, 80 gm	89	<1	10	2	—	58	1.10	559	23	—
JUMBO, 10, 95 gm	105	<1	11	2	—	69	1.30	664	28	—
SLICED, 1 c, 135 gm	174	2	19	4	—	113	2.20	1098	46	—
OLIVES, RIPE, MANZANILLO										
EXTRA LARGE, 10, 55 gm	61	<1	7	1	—	40	.80	385	16	—
LARGE, 10, 46 gm	51	<1	6	1	—	33	.60	322	13	—
MEDIUM, 10, 40 gm	44	<1	5	<1	—	29	.60	280	12	—
SMALL, 10, 34 gm	38	<1	4	<1	—	25	.50	237	10	—
SLICED, 1 c, 135 gm	174	2	19	4	—	113	2.20	1098	46	—
OLIVES, RIPE, MISSION										
EXTRA LARGE, 10, 55 gm	87	<1	10	2	—	50	.80	355	13	—
LARGE, 10, 46 gm	73	<1	8	1	—	42	.70	297	11	—
MEDIUM, 10, 40 gm	63	<1	7	1	—	36	.60	258	9	—
SMALL, 10, 34 gm	54	<1	6	<1	—	31	.50	219	8	—
SLICED, 1 c, 135 gm	248	2	27	4	—	143	2.30	1013	36	—
OLIVES, RIPE, SEVILLANO										
COLOSSAL, 10, 119 gm	95	1	10	3	—	76	1.60	847	45	—
GIANT, 10, 80 gm	64	<1	7	2	—	51	1.10	570	30	—
JUMBO, 10, 95 gm	76	<1	8	2	—	60	1.30	676	36	—
SUPER COLASSAL, 10, 142 gm	114	1	12	3	—	90	2.00	1011	54	—
SLICED, 1 c, 135 gm	126	2	13	4	—	100	2.20	1118	59	—
OLIVES, RIPE, GREEK STYLE, SALT CURED, OIL COATED										
EXTRA LARGE, 10, 33 gm	89	<1	10	2	—	—	—	868	—	—
MEDIUM, 10, 24 gm	65	<1	7	2	—	—	—	631	—	—
PICKLES, BREAD & BUTTER, 2 sl, 1½ × ¼″, 15 gm	11	<1	tr	3	—	5	.30	101	—	—
PICKLES, DILL CUCUMBER										
LARGE, 1, 4 × 1¾″, 135 gm	15	<1	<1	3	—	35	1.40	1928	270	—
MEDIUM, 1, 3¾ × 1¼″, 65 gm	7	<1	<1	1	—	17	.70	928	130	—
SLICES, 2 sl, 13 gm	1	<1	<1	<1	—	3	.10	186	26	—
PICKLES, GHERKINS										
LARGE, 1, 3 × 1″, 35 gm	51	<1	<1	13	—	4	.40	—	—	—
MIDGET, 1, 2⅛ × ⅜″, 6 gm	9	<1	<1	2	—	1	.10	—	—	—
SMALL, 1, 2½ × ¾″, 15 gm	22	<1	<1	6	—	2	.20	—	—	—
CHOPPED, ¼″ cubes, 1 c, 160 gm	234	1	<1	58	—	19	1.90	—	—	—
PICKLES, SOUR, WHOLE										
LARGE, 1, 4 × 1¾″, 135 gm	14	<1	<1	3	—	23	4.30	1827	—	—

FOOD & DESCRIPTION MEASURE OR QUANTITY	CALORIES	PROTEIN (GM)	FAT (GM)	CARBO- HYDRATE (GM)	FIBER (GM)	CALCIUM (MG)	IRON (MG)	SODIUM (MG)	POTASSIUM (MG)	CHOLES- TEROL (MG)
MEDIUM, 1, 3¾ × 1¼", 65 gm	7	<1	<1	1	—	11	2.10	879	—	—
RELISH, SWEET, 1 tbsp, 15 gm	21	<1	<1	5	—	3	.10	107	—	—

Vlasic–Campbell

BREAD & BUTTER SWEET BUTTER STIX, 1 oz, 28 gm	18	0	0	5	—	*	*	110	—	—
BREAD & BUTTER SWEET BUTTER CHIPS, 1 oz, 28 gm	30	0	0	7	—	*	*	160	—	—
DELI BREAD & BUTTER CHUNKS, 1 oz, 28 gm	25	0	0	6	—	*	*	120	—	—
DILL RELISH, 1 oz, 28 gm	2	0	0	1	—	*	*	415	—	—
HALF-THE-SALT CRUNCHY KOSHER DILLS, 1 oz, 28 gm	4	0	0	1	—	*	*	125	—	—
HAMBURGER DILL CHIPS, 1 oz, 28 gm	2	0	0	1	—	*	*	175	—	—
KOSHER DILLS SPEARS, 1 oz, 28 gm	4	0	0	1	—	*	*	120	—	—
SWEET BUTTER CHIPS, 1 oz, 28 gm	30	0	0	7	—	*	*	80	—	—
HAMBURGER RELISH, 1 oz, 28 gm	40	0	0	9	—	*	*	255	—	—
HOT BANANA PEPPER RINGS, 1 oz, 28 gm	4	0	0	1	—	*	.36	465	—	—
HOT DOG RELISH, 1 oz, 28 gm	40	0	1	8	—	*	.36	255	—	—
HOT & SPICY GARDEN MIX, 1 oz, 28 gm	4	0	0	1	—	*	.36	380	—	—
KOSHER BABY DILLS, 1 oz, 28 gm	4	0	0	1	—	*	.36	210	—	—
CRUNCHY DILLS, 1 oz, 28 gm	4	0	0	1	—	*	.36	210	—	—
DELI DILLS, 1 oz, 28 gm	4	0	0	1	—	*	*	290	—	—
DILL GHERKINS, 1 oz, 28 gm	4	0	0	1	—	*	.36	210	—	—
DILL SPEARS, 1 oz, 28 gm	4	0	0	1	—	*	*	175	—	—
LIGHTLY SPICED COCKTAIL ONIONS, 1 oz, 28 gm	4	0	0	1	—	*	*	365	—	—
MEXICAN JALAPENO PEPPERS, 1 oz, 28 gm	8	0	0	2	—	*	.36	380	—	—
MILD CHERRY PEPPERS, 1 oz, 28 gm	8	0	0	2	—	*	.36	410	—	—
MILD GREEK PEPPERONCINI, 1 oz, 28 gm	4	0	0	1	—	*	.36	450	—	—
NO GARLIC DILLS, 1 oz, 28 gm	4	0	0	1	—	*	.36	210	—	—
OLD FASHIONED BREAD & BUTTER CHUNKS, 1 oz, 28 gm	25	0	0	6	—	*	*	120	—	—
OLD FASHIONED SAUERKRAUT, 1 oz, 28 gm	4	0	0	1	—	*	.36	280	—	—
ORIGINAL DILLS, 1 oz, 28 gm	2	0	0	1	—	*	*	375	—	—
SWEET RELISH, 1 oz, 28 gm	30	0	0	8	—	*	*	220	—	—
ZESTY CRUNCHY DILLS, 1 oz, 28 gm	4	0	0	1	—	*	*	250	—	—
DILL SPEARS, 1 oz, 28 gm	4	0	0	1	—	*	*	230	—	—

FOOD & DESCRIPTION MEASURE OR QUANTITY	CALORIES	PROTEIN (GM)	FAT (GM)	CARBO-HYDRATE (GM)	FIBER (GM)	CALCIUM (MG)	IRON (MG)	SODIUM (MG)	POTASSIUM (MG)	CHOLES-TEROL (MG)
Salad Dressings										
Bama–Borden										
MAYONNAISE, 1 tbsp	100	0	11	0	—	*	*	70	0	—
SALAD DRESSING, 1 tbsp	50	0	4	3	—	*	*	120	0	—
Dia-Mel										
BACON AND TOMATO, 1 tbsp	2	0	0	<1	—	—	—	35	—	0
BLUE CHEESE SALAD, 1 tbsp	2	0	<1	<1	—	—	—	20	—	2
CREAMY CUCUMBER, 1 tbsp	2	0	0	<1	—	—	—	30	—	0
CREAMY GARLIC, 1 tbsp	1	0	0	0	—	—	—	10	—	0
CREAMY ITALIAN, 1 tbsp	1	0	0	0	—	—	—	15	—	0
FRENCH, 1 tbsp	1	0	0	0	—	—	—	10	—	0
ITALIAN, 1 tbsp	1	0	0	0	—	—	—	10	—	0
MAYONNAISE, 1 tbsp	106	0	11	0	—	—	—	22	—	—
RED WINE VINEGAR, 1 tbsp	1	0	0	0	—	—	—	10	—	0
TAHITI, 1 tbsp	2	0	0	<1	—	—	—	5	—	0
THOUSAND ISLAND, 1 tbsp	2	<1	0	<1	—	—	—	30	—	5
YOGURT BUTTERMILK, 1 tbsp	2	0	0	<1	—	—	—	10	—	7
Estee										
SALAD DRESSING, 1 tbsp	4–6	0	0	1–2	—	—	—	80–150	—	0
Featherweight										
CREAMY CAESAR, LOW SODIUM, LOW CALORIE, 1 tbsp	14	0	1	2	—	—	—	16	71	—
CREAMY CUCUMBER/ONION, LOW SODIUM, LOW CALORIE, 1 tbsp	12	0	0	2	—	—	—	12	40	—
FRENCH, LOW SODIUM, 1 tbsp	60	0	6	0	—	—	—	4	32	—
FRENCH STYLE, LOW CALORIE, 1 tbsp	6	0	0	1	—	—	—	163	39	—
ITALIAN, LOW CALORIE, 1 tbsp	4	0	0	1	—	—	—	127	24	—
HERB, LOW SODIUM, LOW CALORIE, 1 tbsp	6	0	0	1	—	—	—	5	65	—
NEUBLEU, LOW CALORIE, 1 tbsp	4	0	0	1	—	—	—	125	23	—
RED WINE VINEGAR, LOW CALORIE, 1 tbsp	6	0	0	1	—	—	—	63	18	—
RUSSIAN, LOW CALORIE, 1 tbsp	6	0	0	1	—	—	—	134	27	—
SOY AMAISE, LOW SODIUM, 1 tbsp	60	0	11	0	—	—	—	3	16	—
2 CALORIE, LOW SODIUM, LOW CALORIE, 1 tbsp	2	0	0	0	—	—	—	6	75	—
Good Seasons– General Foods										
ITALIAN, LOW CALORIE, prep, 1 tbsp	8	0	0	2	tr	*	*	160	0	—
Hain										
BLUE CHEESE, NO OIL MIX, prep, 1 tbsp	14	1	1	1	—	*	*	—	—	—
BUTTERMILK										
NO OIL MIX, prep, 1 tbsp	11	1	0	2	—	20	*	—	—	—
POURABLE, 1 tbsp	70	0	7	0	—	—	*	100	20	—

FOOD & DESCRIPTION MEASURE OR QUANTITY	CALORIES	PROTEIN (GM)	FAT (GM)	CARBO-HYDRATE (GM)	FIBER (GM)	CALCIUM (MG)	IRON (MG)	SODIUM (MG)	POTASSIUM (MG)	CHOLES-TEROL (MG)
CAESAR, NO OIL MIX, prep, 1 tbsp	4	1	0	0	—	*	*	—	—	—
CREAMY, 1 tbsp	60	0	6	1	—	*	*	220	10	—
CREAMY FRENCH POURABLE, 1 tbsp	60	0	6	1	—	*	*	80	20	—
CREAMY ITALIAN, 1 tbsp	80	0	8	0	—	*	*	100	10	—
GARLIC & CHEESE, NO OIL MIX, prep, 1 tbsp	6	0	0	1	—	*	*	—	—	—
GARLIC & OIL, 1 tbsp	120	0	14	0	—	*	*	—	—	—
HERB, NO OIL MIX, prep, 1 tbsp	2	0	0	1	—	*	*	—	—	—
ITALIAN										
NO OIL MIX, prep, 1 tbsp	4	0	0	1	—	*	*	—	—	—
TRADITIONAL, 1 tbsp	80	0	8	0	—	—	—	330	10	—
SAVORY HERB, NO SALT ADDED, 1 tbsp	90	0	14	0	—	*	*	25	45	—
1000 ISLAND, POURABLE, 1 tbsp	50	0	5	0	—	*	*	85	30	—

Herb Magic

CREAMY CUCUMBER, 1 tbsp	8	0	0	2	—	*	*	98	—	0
HERB BASKET, 1 tbsp	6	0	0	2	—	*	*	168	—	0
ITALIAN, 1 tbsp	4	0	0	1	—	*	*	122	—	0
SWEET & SOUR, 1 tbsp	18	0	0	5	—	*	.54	82	—	0
THOUSAND ISLAND, 1 tbsp	8	0	0	2	—	*	*	47	—	0
VINAIGRETTE, 1 tbsp	6	0	0	1	—	*	*	167	—	0

Libby

SUPER SLAW DRY MIX, .19 oz	16	0	0	4	—	*	*	—	—	—
SUPER SLAW, READY-TO-SERVE, ½ c	240	1	23	11	—	40	.36	—	—	—

Mrs Filbert

MAYONNAISE										
IMITATION, 1 tbsp, 14 gm	40	0	4	1	—	*	*	110	—	0
REAL, 1 tbsp, 14 gm	100	0	11	0	—	*	*	70	—	10
SALAD DRESSING, 1 tbsp, 15 gm	70	0	6	2	—	*	*	115	—	5
SANDWICH SPREAD, 1 tbsp, 15 gm	60	0	5	2	—	*	*	115	—	5

Seven Seas

BUTTERMILK RECIPE, 1 tbsp	80	0	8	1	—	*	*	130	—	<1
CAPRI FRENCH, 1 tbsp	70	0	6	3	—	*	*	130	—	0
CHUNKY BLUE CHEESE, 1 tbsp	70	1	7	1	—	*	*	195	—	<3
CREAMY BACON, 1 tbsp	60	0	6	1	—	*	*	205	—	<1
CREAMY FRENCH, 1 tbsp	60	0	6	2	—	*	*	265	—	0
CREAMY ITALIAN, 1 tbsp	70	0	7	1	—	*	*	255	—	0
CREAMY RUSSIAN, 1 tbsp	80	0	8	1	—	*	*	115	—	1
CREAMY PARMESAN, 1 tbsp	60	0	6	1	—	*	*	140	—	<2
GREEN GODDESS, 1 tbsp	60	0	7	0	—	*	*	140	—	<1
HERBS AND SPICES, 1 tbsp	60	0	6	1	—	*	*	160	—	0
MILD ITALIAN, 1 tbsp	70	0	7	0	—	*	*	170	—	0
RED WINE VINEGAR & OIL, 1 tbsp	60	0	7	1	—	*	*	265	—	0
THOUSAND ISLAND, 1 tbsp	50	0	5	2	—	*	*	155	—	10
VIVA ITALIAN, 1 tbsp	70	0	7	1	—	*	*	320	—	0
VIVA PARMESAN, 1 tbsp	60	0	6	1	—	*	*	205	—	<1

FOOD & DESCRIPTION MEASURE OR QUANTITY	CALORIES	PROTEIN (GM)	FAT (GM)	CARBO-HYDRATE (GM)	FIBER (GM)	CALCIUM (MG)	IRON (MG)	SODIUM (MG)	POTASSIUM (MG)	CHOLES-TEROL (MG)

USDA

FOOD & DESCRIPTION MEASURE OR QUANTITY	CALORIES	PROTEIN (GM)	FAT (GM)	CARBO-HYDRATE (GM)	FIBER (GM)	CALCIUM (MG)	IRON (MG)	SODIUM (MG)	POTASSIUM (MG)	CHOLES-TEROL (MG)
BLUE CHEESE, 1 tbsp, 15.3 gm	77	<1	8	1	0	12	0	—	—	—
FRENCH										
LOW CALORIE, 1 tbsp, 16.3 gm	22	0	<1	4	0	2	.10	128	13	1
REGULAR, 1 tbsp, 15.6 gm	67	<1	6	3	.1	2	.10	214	12	—
ITALIAN										
LOW CALORIE, 1 tbsp, 15 gm	16	0	2	<1	0	0	0	118	2	1
REGULAR, 1 tbsp, 14.7 gm	69	<1	7	2	0	1	0	116	2	—
MAYONNAISE, 1 tbsp, 13.8 gm	99	<1	11	<1	0	2	.10	78	5	8
SALAD DRESSING, MAYONNAISE TYPE, 1 tbsp, 14.7 gm	57	<1	5	4	0	2	0	104	1	4
RUSSIAN										
LOW CALORIE, 1 tbsp, 16.3 gm	23	<1	<1	5	.1	3	.10	141	26	1
REGULAR, 1 tbsp, 15.3 gm	76	<1	8	2	0	3	.10	133	24	—
SESAME SEED, 1 tbsp, 15.3 gm	68	<1	7	1	.1	—	—	153	—	0
THOUSAND ISLAND										
LOW CALORIE, 1 tbsp, 15.3 gm	24	<1	2	3	.2	2	.10	153	17	2
REGULAR, 1 tbsp, 15.6 gm	59	<1	6	2	.3	2	.10	109	18	—

Weight Watchers

FOOD & DESCRIPTION MEASURE OR QUANTITY	CALORIES	PROTEIN (GM)	FAT (GM)	CARBO-HYDRATE (GM)	FIBER (GM)	CALCIUM (MG)	IRON (MG)	SODIUM (MG)	POTASSIUM (MG)	CHOLES-TEROL (MG)
BLUE CHEESE MIX, 2.1 gm	10	0	1	1	—	—	—	108	—	—
prep, 1 tbsp	14	1	1	1	—	—	—	108	—	—
CREAMY ITALIAN, 1 tbsp, 15 gm	50	0	5	2	—	0	0	120	—	<1
CREAMY ITALIAN MIX, 1.4 gm	4	0	0	1	—	—	—	224	—	—
DIP DRY MIX, 2.8 gm	14	1	1	1	—	—	—	205	—	—
FRENCH STYLE MIX, 1.2 gm	4	0	0	1	—	—	—	164	—	—
ITALIAN MIX, .8 gm	2	0	0	0	—	—	—	175	—	—
MAYONNAISE, REDUCED CALORIE, 1 tbsp, 14 gm	40	0	4	1	—	0	0	120	—	5
LOW SODIUM, 1 tbsp, 14 gm	40	0	4	1	—	0	0	35	—	5
RUSSIAN/THOUSAND ISLAND, 1 tbsp, 15 gm	50	0	5	2	—	—	—	115	—	6
RUSSIAN MIX, .8 gm	2	0	0	0	—	—	—	128	—	—
prep, 1 tbsp	4	0	0	1	—	—	—	128	—	—
SALAD DRESSING, REDUCED CALORIE, 1 tbsp, 14 gm	35	0	3	3	—	0	0	120	—	5
THOUSAND ISLAND MIX, .9 gm	2	0	0	0	—	—	—	265	—	—
prep, 1 tbsp	12	0	1	1	—	—	—	265	—	—

Wishbone–Lipton

FOOD & DESCRIPTION MEASURE OR QUANTITY	CALORIES	PROTEIN (GM)	FAT (GM)	CARBO-HYDRATE (GM)	FIBER (GM)	CALCIUM (MG)	IRON (MG)	SODIUM (MG)	POTASSIUM (MG)	CHOLES-TEROL (MG)
BUTTERMILK LITE, 1 tbsp	50	0	5	2	—	*	*	150	—	<1
CAESAR, 1 tbsp	70	0	8	<1	—	*	*	250	—	<1
CHEDDAR AND BACON, 1 tbsp	70	<1	7	1	—	*	*	110	—	<1
CHUNKY BLUE CHEESE, 1 tbsp	70	0	8	<1	—	*	*	150	—	<1
LITE, 1 tbsp	40	0	4	1	—	*	*	190	—	<1
CREAMY CUCUMBER, 1 tbsp	80	0	8	1	—	*	*	125	—	<1
LITE, 1 tbsp	40	0	4	1	—	*	*	165	—	0
CREAMY GARLIC, 1 tbsp	80	0	8	<1	—	*	*	170	—	0
CREAMY ITALIAN, 1 tbsp	60	0	6	1	—	*	*	145	—	0
LITE, 1 tbsp	30	0	3	1	—	*	*	200	—	0
DELUXE FRENCH, 1 tbsp	50	0	5	2	—	*	*	80	—	0

FOOD & DESCRIPTION MEASURE OR QUANTITY	CALORIES	PROTEIN (GM)	FAT (GM)	CARBO- HYDRATE (GM)	FIBER (GM)	CALCIUM (MG)	IRON (MG)	SODIUM (MG)	POTASSIUM (MG)	CHOLES- TEROL (MG)
FRENCH STYLE LITE, 1 tbsp	30	0	2	2	—	*	*	70	—	0
GARLIC FRENCH, 1 tbsp	60	0	6	2	—	*	*	150	—	0
HERBAL FRENCH, 1 tbsp	60	0	6	2	—	*	*	130	—	0
HERBAL ITALIAN, 1 tbsp	70	0	7	1	—	*	*	240	—	0
ITALIAN, 1 tbsp	70	0	7	1	—	*	*	240	—	0
LITE, 1 tbsp	30	0	3	1	—	*	*	210	—	0
ONION 'N CHIVE LITE, 1 tbsp	40	0	3	3	—	*	*	160	—	0
ROBUSTO ITALIAN, 1 tbsp	80	0	8	1	—	*	*	285	—	0
RUSSIAN, 1 tbsp	45	0	2	6	—	*	*	140	—	0
LITE, 1 tbsp	25	0	<1	5	—	*	*	140	—	0
SOUR CREAM AND BACON, 1 tbsp	70	<1	7	1	—	*	*	95	—	<1
SOUTHERN RECIPE THOUSAND ISLAND, 1 tbsp	70	0	6	3	—	*	*	90	—	10
SOUTHERN RECIPE THOUSAND ISLAND WITH BACON, 1 tbsp	60	0	6	2	—	*	*	95	—	5
SWEET 'N SPICY FRENCH, 1 tbsp	70	0	6	3	—	*	*	150	—	0
LITE, 1 tbsp	30	0	2	4	—	*	*	150	—	0
THOUSAND ISLAND, 1 tbsp	70	0	6	3	—	*	*	130	—	5
LITE, 1 tbsp	40	0	3	3	—	*	*	110	—	10

Spices & Seasonings

Butter Buds

DRY, 1 tsp, 1.75 gm	6	0	0	<1	—	*	*	110	9	0
LIQUID, 1 tbsp, 16.7 gm	6	0	0	<1	—	*	*	110	9	0

Dia-Mel

SALT-IT SALT SUBSTITUTE, ½ tsp	0	0	0	0	—	—	—	1	—	—

Durkee

BUTTER FLAVORED SALT, 1 tsp	—	—	—	—	—	—	—	1362	—	—
CELERY SALT, 1 tsp	—	—	—	—	—	—	—	1646	—	—
CHILI POWDER, 1 tsp	—	—	—	—	—	—	—	54	—	—
CURRY POWDER, 1 tsp	—	—	—	—	—	—	—	63	—	—
GARLIC SALT, 1 tsp	—	—	—	—	—	—	—	2119	—	—
ITALIAN SALAD SEASONING, 1 tsp	—	—	—	—	—	—	—	223	—	—
LEMON PEPPER, 1 tsp	—	—	—	—	—	—	—	312	—	—
MEAT MARINADE MIX, 1 tsp	—	—	—	—	—	—	—	818	—	—
MEAT TENDERIZER, INSTANT, 1 tsp	—	—	—	—	—	—	—	1025	—	—
SEASONED, 1 tsp	—	—	—	—	—	—	—	1172	—	—
MSG, 1 tsp	—	—	—	—	—	—	—	530	—	—
ONION SALT, 1 tsp	—	—	—	—	—	—	—	1841	—	—
POULTRY SEASONING, 1 tsp	—	—	—	—	—	—	—	420	—	—
SEASONED SALT, 1 tsp	—	—	—	—	—	—	—	1466	—	—

Estee

SALT-FREE SEASONINGS, 1 tsp	0	0	0	0	—	—	—	<2	—	0

Featherweight

GARLIC SALT SUBSTITUTE, ¼ tsp	0	0	0	0	—	—	—	<1	520	—

FOOD & DESCRIPTION MEASURE OR QUANTITY	CALORIES	PROTEIN (GM)	FAT (GM)	CARBO-HYDRATE (GM)	FIBER (GM)	CALCIUM (MG)	IRON (MG)	SODIUM (MG)	POTASSIUM (MG)	CHOLES-TEROL (MG)
SALT SUBSTITUTE, ¼ tsp	0	0	0	0	—	—	—	<1	480	—
SEASONED SALT SUBSTITUTE, ¼ tsp	0	0	0	0	—	—	—	<1	420	—

McCormick

CHILI SEASONING MIX, ⅙ pkg, 5.83 gm	18	<1	<1	3	—	12	.51	193	9	—
LEMON & PEPPER SEASONING, 1 tsp, 3.22 gm	7	<1	<1	<1	—	5	.14	618	18	—
MEAT TENDERIZER, 1 tsp, 4.8 gm	2	<1	<1	<1	—	10	.13	1627	2	—
MEAT TENDERIZER, SEASONED, 1 tsp, 4.1 gm	5	<1	<1	<1	—	8	.46	1087	18	—
SALAD SUPREME, 1 tsp, 2.93 gm	11	<1	<1	<1	—	20	.20	2807	23	—
SALT 'N SPICE, 1 tsp, 3.27 gm	3	<1	<1	<1	—	4	.14	939	15	—
SEASON-ALL, 1 tsp, 4 gm	4	<1	<1	<1	—	3	.18	980	17	—
SLOPPY JOE'S SEASONING MIX, ⅙ pkg, 6.17 gm	17	<1	<1	4	—	6	.11	500	36	—
TACO SEASONING MIX, 1/10 pkg, 4.2 gm	12	<1	<1	2	—	—	—	270	53	—

Mrs. Dash– Alberto Culver

EXTRA SPICY SEASONING BLEND, 1 tsp, 3.4 gm	12	<1	<1	2	—	—	—	5	51	—
LEMON & HERB SEASONING BLEND, 1 tsp, 3.4 gm	12	<1	<1	3	—	—	—	4	34	—
LOW PEPPER, NO GARLIC SEASONING BLEND, 1 tsp, 3.4 gm	12	<1	<1	3	—	—	—	4	49	—
ORIGINAL SEASONING BLEND, 1 tsp, 3.4 gm	12	<1	<1	2	—	—	—	4	38	—

R.T. French

BARBECUE SEASONING, 1 tsp, 2.5 gm	6	<1	<1	1	—	*	*	70	—	—
BEEF STEW SEASONING, ⅙ pkg, 8.9 gm	25	0	0	5	—	20	.36	950	—	—
CELERY SALT, 1 tsp, 4.6 gm	2	<1	<1	<1	—	*	*	1430	—	—
CHILI-O, ⅙ pkg, 8.3 gm	25	1	0	5	—	*	*	630	—	—
CINNAMON SUGAR, 1 tsp, 4.3 gm	16	<1	<1	4	—	*	*	0	—	—
ENCHILADA SEASONING, ¼ pkg, 9.8 gm	30	1	1	5	—	20	.36	1130	—	—
GARLIC SALT, 1 tsp, 5.7 gm	4	<1	<1	1	—	*	*	1850	—	—
GARLIC SALT, PARSLIED, 1 tsp, 4.1 gm	6	<1	<1	1	—	*	*	1050	—	—
GROUND BEEF SEASONING WITH ONION, ¼ pkg, 8 gm	25	1	0	6	—	*	*	450	—	—
HAMBURGER SEASONING, ¼ pkg, 7 gm	25	1	0	5	—	*	*	440	—	—
HICKORY SMOKE SALT, 1 tsp, 4.3 gm	2	<1	<1	<1	—	*	*	1170	—	—
LEMON & PEPPER SEASONING, 1 tsp, 3.6 gm	6	<1	<1	1	—	*	*	800	—	—

FOOD & DESCRIPTION MEASURE OR QUANTITY	CALORIES	PROTEIN (GM)	FAT (GM)	CARBO-HYDRATE (GM)	FIBER (GM)	CALCIUM (MG)	IRON (MG)	SODIUM (MG)	POTASSIUM (MG)	CHOLES-TEROL (MG)
MEATBALL SEASONING, ¼ pkg, 10.6 gm	35	1	0	7	—	*	.36	870	—	—
MEATLOAF SEASONING, ⅛ pkg, 5.3 gm	20	1	0	5	—	*	*	655	—	—
MEAT MARINADE, ⅛ pkg, 3.5 gm	10	0	0	2	—	*	*	560	—	—
MEAT TENDERIZER, 1 tsp, 5 gm	2	<1	<1	<1	—	*	*	1760	—	—
SEASONED, 1 tsp, 5 gm	2	<1	<1	<1	—	*	*	1520	—	—
ONION SALT, 1 tsp, 5.3 gm	6	<1	<1	1	—	*	*	1620	—	—
PEPPER, SEASONED, 1 tsp, 2.9 gm	8	<1	<1	1	—	*	*	5	—	—
PIZZA SEASONING, 1 tsp, 3.6 gm	4	<1	<1	1	—	*	*	390	—	—
SALAD LIFT, 1 tsp, 3.6 gm	6	<1	<1	1	—	*	*	640	—	—
SALT, IMITATION BUTTER FLAVORED, 1 tsp, 3.6 gm	8	0	1	0	—	*	*	1090	—	—
SEAFOOD SEASONING, 1 tsp, 5 gm	2	<1	<1	<1	—	*	*	1410	—	—
SEASONING FOR SLOPPY HOT DOGS, ¼ pkg, 10.6 gm	40	2	1	7	—	20	*	55	—	—
SEASONING FOR SLOPPY JOES, ⅛ pkg, 5.3 gm	16	0	0	4	—	*	*	390	—	—
SEASONING SALT, 1 tsp, 4.3 gm	2	<1	<1	1	—	*	*	1230	—	—
TACO SEASONING, ⅙ pkg, 5.9 gm	20	1	0	4	—	*	*	360	—	—

USDA

FOOD & DESCRIPTION MEASURE OR QUANTITY	CALORIES	PROTEIN (GM)	FAT (GM)	CARBO-HYDRATE (GM)	FIBER (GM)	CALCIUM (MG)	IRON (MG)	SODIUM (MG)	POTASSIUM (MG)	CHOLES-TEROL (MG)
ALLSPICE, GROUND, 1 tsp, 1.9 gm	5	<1	<1	1	.41	13	.13	1	20	0
ANISE SEED, 1 tsp, 2.1 gm	7	<1	<1	1	.31	14	.78	tr	30	0
BASIL, GROUND, 1 tsp, 1.4 gm	4	<1	<1	<1	.25	30	.59	tr	48	0
BAY LEAF, CRUMBLED, 1 tsp, .6 gm	2	<1	<1	<1	.16	5	.26	tr	3	0
CARRAWAY SEED, 1 tsp, 2.1 gm	7	<1	<1	1	.27	14	.34	tr	28	0
CARDAMOM, GROUND, 1 tsp, 2 gm	6	<1	<1	1	.23	8	.28	tr	22	0
CELERY SEED, 1 tsp, 2 gm	8	<1	<1	<1	.24	35	.90	3	28	0
CHERVIL, DRIED, 1 tsp, 6 gm	1	<1	<1	<1	.07	8	.19	tr	28	0
CHILI POWDER (with salt), 1 tsp, 2.6 gm	8	<1	<1	1	.58	7	.37	26	50	0
CINNAMON, GROUND, 1 tsp, 2.3 gm	6	<1	<1	2	.56	28	.88	1	11	0
CLOVE, GROUND, 1 tsp, 2.1 gm	7	<1	<1	1	.2	14	.18	5	23	0
CORIANDER LEAF, DRIED, 1 tsp, .6 gm	2	<1	<1	<1	.06	7	.25	1	27	0
CORIANDER SEED, 1 tsp, 1.8 gm	5	<1	<1	<1	.52	13	.29	1	23	0
CUMIN SEED, 1 tsp, 2.1 gm	8	<1	<1	<1	.22	20	1.39	4	38	0
CURRY POWDER, 1 tsp, 2 gm	6	<1	<1	1	.33	10	.59	1	31	0
DILL SEED, 1 tsp, 2.1 gm	6	<1	<1	1	.44	32	.34	tr	25	0
DILL WEED, DRIED, 1 tsp, 1 gm	3	<1	<1	<1	.12	18	.49	2	33	0
FENNEL SEED, 1 tsp, 2 gm	7	<1	<1	1	.31	24	.37	2	34	0
FENUGREEK SEED, 1 tsp, 3.7 gm	12	<1	<1	2	.37	6	1.24	2	28	0
GARLIC POWDER, 1 tsp, 2.8 gm	9	<1	<1	2	.05	2	.08	1	31	0

FOOD & DESCRIPTION MEASURE OR QUANTITY	CALORIES	PROTEIN (GM)	FAT (GM)	CARBO-HYDRATE (GM)	FIBER (GM)	CALCIUM (MG)	IRON (MG)	SODIUM (MG)	POTASSIUM (MG)	CHOLES-TEROL (MG)
GINGER, GROUND, 1 tsp, 1.8 gm	6	<1	<1	1	.11	2	.21	1	24	0
MACE, GROUND, 1 tsp, 1.7 gm	8	<1	<1	<1	.08	4	.24	1	8	0
MARJORAM, DRIED, 1 tsp, .6 gm	2	<1	<1	<1	.11	12	.50	tr	9	0
MUSTARD SEED, YELLOW, 1 tsp, 3.3 gm	15	<1	<1	1	.22	17	.33	tr	23	0
NUTMEG, GROUND, 1 tsp, 2.2 gm	12	<1	<1	1	.09	4	.07	tr	8	0
ONION POWDER, 1 tsp, 2.1 gm	7	<1	<1	2	.12	8	.05	1	20	0
OREGANO, GROUND, 1 tsp, 1.5 gm	5	<1	<1	<1	.22	24	.66	tr	25	0
PAPRIKA, 1 tsp, 2.1 gm	6	<1	<1	1	.44	4	.50	1	49	0
PARSLEY, DRIED, 1 tsp, .3 gm	1	<1	<1	<1	.03	4	.29	1	11	0
PEPPER, BLACK, 1 tsp, 2.1 gm	5	<1	<1	1	.28	9	.61	1	26	0
PEPPER, RED or CAYENNE, 1 tsp, 1.8 gm	6	<1	<1	1	.45	3	.14	1	36	0
PEPPER, WHITE, 1 tsp, 2.4 gm	7	<1	<1	2	.1	6	.34	tr	2	0
POPPY SEEDS, 1 tsp, 2.8 gm	15	<1	1	<1	.18	41	.26	1	20	0
POULTRY SEASONING, 1 tsp, 1.5 gm	5	<1	<1	<1	.17	15	.53	tr	10	0
PUMPKIN PIE SPICE, 1 tsp, 1.7 gm	6	<1	<1	1	.25	12	.34	1	11	0
ROSEMARY, DRIED, 1 tsp, 1.2 gm	4	<1	<1	<1	.21	15	.35	1	11	0
SAFFRON, 1 tsp, .7 gm	2	<1	<1	<1	.03	1	.08	1	12	0
SAGE, GROUND, 1 tsp, .7 gm	2	<1	<1	<1	.13	12	.20	tr	7	0
SAVORY, GROUND, 1 tsp, 1.4 gm	4	<1	<1	<1	.21	30	.53	tr	15	0
SESAME SEED, DECORTICATED, 1 tsp, 2.7 gm	16	<1	1	<1	.08	4	.21	1	11	0
TARRAGON, GROUND, 1 tsp, 1.6 gm	5	<1	<1	<1	.12	18	.52	1	48	0
THYME, GROUND, 1 tsp, 1.4 gm	4	<1	<1	<1	.26	26	1.73	1	11	0
TURMERIC, GROUND, 1 tsp, 2.2 gm	8	<1	<1	1	.15	4	.91	1	56	0

7
DAIRY PRODUCTS

FOOD & DESCRIPTION MEASURE OR QUANTITY	CALORIES	PROTEIN (GM)	FAT (GM)	CARBO- HYDRATE (GM)	FIBER (GM)	CALCIUM (MG)	IRON (MG)	SODIUM (MG)	POTASSIUM (MG)	CHOLES- TEROL (MG)
Cheese										
Armour										
LOWER SALT COLBY, 1 oz, 28 gm	110	7	9	1	—	—	—	120	—	30
LOWER SALT MILD CHEDDAR, 1 oz, 28 gm	110	7	9	1	—	—	—	106	—	30
LOWER SALT MONTEREY JACK, 1 oz, 28 gm	110	7	9	1	—	—	—	111	—	30
Borden										
AMERICAN CHEESE SLICES, PROCESSED, 1 oz, 28 gm	110	6	9	1	—	200	*	445	15	—
AMERICAN CHEESE FOOD, PROCESSED, 1 oz, 28 gm	90	5	7	3	—	150	*	490	60	—
COTTAGE CHEESE, 4% FAT, ½ c	120	14	5	4	—	60	*	465	80	—
SWISS CHEESE, PROCESSED, 1 oz, 28 gm	100	7	8	1	—	350	*	355	25	—
Dorman										
LO-CHOL CHEESE, 1 oz, 28 gm	105	6	9	—	—	120	—	130	—	4
LOW SODIUM MUENSTER, 1 oz, 28 gm	110	6	9	—	—	199	—	92	—	27
NO SALT ADDED SWISS, 1 oz, 28 gm	110	8	8	—	—	280	—	8	—	26
SLIM JACK, 1 oz, 28 gm	90	6	7	1	—	120	—	95	—	—
Easy Cheese—Nabisco										
PASTEURIZED PROCESS CHEESE SPREAD										
AMERICAN, 1 oz	80	4	6	2	—	100	*	350	70	—
CHEDDAR, 1 oz	80	4	6	2	—	100	*	370	70	—
CHEDDAR 'N CHIVE, 1 oz	80	4	6	2	—	100	*	340	70	—
CHEESE N' BACON, 1 oz	80	4	6	2	—	100	*	350	75	—
NACHO, 1 oz	80	4	6	2	—	100	*	340	75	—
SHARP CHEDDAR, 1 oz	80	4	6	2	—	100	*	320	75	—

FOOD & DESCRIPTION MEASURE OR QUANTITY	CALORIES	PROTEIN (GM)	FAT (GM)	CARBO-HYDRATE (GM)	FIBER (GM)	CALCIUM (MG)	IRON (MG)	SODIUM (MG)	POTASSIUM (MG)	CHOLES-TEROL (MG)
Fisher										
CHEEZ-OLA, LOW CHOLESTEROL, 1 oz, 28 gm	90	7	6	<1	—	177	—	417	31	1
REDUCED SODIUM, LOW CHOLESTEROL, 1 oz, 28 gm	90	7	6	<1	—	177	—	156	238	1
COUNT DOWN, 1 oz, 28 gm	40	7	<1	3	—	167	—	405	87	1
Friendship										
COTTAGE CHEESE										
CALIFORNIA STYLE, ½ C, 113 gm	120	14	5	4	—	60	*	390	—	—
LOW FAT, 1% FAT, ½ c, 113 gm	90	14	1	4	—	60	*	360	—	—
LACTOSE REDUCED, ½ c, 113 gm	90	14	1	4	—	60	*	360	—	—
NO SALT ADDED, ½ c, 113 gm	90	14	1	4	—	60	*	31	—	—
POT STYLE, ½ c, 113 gm	100	14	2	4	—	60	*	440	—	—
WITH PINEAPPLE, ½ c, 113 gm	140	11	4	15	—	60	*	270	—	—
HOOP CHEESE, NATURAL, 4 oz, 113 gm	84	18	<1	2	—	20	*	10	—	—
FARMER CHEESE, ½ c, 113 gm	160	16	12	4	—	120	*	356	—	—
NO SALT ADDED, ½ c, 113 gm	160	16	12	4	—	120	*	8	—	—
CREAM CHEESE, SOFT, 1 oz, 28 gm	103	2	<10	<1	—	20	*	70	—	—
Frigo										
BLUE, 1 oz, 28 gm	100	6	8	1	—	150	*	400	70	21
CHEDDAR, 1 oz, 28 gm	110	7	9	1	—	200	*	200	30	—
FETA, 1 oz, 28 gm	100	6	8	1	—	150	*	400	20	—
FONTINA, 1 oz, 28 gm	110	7	9	1	—	150	*	400	70	33
MOZZARELLA, LOW MOISTURE										
PART SKIM, 1 oz, 28 gm	80	7	5	1	—	200	*	190	20	16
WHOLE MILK, 1 oz, 28 gm	90	6	7	1	—	150	*	190	20	26
PARMESAN, GRATED, 1 oz, 28 gm	130	12	9	1	—	400	*	510	30	23
PARMESAN LOAF, 1 oz, 28 gm	110	10	7	1	—	350	*	350	25	20
PARMESAN & ROMANO, GRATED, 1 oz, 28 gm	130	12	9	1	—	400	*	510	30	28
PARMESAN ZEST, 1 oz, 28 gm	130	7	8	8	—	200	.36	460	—	—
PIZZA, 1 oz, 28 gm	90	7	6	1	—	200	*	210	—	—
PROVOLONE, 1 oz, 28 gm	100	7	7	1	—	200	*	230	20	—
RICOTTA										
PART SKIM, 1 oz, 28 gm	45	3	3	1	—	60	*	100	35	10
WHOLE MILK, 1 oz, 28 gm	50	3	4	1	—	60	*	100	30	15
ROMANO, GRATED, 1 oz, 28 gm	130	12	9	1	—	400	*	510	30	35
ROMANO LOAF, 1 oz, 28 gm	110	9	8	1	—	300	*	350	25	30
SWISS, 1 oz, 28 gm	110	8	8	1	—	250	*	80	—	—
TACO, 1 oz, 28 gm	110	7	9	1	—	200	*	200	—	—
Heidi Ann										
COUNTRY STYLE FARMERS, 1 oz, 28 gm	99	8	7	1	—	—	—	105	—	21
FARMER IN THE DILL, 1 oz, 28 gm	99	8	7	1	—	—	—	105	—	21

FOOD & DESCRIPTION MEASURE OR QUANTITY	CALORIES	PROTEIN (GM)	FAT (GM)	CARBO-HYDRATE (GM)	FIBER (GM)	CALCIUM (MG)	IRON (MG)	SODIUM (MG)	POTASSIUM (MG)	CHOLES-TEROL (MG)
LITE 'N CREAMY, 1 oz, 28 gm	103	7	8	—	—	—	—	91	—	18
LOW-FAT CHED-STYLE, 1 oz, 28 gm	83	9	5	1	—	—	—	68	—	14
LOW SODIUM COLBY, 1 oz, 28 gm	112	7	9	1	—	—	—	55	—	27
NATURAL GARDEN VEGETABLE, 1 oz, 28 gm	94	7	7	1	—	—	—	74	—	23
SNAPPY JACK, 1 oz, 28 gm	99	8	7	1	—	—	—	105	—	21
SWISS STYLE, 1 oz, 28 gm	97	9	7	1	—	—	—	32	—	19

Land O'Lakes

FOOD & DESCRIPTION MEASURE OR QUANTITY	CALORIES	PROTEIN (GM)	FAT (GM)	CARBO-HYDRATE (GM)	FIBER (GM)	CALCIUM (MG)	IRON (MG)	SODIUM (MG)	POTASSIUM (MG)	CHOLES-TEROL (MG)
BRICK, 1 oz, 28 gm	110	7	8	1	—	200	*	160	40	25
CHEDDAR, 1 oz, 28 gm	110	7	9	<1	—	200	*	175	30	30
COLBY, 1 oz, 28 gm	110	7	9	1	—	200	*	170	35	25
COTTAGE CHEESE, 4 oz, 113 gm	120	14	5	3	—	60	*	460	95	15
2% FAT, 4 oz, 113 gm	100	16	2	4	—	80	*.	460	110	10
EDAM, 1 oz, 28 gm	100	7	8	<1	—	200	*	275	55	25
GOUDA, 1 oz, 28 gm	100	7	8	1	—	200	*	230	35	30
MONTEREY JACK, 1 oz, 28 gm	110	7	9	<1	—	200	*	150	25	20
MOZZARELLA, LOW MOISTURE PART SKIM, 1 oz, 28 gm	80	8	5	1	—	200	*	150	25	15
MUENSTER, 1 oz, 28 gm	100	7	9	<1	—	200	*	180	40	25
PROCESSED AMERICAN, 1 oz, 28 gm	110	6	9	<1	—	150	*	405	45	25
AMERICAN/SWISS, 1 oz, 28 gm	100	6	9	<1	—	200	*	445	35	25
SALAMI CHEESE FOOD, 1 oz, 28 gm	100	5	8	2	—	150	*	400	—	20
GOLDEN VELVET CHEESE SPREAD, 1 oz, 28 gm	80	5	6	2	—	150	*	380	70	15
JALAPENO CHEESE FOOD, 1 oz, 28 gm	90	6	7	2	—	150	*	360	—	20
LA CHEDDA CHEESE FOOD, 1 oz, 28 gm	90	6	7	2	—	150	*	335	80	20
PEPPERONI CHEESE FOOD, 1 oz, 28 gm	90	6	7	1	—	150	*	395	65	20
ONION CHEESE FOOD, 1oz, 28 gm	90	6	7	2	—	200	*	330	—	15
PROVOLONE, 1 oz, 28 gm	100	7	8	1	—	200	*	250	40	20
SWISS, 1 oz, 28 gm	110	8	8	1	—	250	*	75	30	25

Lite-Line—Borden

FOOD & DESCRIPTION MEASURE OR QUANTITY	CALORIES	PROTEIN (GM)	FAT (GM)	CARBO-HYDRATE (GM)	FIBER (GM)	CALCIUM (MG)	IRON (MG)	SODIUM (MG)	POTASSIUM (MG)	CHOLES-TEROL (MG)
LOW CHOLESTEROL PASTEURIZED PROCESS CHEESE FOOD SUBSTITUTE, 1 oz, 28 gm	90	5	7	2	—	150	*	430	55	5
LOW FAT COTTAGE CHEESE, ½ c	90	14	2	4	—	60	*	375	100	—
PASTEURIZED PROCESS CHEESE PRODUCT, 8% FAT AMERICAN, 1 oz, 28 gm	50	7	2	1	—	200	*	410	20	—
COLBY, 1 oz, 28 gm	50	7	2	1	—	200	*	470	15	—
MONTEREY JACK, 1 oz, 28 gm	50	7	2	1	—	200	*	470	15	—
MEUENSTER, 1 oz, 28 gm	50	7	2	1	—	200	*	470	15	—
SHARP CHEDDAR FLAVOR, 1 oz, 28 gm	50	7	2	1	—	200	*	445	15	—

FOOD & DESCRIPTION MEASURE OR QUANTITY	CALORIES	PROTEIN (GM)	FAT (GM)	CARBO-HYDRATE (GM)	FIBER (GM)	CALCIUM (MG)	IRON (MG)	SODIUM (MG)	POTASSIUM (MG)	CHOLES-TEROL (MG)
SWISS FLAVOR, 1 oz, 28 gm PASTEURIZED PROCESS CHEESE PRODUCT, 15% FAT	50	7	2	1	—	200	*	330	15	—
REDUCED SODIUM, AMERICAN FLAVOR, 1 oz, 28 gm	70	6	4	2	—	200	*	90	310	—
SODIUM LITE, 1 oz, 28 gm	70	6	4	2	—	200	*	200	310	—

Nestle

FOOD & DESCRIPTION	CALORIES	PROTEIN	FAT	CARBO-HYDRATE	FIBER	CALCIUM	IRON	SODIUM	POTASSIUM	CHOLESTEROL
PRICE'S PIMIENTO SPREAD, 1 oz, 28 gm	80	3	6	2	—	100	*	330	30	15
SWISS KNIGHT FONDUE, 1 oz, 28 gm	60	4	5	1	—	150	*	190	—	15
SWISS KNIGHT GRUYERE, 1 oz, 28 gm	100	6	8	<1	—	250	*	360	—	25
WISPRIDE CHEESE FOOD CHEDDAR WITH ONION, SOFT, 1 oz, 28 gm	100	4	7	4	—	150	*	170	120	—
GARLIC AND HERB, SOFT, 1 oz, 28 gm	90	4	7	4	—	100	*	180	120	20
MILD CHEDDAR, SOFT, 1 oz, 28 gm	100	5	7	4	—	150	*	160	120	—
PORT WINE, 1 oz, 28 gm	100	5	9	<1	—	150	*	250	75	20
SOFT, 1 oz, 28 gm	100	5	7	3	—	150	*	190	100	—
SHARP CHEDDAR, 1 oz, 28 gm	90	5	7	4	—	100	*	160	65	20
SOFT, 1 oz, 28 gm	100	5	8	3	—	150	*	180	90	—
SMOKE FLAVOR, 1 oz, 28 gm	90	5	6	3	—	150	*	230	100	20

Polly-O

FOOD & DESCRIPTION	CALORIES	PROTEIN	FAT	CARBO-HYDRATE	FIBER	CALCIUM	IRON	SODIUM	POTASSIUM	CHOLESTEROL
MOZZARELLA LITE, 1 oz, 28 gm	70	7	4	1	—	100	—	200	—	15
LOW-MOISTURE, PART SKIM, STRING CHEESE, 1 oz, 28 gm	90	7	6	2	—	200	—	200	—	15
PART SKIM, 1 oz, 28 gm	80	6	5	1	—	100	—	280	—	15
WHOLE MILK, 1 oz, 28 gm	90	5	6	1	—	100	—	280	—	20
RICOTTA LITE, 2 oz, 57 gm	80	7	4	3	—	200	—	65	—	10
NO SALT ADDED, PART SKIM, 2 oz, 57 gm	90	7	5	2	—	200	—	20	—	15
PART SKIM MILK, 2 oz, 57 gm	90	7	6	2	—	200	—	45	—	20
WHOLE MILK, 2 oz, 57 gm	100	7	7	2	—	150	—	45	—	20

USDA

FOOD & DESCRIPTION	CALORIES	PROTEIN	FAT	CARBO-HYDRATE	FIBER	CALCIUM	IRON	SODIUM	POTASSIUM	CHOLESTEROL
BLUE CHEESE, 1 oz, 28 gm	100	6	8	<1	0	150	.09	396	73	21
BRICK, 1 oz, 28 gm	105	7	8	<1	0	191	.12	159	38	27
BRIE, 1 oz, 28 gm	95	6	8	<1	0	52	.14	178	43	28
CAMEMBERT, 1 oz, 28 gm	85	6	7	<1	0	110	.09	239	53	20
CARAWAY, 1 oz, 28 gm	107	7	8	<1	0	191	—	196	—	—
CHEDDAR, 1 oz, 28 gm	114	7	9	<1	0	204	.19	176	28	30
CHESHIRE, 1 oz, 28 gm	110	7	9	1	0	182	.06	198	27	29
COLBY, 1 oz, 28 gm	112	7	9	<1	0	194	.22	171	36	27
COTTAGE CHEESE CREAMED, 1 c unpacked, 210 gm	217	26	9	6	0	126	.29	850	177	31
DRY CURD, unsalted, 1 c unpacked, 145 gm	123	25	<1	3	0	46	.33	19	47	10
LOW FAT, 2% FAT, 1 c unpacked, 226 gm	203	31	4	8	0	155	.36	918	217	19

111

FOOD & DESCRIPTION MEASURE OR QUANTITY	CALORIES	PROTEIN (GM)	FAT (GM)	CARBO-HYDRATE (GM)	FIBER (GM)	CALCIUM (MG)	IRON (MG)	SODIUM (MG)	POTASSIUM (MG)	CHOLES-TEROL (MG)
LOW FAT, 1% FAT, 1 c unpacked, 226 gm	164	28	2	6	0	138	.32	918	193	10
CREAM CHEESE, 1 oz, 28 gm	99	2	10	<1	0	23	.34	84	34	31
EDAM, 1 oz, 28 gm	101	7	8	<1	0	207	.12	274	53	25
FETA, 1 oz, 28 gm	75	4	6	1	0	140	.18	316	18	25
FONTINA, 1 oz, 28 gm	110	7	9	<1	0	156	.06	—	—	33
GJETOST, 1 oz, 28 gm	132	3	8	12	0	113	—	170	—	—
GOUDA, 1 oz, 28 gm	101	7	8	<1	0	198	.07	232	34	32
GRUYERE, 1 oz, 28 gm	117	8	9	<1	0	287	—	95	23	31
LIMBURGER, 1 oz, 28 gm	93	6	8	<1	0	141	.04	227	36	26
MONTEREY, 1 oz, 28 gm	106	7	9	<1	0	212	.20	152	23	—
MOZZARELLA										
PART SKIM, 1 oz, 28 gm	72	7	5	<1	0	183	.06	132	24	16
LOW MOISTURE, 1 oz, 28 gm	79	8	5	<1	0	207	.07	150	27	15
WHOLE MILK, 1 oz, 28 gm	80	6	6	<1	0	147	.05	106	19	22
LOW MOISTURE, 1 oz, 28 gm	90	6	7	<1	0	163	.06	118	21	25
MUENSTER, 1 oz, 28 gm	104	7	9	<1	0	203	.12	178	38	27
NEUFCHATEL, 1 oz, 28 gm	74	3	7	<1	0	21	.08	113	32	22
PARMESAN										
grated, 1 tbsp, 5 gm	23	2	2	<1	0	69	.05	93	5	4
1 oz, 28 gm	129	12	9	1	0	390	.27	528	30	22
HARD, 1 oz, 28 gm	111	10	7	<1	0	336	.23	454	26	19
PASTEURIZED PROCESS										
AMERICAN, 1 oz, 28 gm	106	6	9	<1	0	174	.11	406	46	27
AMERICAN CHEESE FOOD, 1 oz, 28 gm	93	6	7	2	0	163	.24	337	79	18
COLD PACK, 1 oz, 28 gm	94	6	7	2	0	141	.24	274	103	18
AMERICAN CHEESE SPREAD, 1 oz, 28 gm	82	5	6	2	0	159	.09	381	69	16
PIMIENTO, 1 oz, 28 gm	106	6	9	<1	tr	174	.12	405	46	27
SWISS, 1 oz, 28 gm	95	7	7	<1	0	219	.17	388	61	24
SWISS CHEESE FOOD, 1 oz, 28 gm	92	6	7	1	0	205	.17	440	81	23
PORT DU SALUT, 1 oz, 28 gm	100	7	8	<1	0	184	—	151	—	35
PROVOLONE, 1 oz, 28 gm	100	7	8	<1	0	214	.15	248	39	20
RICOTTA										
PART SKIM, 1 c, 246 gm	340	28	19	13	0	669	1.08	307	308	76
WHOLE MILK, 1 c, 246 gm	428	28	32	7	0	509	.94	207	257	124
ROMANO, SOLID, 1 oz, 28 gm	110	9	8	1	0	302	—	340	—	29
ROQUEFORT, 1 oz, 28 gm	105	6	9	<1	0	188	.16	513	26	26
SWISS, 1 oz, 28 gm	107	8	8	<1	0	272	.05	74	31	26
TILSIT, WHOLE MILK, 1 oz, 28 gm	96	7	7	<1	0	198	.06	213	18	29

Weight Watchers

FOOD & DESCRIPTION MEASURE OR QUANTITY	CALORIES	PROTEIN (GM)	FAT (GM)	CARBO-HYDRATE (GM)	FIBER (GM)	CALCIUM (MG)	IRON (MG)	SODIUM (MG)	POTASSIUM (MG)	CHOLES-TEROL (MG)
COLD PACK CHEESE PRODUCT										
ONION FLAVOR, 1 oz, 2 tbsp	70	5	4	6	—	190	.12	—	—	—
SHARP CHEDDAR FLAVOR, 1 oz, 2 tbsp	70	5	4	6	—	190	.12	—	—	—
SMOKED CHEESE FLAVOR, 1 oz, 2 tbsp	70	5	4	6	—	190	.12	—	—	—
COTTAGE CHEESE, LOW FAT, 1/3 c, 75 gm	60	9	<1	3	—	69	.20	173	60	—
CREAM CHEESE SPREAD, 1/3 c, 75 gm	80	10	3	3	—	62	.23	174	60	—
PART SKIM MILK CHEESE, 1 oz, 28 gm	80	8	5	1	—	223	.10	190	—	—
REDUCED SODIUM, 1 oz, 28 gm	80	8	5	1	—	223	0	105	—	—

FOOD & DESCRIPTION MEASURE OR QUANTITY	CALORIES	PROTEIN (GM)	FAT (GM)	CARBO-HYDRATE (GM)	FIBER (GM)	CALCIUM (MG)	IRON (MG)	SODIUM (MG)	POTASSIUM (MG)	CHOLES-TEROL (MG)
PASTEURIZED PROCESS CHEESE PRODUCT, 2 oz, 57 gm	100	14	4	2	—	450	0	1063	68	16
REDUCED SODIUM, 2 oz, 57 gm	100	14	4	2	—	400	0	450	68	16

Cream, Cream Substitutes & Toppings

Birds Eye–General Foods

COOL WHIP EXTRA CREAMY DAIRY RECIPE, 1 tbsp	16	0	1	1	tr	*	*	0	0	—
COOL WHIP NONDAIRY TOPPING, 1 tbsp	14	0	1	1	0	*	*	0	0	—
DOVER FARMS WHIPPED TOPPING, 1 tbsp	16	0	1	1	0	*	*	0	0	—
DREAM WHIP, DRY MIX, mix to make 1 tbsp	6	0	0	1	tr	*	*	0	0	—
prepared with whole milk, 1 tbsp	8	0	1	1	tr	*	*	0	5	—
DZERTA REDUCED CALORIE WHIPPED TOPPING, prep, 1 tbsp	8	0	1	0	tr	*	*	5	10	—

Borden

CREMORA NONDAIRY CREAMER, 1 tsp	12	0	1	1	—	*	*	5	15	—

Estee

WHIPPED TOPPING, 1 tbsp	4	<1	<1	<1	—	—	—	5	—	0

Featherweight

WHIPPED TOPPING, prep, 1 tbsp	2	0	0	0	—	—	—	4	<1	—

Land O'Lakes

GOURMET HEAVY WHIPPING CREAM, 1 tbsp, 15 gm	60	<1	6	<1	—	*	*	5	10	20
WHIPPING CREAM, 1 tbsp, 15 gm	45	<1	5	<1	—	*	*	5	15	15
HALF AND HALF, 1 tbsp, 15 gm	20	<1	2	1	—	*	*	5	20	5
SOUR CREAM, 1 tbsp, 12 gm	25	<1	3	1	—	*	*	5	15	5

Rich

COFFEE RICH, ½ oz	22	<1	1	2	0	tr	.02	7	5	0
POLY RICH, ½ oz	22	<1	1	2	0	<1	.02	5	11	0
RICH WHIP, LIQUID, ¼ oz	20	—	2	1	0	tr	tr	4	tr	0
PRESSURIZED, ¼ oz	20	<1	2	1	0	tr	tr	3	1	0
PREWHIPPED, 1 tbsp	12	<1	<1	<1	0	tr	.01	1	1	0

USDA

COFFEE WHITENER, NONDAIRY, Liquid, fz, 1 tbsp, 15 gm	20	<1	2	2	0	1	tr	12	29	0
½ c, 120 gm	163	1	12	14	0	11	.04	95	229	0

FOOD & DESCRIPTION MEASURE OR QUANTITY	CALORIES	PROTEIN (GM)	FAT (GM)	CARBO-HYDRATE (GM)	FIBER (GM)	CALCIUM (MG)	IRON (MG)	SODIUM (MG)	POTASSIUM (MG)	CHOLES-TEROL (MG)
powdered, 1 tsp, 2 gm	11	<1	<1	1	0	tr	.02	4	16	0
1 c, 94 gm	514	5	33	52	0	21	1.08	170	763	0
DESSERT TOPPING, NONDAIRY, frz, semisolid, 1 tbsp, 4 gm	13	<1	1	<1	0	tr	tr	1	1	0
1 c, 75 gm	239	<1	19	17	0	5	.09	19	14	0
powdered prep with whole milk, 1 tbsp, 4 gm	8	<1	<1	<1	0	4	tr	3	6	tr
1 c, 80 gm	151	3	10	13	0	72	.03	53	121	8
PRESSURIZED, 1 tbsp, 4 gm	11	<1	<1	<1	0	tr	tr	2	1	0
1 c, 70 gm	184	<1	16	11	0	4	.01	43	13	0
HALF & HALF, 1 tbsp, 15 gm	20	<1	2	<1	0	16	.01	6	19	6
1 c, 242 gm	315	7	28	10	0	254	.17	98	314	89
LIGHT, COFFEE or TABLE CREAM, 1 tbsp, 15 gm	29	<1	3	<1	0	14	.01	6	18	10
1 c, 240 gm	469	6	46	9	0	231	.10	95	292	159
LIGHT WHIPPING CREAM 1 tbsp liquid, 2 tbsp whipped, 15 gm	44	<1	5	<1	0	10	tr	5	15	17
1 c liquid, 2 c whipped, 239 gm	699	5	74	7	0	166	.07	82	231	265
HEAVY WHIPPING CREAM 1 tbsp liquid, 2 tbsp whipped, 15 gm	52	<1	6	<1	0	10	tr	6	11	21
1 c liquid, 2 c whipped, 238 gm	821	5	88	7	0	154	.07	89	179	326
MEDIUM CREAM, 25% fat, 1 tbsp, 15 gm	37	<1	4	<1	0	14	.01	6	17	13
1 c, 239 gm	583	6	60	8	0	216	.10	88	274	209
SOUR CREAM, CULTURED, 1 tbsp, 12 gm	26	<1	3	<1	0	14	.01	6	17	5
1 c, 230 gm	493	7	48	10	0	268	.14	123	331	102
HALF & HALF, CULTURED, 1 tbsp, 15 gm	20	<1	2	<1	0	16	.01	6	19	6
IMITATION, NONDAIRY, 1 oz, 28 gm	59	<1	6	2	0	1	—	29	46	0
1 C, 230 gm	479	6	45	15	0	6	—	235	369	0
WHIPPED CREAM, PRESSURIZED, 1 tbsp	8	<1	<1	<1	0	3	tr	4	4	2
1 c, 60 gm	154	2	13	7	0	61	.03	78	88	46

Eggs & Egg Substitutes

Durkee

SCRAMBLED EGGS, 2 eggs	124	8	10	4	—	—	—	320	173	—
SCRAMBLED EGGS WITH BACON, 2 eggs	181	12	13	6	—	—	—	476	233	—
WESTERN OMELET, 2 eggs	170	11	5	9	—	—	—	489	265	—

Fleischmann's–Nabisco

EGG BEATERS CHOLESTEROL FREE EGG PRODUCT, ¼ c	25	5	0	1	—	20	1.08	80	85	0
WITH CHEEZ, ½ c	130	14	6	3	—	200	1.80	440	110	5

Morning Star Farms

SCRAMBLERS, ¼ c, 57 gm	60	6	3	2	—	40	.36	150	85	0

FOOD & DESCRIPTION MEASURE OR QUANTITY	CALORIES	PROTEIN (GM)	FAT (GM)	CARBO-HYDRATE (GM)	FIBER (GM)	CALCIUM (MG)	IRON (MG)	SODIUM (MG)	POTASSIUM (MG)	CHOLES-TEROL (MG)
USDA										
CHICKEN EGGS										
DRIED										
WHITE POWDER, sifted, 1 c, 107 gm	402	88	<1	5	0	96	.26	1325	1194	0
WHOLE, 1 tbsp, 5 gm	30	2	2	<1	0	11	.39	26	24	96
1 c, sifted, 85 gm	505	39	36	4	0	180	6.70	443	416	1631
YOLK, 1 tbsp, 4 gm	27	1	2	<1	0	11	.42	4	7	117
1 c, sifted, 67 gm	460	20	41	<1	0	189	6.96	61	112	1962
FRIED IN BUTTER, 1 large, 46 gm	83	5	6	<1	0	26	.92	144	58	246
HARD-COOKED										
l large, 50 gm	79	6	6	<1	0	28	1.04	69	65	274
chopped, 1 c, 136 gm	215	17	15	2	0	76	2.84	188	177	745
POACHED, 1 large, 50 gm	79	6	6	<1	0	28	1.04	146	65	273
RAW										
WHOLE										
1 large, 50 gm	79	6	6	<1	0	28	1.04	69	65	274
1 medium, 44 gm	70	5	5	<1	0	25	.92	61	57	241
1 small, 38 gm	59	5	4	<1	0	21	.78	52	49	206
1 c, 243 gm	384	30	27	3	0	136	5.08	336	316	1331
WHITE										
1 large, 33 gm	16	3	tr	<1	0	4	.01	50	45	0
1 medium, 29 gm	14	3	tr	<1	0	3	.01	44	40	0
1 c, 243 gm	118	25	<1	3	0	27	.07	370	334	0
YOLK										
1 large, 17 gm	63	3	6	<1	0	26	.95	8	15	272
1 medium, 15 gm	55	2	5	<1	0	23	.84	7	14	240
1 c, 243 gm	897	40	80	<1	0	368	13.56	118	219	3894
SCRAMBLED WITH BUTTER & MILK										
1 large, 64 gm	95	6	7	1	0	47	.93	155	85	248
1 c, 220 gm	325	21	24	5	0	162	3	534	292	854
DUCK, WHOLE, RAW, 1 egg, 70 gm	130	9	10	1	0	45	2.70	102	156	619
EGG SUBSTITUTE										
FROZEN, ¼ c, 60 gm	96	7	7	2	0	44	1.19	120	128	1
LIQUID, 1½ oz, 47 gm	40	6	2	<1	0	25	.99	83	155	tr
1 c, 251 gm	211	30	8	2	0	133	5.27	444	828	3
POWDER, .7 oz, 19.8 gm	88	11	3	4	0	65	.63	158	147	113
GOOSE, WHOLE, RAW, 1 egg, 144 gm	267	20	19	2	0	—	—	—	—	—
QUAIL, WHOLE, 1 egg, 9 gm	14	1	1	<1	0	6	.33	—	—	76
TURKEY, WHOLE, 1 egg, 79 gm	135	11	9	<1	0	78	3.24	—	—	737

Milk & Milk Substitutes

Borden

EAGLE SWEETENED CONDENSED MILK, ⅓ c	320	7	9	52	—	300	*	120	360	—
MAGNOLIA SWEETENED FILLED DAIRY BLEND, ⅓ c	320	7	9	54	—	300	*	120	360	—

Friendship

BUTTERMILK, LOW FAT, 1 c	120	9	4	12	—	300	*	125	—	—

Land O'Lakes

BUTTERMILK, 8 oz, 245 gm	100	8	2	12	—	300	*	255	370	10

FOOD & DESCRIPTION MEASURE OR QUANTITY	CALORIES	PROTEIN (GM)	FAT (GM)	CARBO-HYDRATE (GM)	FIBER (GM)	CALCIUM (MG)	IRON (MG)	SODIUM (MG)	POTASSIUM (MG)	CHOLES-TEROL (MG)
CHOCOLATE MILK, 8 oz, 250 gm	210	8	8	26	—	300	.72	150	420	30
1% FAT, 8 oz, 250 gm	160	8	3	26	—	300	.72	150	425	5
SKIM MILK, 8 oz, 250 gm	140	8	<1	26	—	300	.72	155	425	5
EGGNOG, 8 oz, 252 gm	300	9	15	32	—	300	*	142	410	123
FLASH INSTANT NONFAT DRY MILK, 8 oz prep, 245 gm	80	8	<1	12	—	300	*	125	390	5
HOMOGENIZED MILK, 8 oz, 244 gm	150	8	8	11	—	300	*	120	370	35
LOWFAT MILK										
1% FAT, 8 oz, 244 gm	100	8	3	12	—	300	*	125	380	10
2% FAT, 8 oz, 244 gm	120	8	5	11	—	300	*	120	375	20
SKIM MILK, 8 oz, 245 gm	90	8	<1	12	—	300	*	125	405	5

Milnot

DAIRY VEGETABLE BLEND, 1 c	293	17	15	24	—	577	.22	275	758	0

USDA

BUTTERMILK, CULTURED										
salted, 1 c, 245 gm	99	8	2	12	0	285	.12	257	371	9
unsalted, 1 c, 245 gm	99	8	2	12	0	285	.12	123	371	9
CHOCOLATE										
WHOLE, 1 c, 250 gm	208	8	8	26	.15	280	.60	149	417	30
1% FAT, 1 c, 250 gm	158	8	3	26	.15	287	.60	152	426	7
2% FAT, 1 c, 250 gm	179	8	5	26	.15	284	.60	150	422	17
CONDENSED, SWEETENED										
cnd, 1 oz, 38 gm	123	3	3	21	0	108	.07	49	142	13
1 c, 306 gm	982	24	27	166	0	868	.58	389	1136	104
DRY										
BUTTERMILK, SWEET CREAM, 1 tbsp, 6.5 gm	25	2	<1	3	0	77	.02	34	103	5
1 c, 120 gm	464	41	7	59	0	1421	.36	621	1910	83
NONFAT										
CALCIUM REDUCED, 1 oz, 28 gm	100	10	<1	15	0	79	—	646	193	1
INSTANT, 1 c, 68 gm	244	24	<1	35	0	837	.21	373	1160	12
WHOLE, 1 c, 128 gm	635	34	34	49	0	1168	.6	475	1702	124
EVAPORATED										
SKIM, 1 oz, 31.9 gm	25	2	<1	4	0	92	.09	37	106	1
½ c, 128 gm	99	10	<1	14	0	369	.37	147	423	5
WHOLE, cnd, 1 oz, 31.5 gm	42	2	2	3	0	82	.06	33	95	9
½ c, 126 gm	169	9	10	13	0	329	.24	133	382	37
FILLED MILK, 1 c, 244 gm	154	8	8	12	0	312	.12	138	339	4
GOAT MILK, WHOLE, 1 c, 244 gm	168	9	10	11	0	326	.12	122	499	28
HUMAN MILK, WHOLE, MATURE, 1 c, 246 gm	171	3	11	17	0	79	.07	42	126	34
IMITATION MILK, 1 c, 244 gm	150	4	8	15	0	79	.95	191	279	tr
INDIAN BUFFALO MILK, WHOLE, 1 c, 244 gm	236	9	17	13	0	412	.29	127	434	46
LOWFAT, 1% FAT, 1 c, 244 gm	102	8	3	12	0	300	.12	123	381	10
NONFAT MILK SOLIDS ADDED, 1 c, 245 gm	104	9	2	12	0	313	.12	128	397	10
PROTEIN FORTIFIED, 1 c, 246 gm	119	10	3	14	0	349	.15	143	444	10
LOWFAT, 2% FAT, 1 c, 244 gm	121	8	5	12	0	297	.12	122	377	18
NONFAT MILK SOLIDS ADDED, 1 c, 245 gm	125	9	5	12	0	313	.12	128	397	18
PROTEIN FORTIFIED, 1 c, 246 gm	137	10	5	14	0	352	.15	145	447	19

FOOD & DESCRIPTION MEASURE OR QUANTITY	CALORIES	PROTEIN (GM)	FAT (GM)	CARBO-HYDRATE (GM)	FIBER (GM)	CALCIUM (MG)	IRON (MG)	SODIUM (MG)	POTASSIUM (MG)	CHOLES-TEROL (MG)
LOW SODIUM, WHOLE, 1 c, 244 gm	149	8	8	11	0	246	—	6	617	33
SHEEP MILK, WHOLE, 1 c, 245 gm	264	15	17	13	0	474	.24	108	334	—
SKIM MILK, 1 c, 245 gm	86	8	<1	12	0	302	.1	126	406	4
PROTEIN FORTIFIED, 1 c, 246 gm	100	10	<1	14	0	352	.15	144	446	5
NONFAT MILK SOLIDS ADDED, 1 c, 245 gm	90	9	<1	12	0	316	.12	130	418	5
WHEY, ACID										
DRY, 1 tbsp, 2.9 gm	10	<1	<1	2	0	59	.04	28	66	—
FLUID, 1 c, 246 gm	59	2	<1	13	0	253	.20	118	352	—
WHEY, SWEET										
DRY, 1 tbsp, 7.5 gm	26	<1	<1	6	0	59	.07	80	155	tr
FLUID, 1 c, 246 gm	66	2	<1	13	0	115	.15	132	396	5
WHOLE MILK, 3.3% FAT, 1 c, 244 gm	150	8	8	11	0	291	.12	120	370	33
3.7% FAT, 1 c, 244 gm	157	8	9	11	0	290	.12	119	368	35

Weight Watchers

SKIM MILK, 1 c, 245 gm	90	9	1	13	—	300	.10	118	329	7

Yogurt

Catelli–Laura Secord

BLUEBERRY, 125 gm	120	4	3	20	.10	158	.15	65	204	—
PEACH, 125 gm	119	4	3	19	.04	156	.13	65	211	—
RASPBERRY, 125 gm	120	4	3	19	.19	158	.15	65	209	—
STRAWBERRY, 125 gm	122	5	3	18	.09	158	.15	89	209	—

Colombo

FLAVORED, 8 oz, 227 gm	272	8	7	43	—	284	.68	136	—	45
FRUITED, 8 oz, 227 gm	249	8	5	45	—	227	.68	159	—	45
PLAIN LITE, 8 oz, 227 gm	109	11	0	17	—	329	1.13	181	340	5
PLAIN WHOLE MILK, 8 oz, 227 gm	150	9	7	12	—	295	1.13	159	306	34

Friendship

BLUEBERRY, STRAWBERRY or PINA COLADA, LOW FAT, 8 oz, 227 gm	230	10	3	44	—	350	*	160	—	—
LOW FAT WITH FRUIT, 8 oz, 227 gm	230	10	3	44	—	350	*	170	—	—
PLAIN, 8 oz, 227 gm	170	10	8	15	—	400	*	160	—	—
VANILLA or COFFEE, LOW FAT, 8 oz, 227 gm	210	11	3	35	—	400	*	170	—	—

Lite-Line–Borden

CHERRY VANILLA, NATURAL FLAVOR, 8 oz	270	9	2	54	—	300	*	160	300	—
LEMON FLAVOR, NATURAL FLAVOR, 8 oz	320	9	2	69	—	300	*	115	300	—
PINEAPPLE, NATURAL FLAVOR, 8 oz	260	9	2	51	—	300	*	115	390	—
PLAIN, LOWFAT, 8 oz	180	11	4	24	—	350	*	145	390	—
STRAWBERRY, NATURAL FLAVOR, 8 oz	230	9	2	46	—	300	*	145	300	—

FOOD & DESCRIPTION MEASURE OR QUANTITY	CALORIES	PROTEIN (GM)	FAT (GM)	CARBO- HYDRATE (GM)	FIBER (GM)	CALCIUM (MG)	IRON (MG)	SODIUM (MG)	POTASSIUM (MG)	CHOLES- TEROL (MG)
USDA										
COFFEE or VANILLA FLAVORED, LOW-FAT, 8 oz, 227 gm	194	11	3	31	0	389	.16	149	498	11
FRUIT FLAVORED, LOW-FAT										
9 gm protein, 8 oz, 227 gm	225	9	3	42	.27	314	.14	121	402	10
10 gm protein, 8 oz, 227 gm	231	10	2	43	.27	345	.16	133	442	10
11 gm protein, 8 oz, 227 gm	239	11	3	42	.27	383	.16	147	491	12
PLAIN										
LOW-FAT, 8 oz, 227 gm	144	12	4	16	0	415	.18	159	531	14
SKIM, 8 oz, 227 gm	127	13	<1	17	0	452	.20	174	579	4
WHOLE, 8 oz, 227 gm	139	8	7	11	0	274	.11	105	351	29
Weight Watchers										
BLUEBERRY, RASPBERRY or STRAWBERRY, 8 oz, 227 gm	150	9	0	29	—	300	1.80	95	—	—
EUROPEAN										
BLUEBERRY, RASPBERRY, STRAWBERRY, 6 oz, 170 gm	150	9	1	27	—	300	.27	—	—	—
PLAIN, 6 oz, 170 gm	90	9	1	12	—	300	.27	—	—	—
NONFAT PLAIN, 8 oz, 227 gm	90	9	0	14	—	300	0	118	—	—
Whitney's										
APPLES & RAISINS, 6 oz, 170 gm	200	7	5	33	—	250	tr	—	—	—
BLUEBERRY, 6 oz, 170 gm	200	7	5	33	—	250	tr	—	—	—
CHERRY, 6 oz, 170 gm	200	7	5	33	—	250	tr	—	—	—
COFFEE, 6 oz, 170 gm	200	8	6	28	—	300	tr	—	—	—
LEMON, 6 oz, 170 gm	200	8	6	28	—	300	tr	—	—	—
PEACH, 6 oz, 170 gm	200	7	5	33	—	250	tr	—	—	—
PLAIN, 6 oz, 170 gm	150	9	7	13	—	350	tr	—	—	—
RASPBERRY, 6 oz, 170 gm	200	7	5	33	—	250	tr	—	—	—
STRAWBERRY, 6 oz, 170 gm	200	7	5	33	—	250	tr	—	—	—
VANILLA, 6 oz, 170 gm	200	8	6	28	—	300	tr	—	—	—
WILD BERRIES, 6 oz, 170 gm	200	7	5	33	—	250	tr	—	—	—
Yoplait										
BREAKFAST STYLE										
APPLE CINNAMON, 6 oz	220	8	4	38	—	200	.36	90	340	—
BERRIES, 6 oz	230	8	4	40	—	200	.36	95	340	—
CHERRY WITH ALMONDS, 6 oz	230	8	4	40	—	200	.36	110	340	—
CITRUS FRUITS, 6 oz	250	8	4	45	—	200	.36	90	360	—
ORCHARD FRUITS, 6 oz	230	8	4	41	—	200	.36	95	380	—
STRAWBERRY BANANA, 6 oz	240	8	4	43	—	200	.36	90	360	—
STRAWBERRY WITH ALMONDS, 6 oz	230	8	4	40	—	200	.36	110	340	—
SUNRISE PEACH, 6 oz	230	8	3	42	—	200	.36	90	350	—
TROPICAL FRUITS, 6 oz	230	8	4	41	—	200	.36	90	360	—
CUSTARD STYLE										
FRUIT FLAVORS, BANANA, BLUEBERRY, LEMON, RASPBERRY or STRAWBERRY, 6 oz	190	7	4	32	—	200	*	95	290	—
MIXED BERRY, 6 oz	180	7	4	30	—	200	*	95	290	—
VANILLA or COFFEE, 6 oz	180	7	4	30	—	250	*	110	300	—
FRUIT ON THE BOTTOM, BLUEBERRY, MIXED BERRY, CHERRY, PINEAPPLE,										

FOOD & DESCRIPTION MEASURE OR QUANTITY	CALORIES	PROTEIN (GM)	FAT (GM)	CARBO- HYDRATE (GM)	FIBER (GM)	CALCIUM (MG)	IRON (MG)	SODIUM (MG)	POTASSIUM (MG)	CHOLES- TEROL (MG)
RASPBERRY, or STRAWBERRY, 6 oz	180	7	2	34	—	250	*	95	350	—
ORIGINAL										
FRUIT FLAVORS, APPLE, BLUEBERRY, BOYSENBERRY, CHERRY, LEMON, MIXED BERRY, ORANGE, PEACH, PINA COLADA, PINEAPPLE, RASPBERRY, STRAWBERRY or STRAWBERRY-BANANA,										
6 oz	190	7	4	32	—	250	*	105	350	—
PLAIN, 6 oz	130	9	5	13	—	300	*	120	370	—

8

DESSERTS

FOOD & DESCRIPTION MEASURE OR QUANTITY	CALORIES	PROTEIN (GM)	FAT (GM)	CARBO-HYDRATE (GM)	FIBER (GM)	CALCIUM (MG)	IRON (MG)	SODIUM (MG)	POTASSIUM (MG)	CHOLES-TEROL (MG)
Frozen										
Baskin-Robbins										
BUTTER PECAN ICE CREAM, 1 scoop, 71 gm	136	4	10	16	—	—	—	81	136	—
CHOCOLATE FUDGE ICE CREAM, 1 scoop, 71 gm	178	3	9	21	—	60	1.24	122	134	—
CHOCOLATE ICE CREAM, 1 scoop, 71 gm	165	3	8	20	—	72	.76	80	171	—
CHOCOLATE MINT ICE CREAM, 1 scoop, 71 gm	162	3	9	17	—	—	—	60	163	—
CHOCOLATE MOUSSE ROYALE ICE CREAM, 1 scoop, 71 gm	183	4	9	23	—	—	—	94	168	—
CONE, CAKE, 1 cone, empty, 4.9 gm	19	<1	<1	4	—	—	—	26	6	—
SUGAR, 1 cone, empty, 14 gm	57	1	1	11	—	—	—	45	21	—
DAIQUIRI ICE, 1 scoop, 71 gm	84	—	—	21	—	—	.07	11	—	—
FRENCH VANILLA ICE CREAM, 1 scoop, 71 gm	181	3	12	16	—	79	.26	60	104	—
JAMOCA ICE CREAM, 1 scoop, 71 gm	146	3	8	16	—	—	—	64	140	—
MOUNTAIN COFFEE, LOW FAT DESSERT, ½ c, 71 gm	90	3	1	17	—	100	*	60	170	4
ORANGE SHERBET, 1 scoop, 71 gm	99	<1	1	21	—	—	—	29	40	—
PINEAPPLE ICE, 1 scoop, 71 gm	94	<1	<1	23	—	—	—	83	36	—
PRALINES 'N CREAM ICE CREAM, 1 scoop, 71 gm	177	2	8	24	—	62	.21	166	—	—
ROCKY ROAD ICE CREAM, 1 scoop, 71 gm	182	3	7	27	—	—	—	77	150	—
STRAWBERRY ICE CREAM, 1 scoop, 71 gm	141	8	6	16	—	63	.14	68	104	—
STRAWBERRY, LOW FAT DESSERT, ½ c, 71 gm	90	3	1	16	—	100	.36	60	160	6
VANILLA ICE CREAM, 1 scoop, 71 gm	147	3	8	16	—	85	.07	57	106	—
Borden										
ALL NATURAL ICE CREAM DUTCH CHOCOLATE ALMOND, ½ c	160	3	9	18	—	100	*	—	—	—
FRENCH VANILLA, ½ c	150	3	8	20	—	100	*	—	—	—

FOOD & DESCRIPTION MEASURE OR QUANTITY	CALORIES	PROTEIN (GM)	FAT (GM)	CARBO- HYDRATE (GM)	FIBER (GM)	CALCIUM (MG)	IRON (MG)	SODIUM (MG)	POTASSIUM (MG)	CHOLES- TEROL (MG)
VANILLA, ½ c	140	3	7	17	—	100	*	—	—	—
ALL NATURAL ICE MILK										
CHOCOLATE, ½ c	110	3	3	17	—	100	*	—	—	—
STRAWBERRY, ½ c	110	2	3	18	—	100	*	—	—	—
VANILLA, ½ c	100	3	3	16	—	100	*	—	—	—
DUTCH CHOCOLATE ICE										
CREAM, ½ c	130	2	6	16	—	80	*	—	—	—
LADY BORDEN ICE CREAM										
BUTTERED PECAN, ½ c	180	3	12	16	—	80	*	—	—	—
CHOCOLATE, ½ c	160	2	10	16	—	80	*	—	—	—
FRENCH VANILLA, ½ c	170	3	9	20	—	100	*	—	—	—
LEMON SHERBET, ½ c	110	1	1	25	—	40	*	—	—	—
ORANGE SHERBET, ½ c	110	1	1	25	—	40	*	—	—	—
STRAWBERRY ICE CREAM, ½ c	120	2	5	17	—	60	*	—	—	—
VANILLA ICE CREAM, ARTIFICIALLY FLAVORED, ½ c	130	2	7	15	—	80	*	—	—	—
Dairy Queen										
CONE										
LARGE, 213 gm	340	9	10	57	—	250	1.44	115	—	25
REGULAR, 142 gm	240	6	7	38	—	150	.72	80	—	15
SMALL, 85 gm	140	3	4	22	—	100	.36	45	—	10
DIPPED CONE, CHOCOLATE										
LARGE, 1 cone, 234 gm	510	9	24	64	—	250	1.44	145	—	30
REGULAR, 1 cone, 156 gm	340	6	16	42	—	150	.72	100	—	20
SMALL, 1 cone, 92 gm	190	3	9	25	—	100	.36	55	—	10
SHAKE, CHOCOLATE										
LARGE, 588 gm	990	19	26	168	—	700	3.60	360	—	70
REGULAR, 418 gm	710	14	19	120	—	450	2.7	260	—	50
SMALL, 291 gm	490	10	13	82	—	350	1.8	180	—	35
SUNDAE, CHOCOLATE										
LARGE, 248 gm	440	8	10	78	—	250	1.44	165	—	30
REGULAR, 177 gm	310	5	8	56	—	200	1.08	120	—	20
SMALL, 106 gm	190	3	4	33	—	100	.36	75	—	10
Dole										
FRUIT 'N CREAM BARS										
BLUEBERRY, 1 bar, 67 gm	90	1	1	19	—	31	.17	20	57	—
PEACH, 1 bar, 67 gm	90	<1	1	19	—	27	.07	19	67	—
STRAWBERRY, 1 bar, 67 gm	90	1	1	19	—	32	.17	22	76	—
FRUIT 'N JUICE BARS										
ORANGE, 1 bar, 2.5 oz, 70 gm	70	<1	<1	16	—	6	.33	6	70	—
PINEAPPLE, 1 bar, 2.5 oz, 70 gm	70	<1	<1	17	—	9	.28	4	51	—
STRAWBERRY, 1 bar, 2.5 oz, 70 gm	70	<1	<1	16	—	6	.20	6	64	—
SORBET										
MANDARIN, 4 oz, 104 gm	110	<1	<1	28	—	—	.38	9	138	—
PEACH, 4 oz, 104 gm	120	<1	<1	30	—	3	.57	11	61	—
PINEAPPLE, 4 oz, 104 gm	120	<1	<1	28	—	9	.47	11	79	—
RASPBERRY, 4 oz, 104 gm	110	<1	<1	28	—	—	.43	12	37	—
STRAWBERRY, 4 oz, 104 gm	110	<1	<1	28	—	8	.52	11	62	—
WHIP										
BANANA, 3 oz	65	0	1	15	—	*	*	18	28	—
LIME, 3 oz	60	0	1	14	—	*	*	17	15	—
ORANGE, 3 oz	60	0	1	14	—	*	*	12	17	—
PINEAPPLE, 3 oz	60	0	1	13	—	*	*	12	32	—
STRAWBERRY, 3 oz	60	0	1	14	—	*	*	12	17	—

FOOD & DESCRIPTION MEASURE OR QUANTITY	CALORIES	PROTEIN (GM)	FAT (GM)	CARBO-HYDRATE (GM)	FIBER (GM)	CALCIUM (MG)	IRON (MG)	SODIUM (MG)	POTASSIUM (MG)	CHOLES-TEROL (MG)
Good Humor–Lipton										
CAL-CONTROL SLICES, VANILLA, 3.2 oz	60	2	1	11	—	60	*	45	—	—
CHIP CRUNCH, 1 bar, 3 oz	200	2	14	16	—	60	*	35	—	—
CHOCOLATE ECLAIR, 1 bar, 3 oz	180	2	9	24	—	40	*	70	—	—
CHOCOLATE FUDGE CAKE, 1 bar, 3 oz	260	3	16	25	—	60	*	95	—	—
CHOCOLATE MALT, 1 bar, 3 oz	190	2	13	16	—	60	*	50	—	—
FAT FROG SHAPED NOVELTY, 3 oz	140	2	7	17	—	80	*	45	—	—
HEART SHAPED NOVELTY, 4 oz	200	3	12	21	—	80	*	60	—	—
ICE CREAM BAR, VANILLA, 1 bar, 3 oz	170	2	11	16	—	60	*	40	—	—
ICE CREAM COOKIE SANDWICH										
4 oz ice cream	400	5	16	59	—	80	1.08	270	—	—
2.7 oz ice cream	290	4	11	42	—	60	.72	195	—	—
ICE CREAM SANDWICH, VANILLA, 2.5 oz	170	3	5	28	—	60	*	120	—	—
ICE CREAM SLICES, VANILLA, 3.2 oz	110	2	6	13	—	60	*	45	—	—
ICE STRIPE, 1.5 oz	40	0	0	10	—	*	*	0	—	—
PUDDING STIX, 1 pop, 1.75 oz	90	4	2	15	—	100	*	65	—	—
SHARK SHAPED NOVELTY, 3 oz	70	0	0	17	—	*	*	0	—	—
TOASTED ALMOND, 1 bar, 3 oz	190	1	8	28	—	40	*	30	—	—
TOASTED CARAMEL, 1 bar, 3 oz	170	2	9	21	—	60	*	55	—	—
WHAMMYS, 1 bar, 1.6 oz	90	1	6	9	—	20	*	25	—	—
Guido's										
ICE JUICEE, 3 oz	60	<1	tr	15	—	7	.50	<1	58	—
Häagen-Dazs										
BUTTER PECAN ICE CREAM, ½ c	316	6	29	27	—	—	—	147	—	—
CAROB ICE CREAM, ½ c	256	6	17	20	—	—	—	101	—	—
CHOCOLATE CHIP ICE CREAM, ½ c	312	7	18	25	—	—	—	223	—	—
CHOCOLATE ICE CREAM, ½ c	280	6	17	25	—	—	—	122	—	—
COFFEE ICE CREAM, ½ c	272	6	17	24	—	—	—	137	—	—
COOKIES & CREAM ICE CREAM, ½ c	272	5	17	24	—	—	—	91	—	—
HONEY ICE CREAM, ½ c	256	5	18	18	—	—	—	96	—	—
LEMON ICE, ½ c	140	<1	0	33	—	—	—	—	—	—
MACADAMIA NUT ICE CREAM, ½ c	260	4	19	20	—	—	—	384	—	—
MAPLE WALNUT ICE CREAM, ½ c	320	6	23	22	—	—	—	68	—	—
MOCHA CHIP ICE CREAM, ½ c	272	5	18	22	—	—	—	68	—	—
ORANGE ICE, ½ c	140	<1	0	33	—	—	—	—	—	—
PEACH ICE CREAM, ½ c	252	5	16	27	—	—	—	103	—	—
PRALINES & CREAM ICE CREAM, ½ c	260	4	16	26	—	—	—	99	—	—
RUM RAISIN ICE CREAM, ½ c	264	4	16	25	—	—	—	224	—	—
STRAWBERRY ICE CREAM, ½ c	268	5	16	25	—	—	—	170	—	—

FOOD & DESCRIPTION MEASURE OR QUANTITY	CALORIES	PROTEIN (GM)	FAT (GM)	CARBO- HYDRATE (GM)	FIBER (GM)	CALCIUM (MG)	IRON (MG)	SODIUM (MG)	POTASSIUM (MG)	CHOLES- TEROL (MG)
SWISS CHOCOLATE ALMOND ICE CREAM, ½ c	292	7	20	25	—	—	—	73	—	—
SWISS VANILLA ALMOND ICE CREAM, ½ c	344	7	24	28	—	—	—	207	—	—
VANILLA CHIP ICE CREAM, ½ c	280	5	17	25	—	—	—	68	—	—
VANILLA ICE CREAM, ½ c	268	5	17	24	—	—	—	112	—	—

Hormel

DULCITA										
APPLE, 4 oz	290	5	10	44	—	—	—	350	—	—
CHERRY, 4 oz	300	5	9	48	—	—	—	345	—	—

Jell-O—General Foods

GELATIN POP BARS, ALL FLAVORS, 1 bar	35	1	0	8	tr	*	*	5	0	—
PUDDING POPS, CHOCOLATE, 1 pop	80	2	2	13	tr	60	*	80	90	—
CHOCOLATE CARAMEL SWIRL, 1 pop	80	2	2	13	tr	60	*	65	70	—
CHOCOLATE COVERED CHOCOLATE, 1 pop	130	2	8	15	tr	60	*	75	105	—
CHOCOLATE COVERED VANILLA, 1 pop	130	2	8	15	tr	60	*	50	80	—
CHOCOLATE VANILLA SWIRL, 1 pop	80	2	2	13	tr	60	*	65	80	—
VANILLA, 1 pop	70	2	2	13	tr	60	*	50	65	—

Land O'Lakes

ICE CREAM, VANILLA, 4 oz	140	2	7	16	—	80	*	60	130	30
ICE MILK, VANILLA, 4 oz	90	3	3	14	—	80	*	50	130	10
SHERBET, FRUIT FLAVORED, 4 oz	130	1	2	27	—	40	*	25	175	5

Life Savers

POPS, all flavors, 1 pop	40	0	0	10	—	*	*	0	0	—

Nestle

CHOCOLATE CHIP ICE CREAM BAR, 1 bar, 66.5 gm	220	3	15	19	—	60	.36	40	140	—
CHOCOLATE CHIP ICE CREAM SANDWICH, 1 bar, 75 gm	220	4	8	32	—	100	.72	95	140	—
CRUNCH ICE CREAM BAR, 1 bar	180	2	13	15	—	80	*	—	—	—

Oreo—Nabisco

COOKIES 'N CREAM										
ICE CREAM, all flavors, 3 oz	140	2	8	16	—	60	.36	100	110	—
ON A STICK, 1 bar	220	3	15	19	—	60	.36	100	120	—
SANDWICH, 1 sandwich	240	4	11	31	—	80	1.08	300	175	—

Salada—Kellogg

DUTCH CHOCOLATE ICE CREAM MIX, 1 oz dry	110	1	0	26	—	*	*	20	48	—
prep, 1 c	310	4	19	31	—	150	*	75	197	—
WILD STRAWBERRY, PEACH or VANILLA MIX, 1 oz dry	110	0	0	27	—	*	*	10	25	—
prep, 1 c	310	4	19	32	—	150	*	60	174	—

FOOD & DESCRIPTION MEASURE OR QUANTITY	CALORIES	PROTEIN (GM)	FAT (GM)	CARBO-HYDRATE (GM)	FIBER (GM)	CALCIUM (MG)	IRON (MG)	SODIUM (MG)	POTASSIUM (MG)	CHOLES-TEROL (MG)
Sunkist–Lipton										
LEMONADE BAR, 1 bar, 3 oz	70	0	0	20	—	*	*	5	—	—
ORANGE JUICE BAR, 1 bar, 3 oz	70	<1	0	18	—	*	*	5	—	—
Tofutti **[hard pack]**										
CHOCOLATE SUPREME, ½ c	210	3	13	20	—	—	—	130	37	0
MAPLE WALNUT, ½ c	230	3	14	20	—	—	—	95	30	0
VANILLA ALMOND BARK, ½ oz	230	3	14	23	—	—	—	95	41	0
WILDBERRY SUPREME, ½ c	210	2	12	22	—	—	—	100	9	0
USDA										
ICE CREAM, 10% FAT, VANILLA, 1 c, 133 gm	269	5	14	32	0	176	.12	116	257	59
16% FAT, VANILLA, 1 c, 148 gm	349	4	24	32	0	151	.10	108	221	88
SOFT-SERVE, FRENCH VANILLA, 1 c, 173 gm	377	7	23	38	0	236	.43	153	338	153
ICE MILK, VANILLA, 1 c, 131 gm	184	5	6	29	0	176	.18	105	265	18
SOFT-SERVE, 1 c, 175 gm	223	8	5	38	0	274	.28	163	412	13
SHERBET, ORANGE, 1 c, 193 gm	270	2	4	59	tr	103	.31	88	198	14
Weight Watchers										
DIETARY FROZEN DESSERT, 4.9 oz, 85 gm	100	4	1	19	—	150	.18	70	200	2
CHOCOLATE DIP BAR, 2.5 oz	100	2	5	11	—	74	0	—	—	—
SUNDAE CONE, 1 cone, 63 gm	150	3	5	22	—	83	.40	—	—	—
FROSTED TREAT/FRAPPE, SOFT-SERVE, all flavors, 6 oz, 119 gm	120	6	1	22	—	210	.05	90	250	2
FROZEN DESSERT SNACK CUPS, 5 oz, 85 gm	100	4	1	19	—	145	.03	70	178	5
SANDWICH BARS, VANILLA or MINT, 1 bar	130	3	2	28	—	100	.58	—	—	—
TREAT BARS, CHOCOLATE, CHOCOLATE MINT, ORANGE or VANILLA, 1 bar, 3 oz, 85 gm	100	4	1	19	—	150	.18	70	200	2
STRAWBERRY VANILLA, 1 bar, 85 gm	100	4	1	19	—	145	—	—	—	—
Gelatin **[All analyses are for** **prepared gelatin]**										
Dia-Mel										
GELATIN DESSERTS, ½ c	8	1	0	<1	—	—	—	10	—	0
READY-TO-EAT GEL-A-THIN, ½ c	2	0	0	<1	—	—	—	0	—	5
Dzerta–General Foods										
all flavors, ½ c	8	2	0	0	0	*	*	5	50	—
Estee										
GELATIN DESSERT, ½ c	8	1	0	<1	—	—	—	10	—	0

FOOD & DESCRIPTION MEASURE OR QUANTITY	CALORIES	PROTEIN (GM)	FAT (GM)	CARBO-HYDRATE (GM)	FIBER (GM)	CALCIUM (MG)	IRON (MG)	SODIUM (MG)	POTASSIUM (MG)	CHOLES-TEROL (MG)
Jell-O–General Foods										
all flavors but those listed below, ½ c	80	2	0	19	0	*	*	50	0	—
BLACK RASPBERRY, ½ c	80	2	0	19	0	*	*	35	0	—
CHERRY, ½ c	80	2	0	19	0	*	*	70	0	—
CONCORD GRAPE, ½ c	80	2	0	19	0	*	*	35	0	—
LEMON, ½ c	80	2	0	19	0	*	*	75	0	—
LIME, ½ c	80	2	0	19	0	*	*	65	0	—
ORANGE-PINEAPPLE, ½ c	80	2	0	19	0	*	*	65	0	—
WILD STRAWBERRY, ½ c	80	2	0	19	0	*	*	75	0	—
SUGAR-FREE										
all flavors but those below, ½ c	8	1	0	0	0	*	*	55	0	—
CHERRY, ½ c	8	1	0	0	0	*	*	80	0	—
LIME, ½ c	8	1	0	0	0	*	*	60	0	—
MIXED FRUIT, ½ c	8	1	0	0	0	*	*	50	0	—
ORANGE, ½ c	8	1	0	0	0	*	*	50	0	—
STRAWBERRY-BANANA, ½ c	8	1	0	0	0	*	*	50	0	—
Royal–Nabisco										
APPLE, ½ c	80	2	0	19	—	*	*	95	0	—
BLACKBERRY, ½ c	80	2	0	19	—	*	*	95	0	—
CHERRY, ½ c	80	2	0	19	—	*	*	95	0	—
LEMON, ½ c	80	2	0	19	—	*	*	100	0	—
LEMON-LIME, ½ c	80	2	0	19	—	*	*	95	0	—
LIME, ½ c	80	2	0	19	—	*	*	90	0	—
ORANGE, ½ c	80	2	0	19	—	*	*	95	0	—
PEACH, ½ c	80	2	0	19	—	*	*	100	0	—
PINEAPPLE, ½ c	80	2	0	19	—	*	*	90	0	—
RASPBERRY, ½ c	80	2	0	19	—	*	*	95	0	—
STRAWBERRY, ½ c	80	2	0	19	—	*	*	100	0	—
SUGAR-FREE										
CHERRY, ½ c	12	2	0	0	—	*	*	70	0	—
LIME, ½ c	12	2	0	0	—	*	*	75	0	—
ORANGE, ½ c	12	2	0	0	—	*	*	70	0	—
RASPBERRY, ½ c	12	2	0	0	—	*	*	70	0	—
STRAWBERRY, ½ c	12	2	0	0	—	*	*	70	0	—
TROPICAL FRUIT, ½ c	80	2	0	19	—	*	*	95	0	—
USDA										
GELATIN MIX, dry, 1 pkg. 3 oz	315	8	0	75	—	—	—	270	—	—
prep, ½ c	71	2	0	17	—	—	—	61	—	—
Pudding										
Del Monte										
PUDDING CUPS										
BANANA, 5 oz, 142 gm	180	3	5	30	—	100	*	285	150	—
BUTTERSCOTCH, 5 oz, 142 gm	180	3	5	31	—	100	*	285	155	—
CHOCOLATE, 5 oz, 142 gm	190	4	6	31	—	100	.36	280	215	—
CHOCOLATE FUDGE, 5 oz, 142 gm	190	4	6	31	—	100	.72	260	295	—
TAPIOCA, 5 oz, 142 gm	180	3	4	30	—	100	*	250	180	—
VANILLA, 5 oz, 142 gm	180	3	5	32	—	100	<2	285	150	—
Dia-Mel										
BUTTERSCOTCH, ½ c	50	4	0	9	—	—	—	80	—	2
CHOCOLATE, ½ c	50	5	<1	9	—	—	—	80	—	2
LEMON, ½ c	14	0	0	4	—	—	—	20	—	0
VANILLA, ½ c	50	4	0	9	—	—	—	80	—	2

FOOD & DESCRIPTION MEASURE OR QUANTITY	CALORIES	PROTEIN (GM)	FAT (GM)	CARBO-HYDRATE (GM)	FIBER (GM)	CALCIUM (MG)	IRON (MG)	SODIUM (MG)	POTASSIUM (MG)	CHOLES-TEROL (MG)
Dzerta–General Foods										
BUTTERSCOTCH, REDUCED										
CALORIE MIX, 1 serving	25	0	0	6	tr	*	*	0	35	—
prep with skim milk, ½ c	70	4	0	12	tr	150	*	65	240	—
CHOCOLATE, REDUCED										
CALORIE MIX, 1 serving	20	0	0	5	tr	*	*	0	120	—
prep with skim milk, ½ c	60	5	0	11	tr	150	*	70	320	—
VANILLA, REDUCED CALORIE										
MIX, 1 serving	25	0	0	6	tr	*	*	0	0	—
prep with skim milk, ½ c	70	4	0	12	tr	150	*	65	200	—
Estee										
BUTTERSCOTCH, ½ c	70	4	<1	13	—	—	—	80	—	2
CHOCOLATE, ½ c	70	5	<1	13	—	—	—	75	—	2
LEMON, ½ c	70	4	<1	12	—	—	—	75	—	2
VANILLA, ½ c	70	4	<1	13	—	—	—	75	—	2
Jell-O–General Foods										
AMERICANA										
GOLDEN EGG CUSTARD MIX,										
1 serving	90	1	1	17	0	40	.36	160	95	—
prep with whole milk, ½ c	160	5	5	23	0	200	.36	220	280	—
RICE PUDDING MIX, 1										
serving	100	1	0	24	tr	*	.36	95	0	—
prep with whole milk, ½ c	170	1	5	30	tr	150	.36	160	190	—
TAPIOCA CHOCOLATE MIX, 1										
serving	90	1	1	22	tr	*	.36	110	120	—
prep with whole milk, ½ c	170	5	5	28	tr	150	.36	170	310	—
TAPIOCA VANILLA MIX, 1										
serving	90	0	0	22	tr	*	*	110	0	—
prep with whole milk, ½ c	160	4	4	27	tr	150	*	170	190	—
BANANA CREAM										
INSTANT MIX, 1 serving	90	0	0	23	tr	*	*	380	0	—
prep with whole milk, ½ c	160	4	4	28	tr	150	*	440	190	—
PUDDING & PIE MIX, 1										
serving	50	0	0	14	tr	*	*	125	0	—
prep with whole mix, filling										
for ⅛ pie	100	3	3	17	tr	100	*	165	125	—
BUTTER PECAN, INSTANT										
MIX, 1 serving	100	0	1	22	tr	*	*	380	10	—
prep with whole milk, ½ c	170	4	5	28	tr	150	*	440	190	—
BUTTERSCOTCH										
INSTANT MIX, 1 serving	90	0	0	23	tr	*	*	420	0	—
prep with whole milk, ½ c	160	4	4	28	tr	150	*	480	190	—
INSTANT, SUGAR-FREE MIX,										
1 serving	30	0	0	7	tr	*	*	360	0	—
prep with 2% fat milk, ½ c	90	4	2	13	tr	150	*	420	190	—
PUDDING & PIE FILLING										
MIX, 1 serving	90	0	0	24	tr	*	*	190	0	—
prep with whole milk, ½ c	170	4	4	30	tr	150	*	250	190	—
CHOCOLATE										
INSTANT MIX, 1 serving	100	0	0	25	tr	*	*	460	110	—
prep with whole milk, ½ c	180	4	4	30	tr	150	*	520	300	—
INSTANT, SUGAR-FREE MIX,										
1 serving	35	0	0	8	tr	*	*	350	95	—
prep with 2% fat milk, ½ c	100	5	3	14	tr	150	*	410	280	—
PUDDING & PIE FILLING										
MIX, 1 serving	90	1	0	22	tr	*	*	110	125	—
prep with whole milk, ½ c	160	5	4	28	tr	150	*	170	310	—
CHOCOLATE FUDGE										
INSTANT MIX, 1 serving	100	1	1	25	tr	*	*	420	170	—
prep with whole milk, ½ c	180	5	5	31	tr	150	.36	480	360	—

FOOD & DESCRIPTION MEASURE OR QUANTITY	CALORIES	PROTEIN (GM)	FAT (GM)	CARBO-HYDRATE (GM)	FIBER (GM)	CALCIUM (MG)	IRON (MG)	SODIUM (MG)	POTASSIUM (MG)	CHOLES-TEROL (MG)
PUDDING & PIE FILLING										
MIX, 1 serving	90	1	0	22	tr	*	*	110	150	—
prep with whole milk, ½ c	160	5	4	28	tr	150	*	170	340	—
CHOCOLATE MOUSSE PIE										
MIX, 1 serving	140	2	5	23	tr	*	.72	310	180	—
prep with whole milk, filling										
for ⅛ pie	220	3	12	26	tr	80	.72	400	260	—
COCONUT CREAM										
INSTANT MIX, 1 serving	100	0	3	20	tr	*	*	300	25	—
prep with whole milk, ½ c	180	4	7	26	tr	150	*	360	210	—
PUDDING & PIE FILLING										
MIX, 1 serving	60	0	2	12	tr	*	*	100	20	—
prep with whole milk, filling										
for ⅛ pie	110	3	4	16	tr	100	*	140	140	—
FRENCH VANILLA										
INSTANT MIX, 1 serving	90	0	0	23	tr	*	*	380	0	—
prep with whole milk, ½ c	160	4	4	28	tr	150	*	440	190	—
PUDDING & PIE FILLING, 1										
serving	90	0	0	24	tr	*	*	140	0	—
prep with whole milk, ½ c	170	4	4	30	tr	150	*	200	190	—
LEMON										
INSTANT MIX, 1 serving	90	0	0	23	tr	*	*	340	0	—
prep with whole milk, ½ c	170	4	4	29	tr	150	*	390	190	—
PUDDING & PIE FILLING, 1										
serving	50	0	0	13	tr	*	*	70	0	—
prep with whole milk, filling										
for ⅛ pie	170	2	2	38	tr	*	*	90	20	—
MILK CHOCOLATE										
INSTANT MIX, 1 serving	100	1	1	25	tr	*	*	450	95	—
prep with whole milk, ½ c	180	5	5	30	tr	150	*	510	280	—
PUDDING & PIE FILLING, 1										
serving	90	0	0	22	tr	*	*	110	65	—
prep with whole milk, ½ c	160	4	4	28	tr	150	*	170	250	—
PINEAPPLE CREAM, INSTANT										
MIX, 1 serving	90	0	0	23	tr	*	*	340	0	—
prep with whole milk, ½ c	160	4	4	29	tr	150	*	390	190	—
PISTACHIO, INSTANT MIX, 1										
serving	100	0	1	22	tr	*	*	380	10	—
prep with whole milk, ½ c	170	4	5	28	tr	150	*	440	190	—
VANILLA										
INSTANT MIX, 1 serving	90	0	0	23	tr	*	*	360	0	—
prep with whole milk, ½ c	170	4	4	29	tr	150	*	420	190	—
INSTANT, SUGAR-FREE MIX,										
1 serving	30	0	0	7	tr	*	*	360	0	—
prep with 2% fat milk, ½ c	90	4	2	13	tr	150	*	420	190	—
PUDDING & PIE FILLING										
MIX, 1 serving	80	0	0	21	tr	*	*	140	0	—
prep with whole milk, ½ c	160	4	4	27	tr	150	*	200	190	—
Junket–Kellogg										
CHOCOLATE RENNET										
CUSTARD										
prep with skim milk, ½ c	90	5	0	15	—	150	.36	70	223	—
prep with whole milk, ½ c	120	5	4	15	—	150	.36	65	205	—
RENNET TABLET, 1 tablet, .8										
gm	1	0	0	0	—	—	—	165	—	—
STRAWBERRY or RASPBERRY										
RENNET CUSTARD										
prep with skim milk, ½ c	90	4	0	16	—	150	*	65	203	—
prep with whole milk, ½ c	120	4	4	16	—	150	*	60	185	—
VANILLA RENNET CUSTARD										
prep with skim milk, ½ c	90	4	0	16	—	150	*	70	203	—
prep with whole milk, ½ c	120	4	4	16	—	150	*	65	185	—

FOOD & DESCRIPTION MEASURE OR QUANTITY	CALORIES	PROTEIN (GM)	FAT (GM)	CARBO-HYDRATE (GM)	FIBER (GM)	CALCIUM (MG)	IRON (MG)	SODIUM (MG)	POTASSIUM (MG)	CHOLES-TEROL (MG)
Laura Secord–Catelli										
BANANA, 5 oz, 142 gm	193	3	7	30	.01	109	.01	156	132	—
BUTTER PECAN, 5 oz. 142 gm	192	3	7	30	.01	109	.01	212	131	—
BUTTERSCOTCH, 5 oz, 142 gm	192	3	7	30	.01	107	.01	156	128	—
CHOCOLATE, 5 oz, 142 gm	199	3	7	32	.20	97	.38	169	132	—
CHOCOLATE FUDGE, 5 oz, 142 gm	199	4	7	33	.30	78	.58	179	298	—
CHOCOLATE MINT, 5 oz, 142 gm	193	4	7	31	.28	98	.58	187	142	—
MAPLE, 5 oz, 142 gm	196	3	7	31	.01	109	.01	158	132	—
MOCHA, 5 oz, 142 gm	189	3	7	30	.11	95	.26	165	128	—
RICE, 5 oz, 142 gm	172	3	7	24	tr	98	.26	206	115	—
TAPIOCA, 5 oz, 142 gm	151	3	5	24	tr	92	.04	149	111	—
VANILLA, 5 oz, 142 gm	192	3	7	29	.01	119	.01	234	203	—
Rich										
BUTTERSCOTCH FLAVORED, ½ c	133	2	6	18	—	26	.20	128	85	—
CHOCOLATE FLAVORED, ½ c	141	2	7	18	—	22	.64	136	111	—
VANILLA FLAVORED, ½ c	129	2	6	18	—	26	.17	162	85	—
Royal–Nabisco										
BANANA CREAM										
INSTANT MIX, 6 tbsp	100	0	1	24	—	*	*	330	5	—
prep with whole milk, ½ c	180	4	5	29	—	150	*	390	190	—
PUDDING & PIE FILLING MIX, 6 tbsp	80	0	1	20	—	*	*	150	5	—
prep with whole milk, ½ c	160	4	4	27	—	150	.36	210	190	—
BUTTERSCOTCH										
INSTANT MIX, 6 tbsp	100	0	1	24	—	*	*	330	5	—
prep with whole milk, ½ c	180	4	5	29	—	150	*	390	190	—
INSTANT, SUGAR-FREE MIX, 6 tbsp	40	0	0	10	—	*	*	410	5	—
prep with 2% fat milk, ½ c	100	4	2	16	—	150	*	470	200	—
PUDDING & PIE FILLING MIX, 6 tbsp	80	0	1	20	—	*	*	150	5	—
prep with whole milk, ½ c	160	4	4	27	—	150	.36	210	190	—
CHOCOLATE										
INSTANT MIX, 6 tbsp	120	1	1	25	—	*	*	330	75	—
prep with whole milk, ½ c	190	4	4	35	—	150	*	390	260	—
INSTANT, SUGAR-FREE MIX, 6 tbsp	50	0	0	11	—	*	*	420	130	—
prep with 2% fat milk, ½ c	110	5	3	17	—	150	*	480	330	—
PUDDING & PIE FILLING MIX, 6 tbsp	120	1	1	25	—	*	.36	90	75	—
prep with whole milk, ½ c	180	5	4	33	—	150	.72	150	260	—
CHOCOLATE CHOCOLATE, INSTANT MIX, 6 tbsp	120	0	1	27	—	*	*	330	35	—
prep with whole milk, ½ c	190	4	4	35	—	150	*	390	220	—
CHOCOLATE MINT, INSTANT MIX, 6 tbsp	120	0	1	27	—	*	*	330	35	—
prep with whole milk, ½ c	190	4	4	35	—	150	*	390	220	—
CUSTARD PUDDING & PIE FILLING MIX, 6 tbsp	60	0	0	15	—	*	*	55	25	—
prep with whole milk, ½ c	150	4	5	22	—	150	*	115	230	—
DARK 'N SWEET INSTANT MIX, 6 tbsp	120	0	1	27	—	*	*	330	35	—
prep with whole milk, ½ c	190	4	4	35	—	150	*	390	220	—
PUDDING & PIE FILLING MIX, 6 tbsp	120	1	1	25	—	*	*	90	125	—
prep with whole milk, ½ c	180	5	4	33	—	150	*	150	310	—

FOOD & DESCRIPTION MEASURE OR QUANTITY	CALORIES	PROTEIN (GM)	FAT (GM)	CARBO-HYDRATE (GM)	FIBER (GM)	CALCIUM (MG)	IRON (MG)	SODIUM (MG)	POTASSIUM (MG)	CHOLES-TEROL (MG)
FLAN WITH CARAMEL SAUCE,										
MIX, 6 tbsp	60	0	0	15	—	*	*	55	25	—
prep with whole milk, ½ c	150	4	5	22	—	150	*	115	230	—
KEY LIME PUDDING & PIE										
FILLING MIX, 6 tbsp	50	0	0	13	—	*	*	100	35	—
prep with whole milk, ½ c	160	1	3	30	—	*	*	120	55	—
LEMON, INSTANT MIX, 6 tbsp	110	0	1	24	—	*	*	290	10	—
prep with whole milk, ½ c	180	1	5	29	—	150	*	350	200	—
LEMON PIE FILLING MIX, 6										
tbsp	50	0	0	13	—	*	*	100	50	—
prep with whole milk, ½ c	160	1	3	30	—	*	.36	120	70	—
PISTACHIO NUT, INSTANT										
MIX, 6 tbsp	100	0	1	23	—	*	*	290	10	—
prep with whole milk, ½ c	170	4	4	30	—	150	*	350	200	—
TEMBLEQUE (COCONUT)										
PUDDING, MIX, 6 tbsp	80	0	1	20	—	*	*	150	5	—
prep with whole milk, ½ c	160	4	4	27	—	150	*	210	190	—
TOASTED BUTTER ALMONDS,										
INSTANT MIX, 6 tbsp	100	0	1	23	—	*	*	290	5	—
prep with whole milk, ½ c	170	4	4	30	—	150	*	350	190	—
TOASTED COCONUT, INSTANT										
MIX, 6 tbsp	100	0	1	23	—	*	*	290	10	—
prep with whole milk, ½ c	170	4	4	30	—	150	*	350	200	—
VANILLA										
INSTANT MIX, 6 tbsp	100	0	1	24	—	*	*	330	5	—
prep with whole milk, ½ c	180	4	5	29	—	150	*	390	200	—
INSTANT, SUGAR-FREE MIX,										
6 tbsp	40	0	0	10	—	*	*	410	5	—
prep with 2% fat milk, ½ c	100	4	2	16	—	150	*	470	200	—
PUDDING & PIE FILLING										
MIX, 6 tbsp	80	0	1	20	—	*	*	150	5	—
prep with whole milk, ½ c	160	4	4	27	—	150	*	210	190	—
VANILLA TAPIOCA MIX, 6 tbsp	80	0	1	20	—	*	*	150	5	—
prep with whole milk, ½ c	160	4	1	27	—	150	*	150	190	—

Sans Sucre–Bernard Foods

CHOCOLATE MOUSSE MIX, 1										
serving	60	1	3	5	—	30	*	54	190	3
½ c, prep	75	3	3	7	—	90	1.44	77	266	4
LEMON MOUSSE MIX, 1										
serving	53	*	3	7	—	*	*	26	37	3
½ c, prep	70	2	3	9	—	70	*	49	114	4

Sweet 'N Low–Bernard Foods

CHOCOLATE CUSTARD MIX, 1										
serving	25	1	<1	4	—	20	1.08	50	110	<5
prep with skim milk, ½ c	70	6	<1	10	—	150	1.08	115	290	5
LEMON CUSTARD MIX, 1										
serving	30	1	<1	5	—	40	.36	80	95	<5
prep with skim milk, ½ c	70	6	<1	11	—	200	.36	145	270	5
VANILLA CUSTARD MIX, 1										
serving	30	1	<1	5	—	40	.36	80	95	<5
prep with skim milk, ½ c	70	6	<1	11	—	200	.36	145	270	5

USDA

BREAD PUDDING WITH										
RAISINS, 1 c	496	15	16	75	—	289	2.90	533	570	180

9

ENTREES

FOOD & DESCRIPTION MEASURE OR QUANTITY	CALORIES	PROTEIN (GM)	FAT (GM)	CARBO-HYDRATE (GM)	FIBER (GM)	CALCIUM (MG)	IRON (MG)	SODIUM (MG)	POTASSIUM (MG)	CHOLES-TEROL (MG)
Canned										
Armour–Dial										
BEEF STEW, 8 oz	210	12	11	16	—	*	1.44	1190	—	—
CHILI MAC, 7.5 oz	220	7	12	20	—	—	—	1190	—	—
CHILI WITH BEANS, 7.5 oz	390	13	26	27	—	80	5.40	1080	—	—
CHILI WITHOUT BEANS, 7.5 oz	390	13	31	14	—	40	1.80	1140	—	—
CORNED BEEF HASH, 7.5 oz	410	18	28	18	—	20	4.50	1420	—	—
HOT CHILI, 7.5 oz	400	14	26	27	—	—	—	1080	—	—
PORK BRAINS IN MILK GRAVY, 2.75 oz	100	7	8	1	—	20	.72	410	—	—
ROAST BEEF HASH, 7.5 oz	350	19	22	21	—	20	3.60	1110	—	—
SLOPPY JOE BEEF, 7.6 oz	360	14	20	28	—	40	2.70	1700	—	—
TEXAS CHILI WITH BEANS, 7.5 oz	360	11	23	28	—	80	3.60	1240	—	—
Catelli										
RAVIOLI, 1 c	378	31	15	51	.80	59	3.99	1112	878	—
SPAGHETTI IN TOMATO AND CHEESE SAUCE, 1 c	245	7	3	47	.54	56	2.39	1291	382	—
Dia-Mel										
BEEF RAVIOLI, 8 oz	260	8	10	35	—	—	—	75	—	—
BEEF STEW, 8 oz	200	13	8	19	—	—	—	70	—	—
CHICKEN STEW, 8 oz	150	11	3	19	—	—	—	65	—	—
CHILI WITH BEANS, 8 oz	360	14	19	31	—	—	—	50	—	—
SPAGHETTI AND MEAT BALLS, 8 oz	220	8	10	24	—	—	—	55	—	—
STUFFED DUMPLINGS, 8 oz	160	10	6	15	—	—	—	70	—	—
Featherweight (Low sodium, ready to serve)										
BEEF RAVIOLI, LOW SODIUM, 8 oz	260	8	10	35	—	—	—	75	312	—
BEEF STEW, 7.5 oz	210	13	8	24	—	—	—	95	295	—
CHICKEN STEW, 7.5 oz	170	10	6	21	—	—	—	55	174	—
CHILI WITH BEANS, 7.5 oz	270	15	13	25	—	—	—	85	1102	—
DUMPLINGS & CHICKEN, 7.5 oz	160	12	5	18	—	—	—	115	760	—
SPAGHETTI WITH MEAT BALLS, 7.5 oz	200	8	5	28	—	—	—	95	863	—
SPANISH RICE, 7.5 oz	140	4	0	30	—	—	—	32	374	—

FOOD & DESCRIPTION MEASURE OR QUANTITY	CALORIES	PROTEIN (GM)	FAT (GM)	CARBO-HYDRATE (GM)	FIBER (GM)	CALCIUM (MG)	IRON (MG)	SODIUM (MG)	POTASSIUM (MG)	CHOLES-TEROL (MG)
Franco-American– Campbell										
BEEF RAVIOLI IN MEAT SAUCE, 7.5 oz	230	9	5	36	—	20	1.80	1090	—	—
BEEF RAVIOLIOS IN MEAT SAUCE, 7.5 oz	250	10	7	35	—	20	1.80	890	—	—
ELBOW MACARONI & CHEESE, 7.38 oz	170	6	6	23	—	80	1.44	910	—	—
MACARONI & CHEESE, 7.38 oz	170	6	5	24	—	80	1.44	960	—	—
SPAGHETTI IN MEAT SAUCE, 7.5 oz	210	8	8	26	—	20	1.80	1110	—	—
IN TOMATO SAUCE WITH CHEESE, 7.38 oz	190	5	2	36	—	40	1.80	810	—	—
WITH MEATBALLS IN TOMATO SAUCE, 7.38 oz	220	9	8	28	—	20	1.80	820	—	—
SPAGHETTIOS IN TOMATO & CHEESE SAUCE, 7.5 oz	170	4	2	34	—	20	1.08	910	—	—
WITH MEATBALLS IN TOMATO SAUCE, 7.38 oz	210	9	8	25	—	20	1.80	910	—	—
WITH BEEF FRANKS, TOMATO SAUCE, 7.38 oz	210	7	7	28	—	20	1.80	990	—	—
UFOS, 7.5 oz	180	5	3	35	—	20	1.80	780	—	—
WITH METEORS (MEATBALLS), 7.5 oz	240	9	9	30	—	20	1.80	790	—	—
Heinz										
BEANS 'N' FRANKS, 7.75 oz	330	14	15	34	—	100	2.70	905	—	—
BEEF GOULASH, 7.5 oz	240	13	11	22	—	*	1.80	920	—	—
BEEF STEW, 7.5 oz	210	12	9	19	—	20	1.80	1245	—	—
CHICKEN STEW WITH DUMPLINGS, 7.5 oz	210	9	9	22	—	40	1.08	850	—	—
CHILI CON CARNE, 7.75 oz	350	15	21	27	—	60	3.60	1000	—	—
CHILI MAC, 7.5 oz	250	10	12	26	—	60	1.80	860	—	—
HOT CHILI WITH BEANS, 7.75 oz	330	15	16	30	—	100	2.70	1140	—	—
MAC 'N' BEEF IN TOMATO SAUCE, 7.25 oz	200	8	8	23	—	20	1.80	850	—	—
MACARONI AND CHEESE, 7.5 oz	190	5	8	26	—	100	1.80	1105	—	—
NOODLES AND BEEF IN SAUCE, 7.5 oz	170	8	8	17	—	20	1.80	825	—	—
NOODLES AND CHICKEN, 7.5 oz	160	6	7	19	—	20	.72	930	—	—
NOODLES AND TUNA, 7.5 oz	170	11	5	20	—	20	1.08	950	—	—
SPAGHETTI IN TOMATO SAUCE WITH CHEESE, 7.75 oz	160	4	2	30	—	20	.72	1105	—	—
SPAGHETTI IN TOMATO SAUCE WITH MEAT, 7.5 oz	170	8	6	21	—	20	1.80	965	—	—
SPANISH RICE, 7.25 oz	150	3	5	26	—	20	1.08	1045	—	—
Hormel										
AU GRATIN POTATOES & BACON, 7.5 oz	240	9	14	20	—	—	—	942	—	—
BEEF GOULASH, individual, 7.5 oz	230	14	12	17	—	—	—	—	—	—
BEEF TAMALES, 2 tamales	140	4	10	8	—	—	—	550	—	—

131

FOOD & DESCRIPTION MEASURE OR QUANTITY	CALORIES	PROTEIN (GM)	FAT (GM)	CARBO-HYDRATE (GM)	FIBER (GM)	CALCIUM (MG)	IRON (MG)	SODIUM (MG)	POTASSIUM (MG)	CHOLES-TEROL (MG)
individual, 7.5 oz	270	8	19	17	—	—	—	1140	—	—
CHILI BEANS IN SAUCE, 5 oz	130	6	3	19	—	—	—	453	—	—
CHILI MAC, individual, 7.5 oz	200	11	10	16	—	—	—	1418	—	—
CHILI NO BEANS, 7.5 oz	370	17	28	12	—	—	—	1012	—	—
individual, 7.5 oz	360	18	27	11	—	—	—	961	—	—
CHILI WITH BEANS, 7.5 oz	310	17	17	23	—	—	—	1127	—	—
individual, 7.5 oz	280	17	14	23	—	—	—	1134	—	—
DINTY MOORE										
BEEF STEW, 8 oz	220	12	12	15	—	—	—	980	—	—
individual, 7.5 oz	180	12	9	14	—	—	—	939	—	—
BRUNSWICK STEW, individual, 7.5 oz	220	11	13	15	—	—	—	—	—	—
CHICKEN STEW, individual, 7.5 oz	240	11	16	14	—	—	—	—	—	—
MEATBALL STEW, 8 oz	240	13	15	15	—	—	—	—	—	—
NOODLES & CHICKEN, individual, 7.5 oz	210	9	12	15	—	—	—	1144	—	—
SLICED POTATOES 'N BEEF, individual, 7.5 oz	250	11	12	25	—	—	—	—	—	—
VEGETABLE STEW, 8 oz	170	5	8	20	—	—	—	1047	—	—
GREAT BEGINNINGS, WITH CHUNKY BEEF, 5 oz	136	12	7	7	—	—	—	904	—	—
CHICKEN, 5 oz	147	14	8	5	—	—	—	567	—	—
PORK, 5 oz	140	14	8	5	—	—	—	567	—	—
TURKEY, 5 oz	138	11	8	7	—	—	—	585	—	—
HOT CHILI NO BEANS, 7.5 oz	370	17	28	12	—	—	—	985	—	—
HOT CHILI WITH BEANS, 7.5 oz	310	16	16	24	—	—	—	1121	—	—
individual, 7.5 oz	300	16	16	23	—	—	—	1086	—	—
HOT 'N SPICY BEEF TAMALES, 2 tamales, 15 oz	140	4	10	9	—	—	—	612	—	—
LASAGNA, individual, 7.5 oz	260	8	14	25	—	—	—	1083	—	—
MARY KITCHEN										
CORNED BEEF HASH, 7.5 oz	360	20	24	19	—	—	—	1386	—	—
individual, 7.5 oz	360	20	24	17	—	—	—	1368	—	—
ROAST BEEF HASH, 7.5 oz	350	20	22	18	—	—	—	1142	—	—
individual, 7.5 oz	360	20	23	18	—	—	—	1156	—	—
NOODLES 'N BEEF, individual, 7.5 oz	230	10	14	16	—	—	—	974	—	—
SCALLOPED POTATOES AND HAM, individual, 7.5 oz	260	9	16	19	—	—	—	1189	—	—
SCALLOPED POTATOES & PEPPERONI, individual, 7.5 oz	246	8	15	21	—	—	—	—	—	—
SPAGHETTI AND BEEF, individual, 7.5 oz	260	8	14	25	—	—	—	1091	—	—
SPAGHETTI AND ITALIAN SAUSAGE, individual, 7.5 oz	187	9	9	19	—	—	—	1369	—	—
SPAGHETTI AND MEATBALLS, individual, 7.5 oz	210	10	8	26	—	—	—	—	—	—
Libby										
BEEF STEW, 7.5 oz	160	12	5	18	—	20	1.44	—	—	—
8 oz	170	12	6	19	—	20	1.80	—	—	—
CHILI NO BEANS, 7.5 oz	390	18	30	11	—	20	3.60	—	—	—
CHILI WITH BEANS, 7.5 oz	270	13	13	25	—	40	2.70	810	390	—
8 oz	290	14	14	27	—	60	3.60	860	410	—
CORNED BEEF HASH, 7.5 oz	400	18	27	20	—	20	1.80	1260	370	—
8 oz	420	19	28	21	—	20	1.80	1330	390	—
Swanson—Campbell										
CHICKEN A LA KING, 5.25 oz	180	10	12	9	—	40	.72	690	—	—

FOOD & DESCRIPTION MEASURE OR QUANTITY	CALORIES	PROTEIN (GM)	FAT (GM)	CARBO-HYDRATE (GM)	FIBER (GM)	CALCIUM (MG)	IRON (MG)	SODIUM (MG)	POTASSIUM (MG)	CHOLES-TEROL (MG)
CHICKEN & DUMPLINGS, 7.5 oz	220	11	12	19	—	20	.72	960	—	—
CHICKEN STEW, 7.63 oz	170	9	7	16	—	20	.72	960	—	—
USDA										
BEANS AND FRANKFURTERS, 1 c	367	19	18	32	—	94	4.80	1374	668	—
CHILI CON CARNE, 15–15.5 oz	572	32	26	53	—	138	7.30	2283	1002	—
1 c	339	19	16	31	—	82	4.30	1354	594	—

Dried

Catelli

MACARONI & CHEESE, prep, 1½ c	425	16	6	77	.28u	246	3.31	582	710	—

Chicken Helper– General Mills

CHICKEN AND DUMPLINGS, ⅕ pkg	220	6	3	41	—	80	1.80	1220	250	—
prep with chicken	530	34	26	41	—	80	2.70	1320	470	—
CHICKEN AND MUSHROOM, ⅕ pkg	160	3	2	32	—	40	1.08	900	170	—
prep with chicken	480	31	25	32	—	40	1.80	1000	390	—
POTATO AND GRAVY, ⅕ pkg	220	5	2	44	—	40	1.08	880	570	—
prep with chicken, milk & butter	600	34	32	45	—	80	1.80	1050	830	—
STUFFING, ⅕ pkg	190	7	1	37	—	40	1.80	1500	170	—
prep with chicken & margarine	590	35	33	37	—	40	2.70	1710	390	—
TERIYAKI CHICKEN, ⅕ pkg	180	4	1	39	—	40	1.44	970	190	—
prep with chicken	500	32	24	39	—	40	2.70	1070	410	—

Hamburger Helper– General Mills

BEEF NOODLE, ⅕ pkg	140	5	2	26	—	20	1.80	1000	90	—
prep with ⅕ lb ground beef	320	20	15	26	—	20	3.60	1050	290	—
BEEF ROMANOFF, ⅕ pkg	170	6	3	30	—	60	1.80	1030	200	—
prep with ⅕ lb ground beef	350	21	16	30	—	60	3.60	1080	400	—
CHEESEBURGER MACARONI, ⅕ pkg	180	6	5	28	—	60	1.08	980	190	—
prep with ⅕ lb ground beef	360	21	18	28	—	60	2.70	1030	390	—
CHILI TOMATO, ⅕ pkg	150	5	1	31	—	20	1.08	1320	220	—
prep with ⅕ ground beef	330	20	14	31	—	20	2.70	1360	420	—
HAMBURGER HASH, ⅕ pkg	140	3	2	27	—	20	.72	970	370	—
prep with ⅕ lb ground beef	320	18	15	27	—	20	2.50	1020	570	—
HAMBURGER PIZZA DISH, ⅕ pkg	180	6	1	37	—	20	1.80	960	290	—
prep with ⅕ lb ground beef	360	21	14	37	—	20	3.60	1010	490	—
HAMBURGER STEW, ⅕ pkg	120	3	1	25	—	40	1.08	960	320	—
prep with ⅕ lb ground beef	300	18	14	25	—	40	2.70	1010	520	—
LASAGNA, ⅕ pkg	170	5	<1	35	—	20	1.80	1020	310	—
prep with ⅕ lb ground beef	340	20	13	35	—	20	3.60	1070	510	—
PIZZA BAKE, ⅙ pkg	150	4	2	29	—	40	1.44	800	180	—
prep with ⅙ lb ground beef	320	19	14	29	—	40	2.70	840	350	—
POTATOES AU GRATIN, ⅕ pkg	150	4	2	28	—	40	.72	860	360	—
prep with ⅕ lb ground beef	320	19	15	28	—	40	2.70	910	560	—
POTATO STROGANOFF, ⅕ pkg	140	3	2	28	—	20	.36	850	320	—
prep with ⅕ lb ground beef	320	18	15	28	—	20	1.80	900	520	—
RICE ORIENTAL, ⅕ pkg	180	4	1	38	—	20	1.08	1070	110	—

FOOD & DESCRIPTION MEASURE OR QUANTITY	CALORIES	PROTEIN (GM)	FAT (GM)	CARBO-HYDRATE (GM)	FIBER (GM)	CALCIUM (MG)	IRON (MG)	SODIUM (MG)	POTASSIUM (MG)	CHOLES-TEROL (MG)
prep with ⅕ lb ground beef	340	19	14	38	—	20	2.70	1120	310	—
SPAGHETTI, ⅕ pkg	170	5	2	32	—	20	1.80	1060	300	—
prep with ⅕ lb ground beef	340	20	15	32	—	20	3.60	1110	500	—
TACO BAKE, ⅙ pkg	170	4	3	31	—	40	.72	900	160	—
prep with ⅙ lb ground beef	310	17	13	31	—	40	2.70	940	330	—
TAMALE PIE, ⅕ pkg	200	4	3	39	—	20	1.08	890	180	—
prep with ⅕ lb ground beef	380	19	16	39	—	20	2.70	940	380	—

Prince

MACARONI & CHEESE, 1.8 oz										
dry	180	7	1	36	—	60	1.80	400	350	—
prep, ¾ c	300	9	12	40	—	80	1.80	500	350	—

Tuna Helper—General Mills

AU GRATIN, ⅕ pkg	180	6	5	27	—	40	1.08	800	100	—
prep with tuna, milk & margarine	300	16	13	29	—	100	1.80	1110	270	—
COLD SALAD, ⅕ pkg	150	5	1	29	—	*	1.08	620	110	—
prep with tuna & mayonnaise	450	14	30	29	—	*	1.44	1060	220	—
CREAMY NOODLES 'N TUNA, ⅕ pkg	230	6	9	32	—	20	1.80	800	190	—
prep with tuna, milk & butter	290	14	12	32	—	20	1.80	960	280	—
NOODLES, CHEESE SAUCE 'N TUNA, ⅕ pkg	190	7	5	30	—	40	1.44	750	160	—
prep with tuna, milk & butter	250	15	8	30	—	40	1.80	910	250	—
TUNA TETRAZZINI, ⅕ pkg	160	7	3	26	—	60	1.44	630	90	—
prep with tuna, milk & butter	270	17	11	26	—	80	1.80	860	200	—

Frozen

Banquet

BARBECUE SAUCE & SLICED BEEF, cooking bag, 4 oz	133	9	5	13	—	16	2	929	234	—
BEANS & FRANKS DINNER, 10.25 oz	500	19	19	64	—	153	5	1377	685	—
BEEF DINNER, EXTRA HELPING, 16 oz	864	40	46	72	—	97	5	1731	904	—
BEEF ENCHILADA cooking bag, 6 oz	215	8	5	34	—	8	1	980	87	—
DINNER, 12 oz	497	19	15	72	—	109	4	1805	419	—
entree, 8 oz	264	11	8	37	—	52	1	1477	92	—
BEEF MEAT PIE, 8 oz	557	15	34	47	—	22	2	964	214	—
BEEF MEAT PIE SUPREME, 8 oz	380	18	17	38	—	17	3	1245	186	—
BEEF STEW, entree, 8 oz	254	12	13	21	—	23	2	977	308	—
BEEF WITH GRAVY DINNER, 10 oz	345	23	19	19	—	59	3	1009	624	—
CHEESE ENCHILADA DINNER, 12 oz	543	22	19	71	—	281	3	2166	429	—
EXTRA HELPING DINNER, 21.25 oz	777	31	27	105	—	411	5	4778	712	—
CHEESE MANICOTTI & MEAT, entree, 5.33 oz	232	14	9	23	—	211	2	891	244	—
CHICKEN ALA KING, cooking bag, 5 oz	159	14	7	10	—	128	1	645	284	—
CHICKEN & DRESSING, EXTRA HELPING DINNER, 19 oz	808	38	34	89	—	109	3	1817	737	—
CHICKEN & DUMPLINGS, EXTRA HELPING DINNER, 19 oz	883	40	40	91	—	241	3	1923	949	—

FOOD & DESCRIPTION MEASURE OR QUANTITY	CALORIES	PROTEIN (GM)	FAT (GM)	CARBO- HYDRATE (GM)	FIBER (GM)	CALCIUM (MG)	IRON (MG)	SODIUM (MG)	POTASSIUM (MG)	CHOLES- TEROL (MG)
CHICKEN MEAT PIE, 8 oz	520	16	30	45	—	36	1	1027	180	—
CHICKEN MEAT PIE										
SUPREME, 8 oz	430	17	22	40	—	36	2	1325	138	—
CHOPPED BEEF DINNER, 11										
oz	434	19	30	23	—	69	3	1199	658	—
EXTRA HELPING DINNER, 18										
oz	1028	40	67	70	—	104	5	1792	872	—
CREAMED CHIP BEEF, cooking										
bag, 4 oz	125	11	5	8	—	112	1	1082	202	—
FISH DINNER, 8.75 oz	553	18	33	45	—	62	6	927	601	—
FISH & CHIPS, EXTRA										
HELPING DINNER, 14 oz	769	28	32	97	—	74	3.	972	1091	—
FRIED CHICKEN DINNER, 11										
oz	359	18	11	46	—	89	2	1831	674	—
EXTRA HELPING DINNER, 17										
oz	744	31	28	92	—	130	3	2780	751	—
GRAVY & SALISBURY STEAK,										
entree, 5.33 oz	235	12	18	5	—	11	1	744	108	—
GRAVY & SLICED BEEF,										
entree, 8 oz	344	13	29	6	—	10	2	890	103	—
GRAVY & SLICED TURKEY										
cooking bag, 5 oz	137	10	8	4	—	17	1	471	119	—
entree, 5.33 oz	134	11	8	4	—	18	1	576	120	—
GRAVY WITH SLICED BEEF,										
cooking bag, 4 oz	136	9	9	4	—	6	1	492	97	—
HAM DINNER, 10 oz	532	21	22	61	—	80	4	1148	530	—
ITALIAN STYLE DINNER, 12 oz	597	21	26	71	—	79	4	1783	527	—
LASAGNA WITH MEAT, entree,										
8 oz	372	21	13	42	—	255	3	1190	338	—
MACARONI & CHEESE										
CASSEROLE, entree, 8 oz	344	11	17	36	—	210	1	930	135	—
cooking bag, 5 oz	227	7	11	25	—	133	0	583	91	—
entree, 8 oz	336	11	16	37	—	198	1	871	134	—
MEAT LOAF										
cooking bag, 5 oz	251	14	17	10	—	24	2	894	254	—
DINNER, 11 oz	437	20	27	30	—	80	3	1525	702	—
EXTRA HELPING DINNER,										
19 oz	984	39	57	80	—	151	5	2396	1042	—
entree, 6 oz	302	17	21	12	—	28	2	1032	296	—
MEXICAN STYLE DINNER, 12										
oz	483	18	18	62	—	110	3	1995	439	—
COMBINATION DINNER, 12										
oz	518	20	17	72	—	194	3	1978	423	—
MOSTACCIOLI & SAUCE,										
entree, 8 oz	251	11	8	34	—	30	2	1421	390	—
SALISBURY STEAK										
cooking bag, 5 oz	251	13	20	5	—	11	1	729	117	—
DINNER, 11 oz	395	17	26	24	—	62	2	1333	514	—
EXTRA HELPING DINNER,										
19 oz	1024	39	65	72	—	127	4	2175	851	—
SPAGHETTI WITH MEAT										
SAUCE CASSEROLE, 8										
oz	270	14	8	35	—	29	3	1242	421	—
TUNA MEAT PIE, 8 oz	510	17	27	48	—	101	1	1305	264	—
TURKEY DINNER, 11 oz	320	19	9	41	—	98	2	1416	639	—
EXTRA HELPING DINNER, 19										
oz	723	31	23	98	—	176	4	2165	946	—
TURKEY MEAT PIE, 8 oz	526	18	32	41	—	56	1	1111	167	—
TURKEY MEAT PIE SUPREME,										
8 oz	430	17	22	41	—	35	3	1370	167	—
VEAL PARMAGIAN										
cooking bag, 5 oz	293	11	17	23	—	144	1	853	173	—
DINNER, 11 oz	413	14	21	43	—	121	3	1310	468	—

FOOD & DESCRIPTION MEASURE OR QUANTITY	CALORIES	PROTEIN (GM)	FAT (GM)	CARBO-HYDRATE (GM)	FIBER (GM)	CALCIUM (MG)	IRON (MG)	SODIUM (MG)	POTASSIUM (MG)	CHOLES-TEROL (MG)
EXTRA HELPING DINNER, 20 oz	1092	30	57	116	—	249	4	2123	545	—
entree, 6.4 oz	277	9	16	25	—	62	1	842	181	—
WESTERN DINNER, 11 oz	513	22	29	43	—	93	4	1548	643	—

Benihana [Numbers are approximate]

BEEF SZECHUAN	398	—	14	—	—	—	—	1650	—	—
CHICKEN IN TERIYAKI SAUCE	373	—	8	—	—	—	—	1050	—	—
ORIENTAL BEEF & BROCCOLI	314	—	6	—	—	—	—	1400	—	—
ORIENTAL CHICKEN & MUSHROOMS	358	—	6	—	—	—	—	1400	—	—
ORIENTAL CHICKEN & SNOW PEAS	258	—	7	—	—	—	—	1100	—	—
ORIENTAL PEPPER STEAK	342	—	6	—	—	—	—	1200	—	—
ROAST PORK & CHINESE VEGETABLES	295	—	5	—	—	—	—	1660	—	—
ROAST PORK LO MEIN	404	—	17	—	—	—	—	1770	—	—
SHRIMP & LOBSTER SAUCE	308	—	6	—	—	—	—	1200	—	—
SHRIMP & VEGETABLES	304	—	5	—	—	—	—	1200	—	—
SLICED BEEF & VEGETABLES	395	—	10	—	—	—	—	1500	—	—
SWEET & SOUR CHICKEN	410	—	3	—	—	—	—	600	—	—

Budget Gourmet

CHICKEN AND COUNTRY VEGETABLES WITH RICE	280	16	10	32	—	—	—	495	—	—
CHICKEN & EGG NOODLES WITH BROCCOLI	450	23	26	31	—	—	—	1110	—	—
CHICKEN WITH FETTUCINE	400	23	21	29	—	—	—	740	—	—
LINGUINI WITH SHRIMP	330	15	15	33	—	—	—	1250	—	—
PASTA SHELLS AND BEEF	340	20	14	35	—	—	—	985	—	—
PEPPER STEAK WITH RICE	300	15	9	39	—	—	—	800	—	—
SIRLOIN TIPS WITH COUNTRY STYLE VEGETABLES	310	16	18	21	—	—	—	570	—	—
SPAGHETTI AND SAUCE WITH VEAL & MUSHROOM	320	13	14	33	—	—	—	1010	—	—
SWEDISH MEATBALLS	600	23	39	40	—	—	—	1085	—	—
SWEET & SOUR CHICKEN WITH RICE	350	18	7	53	—	—	—	640	—	—
THREE CHEESE LASAGNA	400	22	17	38	—	—	—	760	—	—
TURKEY A LA KING WITH RICE	390	20	18	36	—	—	—	740	—	—

Celentano

BROCCOLI STUFFED SHELLS WITH SAUCE, 11.5 oz	385	24	14	44	—	300	3.60	670	—	—
CANNELLONI FLORENTINE WITH SAUCE, 12 oz	370	18	17	36	—	300	2.70	540	—	—
CAVATELLI, 3.2 oz	270	12	1	57	—	20	4.14	100	—	—
CHICKEN CUTLETS PARMIGIANA WITH SAUCE, 9 oz	330	30	18	13	—	500	7.20	555	—	—
CHICKEN PRIMAVERA, 11.5 oz	270	25	10	18	—	150	12.60	580	—	—
EGGPLANT PARMIGIANA, 7 oz	270	9	12	32	—	130	2.88	330	—	—
WITH SAUCE, 8 oz	330	12	22	22	—	150	4.14	405	—	—
EGGPLANT ROLLETTES WITH SAUCE, 11 oz	420	18	30	18	—	250	2.70	510	—	—
LASAGNA, 6.25 oz	250	15	7	58	—	300	4.50	325	—	—
WITH SAUCE, 8 oz	320	14	16	30	—	200	2.88	410	—	—
LASAGNA PRIMAVERA, 11 oz	300	17	9	36	—	250	2.70	500	—	—
MANICOTTI, 7 oz	380	24	18	34	—	500	7.20	420	—	—

FOOD & DESCRIPTION MEASURE OR QUANTITY	CALORIES	PROTEIN (GM)	FAT (GM)	CARBO-HYDRATE (GM)	FIBER (GM)	CALCIUM (MG)	IRON (MG)	SODIUM (MG)	POTASSIUM (MG)	CHOLES-TEROL (MG)
WITH SAUCE, 8 oz	300	18	15	22	—	210	3.34	435	—	—
MINI ROUND CHEESE RAVIOLI, 4 oz	250	13	6	37	—	80	1.62	180	—	—
ROUND CHEESE RAVIOLI, 6.5 oz	410	22	12	51	—	230	3.96	360	—	—
STUFFED SHELLS, 4 shells, 6.25 oz	350	20	15	33	—	350	5.40	265	—	45
WITH SAUCE, 8 oz	320	19	14	30	—	210	3.42	425	—	—

Classic Lite—Armour

BABY BAY SHRIMP IN SHERRIED CREAM SAUCE, 10.5 oz	280	17	8	34	—	150	.72	1220	490	105
BEEF PEPPER STEAK, 10 oz	240	16	7	28	1.40	20	2.70	1020	380	55
CHICKEN BURGUNDY, 11.25 oz	230	21	5	26	1.60	60	2.70	1220	530	75
CHICKEN CHOW MEIN, 10.5 oz	220	20	4	25	—	20	1.08	1180	240	—
CHICKEN ORIENTAL, 10.5 oz	250	24	6	26	.60	20	1.44	880	330	75
MEDALLIONS OF CHICKEN BREAST MARSALA, 11 oz	270	22	7	28	—	60	1.08	970	470	80
ROAST BREAST OF CHICKEN, 11 oz	270	22	9	26	—	100	.72	1220	560	—
SALISBURY STEAK, 10 oz	290	20	13	25	—	40	2.70	870	780	—
SEAFOOD, NATURAL HERBS, 11.5 oz	250	12	6	38	1.90	150	1.44	1240	340	25
STEAK DIANE MIGNONETTES, 10 oz	290	29	9	23	—	80	2.70	770	760	85
STUFFED CABBAGE, 12 oz	290	13	8	43	—	100	2.70	600	780	—
SWEET AND SOUR CHICKEN, 11 oz	250	23	3	33	—	60	1.80	640	400	70
SZECHUAN BEEF, 10 oz	280	23	9	26	—	40	2.70	1010	520	—
TURF & SURF, 10 oz	250	31	7	14	1.20	60	1.80	890	520	105
TURKEY PARMESAN, 11 oz	240	19	8	25	1.60	100	1.80	480	770	75

Dinner Classics—Armour

BEEF BURGUNDY, 10.5 oz	330	30	14	23	.90	40	3.60	990	510	95
BEEF STROGANOFF, 11.25 oz	370	31	17	23	1.40	100	2.70	1330	570	90
BONELESS BEEF SHORT RIBS, 10.5 oz	460	26	25	31	1.60	100	3.60	1180	580	95
CHICKEN FRICASSEE, 11.75 oz	330	23	12	32	1.60	100	1.80	1210	420	75
CHICKEN HAWAIIAN, 11.5 oz	360	24	9	46	—	40	1.80	700	—	—
CHICKEN MILANO, 11.5 oz	380	25	12	42	—	80	3.60	1360	—	—
COD ALMONDINE, 12 oz	360	23	15	33	1.40	60	1.80	1440	550	75
LASAGNA, 10 oz	380	18	17	39	1.40	200	1.44	1120	510	75
SALISBURY STEAK, 11 oz	470	20	26	39	1.60	80	2.70	1400	580	105
SEAFOOD NEWBURG, 10.5 oz	270	12	10	33	1.00	200	1.80	1500	260	65
SIRLOIN TIPS, 11 oz	380	33	17	28	1.00	100	1.80	1180	740	100
SPAGHETTI WITH MEATBALLS, 11 oz	380	17	24	25	—	100	3.60	1300	—	—
STUFFED GREEN PEPPERS, 12 oz	360	16	16	37	2.50	80	2.70	1750	600	70
SWEDISH MEATBALLS, 11.5 oz	470	23	28	32	1.20	100	2.70	1560	670	125
SWEET & SOUR CHICKEN, 11 oz	410	14	17	50	1.30	80	1.08	1240	420	65
SWEET & SOUR PORK, 12 oz	490	36	18	48	1.60	100	1.80	870	490	95
TERIYAKI CHICKEN, 10.5 oz	340	14	15	38	.90	60	1.08	1340	400	70
TERIYAKI STEAK, 10 oz	360	24	16	33	1.00	40	1.80	1440	520	95

FOOD & DESCRIPTION MEASURE OR QUANTITY	CALORIES	PROTEIN (GM)	FAT (GM)	CARBO-HYDRATE (GM)	FIBER (GM)	CALCIUM (MG)	IRON (MG)	SODIUM (MG)	POTASSIUM (MG)	CHOLES-TEROL (MG)
VEAL PARMIGIANA, 10.75 oz	380	17	20	36	1.50	100	2.70	1430	440	85
YANKEE POT ROAST, 11 oz	370	31	12	34	—	40	4.50	820	—	—

Green Giant—Pillsbury

FOOD & DESCRIPTION MEASURE OR QUANTITY	CALORIES	PROTEIN (GM)	FAT (GM)	CARBO-HYDRATE (GM)	FIBER (GM)	CALCIUM (MG)	IRON (MG)	SODIUM (MG)	POTASSIUM (MG)	CHOLES-TEROL (MG)
BEEF BURGUNDY WITH RICE AND CARROTS, 9 oz	270	18	6	36	—	20	1.44	860	235	—
BEEF CHOW MEIN WITH RICE AND VEGETABLES, 10 oz	240	14	6	33	—	40	1.44	1050	280	—
BEEF STEW, boiling bag, 9 oz	180	18	3	20	—	20	2.70	275	220	—
BEEF STROGANOFF WITH NOODLES, 9 oz	370	21	16	34	—	60	3.60	870	250	—
BEEF TERIYAKI STIR FRY, 10 oz	330	20	10	40	—	20	1.80	760	440	—
BONELESS BEEF RIBS IN BBQ SAUCE WITH CORN ON COB, 1 pkg	400	31	10	46	—	40	2.70	1220	890	—
CASHEW CHICKEN STIR FRY, 10 oz	350	20	14	37	—	20	1.80	1025	435	—
CHICKEN ALA KING WITH BISCUITS, 9 oz	370	20	15	38	—	100	1.80	1500	275	—
CHICKEN AND BROCCOLI WITH RICE IN CHEESE SAUCE, 9.5 oz	340	23	15	28	—	200	.72	890	325	—
CHICKEN AND GARDEN VEGETABLES STIR FRY, 10 oz	240	17	6	29	—	40	1.80	670	500	—
CHICKEN AND NOODLES WITH VEGETABLES, 9 oz	370	22	16	34	—	150	1.80	1045	265	—
CHICKEN AND PEA PODS IN SAUCE WITH RICE AND VEGETABLES, 10 oz	320	15	13	36	—	20	.72	1005	225	—
CHICKEN CACCIATORE, 9 oz	320	22	13	28	—	60	2.70	740	470	—
CHICKEN CHOW MEIN WITH RICE AND VEGETABLES, 9 oz	240	18	5	30	—	20	.72	1070	225	—
CHICKEN IN BBQ SAUCE WITH CORN ON COB, 1 pkg	330	29	5	42	—	40	1.80	730	920	—
CHICKEN IN HERB BUTTER WITH STUFFED POTATO, 1 pkg	430	32	26	31	—	60	1.08	860	910	—
CHICKEN LASAGNA, 12 oz	640	39	32	47	—	800	2.70	1220	370	—
CHICKEN PROVENCALE, 10 oz	300	21	10	31	—	60	1.80	670	500	—
LASAGNA, boiling bag, 9.5 oz	290	16	6	42	—	150	2.70	1145	475	—
LASAGNA WITH MEAT SAUCE, 10.5 oz	430	26	16	45	—	450	3.60	1515	580	—
single serving	490	33	20	44	—	500	3.60	1660	610	—
MACARONI AND CHEESE, boiling bag, 9 oz	290	13	10	36	—	200	1.44	1115	385	—
MY CLASSIC LASAGNA, 10.5 oz	430	28	17	40	—	400	1.80	1210	630	—
SALISBURY STEAK WITH CREOLE SAUCE, boiling bag, 9 oz	410	31	26	11	—	20	4.50	910	675	—
SALISBURY STEAK WITH GRAVY, 7 oz	280	15	19	11	—	20	1.80	1095	285	—
SALISBURY STEAK WITH MASHED POTATOES, 11 oz	430	20	27	26	—	100	2.70	1600	560	—
SHRIMP CREOLE, 9 oz	230	11	5	35	—	60	2.70	370	370	—
SHRIMP IN CREAMY HERB SAUCE WITH LINGUINE, 9.5 oz	330	13	16	34	—	80	1.80	780	140	—

FOOD & DESCRIPTION MEASURE OR QUANTITY	CALORIES	PROTEIN (GM)	FAT (GM)	CARBO-HYDRATE (GM)	FIBER (GM)	CALCIUM (MG)	IRON (MG)	SODIUM (MG)	POTASSIUM (MG)	CHOLES-TEROL (MG)
SHRIMP FRIED RICE STIR FRY, 10 oz	300	14	5	49	—	60	1.08	1130	420	—
SPINACH LASAGNA, 12 oz	540	20	14	41	—	450	4.50	1455	445	—
STEAK & GREEN PEPPERS IN SAUCE WITH RICE AND VEGETABLES, 9 oz	260	17	6	34	—	20	1.80	1140	335	—
STUFFED CABBAGE ROLLS WITH BEEF IN TOMATO SAUCE, ½ pkg	220	8	12	19	—	40	1.08	800	365	—
STUFFED GREEN PEPPERS, ½ pkg	200	9	10	18	—	20	1.44	725	400	—
SWEET AND SOUR CHICKEN STIR FRY, 10 oz	300	15	6	47	—	40	1.08	585	395	—
SWEET AND SOUR MEATBALLS WITH RICE AND VEGETABLES, 9.4 oz	350	13	8	56	—	20	1.80	855	305	—
SWISS STEAK IN GRAVY WITH STUFFED POTATO, 1 pkg	360	25	12	38	—	60	3.60	1010	1120	—
SZECHUWUAN BEEF STIR FRY, 10 oz	280	21	10	26	—	60	2.70	580	520	—
TURKEY BREAST SLICES WITH WHITE AND WILD RICE STUFFING, 9 oz	460	18	28	34	—	40	1.44	1235	240	—

Hormel

BEEF BURRITOS, 1 burrito	205	9	8	31	—	—	—	780	—	—
BEEF ENCHILADAS, 1 enchilada	140	6	5	17	—	—	—	573	—	—
BEEF TAMALES, 1 tamale	140	6	7	13	—	—	—	555	—	—
BURRITO GRANDE, 5.5 oz	380	14	16	45	—	—	—	877	—	—
CHEESE BURRITO, 1 burrito	210	9	5	32	—	—	—	792	—	—
CHEESE ENCHILADAS, 1 enchilada	151	6	6	18	—	—	—	676	—	—
CHICKEN & RICE BURRITOS, 1 burrito	200	9	4	32	—	—	—	594	—	—
HOT CHILI BURRITOS, 1 burrito	240	9	8	33	—	—	—	619	—	—

Land O'Lakes

POUR-A-QUICHE

BACON & ONION, 4.33 oz	230	13	18	6	—	300	1.08	380	190	240
SPINACH & ONION, 4.33 oz	220	12	16	6	—	300	1.08	365	210	230
HAM, 4.33 oz	230	13	17	4	—	250	1.08	360	165	235
3 CHEESE, 4.33 oz	230	13	18	4	—	300	.72	385	170	250

Le Menu–Campbell

BEEF SIRLOIN TIPS, 11.5 oz	390	30	18	26	—	80	4.50	840	—	—
BEEF STROGANOFF, 9.25 oz	430	28	24	24	—	150	4.50	930	—	—
BREAST OF CHICKEN PARMIGIANA, 11.5 oz	380	27	18	28	—	150	2.70	890	—	—
CHICKEN A LA KING, 10.25 oz	320	22	13	29	—	60	1.80	1050	—	—
CHICKEN CORDON BLEU, 11 oz	460	26	19	47	—	100	2.70	870	—	—
CHICKEN FLORENTINE, 12.5 oz	480	28	23	40	—	150	3.60	880	—	—
CHOPPED SIRLOIN BEEF, 12.25 oz	410	26	23	28	—	150	4.50	1080	—	—
FLOUNDER FILLET WITH SALMON MOUSSE, 10.5 oz	340	20	18	26	—	100	2.70	1060	—	—
HAM STEAK, 9.25 oz	320	19	12	35	—	60	1.80	1510	—	—

FOOD & DESCRIPTION MEASURE OR QUANTITY	CALORIES	PROTEIN (GM)	FAT (GM)	CARBO-HYDRATE (GM)	FIBER (GM)	CALCIUM (MG)	IRON (MG)	SODIUM (MG)	POTASSIUM (MG)	CHOLES-TEROL (MG)
PEPPER STEAK, 11.5 oz	360	27	14	32	—	40	4.50	1110	—	—
SLICED BREAST OF TURKEY WITH MUSHROOMS, 11.25 oz	460	28	24	34	—	40	1.80	1140	—	—
SWEET AND SOUR CHICKEN, 11.25 oz	450	22	22	43	—	80	2.70	980	—	—
VEGETABLE LASAGNA, 11 oz	360	14	20	32	—	200	3.60	1010	—	—
YANKEE POT ROAST, 11 oz	360	28	15	28	—	40	4.50	810	—	—

Lean Cuisine–Stouffer's

BEEF & PORK CANNELLONI WITH MORNAY SAUCE, 9.63 oz	260	18	10	25	—	200	1.44	940	390	50
CHEESE CANNELLONI WITH TOMATO SAUCE, 9.13 oz	270	22	10	24	—	300	.72	950	310	45
CHICKEN A L'ORANGE WITH ALMOND RICE, 8 oz	280	27	5	32	—	20	.72	460	430	45
CHICKEN AND VEGETABLES WITH VERMICELLI, 12.75 oz	260	22	7	28	—	100	1.44	1250	360	40
CHICKEN CACCIATORE WITH VERMICELLI, 10.88 oz	280	23	10	25	—	40	1.80	1040	420	40
CHICKEN CHOW MEIN WITH RICE, 11.25 oz	250	16	5	36	—	20	1.08	1160	260	25
FILLET OF FISH DIVAN, 12.38 oz	270	31	9	17	—	200	1.08	770	820	85
FILLET OF FISH FLORENTINE, 9 oz	240	27	9	13	—	150	1.08	800	600	100
FILLET OF FISH JARDINIERE WITH SOUFFLEED POTATOES, 11.25 oz	280	30	10	18	—	150	.72	810	830	100
GLAZED CHICKEN WITH VEGETABLE RICE, 8.5 oz	270	26	8	23	—	20	.72	840	390	55
LINGUINI WITH CLAM SAUCE, 9.63 oz	260	16	7	32	—	20	1.80	860	120	40
MEATBALL STEW, 10 oz	250	22	9	20	—	40	2.70	1150	420	65
ORIENTAL BEEF WITH VEGETABLES AND RICE, 8.63 oz	260	18	8	30	—	20	1.44	1270	280	35
ORIENTAL SCALLOPS AND VEGETABLES WITH RICE, 11 oz	220	15	3	32	—	60	.72	1200	340	20
SALISBURY STEAK WITH ITALIAN STYLE SAUCE AND VEGETABLES, 9.5 oz	270	25	13	14	—	150	2.70	820	680	95
SPAGHETTI WITH BEEF & MUSHROOM SAUCE, 11.5 oz	280	15	7	38	—	60	2.70	1400	560	20
STUFFED CABBAGE WITH MEAT IN TOMATO SAUCE, 10.75 oz	210	14	9	19	—	60	1.80	830	560	40
ZUCCHINI LASAGNA, 11 oz	260	22	7	28	—	300	1.44	1050	550	20

Light and Elegant–Banquet

BEEF BURGUNDY WITH PARSLEY NOODLES, 9 oz	230	23	4	25	—	14	3.10	1235	200	—

FOOD & DESCRIPTION MEASURE OR QUANTITY	CALORIES	PROTEIN (GM)	FAT (GM)	CARBO-HYDRATE (GM)	FIBER (GM)	CALCIUM (MG)	IRON (MG)	SODIUM (MG)	POTASSIUM (MG)	CHOLES-TEROL (MG)
BEEF JULIENNE WITH RICE AND PEPPERS, 8.5 oz	260	21	7	27	—	27	4.90	990	240	—
BEEF STROGANOFF WITH PARSLEY NOODLES, 9 oz	260	24	6	27	—	45	3.00	785	230	—
BEEF TERIYAKI WITH RICE AND PEA PODS, 8 oz	240	18	3	37	—	30	5.60	625	215	—
CHICKEN IN BARBEQUE SAUCE WITH CORN & PECAN RICE, 8 oz	300	26	6	35	—	22	1.50	900	450	—
CHICKEN IN CHEESE SAUCE WITH RICE AND BROCCOLI, 9.5 oz	290	19	11	30	—	204	1.60	805	180	—
CHICKEN PARMIGIANA WITH PARSLEY NOODLES, 8 oz	260	28	6	23	—	73	2.80	685	310	—
GLAZED CHICKEN WITH VEGETABLE RICE, 8 oz	230	24	4	25	—	18	4.80	655	300	—
LASAGNA FLORENTINE, 11.25 oz	280	24	5	34	—	280	3.60	975	720	—
MACARONI & CHEESE WITH BREAD CRUMB TOPPING, 9 oz	300	15	9	37	—	238	2.00	1015	210	—
SHRIMP CREOLE WITH RICE AND PEPPERS, 10 oz	200	11	2	31	—	54	2.50	1045	200	—
SLICED TURKEY & GRAVY WITH WHITE AND WILD RICE STUFFING, 8 oz	230	20	5	25	—	18	1.00	1020	280	—
SPAGHETTI WITH MEAT SAUCE, 10.25 oz	290	16	8	40	—	100	6.00	700	273	—

Mrs. Paul's—Campbell

FOOD & DESCRIPTION MEASURE OR QUANTITY	CALORIES	PROTEIN (GM)	FAT (GM)	CARBO-HYDRATE (GM)	FIBER (GM)	CALCIUM (MG)	IRON (MG)	SODIUM (MG)	POTASSIUM (MG)	CHOLES-TEROL (MG)
FISH DIJON, 8.5 oz	250	24	14	7	—	80	1.44	650	—	—
FISH FLORENTINE, 9 oz	200	23	5	16	—	250	1.44	1025	—	—
FISH MORNAY, 10 oz	230	25	10	11	—	150	.72	665	—	—
SCALLOPS MEDITERRANEAN, 11 oz	250	17	5	36	—	60	2.70	775	—	—
SEAFOOD NEWBURG, 8.5 oz	310	14	13	34	—	80	1.44	610	—	—
SHRIMP ORIENTAL, 11 oz	230	11	2	42	—	80	1.08	940	—	—
SHRIMP PRIMAVERA, 11 oz	310	16	9	42	—	80	1.80	1185	—	—

Sara Lee

FOOD & DESCRIPTION MEASURE OR QUANTITY	CALORIES	PROTEIN (GM)	FAT (GM)	CARBO-HYDRATE (GM)	FIBER (GM)	CALCIUM (MG)	IRON (MG)	SODIUM (MG)	POTASSIUM (MG)	CHOLES-TEROL (MG)
BROCCOLI & CHEESE LE SAN*WICH, 1	320	10	18	30	—	100	1.44	610	—	—
CHICKEN & BROCCOLI LE SAN*WICH, 1	360	17	19	29	—	100	1.80	660	—	—
HAM & CHEESE LE SAN*WICH, 1	320	14	17	25	—	100	1.80	760	—	—
ROAST BEEF IN WINE LE SAN*WICH, 1	300	14	15	26	—	40	1.80	570	—	—

Stouffer's

FOOD & DESCRIPTION MEASURE OR QUANTITY	CALORIES	PROTEIN (GM)	FAT (GM)	CARBO-HYDRATE (GM)	FIBER (GM)	CALCIUM (MG)	IRON (MG)	SODIUM (MG)	POTASSIUM (MG)	CHOLES-TEROL (MG)
BEEF CHOP SUEY WITH RICE, 12 oz	340	19	12	38	—	20	1.80	1590	260	—
BEEF PIE, 10 oz	560	21	37	36	—	40	3.60	1300	180	—
BEEF & SPINACH STUFFED PASTA SHELLS WITH TOMATO SAUCE, 9 oz	300	21	12	27	—	150	1.80	1100	480	—
BEEF STEW, 10 oz	310	22	16	19	—	20	1.80	1460	530	—
BEEF STROGANOFF WITH PARSLIED NOODLES, 9.75 oz	410	25	21	2\'	—	60	2.70	1180	190	—

FOOD & DESCRIPTION MEASURE OR QUANTITY	CALORIES	PROTEIN (GM)	FAT (GM)	CARBO-HYDRATE (GM)	FIBER (GM)	CALCIUM (MG)	IRON (MG)	SODIUM (MG)	POTASSIUM (MG)	CHOLES-TEROL (MG)
BEEF TERIYAKI IN SAUCE WITH RICE & VEGETABLES, 9.75 oz	330	22	9	35	—	40	1.80	1260	300	—
CASHEW CHICKEN IN SAUCE WITH RICE, 9.5 oz	410	31	17	33	—	20	2.70	1240	580	—
CHEESE SOUFFLE, 6 oz	380	18	29	12	—	300	1.44	950	260	—
CHEESE STUFFED PASTA SHELLS WITH MEAT SAUCE, 9 oz	340	23	16	25	—	400	1.80	1200	500	—
CHICKEN A LA KING WITH RICE, 9.5 oz	320	20	11	36	—	80	1.08	840	200	—
CHICKEN CHOW MEIN WITHOUT NOODLES, 8 oz	140	12	5	11	—	20	.72	1170	200	—
CHICKEN CREPES WITH MUSHROOM SAUCE, 8.25 oz	370	27	21	18	—	150	1.44	930	400	—
CHICKEN DIVAN, 8.5 oz	350	23	22	14	—	200	1.08	850	420	—
CHICKEN PAPRIKASH WITH EGG NOODLES, 10.5 oz	390	32	15	31	—	60	1.80	1250	200	—
CHICKEN PIE, 10 oz	530	21	34	34	—	80	2.70	1210	250	—
CHICKEN STUFFED PASTA SHELLS WITH CHEESE SAUCE, 9 oz	420	29	24	21	—	350	1.08	810	190	—
CHILI CON CARNE WITH BEANS, 8.75 oz	280	21	11	23	—	80	3.60	1190	730	—
CREAMED CHICKEN, 6.5 oz	320	19	24	7	—	60	.36	700	200	—
CREAMED CHIP BEEF, 5.5 oz	230	12	17	8	—	100	1.08	890	300	—
ESCALLOPED CHICKEN & NOODLES, 5.75 oz	260	12	16	16	—	40	.72	720	150	—
GREEN PEPPER STEAK WITH RICE, 10.5 oz	330	22	10	38	—	20	1.80	1500	400	—
HAM & ASPARAGUS CREPES, 6.25 oz	310	14	18	24	—	150	1.08	750	350	—
HAM & SWISS CHEESE CREPES WITH CREAM SAUCE, 7.5 oz	410	23	26	21	—	400	1.08	980	370	—
LASAGNA, 10.5 oz	380	28	14	35	—	250	1.80	1020	630	—
LOBSTER NEWBURG, 6.5 oz	360	15	30	8	—	100	.36	840	150	—
MACARONI & BEEF WITH TOMATOES, 11.5 oz	360	21	16	32	—	60	2.70	1600	640	—
MACARONI & CHEESE, 6 oz	250	11	12	24	—	200	.36	750	140	—
ROAST BEEF HASH, 5.75 oz	250	18	15	11	—	*	1.80	710	350	—
SALISBURY STEAK WITH ONION GRAVY, 6 oz	230	20	14	6	—	20	2.70	1120	300	—
SCALLOPS & SHRIMP MARINER WITH RICE, 10.25 oz	390	21	18	35	—	150	.72	850	300	—
SHORT RIBS OF BEEF WITH VEGETABLE GRAVY, 5.75 oz	280	24	20	2	—	*	2.70	510	280	—
SPAGHETTI WITH MEATBALLS, 12.63 oz	390	21	14	44	—	150	1.80	1800	600	—
SPAGHETTI WITH MEAT SAUCE, 14 oz	440	22	15	53	—	100	4.50	1730	850	—
SPINACH CREPES WITH CHEDDAR CHEESE SAUCE, 9.5 oz	420	17	27	27	—	300	2.70	1100	470	—
STUFFED GREEN PEPPER WITH BEEF IN TOMATO SAUCE, 7.75 oz	220	11	11	18	—	150	1.08	870	310	—
SWEDISH MEATBALLS IN GRAVY WITH PARSLIED NOODLES, 11 oz	470	25	25	36	—	60	3.60	1460	350	—

FOOD & DESCRIPTION MEASURE OR QUANTITY	CALORIES	PROTEIN (GM)	FAT (GM)	CARBO-HYDRATE (GM)	FIBER (GM)	CALCIUM (MG)	IRON (MG)	SODIUM (MG)	POTASSIUM (MG)	CHOLES-TEROL (MG)
TUNA NOODLE CASSEROLE, 5.75 oz	190	11	8	18	—	80	.72	680	200	—
TURKEY CASSEROLE WITH GRAVY & DRESSING, 9.75 oz	380	24	19	28	—	100	1.80	1250	450	—
TURKEY PIE, 10 oz	540	20	35	36	—	80	1.80	1260	200	—
TURKEY TETRAZZINI, 6 oz	230	13	14	14	—	60	.72	650	200	—
VEGETABLE LASAGNA, 10.5 oz	450	26	25	29	—	500	1.08	910	460	—
WELSH RAREBIT, 5 oz	360	13	30	9	—	400	.36	700	150	—

Swanson–Campbell

FOOD & DESCRIPTION MEASURE OR QUANTITY	CALORIES	PROTEIN (GM)	FAT (GM)	CARBO-HYDRATE (GM)	FIBER (GM)	CALCIUM (MG)	IRON (MG)	SODIUM (MG)	POTASSIUM (MG)	CHOLES-TEROL (MG)
BEAN & BEEF BURRITO DINNER, 15.25 oz	720	21	32	88	—	150	4.50	1630	—	—
BEEF DINNER, 11.5 oz	320	27	8	35	—	20	4.50	870	—	—
BEEF ENCHILADAS ENTREE, 11.25 oz	440	16	20	49	—	100	3.60	1190	—	—
HUNGRY MAN, 16 oz	660	21	35	65	—	200	6.30	2010	—	—
DINNER, 15 oz	510	18	23	57	—	150	3.60	1400	—	—
BEEF MEAT PIE, 8 oz	400	11	21	42	—	20	2.70	900	—	—
HUNGRY MAN, 16 oz	670	23	34	68	—	20	5.40	1750	—	—
BONELESS CHICKEN, HUNGRY MAN DINNER, 17.5 oz ep	670	47	27	60	—	80	6.30	1640	—	—
CHICKEN NIBBLES, 5 oz ep	390	13	25	28	—	20	3.60	880	—	—
CHICKEN MEAT PIE, 8 oz	420	13	24	39	—	20	1.80	840	—	—
HUNGRY MAN, 16 oz	700	26	37	64	—	60	4.50	1670	—	—
CHICKEN PARMIGIANA, HUNGRY MAN, 20 oz	810	34	51	53	—	300	2.70	2080	—	—
CHOPPED BEEF STEAK, HUNGRY MAN, 17.25 oz	600	36	29	48	—	60	7.20	1640	—	—
CHOPPED SIRLOIN OF BEEF DINNER, 11.5 oz	350	21	17	29	—	80	4.50	930	—	—
CHUNKY BEEF MEAT PIE, 10 oz	530	19	28	53	—	20	3.60	900	—	—
CHUNKY CHICKEN MEAT PIE, 10 oz	580	19	33	53	—	40	2.70	850	—	—
CHUNKY TURKEY MEAT PIE, 10 oz	530	19	31	45	—	20	1.80	950	—	—
FISH 'N' CHIPS, DINNER, 10.5 oz	570	21	28	58	—	40	3.60	970	—	—
HUNGRY MAN, 14.75 oz	770	36	36	73	—	100	3.60	1350	—	—
ENTREE, 5.5 oz	320	11	17	32	—	20	1.80	600	—	—
FRIED CHICKEN DINNER, BARBECUE FLAVORED, 9.25 oz ep	560	24	30	49	—	150	3.60	960	—	—
BREAST PORTION DINNER, 10.75 oz ep	650	26	33	63	—	60	5.40	1580	—	—
HUNGRY MAN, 14 oz ep	880	37	49	73	—	60	4.50	2120	—	—
ENTREE, HUNGRY MAN, 11.75 oz ep	670	34	37	50	—	100	4.50	1760	—	—
DARK MEAT DINNER, 10.25 oz	610	24	32	55	—	60	4.50	1390	—	—
HUNGRY MAN, 14 oz ep	860	37	46	75	—	60	5.40	1680	—	—
ENTREE, DARK MEAT, 7.25 oz ep	390	19	21	30	—	40	2.70	1070	—	—
HUNGRY MAN, 11 oz ep	620	33	36	42	—	60	4.50	1370	—	—
GRAVY AND SLICED BEEF ENTREE, 8 oz	200	18	6	18	—	20	2.70	760	—	—
LASAGNA DINNER, 13 oz	410	12	16	55	—	150	2.70	800	—	—
LASAGNA WITH MEAT ENTREE, 13.25 oz	450	23	18	50	—	300	3.60	1120	—	—
HUNGRY MAN DINNER,										

FOOD & DESCRIPTION MEASURE OR QUANTITY	CALORIES	PROTEIN (GM)	FAT (GM)	CARBO-HYDRATE (GM)	FIBER (GM)	CALCIUM (MG)	IRON (MG)	SODIUM (MG)	POTASSIUM (MG)	CHOLES-TEROL (MG)
18.75 oz	730	25	26	99	—	300	7.20	1510	—	—
LOIN OF PORK DINNER, 11.25 oz	290	22	11	26	—	20	1.80	710	—	—
MACARONI AND BEEF DINNER, 12 oz	360	11	14	46	—	100	2.70	850	—	—
MACARONI AND CHEESE DINNER, 12.25 oz	380	13	15	46	—	200	1.80	980	—	—
ENTREE, 12 oz	380	15	16	45	—	250	2.70	1850	—	—
POT PIE, 7 oz	210	8	9	26	—	150	1.08	880	—	—
MEATBALLS WITH BROWN GRAVY ENTREE, 8.5 oz	290	14	18	19	—	40	2.70	900	—	—
MEAT LOAF DINNER, 11 oz	500	19	26	48	—	100	3.60	970	—	—
MEAT LOAF WITH TOMATO SAUCE ENTREE, 9 oz	310	16	15	28	—	60	1.80	950	—	—
MEXICAN DINNER, HUNGRY MAN, 22 oz	920	28	46	99	—	350	5.40	2430	—	—
MEXICAN STYLE COMBINATION DINNER, 16 oz	580	20	26	67	—	150	4.50	1780	—	—
NOODLES AND CHICKEN DINNER, 10.5 oz	270	11	9	37	—	40	1.80	820	—	—
POLYNESIAN STYLE DINNER, 12 oz	360	21	8	52	—	60	2.70	1430	—	—
SALISBURY STEAK DINNER, 11 oz	460	21	22	44	—	80	4.50	1050	—	—
HUNGRY MAN, 16.5 oz	690	40	40	42	—	200	6.30	1630	—	—
ENTREE, 5.5 oz	340	18	21	19	—	40	2.70	650	—	—
HUNGRY MAN, 11.75 oz	610	39	38	29	—	100	7.20	1340	—	—
MAIN COURSE, 10 oz	380	26	21	26	—	40	3.60	1400	—	—
SLICED BEEF DINNER, HUNGRY MAN, 16 oz	470	40	12	49	—	40	5.40	1150	—	—
ENTREE, HUNGRY MAN, 12.25 oz	330	40	8	24	—	20	4.50	1040	—	—
SPAGHETTI AND MEATBALLS DINNER, 12.5 oz	360	12	15	44	—	100	2.70	1040	—	—
SPAGHETTI IN TOMATO SAUCE WITH BREADED VEAL ENTREE, 8.25 oz	280	15	12	29	—	40	2.70	810	—	—
STEAKBURGER MEAT PIE, HUNGRY MAN, 16 oz	750	27	44	61	—	40	4.50	1520	—	—
SWISS STEAK DINNER, 10 oz	350	23	14	33	—	40	4.50	830	—	—
TURKEY DINNER, 11.5 oz	330	21	10	39	—	40	2.70	1260	—	—
HUNGRY MAN, 18.5 oz	590	40	18	66	—	80	5.40	2150	—	—
ENTREE, 8.75 oz	250	17	10	24	—	20	1.80	1090	—	—
HUNGRY MAN, 13.25 oz	390	30	14	36	—	40	3.60	1740	—	—
MEAT PIE, 8 oz	430	12	24	41	—	20	1.80	800	—	—
HUNGRY MAN, 16 oz	740	27	41	66	—	40	4.50	1590	—	—
TURKEY WITH GRAVY ENTREE, 9.25 oz	300	28	10	24	—	20	2.70	1120	—	—
VEAL PARMIGIANA DINNER, 12.75 oz	470	22	21	49	—	150	3.60	1120	—	—
HUNGRY MAN, 20 oz	640	35	28	62	—	200	4.50	2010	—	—
WESTERN STYLE DINNER, 12.25 oz	440	23	19	45	—	60	4.50	1150	—	—
HUNGRY MAN, 17.5 oz	750	41	34	71	—	80	9.00	1930	—	—

Tyson

CHICKEN A L'ORANGE WITH FRUITED RICE PILAF, 8.25 oz	300	26	8	31	—	—	—	440	—	—

FOOD & DESCRIPTION MEASURE OR QUANTITY	CALORIES	PROTEIN (GM)	FAT (GM)	CARBO-HYDRATE (GM)	FIBER (GM)	CALCIUM (MG)	IRON (MG)	SODIUM (MG)	POTASSIUM (MG)	CHOLES-TEROL (MG)
CHICKEN CACCIATORE WITH PASTA PRIMAVERA, 10.5 oz	300	30	12	18	—	—	—	770	—	—
CHICKEN FIESTA WITH SPANISH RICE, 11 oz	420	32	20	27	—	—	—	1510	—	—
CHICKEN FRANCAIS WITH GREEN BEANS ALMONDINE, 8.75 oz	320	28	16	16	—	—	—	940	—	—
CHICKEN MARSALA WITH BROCCOLI/CHEESE POTATO SHELL, 10.5 oz	300	26	11	24	—	—	—	760	—	—
CHICKEN ORIENTAL, ORIENTAL VEGETABLES WITH RICE, 10.25 oz	300	26	8	31	—	—	—	1050	—	—
CHICKEN PARMIGIANA, PASTA WITH BUTTER SAUCE, 11.75 oz	450	34	18	38	—	—	—	1100	—	—
CHICKEN PICATTA, PARSLIED NEW POTATOES & BROCCOLI FLORETS, 9 oz	280	26	9	24	—	—	—	660	—	—
CHICKEN SWEET N' SOUR, RICE WITH CARROTS AND ALMONDS, 11 oz	440	29	17	42	—	—	—	840	—	—

Van de Kamp

FOOD & DESCRIPTION MEASURE OR QUANTITY	CALORIES	PROTEIN (GM)	FAT (GM)	CARBO-HYDRATE (GM)	FIBER (GM)	CALCIUM (MG)	IRON (MG)	SODIUM (MG)	POTASSIUM (MG)	CHOLES-TEROL (MG)
ALMOND CHICKEN CANTONESE WITH RICE, 11 oz	440	23	16	50	—	80	4.50	1220	—	—
BEEF AND MUSHROOM LASAGNA, 11 oz	430	26	23	30	—	450	3.60	970	—	—
BEEF AND VEGETABLES SZECHWAN WITH RICE, 11 oz	370	21	15	37	—	30	1.08	940	—	—
BEEF CHOW MEIN MANDARIN, 11 oz	310	20	9	40	—	100	5.40	1700	—	—
BEEF ENCHILADAS										
1 enchilada, 7.5 oz	250	12	13	21	—	160	1.80	1201	—	—
2 enchiladas, 5.5 oz	230	10	9	3	—	100	.72	664	—	—
4 enchiladas, 8.5 oz	340	16	16	33	—	240	4.86	1481	—	—
DINNER, 12 oz	390	18	15	45	—	190	3.42	2177	—	—
BEEF/CHEESE ENCHILADA WITH RICE & BEANS, 14.75 oz	540	27	22	59	—	350	3.60	1380	—	—
BEEF TOSTADA SUPREME, 8.5 oz	530	24	30	40	—	350	2.70	900	—	—
CHEESE ENCHILADAS										
1 enchilada, 7.5 oz	270	11	15	23	—	320	1.62	963	—	—
2 enchiladas, 5.5 oz	245	9	13	22	—	190	1.62	615	—	—
4 enchiladas, 8.5 oz	370	15	21	29	—	430	1.98	1177	—	—
DINNER, 12 oz	450	19	22	44	—	230	2.70	1664	—	—
RANCHERO, 5.5 oz	250	11	14	22	—	250	.72	540	—	—
WITH RICE & BEANS, 14.75 oz	620	24	31	60	—	500	2.88	1460	—	—
CHICKEN CHOW MEIN MANDARIN, 11 oz	340	21	9	42	—	100	7.20	1180	—	—
CHICKEN ENCHILADA, 7.5 oz	250	14	11	24	—	190	1.62	1108	—	—
CHICKEN ENCHILADA SUIZA, 5.5 oz	220	11	10	21	—	300	.72	590	—	—
CHICKEN SUIZA WITH RICE & BEANS, 14.75 oz	550	28	20	64	—	450	2.16	1210	—	—
CRISPY FRIED BURRITO, 6 oz	365	12	16	42	—	60	4.50	823	—	—

FOOD & DESCRIPTION MEASURE OR QUANTITY	CALORIES	PROTEIN (GM)	FAT (GM)	CARBO-HYDRATE (GM)	FIBER (GM)	CALCIUM (MG)	IRON (MG)	SODIUM (MG)	POTASSIUM (MG)	CHOLES-TEROL (MG)
EGG ROLLS CANTONESE, 5.25 oz	280	11	7	41	—	150	1.08	550	—	—
FILLET OF FISH DINNER, 12 oz	300	25	11	27	—	250	3.60	1820	—	—
GRANDE BURRITO WITH RICE & CORN, 14.75 oz	530	19	20	69	—	200	1.80	1210	—	—
GUACAMOLE PACKET, 1.25 oz	45	0	4	1	—	0	.36	85	—	—
ITALIAN SAUSAGE LASAGNA, 11 oz	440	25	23	34	—	450	3.60	1190	—	—
MEXICAN STYLE DINNER, 11.5 oz	420	19	20	43	—	160	1.08	1040	—	—
SHREDDED BEEF ENCHILADA, 5.5 oz	180	11	8	16	—	180	1.44	930	—	—
WITH RICE & CORN, 14.75 oz	490	28	15	60	—	150	1.08	1170	—	—
SHREDDED BEEF TAQUITOS WITH GUACAMOLE, 8 oz	490	17	26	47	—	100	4.50	990	—	—
SIRLOIN BURRITO GRANDE, 11 oz	440	25	18	45	—	200	3.60	1120	—	—
SWEET & SOUR PORK WITH RICE, 11 oz	430	13	13	67	—	60	1.08	790	—	—

Weight Watchers

FOOD & DESCRIPTION MEASURE OR QUANTITY	CALORIES	PROTEIN (GM)	FAT (GM)	CARBO-HYDRATE (GM)	FIBER (GM)	CALCIUM (MG)	IRON (MG)	SODIUM (MG)	POTASSIUM (MG)	CHOLES-TEROL (MG)
BAKED CHEESE RAVIOLI, 8.06 oz, 228 gm	290	16	11	32	—	200	1.80	685	605	
BEEFSTEAK IN GREEN PEPPER AND MUSHROOM SAUCE WITH CARROTS, 9.75 oz, 276 gm	320	22	21	15	—	100	1.80	1115	—	—
BEEF ORIENTAL WITH VEGETABLES AND RICE, 10 oz, 283 gm	260	22	4	32	—	80	3.60	1130	—	—
CHICKEN ALA KING, 9 oz, 255 gm	230	26	7	15	—	200	1.40	977	348	
CHICKEN CACCIATORE WITH SPAGHETTI, 10 oz, 283 gm	290	23	8	30	—	80	3.60	925	526	—
CHICKEN PARMIGIANA WITH VEGETABLE MEDLEY, 8 oz, 226 gm	290	21	16	13	—	250	.90	414	406	—
FILLET OF FISH AU GRATIN, BROCCOLI, 9.25 oz, 262 gm	200	23	7	14	—	150	1.80	835	386	—
ITALIAN CHEESE LASAGNA, 11 oz, 311 gm	350	19	16	33	—	400	1.80	1129	446	—
ITALIAN STYLE FISH FILLET IN TOMATO SAUCE WITH CHEESE, VEGETABLE MEDLEY, 9 oz, 255 gm	180	25	7	6	—	150	1.80	540	392	—
LASAGNA WITH MEAT, TOMATO SAUCE & CHEESE, 12 oz, 340 gm	360	22	13	38	—	200	1.80	1345	821	—
OVEN FRIED FISH, VEGETABLE MEDLEY, 6.75 oz, 191 gm	220	19	12	8	—	40	1.80	390	—	—
SIRLOIN OF BEEF, MUSHROOM SAUCE, GREEN BEANS, CAULIFLOWER, 13 oz, 369 gm	410	30	25	16	—	100	1.80	1425	620	—
SLICED TURKEY, GRAVY, AND STUFFING, CARROTS, BROCCOLI, 15.25 oz, 431 gm	380	36	12	32	—	150	2.70	1775	700	—

FOOD & DESCRIPTION MEASURE OR QUANTITY	CALORIES	PROTEIN (GM)	FAT (GM)	CARBO-HYDRATE (GM)	FIBER (GM)	CALCIUM (MG)	IRON (MG)	SODIUM (MG)	POTASSIUM (MG)	CHOLES-TEROL (MG)
SOLE IN LEMON SAUCE, PEAS & ONIONS, 9.13 oz, 259 gm	200	22	5	17	—	100	1.08	835	475	—
SOUTHERN FRIED CHICKEN PATTY, VEGETABLE MEDLEY, 6.75 oz, 191 gm	260	20	15	11	—	40	1.08	785	234	—
SPAGHETTI WITH MEAT SAUCE, 10.5 oz, 297 gm	280	16	8	36	—	60	2.70	835	606	—
SWEET N' SOUR CHICKEN, ORIENTAL VEGETABLES, 9 oz, 255 gm	210	18	4	26	—	40	1.08	535	336	—
VEAL PATTY PARMIGIANA, ZUCCHINI IN TOMATO SAUCE, 8.13 oz, 230 gm	230	24	11	9	—	150	1.80	605	519	—
VEAL STUFFED PEPPER, TOMATO SAUCE, 11.75 oz, 333 gm	240	24	6	22	—	40	1.80	1125	762	—
ZITI MACARONI WITH MEAT, TOMATO SAUCE AND CHEESE, 11.25 oz, 318 gm	290	21	9	30	—	150	1.80	1345	543	—

Pizzas

Applan Way–Armour

REGULAR, 3.13 oz	190	5	4	36	—	20	2.70	510	—	—
THICK CRUST, 5.25 oz	370	13	8	65	—	150	5.40	980	—	—

Celentano

NINE SLICE PIZZA WITH MOZZARELLA, 2.67 oz	157	9	5	20	—	60	.72	166	—	—
THICK CRUST PIZZA WITH MOZZARELLA, 4.3 oz	238	13	7	31	—	90	1.26	252	—	—

Celeste

CANADIAN STYLE BACON PIZZA										
7.75 oz pizza	541	27	26	50	.70	491	1.89	1593	444	—
19 oz, ¼ pizza, 4.75 oz piece	329	17	17	28	.50	301	1.21	976	290	—
CHEESE PIZZA										
6.5 oz pizza	497	21	25	48	.70	375	1.36	828	342	—
17.75 oz, ¼ pizza, 4.44 oz piece	317	14	17	28	.50	204	1.00	673	268	—
DELUXE PIZZA										
8.25 oz pizza	582	23	32	51	1.20	332	2.57	1308	498	—
22.25 oz, ¼ pizza, 5.56 oz piece	378	16	22	29	.80	267	1.85	953	352	—
PEPPERONI PIZZA										
6.75 oz pizza	546	20	30	50	.80	336	2.04	1417	416	—
19 oz, ¼ pizza, 5 oz piece	368	15	21	29	.50	186	1.42	1061	284	—
SAUSAGE PIZZA										
7.5 oz pizza	571	23	32	49	1.10	371	2.28	1374	456	—
20 oz, ¼ pizza, 5 oz piece	376	16	22	30	.70	322	1.52	988	311	—
SAUSAGE AND MUSHROOM PIZZA										
8.5 oz pizza	592	24	32	51	1.20	362	2.41	1347	549	—
22.5 oz, ¼ pizza, 6.25 oz piece	387	17	22	29	1.00	310	1.61	1033	361	—
SUPREME PIZZA										
9 oz pizza	678	27	39	54	1.30	454	2.73	1693	528	—
23 oz, ¼ pizza, 5.75 oz piece	381	17	24	29	.80	295	1.78	1043	342	—

FOOD & DESCRIPTION MEASURE OR QUANTITY	CALORIES	PROTEIN (GM)	FAT (GM)	CARBO-HYDRATE (GM)	FIBER (GM)	CALCIUM (MG)	IRON (MG)	SODIUM (MG)	POTASSIUM (MG)	CHOLES-TEROL (MG)
Fox Deluxe—Pillsbury										
CHEESE, ⅓ pizza	160	8	4	24	—	150	1.08	430	115	—
HAMBURGER, ⅓ pizza	190	8	7	24	—	80	1.80	510	160	—
PEPPERONI, ⅓ pizza	190	7	7	24	—	60	1.44	580	130	—
SAUSAGE, ⅓ pizza	190	7	7	24	—	80	1.44	590	140	—
SAUSAGE/PEPPERONI COMBINATION, ⅓ pizza	190	7	7	24	—	80	1.44	590	140	—
Ragu										
PIZZA QUICK MIX FOR HOMEMADE PIZZA CRUST, 1.6 oz	170	6	2	31	—	20	1.80	—	—	0
Stouffer's										
FRENCH BREAD PIZZA										
CHEESE, 5.19 oz serving	340	15	13	41	—	200	2.70	840	270	—
DELUXE, 6.19 oz serving	430	18	21	41	—	200	3.60	1130	360	—
HAMBURGER, 6.13 oz serving	410	21	18	40	—	200	3.60	1040	340	—
PEPPERONI, 5.63 oz serving	390	17	18	41	—	200	3.60	1040	310	—
SAUSAGE, 6 oz serving	420	18	20	42	—	200	2.70	1080	380	—
SAUSAGE & MUSHROOM, 6.25 oz serving	400	18	17	44	—	100	3.60	1160	380	—
Totino—Pillsbury										
EXTRA PIZZA										
CHEESE, ¼ pizza	250	11	12	24	—	200	1.08	450	110	—
PEPPERONI, ¼ pizza	260	10	14	24	—	150	1.44	700	170	—
SAUSAGE, ¼ pizza	280	10	16	24	—	150	1.44	770	200	—
SAUSAGE AND PEPPERONI COMBINATION, ¼ pizza	290	11	16	25	—	150	1.44	800	200	—
HEAT 'N EAT MICROWAVE PIZZA										
CHEESE, 4.1 oz	270	13	11	31	—	250	1.08	670	200	—
COMBINATION, 4.9 oz	380	14	21	31	—	200	1.80	1190	270	—
PEPPERONI, 4.6 oz	350	13	18	31	—	200	1.80	1070	230	—
SAUSAGE, 4.8 oz	360	13	20	31	—	200	1.80	1130	260	—
MICROWAVE PIZZA										
CHEESE, 3.9 oz	250	11	9	31	—	200	1.08	630	200	—
PEPPERONI, 4 oz	290	10	14	31	—	100	1.80	1270	190	—
SAUSAGE, 4.2 oz	300	10	15	31	—	100	1.44	920	240	—
SAUSAGE AND PEPPERONI COMBINATION, 4.2 oz	310	11	15	31	—	150	1.80	1090	230	—
MY CLASSIC										
CANADIAN STYLE BACON, ¼ pizza	320	16	12	38	—	200	1.80	830	230	—
DELUXE CHEESE, ¼ pizza	350	15	15	39	—	300	1.44	810	270	—
DELUXE COMBINATION, ¼ pizza	460	18	25	40	—	250	1.80	1040	350	—
DELUXE PEPPERONI, ¼ pizza	410	17	20	40	—	250	1.80	1090	330	—
DELUXE SAUSAGE, ¼ pizza	440	16	24	41	—	250	1.80	980	370	—
PARTY PIZZA										
CANADIAN STYLE BACON, ⅓ pizza	230	10	9	27	—	100	1.44	640	160	—
CHEESE, ⅓ pizza	240	10	10	28	—	200	1.08	480	120	—
HAMBURGER, ⅓ pizza	280	11	14	27	—	100	1.80	630	180	—
MEXICAN STYLE, ⅓ pizza	250	7	15	21	—	100	1.80	580	160	—
NACHO, ⅓ pizza	230	8	14	20	—	200	1.44	440	85	—
PEPPERONI, ⅓ pizza	260	9	12	28	—	100	1.44	700	140	—
SAUSAGE, ⅓ pizza	270	9	14	27	—	100	1.44	750	160	—
SAUSAGE AND PEPPERONI COMBINATION, ⅓ pizza	270	10	13	27	—	100	1.44	740	160	—

FOOD & DESCRIPTION MEASURE OR QUANTITY	CALORIES	PROTEIN (GM)	FAT (GM)	CARBO- HYDRATE (GM)	FIBER (GM)	CALCIUM (MG)	IRON (MG)	SODIUM (MG)	POTASSIUM (MG)	CHOLES- TEROL (MG)
SINGLE SERVE MICROWAVE PIZZA										
CHEESE, 7.1 oz	490	20	21	56	—	400	1.80	1170	340	—
COMBINATION, 9 oz	690	24	39	59	—	350	3.60	1750	460	—
PEPPERONI, 8.5 oz	610	23	31	59	—	350	3.60	1760	420	—
SAUSAGE, 8.75 oz	660	22	37	59	—	350	3.60	1620	440	—
Weight Watchers										
CHEESE PIZZA, 6 oz, 170 gm	350	20	14	37	—	350	1.80	740	1269	—
DELUXE COMBINATION PIZZA, 7.25 oz, 205 gm	340	20	12	38	—	250	1.80	850	—	—
PEPPERONI PIZZA, 6.25 oz, 177 gm	370	21	15	38	—	100	1.10	685	—	—
VEAL SAUSAGE PIZZA, 6.75 oz, 191 gm	350	24	12	35	—	250	1.80	930	—	—

10

FAST FOODS

FOOD & DESCRIPTION MEASURE OR QUANTITY	CALORIES	PROTEIN (GM)	FAT (GM)	CARBO-HYDRATE (GM)	FIBER (GM)	CALCIUM (MG)	IRON (MG)	SODIUM (MG)	POTASSIUM (MG)	CHOLES-TEROL (MG)
Beverages										
Arby's										
CHOCOLATE SHAKE, 10.6 oz, 300 gm	384	9	11	62	—	300	1.08	300	—	32
JAMOCHA SHAKE, 10.8 oz, 305 gm	424	8	10	76	—	300	1.08	280	—	31
VANILLA SHAKE, 8.8 oz, 250 gm	295	8	10	44	—	300	.72	245	—	30
Burger King										
CHOCOLATE SHAKE, 10 oz, 273 gm	320	8	12	46	—	—	—	202	567	—
with syrup added, 284 gm	374	8	11	60	—	—	—	225	590	—
VANILLA SHAKE, 10 oz, 273 gm	321	9	10	49	—	—	—	205	505	—
with syrup added, 284 gm	334	9	10	51	—	—	—	213	524	—
Dairy Queen										
FLOAT, 397 gm	410	5	7	82	—	200	1.08	85	—	20
FREEZE, 397 gm	500	9	12	89	—	300	1.80	180	—	30
MALT										
LARGE, 588 gm	1060	20	25	187	—	700	5.40	360	—	70
REGULAR, 418 gm	760	14	18	134	—	450	4.50	260	—	50
SMALL, 291 gm	520	10	13	91	—	350	2.70	180	—	35
MR. MISTY										
LARGE, 439 gm	340	0	0	84	—	*	*	<10	—	0
REGULAR, 330 gm	250	0	0	63	—	*	*	<10	—	0
SMALL, 248 gm	190	0	0	48	—	*	*	<10	—	0
FLOAT, 411 gm	390	5	7	74	—	200	.72	95	—	20
FREEZE, 411 gm	500	9	12	91	—	300	1.44	140	—	30
KISS, 89 gm	70	0	0	17	—	*	*	<10	—	0
SHAKE										
LARGE, 588 gm	990	19	26	168	—	700	3.60	360	—	70
REGULAR, 418 gm	710	14	19	120	—	450	2.70	260	—	50
SMALL, 291 gm	490	10	13	82	—	350	1.80	180	—	35
Hardee's										
MILKSHAKE, 326 gm	391	11	10	63	—	450	<1	—	652	42
McDonald's										
CHOCOLATE SHAKE, 291 gm	383	10	9	66	—	320	.84	300	—	30
STRAWBERRY SHAKE, 290 gm	362	9	9	62	—	322	.17	207	—	32
VANILLA SHAKE, 291 gm	352	9	8	60	—	329	.18	201	—	31

FOOD & DESCRIPTION MEASURE OR QUANTITY	CALORIES	PROTEIN (GM)	FAT (GM)	CARBO-HYDRATE (GM)	FIBER (GM)	CALCIUM (MG)	IRON (MG)	SODIUM (MG)	POTASSIUM (MG)	CHOLES-TEROL (MG)
Roy Rogers										
CHOCOLATE SHAKE, 319 gm	358	8	10	61	—	290	.47	290	—	37
HOT CHOCOLATE, 6 oz	123	3	2	22	—	80	*	125	—	35
STRAWBERRY SHAKE, 312 gm	315	8	10	49	—	284	.47	261	—	37
VANILLA SHAKE, 306 gm	306	8	11	45	—	300	.50	282	—	40

Breakfast Foods

Burger King

BREAKFAST CROISSAN'WICH individual ingredients										
BACON	51	3	5	0	—	—	—	125	33	6
CHEESE	42	2	3	1	—	—	—	142	12	11
CROISSANT	187	4	11	18	—	—	—	297	60	5
EGG MIX	75	5	5	1	—	—	—	198	77	227
HAM	31	6	1	0	—	—	—	350	107	19
SAUSAGE	234	9	22	0	—	—	—	405	136	50
BACON, total, 120 gm	355	14	24	20	—	—	—	762	182	249
HAM, total, 145 gm	335	17	20	20	—	—	—	987	256	262
SAUSAGE, total, 163 gm	538	20	41	20	—	—	—	1042	285	293
FRENCH TOAST PLATTER individual ingredients										
BACON	68	4	6	0	—	—	—	167	45	8
FRENCH TOAST	401	7	24	41	—	—	—	281	106	65
SAUSAGE	234	9	22	0	—	—	—	405	136	50
WITH BACON, total, 117 gm	469	11	30	41	—	—	—	448	151	73
WITH SAUSAGE, total, 158 gm	635	16	46	41	—	—	—	686	242	115
SCRAMBLED EGG PLATTER individual ingredients										
BACON	68	4	6	0	—	—	—	167	45	8
CROISSANT	187	4	11	18	—	—	—	298	60	5
EGG MIX	119	9	8	2	—	—	—	317	122	363
HASH BROWNS	162	2	11	13	—	—	—	193	305	2
SAUSAGE	234	9	22	0	—	—	—	405	136	50
WITH BACON, total, 206 gm	536	19	36	33	—	—	—	975	532	378
WITH SAUSAGE, total, 247 gm	702	24	52	33	—	—	—	1213	623	420

Hardee's

BACON & EGG BISCUIT, 114 gm	405	13	26	30	—	144	3	823	12	114
BISCUIT, 82 gm	275	5	13	35	—	149	2	650	117	82
WITH EGG, 158 gm	383	11	22	35	—	179	4	819	187	158
WITH JELLY, 100 gm	324	5	13	47	—	153	3	653	131	100
BISCUIT GRAVY, 195 gm	419	10	22	44	—	168	4	1090	238	21
EGG, FRIED, 1 medium, 50 gm	108	6	7	<1	—	30	<2	169	70	50
HAM & EGG BISCUIT, 184 gm	458	19	26	37	—	211	4	1585	305	184
HAM BISCUIT, 108 gm	349	12	17	37	—	181	3	1415	235	108
HASH ROUNDS, 71 gm	200	2	13	20	—	*	<1	310	300	10
SAUSAGE & EGG BISCUIT, 162 gm	521	16	35	34	—	169	<4	1033	287	162
SAUSAGE BISCUIT, 112 gm	413	10	26	34	—	134	<3	864	217	112
STEAK & EGG BISCUIT, 162 gm	527	20	31	41	—	151	<6	973	335	162
STEAK BISCUIT, 112 gm	419	14	23	41	—	121	<5	804	265	134

FOOD & DESCRIPTION MEASURE OR QUANTITY	CALORIES	PROTEIN (GM)	FAT (GM)	CARBO-HYDRATE (GM)	FIBER (GM)	CALCIUM (MG)	IRON (MG)	SODIUM (MG)	POTASSIUM (MG)	CHOLES-TEROL (MG)
McDonald's										
BISCUIT										
plain, 85 gm	330	5	18	37	—	74	1.30	786	—	9
WITH BACON, EGG & CHEESE, 145 gm	483	17	32	33	—	2	2.57	1269	—	263
WITH SAUSAGE, 121 gm	467	12	31	35	—	82	2.05	1147	—	48
WITH SAUSAGE & EGG, 175 gm	585	20	40	36	—	119	3.43	1301	—	285
EGG MCMUFFIN, 138 gm	340	19	16	31	—	226	2.93	885	—	259
ENGLISH MUFFIN WITH BUTTER, 63 gm	186	5	5	30	—	117	1.51	310	—	15
HASH BROWN POTATOES, 55 gm	125	2	7	14	—	5	.40	325	—	7
HOT CAKES WITH BUTTER & SYRUP, 214 gm	500	8	10	94	—	103	2.23	1070	—	47
SAUSAGE, 53 gm	210	10	19	<1	—	16	.82	423	—	39
SAUSAGE MCMUFFIN, 115 gm	427	18	26	30	—	168	2.25	942	—	59
WITH EGG, 165 gm	517	23	33	32	—	196	3.47	1044	—	287
SCRAMBLED EGGS, 98 gm	180	13	13	3	—	61	2.53	205	—	514
Roy Rogers										
BISCUIT, 63 gm	231	4	12	26	—	64	.34	575	—	<5
BREAKFAST CRESCENT SANDWICH, 127 gm	401	13	27	25	—	161	1.58	867	—	148
WITH BACON, 133 gm	431	15	30	26	—	164	1.66	1035	—	156
WITH HAM, 165 gm	557	20	42	25	—	167	2.14	1192	—	189
WITH SAUSAGE, 162 gm	449	20	29	26	—	163	1.85	1289	—	168
CRESCENT ROLL, 70 gm	287	5	18	27	—	52	.65	547	—	<5
DANISH										
APPLE, 71 gm	249	5	12	32	—	100	1.24	255	—	15
CHEESE, 71 gm	254	5	12	31	—	37	1.13	260	—	11
CHERRY, 71 gm	271	4	14	32	—	39	1.04	242	—	11
EGG AND BISCUIT PLATTER, 165 gm	394	17	27	22	—	117	2.30	734	—	284
WITH BACON, 173 gm	435	20	30	22	—	120	2.38	957	—	294
WITH HAM, 200 gm	442	24	29	23	—	120	2.57	1156	—	304
WITH SAUSAGE, 203 gm	550	23	41	22	—	123	2.86	1059	—	325
PANCAKES, SYRUP & BUTTER PLATTER, 165 gm	452	8	15	72	—	91	2.02	842	—	53
WITH BACON, 173 gm	493	10	18	72	—	94	2.11	1065	—	63
WITH HAM, 200 gm	506	14	17	72	—	94	2.29	1264	—	73
WITH SAUSAGE, 203 gm	608	14	30	72	—	97	2.57	1167	—	94
Wendy's										
BACON, 2 strips, 18 gm	110	5	10	<1	—	*	*	445	65	15
BREAKFAST SANDWICH, 129 gm	370	17	19	33	—	150	3.60	770	155	200
DANISH, 1 piece, 85 gm	360	6	18	44	—	20	1.80	340	—	—
FRENCH TOAST, 2 sl, 135 gm	400	11	19	45	—	80	1.80	850	175	115
HOME FRIES, 103 gm	360	4	22	37	—	20	.72	745	615	20
OMELETS										
#1, HAM & CHEESE, 114 gm	250	18	17	6	—	100	2.70	405	180	450
#2, HAM, CHEESE & MUSHROOM, 118 gm	290	18	21	7	—	100	2.70	570	190	355
#3, HAM, CHEESE, ONION, GREEN PEPPER, 128 gm	280	19	19	7	—	150	2.70	485	200	525
#4, MUSHROOM, ONION, GREEN PEPPER, 114 gm	210	14	15	7	—	60	2.70	200	190	460
SAUSAGE, 1 patty, 45 gm	200	9	18	<1	—	*	.72	410	125	30
SCRAMBLED EGG, 91 gm	190	14	12	7	—	60	2.70	160	130	450
TOAST WITH MARGARINE, 2 sl, 69 gm	250	6	9	35	—	20	2.70	410	80	0

FOOD & DESCRIPTION MEASURE OR QUANTITY	CALORIES	PROTEIN (GM)	FAT (GM)	CARBO-HYDRATE (GM)	FIBER (GM)	CALCIUM (MG)	IRON (MG)	SODIUM (MG)	POTASSIUM (MG)	CHOLES-TEROL (MG)
Desserts										
Arthur Treacher Fish and Chips										
LEMON LUVS, 3 oz	276	3	14	35	—	10	.85	314	—	<1
Burger King										
APPLE PIE, 125 gm	305	3	12	44	—	—	—	412	122	4
CHERRY PIE, 128 gm	357	4	13	55	—	—	—	204	166	6
PECAN PIE, 113 gm	459	5	20	64	—	—	—	374	204	4
Dairy Queen										
BANANA SPLIT, 383 gm	540	9	11	103	—	250	1.80	150	—	30
BUSTER BAR, 149 gm	460	10	29	41	—	100	1.08	175	—	10
CONE, LARGE, 213 gm	340	9	10	57	—	250	1.44	115	—	25
REGULAR, 142 gm	240	6	7	38	—	150	.72	80	—	15
SMALL, 85 gm	140	3	4	22	—	100	.36	45	—	10
CONE, CHOCOLATE DIPPED, LARGE, 234 gm	510	9	24	64	—	250	1.44	145	—	30
REGULAR, 156 gm	340	6	16	42	—	150	.72	100	—	20
SMALL, 92 gm	190	3	9	25	—	100	.36	55	—	10
DILLY BAR, 85 gm	210	3	13	21	—	100	.36	50	—	10
DOUBLE DELIGHT PARFAIT, 255 gm	490	9	20	69	—	200	1.44	150	—	25
DQ SANDWICH, 60 gm	140	3	4	24	—	60	*	40	—	5
HOT FUDGE BROWNIE DELIGHT, 266 gm	600	9	25	85	—	200	1.80	225	—	20
PARFAIT, 283 gm	430	8	8	76	—	250	1.44	140	—	30
PEANUT BUSTER PARFAIT, 305 gm	740	16	34	94	—	250	1.80	250	—	30
STRAWBERRY SHORTCAKE, 312 gm	540	10	11	100	—	250	1.80	215	—	25
SUNDAE, CHOCOLATE, LARGE, 248 gm	440	8	10	78	—	250	1.44	165	—	30
REGULAR, 177 gm	310	5	8	56	—	200	1.08	120	—	20
SMALL, 106 gm	190	3	4	33	—	100	.36	75	—	10
Hardee's										
APPLE TURNOVER, 87 gm	282	3	14	37	—	19	1	—	17	5
BIG COOKIE, 54 gm	278	3	15	33	—	16	1	258	64	9
McDonald's										
APPLE PIE, 85 gm	253	2	14	29	—	14	.62	398	—	12
CARAMEL SUNDAE, 165 gm	361	7	10	608	—	200	.23	145	—	31
CHERRY PIE, 88 gm	260	2	14	32	—	12	.59	427	—	13
CHOCOLATY CHIP COOKIES, 69 gm	342	4	16	45	—	29	1.56	313	—	18
HOT FUDGE SUNDAE, 164 gm	357	7	11	58	—	215	.61	170	—	27
ICE CREAM CONE, 115 gm	185	4	5	30	—	183	.12	109	—	24
MCDONALDLAND COOKIES, 67 gm	308	4	11	49	—	12	1.47	358	—	10
STRAWBERRY SUNDAE, 164 gm	320	6	9	54	—	174	.38	90	—	25
Roy Rogers										
BROWNIE, 64 gm	264	3	11	37	—	25	2.70	150	—	10
CARAMEL SUNDAE, 145 gm	293	7	9	52	—	204	.47	193	—	23
HOT FUDGE SUNDAE, 151 gm	337	7	13	53	—	264	.97	186	—	23
STRAWBERRY SHORTCAKE, 205 gm	447	10	19	59	—	274	.81	674	—	28

FOOD & DESCRIPTION MEASURE OR QUANTITY	CALORIES	PROTEIN (GM)	FAT (GM)	CARBO-HYDRATE (GM)	FIBER (GM)	CALCIUM (MG)	IRON (MG)	SODIUM (MG)	POTASSIUM (MG)	CHOLES-TEROL (MG)
STRAWBERRY SUNDAE, 142 gm	216	6	7	33	—	210	.47	99	—	23

Wendy's

FROSTY DAIRY DESSERT, 12 oz, 243 gm	400	8	14	59	—	300	1.08	220	585	50

Entrees
[For individual condiments, see Salads and Salad Bar Items]

Arby's

BAC'N CHEDDAR DELUXE, 8 oz, 225 gm	561	28	34	36	—	100	2.70	1385	—	78
BEEF 'N CHEDDAR, 6.7 oz, 190 gm	490	24	21	51	—	80	5.40	1520	—	51
CHICKEN BREAST SANDWICH, 7.4 oz, 210 gm	592	28	27	56	—	100	3.60	1340	—	57
HOT HAM 'N CHEESE SANDWICH, 5.7 oz, 161 gm	353	26	13	33	—	200	1.80	1655	—	50
ROAST BEEF SANDWICHES										
JUNIOR, 3 oz, 86 gm	218	12	8	22	—	40	1.80	345	—	20
KING, 6.7 oz, 192 gm	467	27	19	44	—	100	4.50	765	—	49
REGULAR, 5.2 oz, 147 gm	353	22	15	32	—	80	3.60	590	—	39
SUPER, 8.3 oz, 234 gm	501	25	22	50	—	100	4.50	800	—	40
TURKEY DELUXE, 7 oz, 197 gm	375	24	17	32	—	80	2.70	850	—	39

Arthur Treacher Fish and Chips

BROILED FISH, 5 oz	245	20	14	10	—	—	—	144	—	—
FISH, 5.2 oz	355	19	20	25	—	15	.57	450	—	56
FISH SANDWICH, 5.5 oz	440	16	24	39	—	89	1.49	836	—	42
SHRIMP, 4 oz	381	13	24	27	—	57	.64	538	—	93

Burger King

BACON DOUBLE CHEESE-BURGER, 159 gm	510	33	31	27	—	—	—	728	363	104
individual ingredients										
BACON	46	3	4	0	—	—	—	113	30	6
BEEF	238	20	17	0	—	—	—	68	256	75
BUN	143	5	3	26	—	—	—	263	54	—
CHEESE	83	5	7	1	—	—	—	284	23	23
CHICKEN SPECIALTY SANDWICH, 230 gm	688	26	40	56	—	—	—	1423	375	82
individual ingredients										
BUN	220	7	4	40	—	—	—	467	85	—
CHICKEN	272	19	16	14	—	—	—	813	261	66
LETTUCE	2	0	0	0	—	—	—	1	25	0
MAYONNAISE	194	0	20	2	—	—	—	142	4	16
CHICKEN TENDERS, 6 pieces, 95 gm	204	20	10	10	—	—	—	636	200	47
HAM & CHEESE SPECIALTY SANDWICH, 230 gm	471	24	23	44	—	—	—	1534	419	70
individual ingredients										
BUN	220	7	4	40	—	—	—	467	85	—
CHEESE	83	5	7	1	—	—	—	284	23	23

FOOD & DESCRIPTION MEASURE OR QUANTITY	CALORIES	PROTEIN (GM)	FAT (GM)	CARBO-HYDRATE (GM)	FIBER (GM)	CALCIUM (MG)	IRON (MG)	SODIUM (MG)	POTASSIUM (MG)	CHOLES-TEROL (MG)
HAM	62	12	2	0	—	—	—	710	217	39
LETTUCE	3	0	0	1	—	—	—	1	22	0
MAYONNAISE	97	0	10	1	—	—	—	71	2	8
TOMATO	6	0	0	1	—	—	—	1	70	0
HAMBURGER, 109 gm	275	15	12	29	—	—	—	509	235	37
CHEESEBURGER, total, 120 gm	317	17	15	30	—	—	—	651	247	48
individual ingredients										
BEEF	119	10	9	0	—	—	—	34	129	37
BUN	143	5	3	26	—	—	—	263	54	—
CHEESE	42	2	3	1	—	—	—	142	12	11
KETCHUP	11	0	0	3	—	—	—	121	46	0
MUSTARD	2	0	0	0	—	—	—	31	4	0
PICKLES	0	0	0	0	—	—	—	60	2	0
WHALER, 190 gm	488	19	27	45	—	—	—	592	369	84
WITH CHEESE, 201 gm	530	21	30	46	—	—	—	734	381	95
individual ingredients										
BUN	143	5	3	26	—	—	—	263	54	—
CHEESE	42	2	3	1	—	—	—	142	12	11
FISH	210	14	10	17	—	—	—	126	283	64
LETTUCE	1	0	0	0	—	—	—	1	19	0
TARTAR SAUCE	134	0	14	2	—	—	—	202	13	20
WHOPPER, 265 gm	640	25	41	42	—	—	—	842	547	94
WITH CHEESE, 288 gm	723	30	48	43	—	—	—	1126	570	117
individual ingredients										
BEEF	275	19	22	0	—	—	—	80	268	82
BUN	189	6	4	34	—	—	—	349	73	—
CHEESE	83	5	7	1	—	—	—	284	23	23
KETCHUP	17	0	0	4	—	—	—	183	69	0
LETTUCE	1	0	0	0	—	—	—	2	38	0
MAYONNAISE	146	0	15	2	—	—	—	107	3	12
ONION	5	0	0	1	—	—	—	1	22	0
PICKLES	1	0	0	0	—	—	—	119	4	0
TOMATO	6	0	0	1	—	—	—	1	70	0
WHOPPER JR, 136 gm	322	15	17	30	—	—	—	486	275	41
WITH CHEESE, 147 gm	364	17	20	31	—	—	—	628	287	52
individual ingredients										
BEEF	119	10	9	0	—	—	—	34	129	37
BUN	143	5	3	26	—	—	—	263	54	—
KETCHUP	8	0	0	2	—	—	—	91	35	0
CHEESE	42	2	3	1	—	—	—	142	12	11
LETTUCE	1	0	0	0	—	—	—	1	19	0
MAYONNAISE	48	0	5	1	—	—	—	36	1	4
PICKLES	0	0	0	0	—	—	—	60	2	0
TOMATO	3	0	0	1	—	—	—	1	35	0

Church's

FOOD & DESCRIPTION MEASURE OR QUANTITY	CALORIES	PROTEIN (GM)	FAT (GM)	CARBO-HYDRATE (GM)	FIBER (GM)	CALCIUM (MG)	IRON (MG)	SODIUM (MG)	POTASSIUM (MG)	CHOLES-TEROL (MG)
CATFISH, .75 oz, 21 gm	67	4	4	4	.1	—	—	151	—	—
FRIED CHICKEN										
BREAST, 4.3 oz, 121 gm	278	21	17	9	0	—	—	560	—	—
LEG, 2.9 oz, 83 gm	147	13	9	5	0	—	—	286	—	—
THIGH, 4.2 oz, 120 gm	306	19	22	9	0	—	—	448	—	—
WING, 4.8 oz, 136 gm	303	22	20	9	0	—	—	583	—	—
HUSHPUPPY, 1 piece, 23 gm	78	1	3	12	0	—	—	55	—	—
NUGGETS										
REGULAR, .63 oz, 18 gm	55	3	3	4	0	—	—	125	—	—
SPICY, .63 oz, 18 gm	52	3	3	3	0	—	—	91	—	—

Dairy Queen/Brazier

FOOD & DESCRIPTION MEASURE OR QUANTITY	CALORIES	PROTEIN (GM)	FAT (GM)	CARBO-HYDRATE (GM)	FIBER (GM)	CALCIUM (MG)	IRON (MG)	SODIUM (MG)	POTASSIUM (MG)	CHOLES-TEROL (MG)
CHICKEN SANDWICH, 220 gm	670	29	41	46	—	*	.36	870	—	75
FISH SANDWICH, 170 gm	400	20	17	41	—	60	.72	875	—	50
WITH CHEESE, 177 gm	440	24	21	39	—	150	.36	1035	—	60

FOOD & DESCRIPTION MEASURE OR QUANTITY	CALORIES	PROTEIN (GM)	FAT (GM)	CARBO-HYDRATE (GM)	FIBER (GM)	CALCIUM (MG)	IRON (MG)	SODIUM (MG)	POTASSIUM (MG)	CHOLES-TEROL (MG)
HAMBURGER										
DOUBLE, 210 gm	530	36	28	33	—	100	6.30	660	—	85
WITH CHEESE, 239 gm	650	43	37	34	—	350	6.30	980	—	95
SINGLE, 148 gm	360	21	16	33	—	100	3.60	630	—	45
WITH CHEESE, 162 gm	410	24	20	33	—	200	3.60	790	—	50
TRIPLE, 272 gm	710	51	45	33	—	100	9.00	690	—	135
WITH CHEESE, 301 gm	820	58	50	34	—	350	9.00	1010	—	145
HOT DOG, 100 gm	280	11	16	21	—	80	1.44	830	—	45
WITH CHEESE, 114 gm	330	15	21	21	—	150	1.44	990	—	55
WITH CHILI, 128 gm	320	13	20	23	—	80	1.80	985	—	55
SUPER HOT DOGS, 175 gm	520	17	27	44	—	150	2.70	1365	—	80
WITH CHEESE, 196 gm	580	22	34	45	—	250	1.44	1605	—	100
WITH CHILI, 218 gm	570	21	32	47	—	150	2.70	1595	—	100
Hardee's										
BACON CHEESEBURGER, 244 gm	686	35	42	42	—	152	6	1074	33	295
BIG DELUXE, 248 gm	546	29	26	48	—	98	7	1083	594	77
BIG ROAST BEEF, 167 gm	418	28	19	34	—	74	8	1770	470	60
CHEESEBURGER, 116 gm	335	17	17	29	—	48	3	789	197	—
CHICKEN FILLET, 192 gm	510	27	26	42	—	83	5	360	334	57
FISHERMAN'S FILLET, 196 gm	469	25	20	47	—	139	2	1013	465	80
HAMBURGER, 110 gm	305	17	13	29	—	23	4	682	231	—
HOT DOG, 120 gm	346	11	22	26	—	43	<3	744	120	42
HOT HAM 'N' CHEESE, 148 gm	376	23	15	37	—	207	4	1067	317	59
MUSHROOM 'N' SWISS, 205 gm	512	32	23	46	—	111	4	1051	437	86
ROAST BEEF SANDWICH, 143 gm	377	20	17	36	—	56	6	1030	205	57
TURKEY CLUB, 194 gm	426	24	22	32	—	39	2	1185	444	45
Kentucky Fried Chicken										
FRIED CHICKEN PIECES [figures reflect edible portion only]										
DRUMSTICK										
EXTRA CRISPY, 60 gm	173	13	11	6	—	15	.61	346	—	65
ORIGINAL RECIPE, 58 gm	147	14	9	3	—	13	.60	269	—	81
CENTER BREAST										
EXTRA CRISPY, 120 gm	353	27	21	14	—	35	.86	842	—	93
ORIGINAL RECIPE, 107 gm	257	26	14	8	—	39	.63	532	—	93
SIDE BREAST										
EXTRA CRISPY, 98 gm	354	18	24	17	—	32	.86	797	—	66
ORIGINAL RECIPE, 95 gm	276	20	17	10	—	48	.79	654	—	96
THIGH										
EXTRA CRISPY, 112 gm	371	20	26	14	—	46	1.21	766	—	121
ORIGINAL RECIPE, 96 gm	278	18	19	8	—	28	1.05	517	—	122
WING										
EXTRA CRISPY, 57 gm	218	12	16	8	—	21	.52	437	—	63
ORIGINAL RECIPE, 56 gm	181	12	12	6	—	38	.45	387	—	67
KENTUCKY NUGGETS, 6 nuggets, 97 gm	275	17	17	13	—	14	.78	839	—	71
BARBEQUE SAUCE, 1 oz	35	<1	<1	7	—	6	.24	450	—	<1
HONEY, .5 oz	49	0	<1	12	—	<1	.11	<15	—	0
MUSTARD SAUCE, 1 oz	36	<1	<1	6	—	10	.26	346	—	<1
SWEET & SOUR SAUCE, 1 oz	58	<1	<1	13	—	5	.16	148	—	<1
McDonald's										
BIG MAC, 200 gm	570	25	35	39	—	203	4.90	979	—	83
CHEESEBURGER, 114 gm	318	15	16	29	—	169	2.84	743	—	41

FOOD & DESCRIPTION MEASURE OR QUANTITY	CALORIES	PROTEIN (GM)	FAT (GM)	CARBO- HYDRATE (GM)	FIBER (GM)	CALCIUM (MG)	IRON (MG)	SODIUM (MG)	POTASSIUM (MG)	CHOLES- TEROL (MG)
CHICKEN MCNUGGETS, 109 gm	323	19	21	14	—	11	1.25	512	—	73
BARBECUE SAUCE, 32 gm	60	<1	<1	14	—	4	.12	309	—	<1
HONEY, 14 gm	50	<1	<1	12	—	1	.02	2	—	0
HOT MUSTARD SAUCE, 30 gm	63	<1	2	11	—	8	.17	259	—	3
SWEET & SOUR SAUCE, 32 gm	64	<1	<1	15	—	2	.08	186	—	<1
FILLET OF FISH, 143 gm	435	15	26	36	—	133	2.47	799	—	45
HAMBURGER, 100 gm	263	12	11	28	—	84	2.85	506	—	29
QUARTER POUNDER, 160 gm	427	25	24	29	—	98	4.30	718	—	81
WITH CHEESE, 186 gm	525	30	32	31	—	255	4.84	1220	—	107

Roy Rogers

FOOD & DESCRIPTION MEASURE OR QUANTITY	CALORIES	PROTEIN (GM)	FAT (GM)	CARBO- HYDRATE (GM)	FIBER (GM)	CALCIUM (MG)	IRON (MG)	SODIUM (MG)	POTASSIUM (MG)	CHOLES- TEROL (MG)
BACON CHEESEBURGER, 180 gm	581	32	39	25	—	343	4.41	1536	—	103
CHEESEBURGER, 173 gm	563	30	37	27	—	340	3.53	1404	—	95
FRIED CHICKEN PIECES										
BREAST, 126 gm	324	32	19	7	—	35	1.04	601	—	324
BREAST & WING, 169 gm	466	42	29	11	—	52	1.57	867	—	376
LEG, 47 gm	117	12	7	2	—	8	.50	162	—	64
THIGH, 98 gm	282	20	20	7	—	19	.97	505	—	89
THIGH & LEG, 146 gm	399	32	26	9	—	27	1.48	667	—	153
WING, 43 gm	142	10	10	3	—	17	.52	266	—	52
HAMBURGER, 143 gm	456	24	28	27	—	90	3.42	495	—	73
ROAST BEEF, 154 gm	317	27	10	29	—	87	4.14	785	—	55
WITH CHEESE, 182 gm	424	33	19	30	—	337	4.25	1694	—	77
LARGE, 182 gm	360	34	12	30	—	89	4.70	1044	—	73
WITH CHEESE, 211 gm	467	40	21	30	—	339	4.81	1953	—	95
RR BAR BURGER, 208 gm	611	36	39	28	—	343	3.80	1826	—	115

Taco Bell

FOOD & DESCRIPTION MEASURE OR QUANTITY	CALORIES	PROTEIN (GM)	FAT (GM)	CARBO- HYDRATE (GM)	FIBER (GM)	CALCIUM (MG)	IRON (MG)	SODIUM (MG)	POTASSIUM (MG)	CHOLES- TEROL (MG)
BEAN BURRITO, 203 gm	440	17	15	58	—	171	4.70	935	—	19
BEEF BURRITO, 187 gm	430	23	19	41	—	147	3.70	989	—	54
BEEFY TOSTADA, 210 gm	360	18	19	29	—	204	5.00	714	—	49
BELLBEEFER, 142 gm	280	15	9	34	—	92	3.10	710	—	23
WITH CHEESE & TOMATO, 156 gm	305	16	12	34	—	156	3.10	670	—	27
BURRITO SUPREME, 237 gm	420	19	19	43	—	166	1.70	855	—	28
COMBINATION BURRITO, 159 gm	350	15	13	41	—	124	5.10	777	—	29
ENCHIRITO, 184 gm	325	20	11	35	—	267	2.20	1030	—	40
NACHOS, 94 gm	355	7	19	37	—	169	1.50	319	—	11
NACHOS BELLGRANDE, 300 gm	725	22	38	69	—	330	6.30	1140	—	44
PINTOS & CHEESE, 144 gm	225	11	10	22	—	180	2.20	732	—	7
TACO, 87 gm	210	11	12	14	—	96	1.00	279	—	34
BELLGRANDE, 147 gm	310	17	19	19	—	147	1.90	353	—	36
LIGHT, 142 gm	345	15	22	19	—	105	2.00	426	—	39
TOSTADA, 162 gm	270	10	13	28	—	186	3.10	534	—	10

Wendy's

FOOD & DESCRIPTION MEASURE OR QUANTITY	CALORIES	PROTEIN (GM)	FAT (GM)	CARBO- HYDRATE (GM)	FIBER (GM)	CALCIUM (MG)	IRON (MG)	SODIUM (MG)	POTASSIUM (MG)	CHOLES- TEROL (MG)
BACON CHEESEBURGER, WHITE BUN, 5 oz, 147 gm	460	29	28	23	—	150	3.60	860	330	65
CHICKEN SANDWICH, MULTIGRAIN BUN, 5 oz, 128 gm	320	25	10	31	—	20	1.44	500	320	59
CHILI, 8 oz, 256 gm	260	21	8	26	—	80	4.50	1070	585	30
CONDIMENTS [in addition to sandwich]										

157

FOOD & DESCRIPTION MEASURE OR QUANTITY	CALORIES	PROTEIN (GM)	FAT (GM)	CARBO-HYDRATE (GM)	FIBER (GM)	CALCIUM (MG)	IRON (MG)	SODIUM (MG)	POTASSIUM (MG)	CHOLES-TEROL (MG)
AMERICAN CHEESE, 1 sl, 17.8 gm	70	4	6	<1	—	100	*	260	30	15
BACON, 3 half sl, 13.5 gm	90	4	8	<1	—	*	*	335	50	10
DILL PICKLES, 4 sl, 9 gm	1	<1	<1	<1	—	*	*	125	15	0
KETCHUP, 1 tsp, 5 gm	6	<1	<1	1	—	*	*	65	25	0
LETTUCE, 1 piece, 13 gm	2	<1	<1	<1	—	*	*	0	25	0
MAYONNAISE, 1 tbsp, 14 gm	100	<1	11	<1	—	*	*	80	0	10
MUSTARD, 1 tsp, 5 gm	4	<1	<1	<1	—	*	*	50	5	0
ONION RINGS, 9.5 gm	4	<1	<1	<1	—	*	*	0	15	0
RELISH, ⅓ oz, 9 gm	14	<1	<1	3	—	*	*	70	—	0
TOMATOES, 1 sl, 13.5 gm	2	<1	<1	<1	—	*	*	0	30	0
HAMBURGER										
DOUBLE, WHITE BUN, 7 oz, 197 gm	560	41	34	24	—	40	6.30	575	485	125
SINGLE, MULTIGRAIN BUN, 4 oz, 119 gm	340	25	17	20	—	20	2.70	290	310	67
SINGLE, WHITE BUN, 4 oz, 117 gm	350	21	18	27	—	40	4.50	410	275	65
KID'S MEAL HAMBURGER, 3 oz, 75 gm	220	13	8	11	—	20	1.80	265	150	20

Potatoes & Accompaniments

Arby's

BAKED POTATO, PLAIN, 11 oz, 312 gm	290	8	<1	66	—	20	1.80	12	—	0
FRENCH FRIES, 2.5 oz, 71 gm	211	2	8	33	—	*	1.08	30	—	6
POTATO CAKES, 3 oz, 85 gm	201	2	14	22	—	*	.72	425	—	13
SUPERSTUFFED POTATO										
BROCCOLI AND CHEDDAR, 12 oz, 340 gm	541	13	22	72	—	150	2.70	475	—	24
DELUXE, 11 oz, 312 gm	648	18	38	59	—	300	2.70	475	—	72
MUSHROOM AND CHEESE, 10.5 oz, 300 gm	506	16	22	61	—	300	2.70	635	—	21
TACO, 15 oz, 425 gm	619	23	27	73	—	450	3.60	1065	—	145

Arthur Treacher Fish and Chips

CHIPS, 4 oz	276	4	13	35	—	12	.47	39	—	<1
CHOWDER, 6 oz	112	5	5	11	—	61	.09	835	—	9
KRUNCH PUP, 2 oz	203	5	15	12	—	8	.60	446	—	25

Burger King

FRENCH FRIES, REGULAR, 74 gm	227	3	13	24	—	—	—	160	360	14
ONION RINGS, REGULAR, 79 gm	274	4	16	28	—	—	—	665	173	0

Dairy Queen/Brazier

FRENCH FRIES, REGULAR, 71 gm	200	2	10	25	—	*	1.08	115	—	10
LARGE, 113 gm	320	3	16	40	—	20	.72	185	—	15
ONION RINGS, 85 gm	280	4	16	31	—	100	4.50	140	—	15

Hardee's

FRENCH FRIES, LARGE, 113 gm	381	5	21	44	—	21	1	192	689	6
SMALL, 71 gm	239	3	13	28	—	13	1	121	433	4

FOOD & DESCRIPTION MEASURE OR QUANTITY	CALORIES	PROTEIN (GM)	FAT (GM)	CARBO-HYDRATE (GM)	FIBER (GM)	CALCIUM (MG)	IRON (MG)	SODIUM (MG)	POTASSIUM (MG)	CHOLES-TEROL (MG)
Kentucky Fried Chicken										
BUTTERMILK BISCUIT, 75 gm	269	5	14	32	—	77	1.22	521	—	<1
CORN, 1 ear, 5.5″, 143 gm	176	5	3	32	—	7	.79	<21	—	<1
GRAVY, 78 gm	59	2	4	4	—	9	.48	398	—	2
KENTUCKY FRIES, 119 gm	268	5	13	33	—	24	.94	81	—	2
MASHED POTATOES, 80 gm	59	2	<1	12	—	21	.28	228	—	<1
MASHED POTATOES WITH GRAVY, 86 gm	62	2	1	10	—	19	.35	297	—	<1
POTATO SALAD, 90 gm	141	2	9	13	—	10	.32	396	—	11
McDonald's										
REGULAR FRIES, 68 gm	220	3	12	26	—	9	.61	109	—	9
Roy Rogers										
FRENCH FRIES, 85 gm	268	4	14	32	—	18	.59	165	—	42
LARGE, 113 gm	357	5	18	43	—	25	.79	221	—	56
HOT TOPPED POTATO, PLAIN, 227 gm	211	6	<1	48	—	20	1.60	65	—	0
POTATO WITH BACON 'N CHEESE, 248 gm	397	17	22	33	—	150	2.16	778	—	34
BROCCOLI 'N CHEESE, 312 gm	376	14	18	40	—	210	2.52	523	—	<19
OLEO, 236 gm	274	6	7	48	—	23	1.60	161	—	0
SOUR CREAM 'N CHIVES, 297 gm	408	7	21	48	—	96	2.34	138	—	31
TACO BEEF 'N CHEESE, 359 gm	463	22	22	45	—	150	3.78	726	—	37
Wendy's										
HOT STUFFED BAKED POTATOES BACON & CHEESE, 12.4 oz, 350 gm	570	19	30	57	—	200	2.70	1180	1380	22
BROCCOLI & CHEESE, 12.9 oz, 365 gm	500	13	25	54	—	250	2.70	430	1550	22
CHEESE, 12.4 oz, 350 gm	590	17	34	55	—	350	2.70	450	1380	22
CHICKEN A LA KING, 12.6 oz, 358 gm	350	15	6	59	—	60	2.70	820	1550	20
CHILI & CHEESE, 14.1 oz, 400 gm	510	22	20	63	—	250	3.60	610	1590	22
PLAIN, 8.8 oz, 250 gm	250	6	2	52	—	20	2.70	60	1360	tr
SOUR CREAM & CHIVE, 10.9 oz, 310 gm	460	6	24	53	—	40	2.70	230	1420	15
STROGANOFF & SOUR CREAM, 14 oz, 406 gm	490	14	21	60	—	80	3.60	910	1920	43
FRENCH FRIES, SALTED, 3.4 oz, 98 gm	280	4	14	35	—	*	1.08	95	635	15
Salads & Salad Bar Items										
Arthur Treacher Fish and Chips										
COLE SLAW, 3 oz	123	1	8	11	—	24	.19	266	—	7
Burger King										
TYPICAL SALAD without dressing, 148 gm	28	2	0	5	—	—	—	23	382	0

FOOD & DESCRIPTION MEASURE OR QUANTITY	CALORIES	PROTEIN (GM)	FAT (GM)	CARBO-HYDRATE (GM)	FIBER (GM)	CALCIUM (MG)	IRON (MG)	SODIUM (MG)	POTASSIUM (MG)	CHOLES-TEROL (MG)
DRESSINGS										
BLUE CHEESE, 28 gm	156	1	16	2	—	—	—	309	—	22
FRENCH, 28 gm	123	0	11	8	—	—	—	309	30	0
GOLDEN ITALIAN, 28 gm	134	0	14	2	—	—	—	268	7	0
HOUSE, 28 gm	130	1	13	3	—	—	—	269	20	11
REDUCED CALORIE										
ITALIAN, 28 gm	14	0	0	2	—	—	—	426	6	0
THOUSAND ISLAND, 28 gm	117	0	12	4	—	—	—	228	22	17

Hardee's

CHEF SALAD, 329 gm	277	23	16	10	—	212	2	517	414	179
SHRIMP SALAD, 336 gm	362	14	29	11	—	104	3	941	696	293

Kentucky Fried Chicken

COLE SLAW, 79 gm	103	1	6	12	—	29	.19	171	—	4

Roy Rogers

BACON BITS, 1 tbsp	24	4	1	—	—	—	—	210	—	—
BEETS, sliced, ¼ c	16	<1	0	4	—	—	—	100	—	—
BROCCOLI, ½ c	20	3	0	4	—	—	—	7	—	—
CARROTS, shredded, ¼ c	12	<1	0	—	—	—	—	7	—	—
CHEDDAR CHEESE, ¼ c	112	6	9	<1	—	—	—	195	—	—
CHINESE NOODLES, ¼ c	55	2	3	7	—	—	—	100	—	—
COLE SLAW, 99 gm	110	1	7	11	—	34	.22	261	—	<5
CROUTONS, 2 tbsp	132	6	0	31	—	—	—	453	—	—
CUCUMBERS, 5–6 sl	4	—	0	1	—	—	—	2	—	—
DRESSINGS										
BACON 'N TOMATO, 2 tbsp	136	—	12	6	—	—	—	150	—	—
BLUE CHEESE, 2 tbsp	150	2	16	2	—	—	—	153	—	—
LO-CAL ITALIAN, 2 tbsp	70	—	6	2	—	—	—	100	—	—
RANCH, 2 tbsp	155	—	14	4	—	—	—	100	—	—
THOUSAND ISLAND, 2 tbsp	160	—	16	4	—	—	—	150	—	—
EGG, chopped, 2 tbsp	55	4	4	<1	—	—	—	41	—	—
LETTUCE, 1 c	10	—	0	4	—	—	—	7	—	—
MACARONI SALAD, 2 tbsp	60	1	4	6	—	—	—	301	—	—
100 gm	186	3	11	19	—	10	.41	603	—	<5
MUSHROOMS, ¼ c	5	<1	0	<1	—	—	—	3	—	—
PEAS, GREEN, ¼ c	7	1	—	1	—	—	—	66	—	—
PEPPERS, GREEN, 2 tbsp	4	<1	0	1	—	—	—	2	—	—
POTATO SALAD, 2 tbsp	50	1	3	6	—	—	—	350	—	—
100 gm	107	2	6	11	—	13	.34	696	—	<5
SUN FLOWER SEEDS, 2 tbsp	101	4	9	5	—	—	—	7	—	—
TOMATOES, 3 sl	20	<1	0	5	—	—	—	3	—	—

Taco Bell

TACO SALAD, 520 gm	910	36	57	63	—	374	10.90	1455	—	69

Wendy's

ALFALFA SPROUTS, 2 oz, 56 gm	20	2	<1	2	—	*	.72	—	—	0
AMERICAN CHEESE, IMITATION, 1 oz, 28 gm	70	6	5	1	—	200	*	—	—	0
BACON BITS, ⅛ oz, 3.5 gm	10	1	<1	<1	—	*	*	95	20	5
BELL PEPPER, ¼ c, 20 gm	4	<1	<1	1	—	*	*	5	45	0
BLUEBERRIES, fresh, 1 tbsp, 14 gm	8	<1	<1	2	—	*	*	0	10	—
BREAD STICK, 1 piece, 3.5 gm	20	<1	1	2	—	*	*	—	—	0
BROCCOLI, ½ c, 44 gm	14	1	<1	2	—	20	*	10	140	0
CANTALOUPE, fresh, 2 pieces, 57 gm	4	<1	<1	1	—	*	*	0	35	0
CARROTS, ¼ c, 27.5 gm	12	<1	<1	3	—	*	*	15	95	0

FOOD & DESCRIPTION MEASURE OR QUANTITY	CALORIES	PROTEIN (GM)	FAT (GM)	CARBO-HYDRATE (GM)	FIBER (GM)	CALCIUM (MG)	IRON (MG)	SODIUM (MG)	POTASSIUM (MG)	CHOLES-TEROL (MG)
CAULIFLOWER, ½ c, 50 gm	14	1	<1	3	—	*	.36	5	150	0
CHEDDAR CHEESE, IMITATION, 1 oz, 28 gm	90	6	6	1	—	200	*	450	—	0
CHOW MEIN NOODLES, ¼ c, 11 gm	60	1	3	6	—	*	.36	80	20	0
COLE SLAW, ½ c, 60 gm	90	<1	8	3	—	20	*	70	120	0
COTTAGE CHEESE, ½ c, 105 gm	110	13	5	3	—	60	*	425	90	15
CROUTONS, 18 pieces, 7 gm	30	1	1	4	—	*	*	90	—	—
CUCUMBERS, ¼ c, 26 gm	4	<1	<1	1	—	*	*	0	40	0
DRESSINGS BLUE CHEESE, 1 tbsp, 15 gm	60	1	7	<1	—	*	*	85	10	12
CELERY SEED, 1 tbsp, 14 gm	70	<1	6	3	—	*	*	65	5	3
GOLDEN ITALIAN, 1 tbsp, 15 gm	45	<1	4	3	—	*	*	260	10	0
OIL, 1 tbsp, 15 gm	130	<1	15	<1	—	*	*	0	0	0
RANCH, 1 tbsp, 15 gm	80	<1	9	<1	—	*	*	155	10	0
RED FRENCH, 1 tbsp, 15 gm	70	<1	5	5	—	*	*	130	20	0
REDUCED CALORIE BACON & TOMATO, 1 tbsp, 15 gm	45	<1	4	2	—	*	*	160	25	0
CREAMY CUCUMBER, 1 tbsp, 15 gm	50	<1	5	2	—	*	*	140	10	0
ITALIAN, 1 tbsp, 15 gm	25	<1	2	2	—	*	*	180	10	0
THOUSAND ISLAND, 1 tbsp, 15 gm	45	<1	4	2	—	*	*	125	20	5
THOUSAND ISLAND, 1 tbsp, 15 gm	70	<1	7	2	—	*	*	115	15	8
WINE VINEGAR, 1 tbsp, 15 gm	2	<1	<1	<1	—	*	*	5	10	0
EGGS, 1 tbsp, 8.5 gm	14	1	1	<1	—	*	*	10	10	40
LETTUCE, ICEBERG, 1 c, 55 gm	8	<1	<1	2	—	*	*	5	95	0
ROMAINE, 1 c, 55 gm	10	<1	<1	2	—	*	.72	5	145	0
MOZZARELLA CHEESE, IMITATION, 1 oz, 28 gm	90	6	7	<1	—	*	*	320	—	1
MUSHROOMS, ¼ c, 17.5 gm	6	<1	<1	<1	—	*	*	5	60	0
ORANGE, fresh, 2 pieces, 57 gm	10	<1	—	3	—	*	*	0	45	0
PASTA SALAD, ½ c, 99 gm	134	4	6	17	—	20	.72	400	85	—
PEACHES IN SYRUP, 2 pieces, 57 gm	17	<1	<1	4	—	*	*	0	40	0
PEAS, GREEN, ½ c, 80 gm	60	4	<1	9	—	*	1.44	90	110	0
PEPPERONCINI or BANANA PEPPER, 1 tbsp, 14 gm	18	<1	<1	4	—	*	*	—	6	0
PEPPERS, JALAPENO, 1 tbsp, 14 gm	9	<1	<1	2	—	*	*	4	80	0
PICK-UP WINDOW SIDE DISH, 18 oz, 510 gm	110	8	6	5	—	100	1.08	540	320	15
PINEAPPLE CHUNKS IN JUICE, ½ c, 125 gm	80	<1	<1	20	—	*	*	0	150	0
RED ONIONS, 1 tbsp, 10 gm	4	<1	<1	<1	—	*	*	0	15	0
SALTINE CRACKERS, 4 pieces, 12 gm	45	1	2	8	—	—	—	150	15	4
SWISS CHEESE, IMITATION, 1 oz, 1 gm	80	6	6	<1	—	*	*	450	—	1
SUNFLOWER SEEDS & RAISINS, ¼ c, 36 gm	180	7	13	12	—	40	2.70	10	320	0
TACO SALAD, 12.6 oz, 357 gm	390	23	18	36	—	200	4.50	1100	790	40
TOMATOES, 1 oz, 28 gm	6	<1	<1	1	—	*	*	0	60	0
TURKEY HAM, ¼ c, 36 gm	46	7	2	1	—	—	—	—	—	27
WATERMELON, fresh, 2 pieces, 57 gm	3	<1	<1	<1	—	*	*	0	15	0

11

FATS & OILS

FOOD & DESCRIPTION MEASURE OR QUANTITY	CALORIES	PROTEIN (GM)	FAT (GM)	CARBO-HYDRATE (GM)	FIBER (GM)	CALCIUM (MG)	IRON (MG)	SODIUM (MG)	POTASSIUM (MG)	CHOLES-TEROL (MG)
Animal Fats										
Hain										
COD LIVER OIL, high potency, 1 tbsp, 14 gm	120	0	14	0	—	*	*	—	—	—
CHERRY, 1 tbsp, 14 gm	120	0	14	0	—	*	*	—	—	—
LEMON , 1 tbsp, 14 gm	120	0	14	0	—	*	*	—	—	—
MINT, 1 tbsp, 14 gm	120	0	14	0	—	*	*	—	—	—
ORANGE, 1 tbsp, 14 gm	120	0	14	0	—	*	*	—	—	—
Land O'Lakes										
SWEET CREAM BUTTER LIGHTLY SALTED, 1 tbsp, 14 gm	100	0	11	0	—	*	*	115	4	30
UNSALTED, 1 tbsp, 14 gm	100	0	11	0	—	*	*	2	4	30
WHIPPED LIGHTLY SALTED, 1 tbsp, 9 gm	60	0	7	0	—	*	*	75	2	20
UNSALTED, 1 tbsp, 9 gm	60	0	7	0	—	*	*	1	2	20
USDA										
BEEF TALLOW, 1 tbsp, 12.8 gm	116	0	13	0	0	—	—	0	0	14
BUTTER, 1 pat, 5 gm	36	<1	4	0	0	1	.01	41	1	11
BUTTER, unsalted, 1 pat, 5 gm	36	<1	4	0	0	1	.01	<1	1	11
CHICKEN FAT, 1 tbsp, 12.8 gm	115	0	13	0	0	—	—	—	—	11
DUCK FAT, 1 tbsp, 12.8 gm	115	0	13	0	0	—	—	—	—	13
GOOSE FAT, 1 tbsp, 12.8 gm	115	0	13	0	0	—	—	—	—	13
LARD, pork, 1c, 205 gm	1849	0	205	0	0	<1	—	<1	<1	195
1 tbsp, 12.8 gm	116	0	13	0	0	<1	—	0	0	12
MUTTON TALLOW, 1 tbsp, 12.8 gm	116	0	13	0	0	—	—	—	—	13
PORK CURED heated, 1 oz, 28 gm	167	2	18	0	0	2	.17	177	46	24
unheated, 1 oz, 28 gm	164	2	17	<1	0	1	.11	143	30	19
TURKEY FAT, 1 tbsp, 12.8 gm	115	0	13	0	0	—	—	—	—	13
Vegetable Fats										
Margarines										

FOOD & DESCRIPTION MEASURE OR QUANTITY	CALORIES	PROTEIN (GM)	FAT (GM)	CARBO-HYDRATE (GM)	FIBER (GM)	CALCIUM (MG)	IRON (MG)	SODIUM (MG)	POTASSIUM (MG)	CHOLES-TEROL (MG)
Blue Bonnet–Nabisco										
BUTTER BLEND SOFT, 1 tbsp	90	0	11	0	—	*	*	95	10	5
STICK, 1 tbsp	90	0	11	0	—	*	*	95	10	5
UNSALTED, 1 tbsp	90	0	11	0	—	*	*	0	0	5
DIET MARGARINE, 1 tbsp	50	0	6	0	—	*	*	100	5	0
LIGHT TASTY SPREAD, 52% vegetable oil, 1 tbsp	60	0	7	0	—	*	*	100	10	0
SOFT MARGARINE, 1 tbsp	100	0	11	0	—	*	*	95	5	0
WHIPPED, 1 tbsp	70	0	7	0	—	*	*	70	5	0
SPREAD, 52% FAT, 1 tbsp	80	0	8	0	—	*	*	110	15	0
SPREAD STICK, 70% FAT, 1 tbsp	90	0	10	0	—	*	*	95	10	0
SPREAD STICK, 75% FAT, 1 tbsp	90	0	11	0	—	*	*	95	10	0
STICK, 1 tbsp	100	0	11	0	—	*	*	95	5	0
WHIPPED, 1 tbsp	70	0	7	0	—	*	*	70	5	0
WHIPPED SPREAD, 60%FAT, 1 tbsp	50	0	6	0	—	*	*	55	5	0
Chiffon										
SOFT REGULAR, 1 tbsp, 13 gm	90	0	10	0	—	*	*	105	—	0
UNSALTED, 1 tbsp, 13 gm	90	0	10	0	—	*	*	<10	—	0
SOFT WHIPPED, 1 tbsp, 10 gm	70	0	8	0	—	*	*	80	—	0
STICK, 1 tbsp, 14 gm	100	0	11	0	—	*	*	110	—	0
Fleischmann–Nabisco										
DIET, 1 tbsp	50	0	6	0	—	*	*	100	5	0
WITH LIGHT SALT, 1 tbsp	50	0	6	0	—	*	*	50	5	0
LIGHT CORN OIL SPREAD, SOFT, 1 tbsp	80	0	8	0	—	*	*	70	10	0
STICK, 1 tbsp	80	0	8	0	—	*	*	70	10	0
LIQUID CORN OIL, 1 tbsp	120	0	14	0	—	*	*	0	0	0
SOFT, 1 tbsp	100	0	11	0	—	*	*	95	5	0
SWEET UNSALTED, 1 tbsp	100	0	11	0	—	*	*	0	5	0
STICK, 1 tbsp	100	0	11	0	—	*	*	95	5	0
SWEET UNSALTED, 1 tbsp	100	0	11	0	—	*	*	0	5	0
SQUEEZE, 1 tbsp	100	0	11	0	—	*	*	85	5	0
WHIPPED										
LIGHTLY SALTED, 1 tbsp	70	0	7	0	—	*	*	60	5	0
UNSALTED, 1 tbsp	70	0	7	0	—	*	*	0	5	0
Hain										
SAFFLOWER OIL MARGARINE, 1 tbsp, 14 gm	100	0	11	0	—	*	*	—	—	0
UNSALTED, 1 tbsp, 14 gm	100	0	11	0	—	*	*	—	—	0
Land O'Lakes										
COUNTRY MORNING BLEND STICK										
LIGHTLY SALTED, 1 tbsp, 14 gm	100	0	11	0	—	*	*	115	5	10
UNSALTED, 1 tbsp, 14 gm	100	0	11	0	—	*	*	1	5	10
SOFT TUB										
LIGHTLY SALTED, 1 tbsp, 12 gm	90	0	10	0	—	*	*	85	2	10
UNSALTED, 1 tbsp, 12 gm	90	0	10	0	—	*	*	1	2	10
PREMIUM CORN OIL, stick, 1 tbsp, 14 gm	100	0	11	0	—	*	*	115	2	0
REGULAR										

FOOD & DESCRIPTION MEASURE OR QUANTITY	CALORIES	PROTEIN (GM)	FAT (GM)	CARBO-HYDRATE (GM)	FIBER (GM)	CALCIUM (MG)	IRON (MG)	SODIUM (MG)	POTASSIUM (MG)	CHOLES-TEROL (MG)
STICK, soy oil, 1 tbsp, 14 gm	100	0	11	0	—	*	*	115	2	0
SOFT TUB, soy oil, 1 tbsp, 14 gm	100	0	11	0	—	*	*	115	2	0

Lever Brothers

AUTUMN SPREAD, stick, 1 tbsp, 14 gm	74	<1	8	<1	—	1	*	109	5	0
SOFT TUB, 1 tbsp, 14 gm	74	tr	8	tr	—	<1	*	95	4	0
IMPERIAL										
DIET, 1 tbsp, 14 gm	49	0	6	0	—	<1	*	136	4	0
LIGHT SPREAD, 1 tbsp, 14 gm	65	<1	7	<1	—	1	*	109	5	0
LIGHT STICK, 1 tbsp, 14 gm	74	<1	8	<1	—	1	*	109	5	0
SOFT, 1 tbsp, 14 gm	100	<1	11	<1	—	2	*	96	5	0
SOFT SPREAD, 43% VEGETABLE OIL, 1 tbsp, 14 gm	56	tr	6	0	—	<1	*	109	4	0
SPREAD STICK, 52% VEGETABLE OIL, 1 tbsp, 14 gm	64	tr	7	<1	—	<1	*	109	4	0
STICK, 1 tbsp, 14 gm	100	<1	11	<1	—	2	*	112	4	0
WHIPPED SPREAD, 1 tbsp, 10 gm	46	tr	5	tr	—	<1	*	78	3	0
PROMISE										
SOFT, 1 tbsp, 14 gm	90	<1	10	<1	—	2	*	96	5	0
SPREAD SOFT, EXTRA LIGHT, 53% VEGETABLE OIL, 1 tbsp, 14 gm	66	tr	7	<1	—	<1	*	66	4	0
STICK, 1 tbsp, 14 gm	90	<1	10	<1	—	2	*	111	3	0
STICK, EXTRA LIGHT SPREAD, 53% VEGETABLE OIL, 1 tbsp, 14 gm	66	tr	7	<1	—	<1	*	71	4	0

Mazola–Best Foods

DIET REDUCED CALORIE, 1 tbsp, 14.5 gm	50	0	6	0	0	*	*	130	—	0
MARGARINE, 1 tbsp, 14 gm	100	<1	11	<1	—	*	*	100	—	0
UNSALTED, 1 tbsp, 14 gm	100	0	11	0	0	*	*	<1	—	0

Mother's

PURE CORN OIL SPREAD (100%), SOFT, UNSALTED, 1 tbsp, 14 gm	70	0	7	0	—	*	*	<10	—	0
SOFT										
SALTED, 1 tbsp, 14 gm	100	0	11	0	—	*	*	—	—	0
UNSALTED, 1 tbsp, 14 gm	100	0	11	0	—	*	*	<10	—	0
STICK										
SALTED, 1 tbsp, 14 gm	100	0	11	0	—	*	*	—	—	0
UNSALTED, 1 tbsp, 14 gm	100	0	11	0	—	*	*	<10	—	0

Mrs. Filbert's

CORN OIL QUARTERS, 1 tbsp, 14 gm	100	0	11	0	—	*	*	110	—	0
FAMILY SPREAD										
QUARTERS, 1 tbsp, 14 gm	80	0	8	0	—	*	*	95	—	0
SOFT, 1 tbsp, 14 gm	70	0	7	0	—	*	*	85	—	0
"I CAN'T BELIEVE IT'S NOT BUTTER"										
QUARTERS, 1 tbsp, 14 gm	90	0	10	0	—	*	*	95	—	0
SOFT, 1 tbsp, 14 gm	90	0	10	0	—	*	*	90	—	0

FOOD & DESCRIPTION MEASURE OR QUANTITY	CALORIES	PROTEIN (GM)	FAT (GM)	CARBO- HYDRATE (GM)	FIBER (GM)	CALCIUM (MG)	IRON (MG)	SODIUM (MG)	POTASSIUM (MG)	CHOLES- TEROL (MG)
REDUCED CALORIE, 1 tbsp, 14 gm	50	0	6	0	—	*	*	110	—	0
SOFT CORN OIL, 1 tbsp, 14 gm	100	0	11	0	—	*	*	110	—	0
SOFT GOLDEN, 1 tbsp, 14 gm	100	0	11	0	—	*	*	110	—	0
SPREAD 25, 1 tbsp, 14 gm	80	0	8	0	—	*	*	105	—	0

Nucoa–Best Foods

MARGARINE, 1 tbsp, 14 gm	100	0	11	0	0	*	*	160	—	0
SOFT, 1 tbsp, 13 gm	90	0	11	<1	0	*	*	150	—	0

Shedd's Spreads– Lever Brothers

BUTTERMATCH, LIGHTLY SALTED, 1 tbsp, 14 gm	91	<1	10	<1	—	<1	—	115	3	4
UNSALTED, 1 tbsp, 14 gm	91	0	10	0	—	0	—	<1	4	4
CORN OIL, STICK, SPREAD, 1 tbsp, 14 gm	66	0	7	0	—	<1	—	100	3	0
CORN OIL, SOFT, SPREAD, 1 tbsp	66	0	7	0	—	<1	—	100	3	0
COUNTRY CROCK, SOFT, 1 tbsp, 14 gm	66	0	7	0	—	<1	—	100	3	0
SOFT VEGETABLE OIL, SPREAD, 1 tbsp, 14 gm	66	0	7	0	—	<1	—	100	3	0
WHIPPED, SPREAD, 1 tbsp, 10 gm	70	0	7	0	—	<1	—	100	3	0

USDA

CORN & CORN HYDROGENATED										
SALTED, 1 tsp, 4.7 gm	34	0	4	0	—	1	—	44	2	—
UNSALTED, 1 tsp, 4.7 gm	34	0	4	0	—	<1	—	<1	1	—
IMITATION 40% FAT, 1 tsp, 4.8 gm	17	0	2	0	—	<1	—	46	1	0
REGULAR SOFT TUB										
SALTED, 1 tsp, 4.7 gm	34	0	4	0	—	1	—	51	2	—
UNSALTED, 1 tsp, 4.7 gm	34	0	4	0	—	1	—	1	2	—
SPREAD MARGARINELIKE, approximately 60% fat										
STICK, 1 tsp, 4.8 gm	26	0	3	0	—	1	—	48	1	—
TUB, 1 tsp, 4.8 gm	26	0	3	0	—	1	—	48	1	—

Weight Watchers

REDUCED CALORIE										
STICK, 1 tbsp, 14 gm	50	0	6	0	—	0	0	110	—	0
TUB, 1 tbsp, 14 gm	50	0	6	0	—	—	—	110	—	—
TUB, unsalted, 1 tbsp, 14 gm	50	0	6	0	—	—	—	<10	—	—

Oils

Arrowhead Mills

CORN GERM OIL, unrefined, 1 tbsp	120	0	14	0	—	—	—	—	—	0
OLIVE OIL, unrefined, 1 tbsp	120	0	14	0	—	—	—	—	—	0
PEANUT OIL, unrefined, 1 tbsp	120	0	14	0	—	—	—	—	—	0
SAFFLOWER OIL, unrefined, 1 tbsp	120	0	14	0	—	—	—	—	—	0
SESAME OIL, unrefined, 1 tbsp	120	0	14	0	—	—	—	—	—	0
SOYBEAN OIL, unrefined, 1 tbsp	120	0	14	0	—	—	—	—	—	0

FOOD & DESCRIPTION MEASURE OR QUANTITY	CALORIES	PROTEIN (GM)	FAT (GM)	CARBO- HYDRATE (GM)	FIBER (GM)	CALCIUM (MG)	IRON (MG)	SODIUM (MG)	POTASSIUM (MG)	CHOLES- TEROL (MG)
SUNFLOWER OIL, refined, 1 tbsp	120	0	14	0	—	—	—	—	—	0
WHEAT GERM OIL, refined, 1 tbsp	120	0	14	0	—	—	—	—	—	0

Hain

ALL BLEND OIL, 1 tbsp, 14 gm	120	0	14	0	—	*	*	—	—	0
ALMOND OIL, 1 tbsp, 14 gm	120	0	14	0	—	*	*	—	—	0
APRICOT KERNEL OIL, 1 tbsp, 14 gm	120	0	14	0	—	*	*	—	—	0
CORN OIL, 1 tbsp, 14 gm	120	0	14	0	—	*	*	—	—	0
COTTON SEED OIL, 1 tbsp, 14 gm	120	0	14	0	—	*	*	—	—	0
PEANUT OIL, 1 tbsp, 14 gm	120	0	14	0	—	*	*	—	—	0
SAFFLOWER OIL, SUPER E, 1 tbsp, 14 gm	120	0	14	0	—	*	*	—	—	0
SESAME OIL, 1 tbsp, 14 gm	120	0	14	0	—	*	*	—	—	0
SOY OIL, 1 tbsp, 14 gm	120	0	14	0	—	*	*	—	—	0
SUNFLOWER OIL, 1 tbsp, 14 gm	120	0	14	0	—	*	*	—	—	0
WALNUT OIL, 1 tbsp, 14 gm	120	0	14	0	—	*	*	—	—	0
WHEAT GERM OIL, 1 tbsp, 14 gm	120	0	14	0	—	*	*	—	—	0

Mazola—Best Foods

CORN OIL, 1 tbsp, 14 gm	125	0	14	0	0	*	*	0	—	0
NO STICK, 2.5-second spray	6	0	<1	0	0	*	*	0	—	0

Planters—Nabisco

PEANUT OIL, 1 tbsp	130	0	14	0	—	*	*	0	0	0
POPCORN OIL, 1 tbsp	130	0	14	0	—	*	*	0	0	0

Procter & Gamble

CRISCO OIL, 1 tbsp	120	0	14	0	—	*	*	0	—	0
PURITAN, 1 tbsp	120	0	14	0	—	*	*	0	—	0

USDA

ALMOND OIL, 1 tbsp, 13.6 gm	120	0	14	0	0	—	—	—	—	0
APRICOT KERNEL, 1 tbsp, 13.6 gm	120	0	14	0	0	—	—	—	—	0
COCOA BUTTER, 1 tbsp, 13.6 gm	120	0	14	0	0	—	—	—	—	0
COCONUT OIL, 1 tbsp, 13.6 gm	120	0	14	0	0	—	.01	—	—	0
CORN OIL, 1 tbsp, 13.6 gm	120	0	14	0	0	—	—	—	—	0
COTTONSEED OIL, 1 tbsp, 13.6 gm	120	0	14	0	0	—	—	—	—	0
HAZELNUT OIL, 1 tbsp, 13.6 gm	120	0	14	0	0	—	—	—	—	0
LINSEED OIL, 1 tbsp, 13.6 gm	120	0	14	0	0	<1	—	—	—	0
NUTMEG BUTTER, 1 tbsp, 13.6 gm	120	0	14	0	0	—	—	—	—	0
OLIVE OIL, 1 tbsp, 13.5 gm	119	0	14	0	0	<1	.05	0	—	0
PALM OIL, 1 tbsp, 13.6 gm	120	0	14	0	0	—	0	—	—	0
PALM KERNEL, 1 tbsp, 13.6 gm	120	0	14	0	0	—	—	—	—	0
PEANUT OIL, 1 tbsp, 13.5 gm	119	0	14	0	0	<1	0	<1	0	0
POPPY SEED OIL, 1 tbsp, 13.6 gm	120	0	14	0	0	—	—	—	—	0
RAPESEED OIL, 1 tbsp, 13.6 gm	120	0	14	0	0	—	—	—	—	0

FOOD & DESCRIPTION MEASURE OR QUANTITY	CALORIES	PROTEIN (GM)	FAT (GM)	CARBO- HYDRATE (GM)	FIBER (GM)	CALCIUM (MG)	IRON (MG)	SODIUM (MG)	POTASSIUM (MG)	CHOLES- TEROL (MG)
RICE BRAN OIL, 1 tbsp, 13.6 gm	120	0	14	0	0	<1	—	—	—	0
SAFFLOWER OIL, 1 tbsp, 13.6 gm	120	0	14	0	0	—	—	—	—	0
SESAME OIL, 1 tbsp, 13.6 gm	120	0	14	0	0	—	—	—	—	0
SOYBEAN OIL, 1 tbsp, 13.6 gm	120	0	14	0	0	<1	0	0	—	0
SUNFLOWER OIL, 1 tbsp, 13.6 gm	120	0	14	0	0	<1	0	<1	—	0
WALNUT OIL, 1 tbsp, 13.6 gm	120	0	14	0	0	—	—	—	—	0
WHEAT GERM OIL, 1 tbsp, 13.6 gm	120	0	14	0	0	—	—	—	—	0

Weight Watchers

COOKING SPRAY, 1-second spray	2	0	<1	0	—	0	0	<10	0	—

Shortenings

Procter & Gamble

CRISCO, 1 tbsp	110	0	12	0	—	*	*	0	—	0
BUTTER FLAVOR, 1 tbsp	110	0	12	0	—	*	*	0	—	0

Rokeach

NEUTRAL NYAFAT, 1 tbsp, 11 gm	99	0	11	0	—	—	—	0	—	0

USDA

VEGETABLE SHORTENING										
1 c, 205 gm	1812	0	205	0	—	—	—	—	—	0
1 tbsp, 12.8 gm	113	0	13	0	—	—	—	—	—	0

12

FISH & SEAFOOD

FOOD & DESCRIPTION MEASURE OR QUANTITY	CALORIES	PROTEIN (GM)	FAT (GM)	CARBO-HYDRATE (GM)	FIBER (GM)	CALCIUM (MG)	IRON (MG)	SODIUM (MG)	POTASSIUM (MG)	CHOLES-TEROL (MG)
Bumble Bee–Dole										
OYSTERS, without shell, ½ c, 120 gm	109	13	3	8	—	102	8.70	160	264	—
SALMON [bones included in analyses]										
KETA, salt added, ½ c, 110 gm	153	24	6	0	—	274	.70	536	370	—
PINK, salt added, ½ c, 110 gm	155	23	7	0	—	216	.90	542	397	—
RED SOCKEYE, salt added, ½ c, 110 gm	188	22	10	0	—	285	1.30	455	379	—
TUNA										
CHUNK LIGHT, undrained										
OIL PACK, ½ c, 92 gm	265	22	19	0	—	6	1.00	327	277	—
WATER PACK, ½ c, 92 gm	117	26	<1	0	—	15	1.40	311	257	—
SOLID WHITE, undrained										
OIL PACK, ½ c, 99 gm	285	24	20	0	—	6	1.10	414	298	—
WATER PACK, ½ c, 99 gm	126	28	<1	0	—	16	1.60	333	276	—
Celentano										
FILLET OF FISH FLORENTINE WITH SAUCE, MICROWAVEABLE, 10 oz	290	25	18	7	—	250	4.50	410	—	—
DelicaSeas–Kibun										
SEA BITES, lightly breaded, 4 oz	140	16	2	17	—	20	.36	750	—	—
SEA STIX,										
salad style, 4 oz	100	14	1	9	—	40	1.08	705	—	—
whole leg, 4 oz	100	14	1	9	—	40	1.08	705	—	—
SEA TAILS, whole, 4 oz	100	17	<1	8	—	20	.72	720	—	—
Del Monte										
SALMON, PINK, cnd, ½ c, 113.5 gm	160	22	7	0	—	200	.72	660	370	—
SALMON, RED, cnd, ½ c, 113.5 gm	180	23	9	0	—	250	.72	660	405	—
SARDINES IN TOMATO SAUCE, ½ c, 113.5 gm	360	19	12	45	—	300	3.60	540	415	—
Durkee										
GRANADAISA FLAT FILETS OF ANCHOVIES,										

FOOD & DESCRIPTION MEASURE OR QUANTITY	CALORIES	PROTEIN (GM)	FAT (GM)	CARBO-HYDRATE (GM)	FIBER (GM)	CALCIUM (MG)	IRON (MG)	SODIUM (MG)	POTASSIUM (MG)	CHOLES-TEROL (MG)
cnd, 2 oz, 57 gm	80	9	5	<1	—	—	—	3175	—	—
SARDINES IN OLIVE OIL, skinless & cnd, 3¾ oz, 106 gm	277	24	19	0	—	—	—	526	273	—
SARDINES IN TOMATO SAUCE, Norwegian, cnd, 3¾ oz, 106 gm	195	19	13	0	—	—	—	434	340	—
KING DAVID BRISLING SARDINES IN OLIVE OIL, Norwegian, cnd, 3¾ oz, 106 gm	293	21	23	0	—	—	—	842	273	—
KIPPER SNACKS, Norwegian, cnd, 3¼ oz, 92 gm	195	20	12	0	—	—	—	—	—	—
QUEEN HELGA SILD SARDINES IN OIL, Norwegian, cnd, 3¾ oz	310	20	26	0	—	—	—	603	273	—

Featherweight

SALMON, PINK, 3 oz	120	17	6	0	—	—	—	60	307	—
SARDINES										
IN TOMATO SAUCE, 1⅞ oz	—	13	6	—	—	—	—	65	133	—
IN WATER, 1⅞ oz	109	13	6	0	—	—	—	65	96	—
TUNA, CHUNK LIGHT, 3 oz	97	20	2	0	—	—	—	44	237	—

Gorton

LIGHT RECIPE, fz										
BAKED STUFFED SCROD, 1 pkg, 6 oz	260	26	15	4	—	20	*	490	—	—
CRAB AU GRATIN WITH ASPARAGUS, 1 pkg, 9 oz	280	22	13	18	—	300	1.08	810	—	—
FILLET OF FLOUNDER, ½ pkg, 5 oz	260	18	11	23	—	*	.72	710	—	—
FILLET OF HADDOCK, ½ pkg, 5 oz	270	19	12	22	—	40	.72	—	—	—
WITH LEMON BUTTER SAUCE, 1 pkg, 6 oz	240	26	11	8	—	20	.36	570	—	—
FILLET OF SOLE, ½ pkg, 5 oz	260	20	11	20	—	*	*	—	—	—
WITH LEMON BUTTER SAUCE, 1 pkg, 6 oz	250	24	13	8	—	20	.36	730	—	—
FISH FILLET, ½ pkg, 5 oz	260	19	11	22	—	20	1.80	—	—	—
IN TEMPURA BATTER, ½ pkg, 5 oz	280	17	16	16	—	*	1.44	—	—	—
FOUR FISH FILLETS, 1 fillet, 3 oz	170	11	7	16	—	*	.36	380	—	—
FOUR FISH FILLETS IN TEMPURA BATTER, 1 fillet, 3 oz	190	10	12	10	—	*	.36	400	—	—
FISH STICKS, lightly breaded, 3 sticks	200	10	11	15	—	*	.36	—	—	—
FISH STICKS TEMPURA, 3 sticks, 3.33 oz	200	10	13	11	—	*	*	—	—	—
SHRIMP ORIENTAL, 1 pkg, 10 oz	350	11	2	72	—	40	1.44	740	—	—
SHRIMP SCAMPI WITH LEMON BUTTER SAUCE AND GARLIC, 1 pkg, 6 oz	350	20	25	11	—	60	.72	410	—	—
STUFFED FLOUNDER STUFFED WITH SHRIMP AND CRABMEAT, 1 pkg, 6.5 oz	250	22	13	11	—	60	1.08	980	—	—

FOOD & DESCRIPTION MEASURE OR QUANTITY	CALORIES	PROTEIN (GM)	FAT (GM)	CARBO-HYDRATE (GM)	FIBER (GM)	CALCIUM (MG)	IRON (MG)	SODIUM (MG)	POTASSIUM (MG)	CHOLES-TEROL (MG)
Libby										
PINK SALMON, 7.75 oz	310	45	13	0	—	400	1.44	—	—	—
SOCKEYE RED SALMON, 7.75 oz	380	45	21	0	—	550	2.70	—	—	—
Mother's										
GEFILTE FISH										
OLD WORLD, JELLED, 1 piece fish, 78 gm; 35 gm jell	70	8	1	7	—	33	.43	—	—	—
OLD FASHIONED IN LIQUID BROTH, 1 piece fish, 78 gm; 35 gm liquid	70	9	1	7	—	48	.55	—	—	—
UNSALTED IN JELLED BROTH, 1 fishball, 50 gm	45	5	1	2	—	20	.36	10	—	—
WHITEFISH & PIKE, JELLED, 1 piece fish, 78 gm; 35 gm jell	60	9	1	4	—	34	.39	—	—	—
Mrs. Pauls–Campbell										
BATTER DIPPED FISH FILLETS, 2 fillets	360	20	19	27	—	20	1.80	830	—	—
BUTTERED FISH FILLETS, 2 fillets	210	22	13	0	—	20	.36	780	—	—
COMBINATION SEAFOOD PLATTER, 9 oz	510	22	25	49	—	80	1.80	1340	—	—
CRISPY CRUNCHY										
FISH FILLETS, 2 fillets	290	14	16	22	—	20	.36	650	—	—
FISH STICKS, 4 sticks	200	11	10	17	—	20	.36	455	—	—
FLOUNDER, 2 fillets	280	12	15	25	—	40	.72	800	—	—
HADDOCK FILLETS, 2 fillets	280	12	15	25	—	40	.72	800	—	—
PERCH FILLETS, 2 fillets	290	13	17	21	—	20	.36	480	—	—
CRUNCHY LIGHT BATTER										
FISH FILLETS, 2 fillets	310	14	16	27	—	40	.36	855	—	—
FISH STICKS, 4 sticks	240	9	13	21	—	20	.36	795	—	—
FLOUNDER FILLETS, 2 fillets	310	14	17	26	—	40	.36	1110	—	—
HADDOCK FILLETS, 2 fillets	320	13	17	28	—	40	.36	935	—	—
DEVILED CRABS, 1 piece	170	8	6	20	—	100	.72	385	—	—
MINIATURES, 3.5 oz	220	15	10	18	—	100	1.44	195	—	—
FISH CAKES, 2 cakes	220	11	8	24	—	40	1.08	670	—	—
THINS, 2 cakes	300	14	15	25	—	20	1.80	1020	—	—
FISH PARMESAN, 5 oz	220	15	11	16	—	100	.72	540	—	—
FRENCH FRIED SCALLOPS, 3.5 oz	210	13	7	23	—	60	1.08	545	—	—
FRIED CLAMS IN A LIGHT BATTER, 2.5 oz	230	9	13	20	—	*	1.08	385	—	—
FRIED SHRIMP, 3 oz	190	9	10	15	—	40	1.08	525	—	—
LIGHT BREADED										
FISH FILLETS, 1 fillet	290	22	13	21	—	20	.36	770	—	—
FLOUNDER FILLETS, 1 fillet	320	21	16	24	—	40	.72	975	—	—
HADDOCK FILLETS, 1 fillet	320	23	14	25	—	40	1.08	960	—	—
SOLE FILLETS, 1 fillet	280	21	13	19	—	40	1.08	700	—	—
SUPREME LIGHT BATTER FISH FILLETS, 1 fillet	220	11	10	19	—	60	.72	505	—	—
Nouvelle–Homarus										
POACHED NORWEGIAN SALMON IN BUTTER DILL SAUCE, 6.5 oz	270	36	11	9	—	—	—	326	—	—
POACHED RAINBOW TROUT ALMONDINE, 7 oz	380	38	24	2	—	—	—	631	—	—

FOOD & DESCRIPTION MEASURE OR QUANTITY	CALORIES	PROTEIN (GM)	FAT (GM)	CARBO-HYDRATE (GM)	FIBER (GM)	CALCIUM (MG)	IRON (MG)	SODIUM (MG)	POTASSIUM (MG)	CHOLES-TEROL (MG)
SHRIMP IN SCAMPI SAUCE, 5.5 oz	170	32	4	2	—	—	—	142	—	—
Rokeach										
GEFILTE FISH, ls, 1 fishball, 2 oz, 57 gm	50	6	2	3	—	20	.36	15	—	—
GEFILTE FISH, REDI JELLED, 1 piece fish & jell, 113 gm	60	8	1	4	—	42	.36	835	—	—
OLD VIENNA, 1 piece fish & jell, 113 gm	70	8	1	8	—	44	.29	—	—	—
NATURAL BROTH, 1 piece fish & jell, 113 gm	50	7	1	4	—	39	.29	—	—	—
WHITEFISH-PIKE, 1 piece fish & jell, 113 gm	60	9	1	4	—	42	.29	—	—	—
Snow—Borden										
SNOW CLAM JUICE, 3 oz	14	1	0	2	—	*	.36	470	45	—
SNOW MINCED CLAMS, 6.5 oz	100	18	1	4	—	40	2.70	920	140	—
Star-Kist **[All tuna is undrained]**										
CHUNK LIGHT TUNA										
PACKED IN OIL, 2 oz	150	13	13	<1	—	*	.72	310	—	—
60% LESS SALT, 2 oz	170	14	13	<1	—	*	.72	135	—	—
PACKED IN SPRING WATER, 2 oz	60	13	<1	<1	—	*	.72	310	—	—
60% LESS SALT, 2 oz	65	14	1	<1	—	*	.72	135	—	—
CHUNK WHITE TUNA										
PACKED IN OIL, 2 oz	140	14	10	<1	—	*	*	310	—	—
DIETETIC, IMPORTED ALBACORE, 2 oz	70	15	1	<1	—	*	*	30	—	—
SOLID LIGHT TUNA										
PACKED IN OIL, 2 oz	150	13	13	<1	—	*	.72	310	—	—
PACKED IN SPRING WATER, 2 oz	60	14	<1	<1	—	*	.72	310	—	—
IMPORTED ALBACORE, 2 oz	70	15	1	<1	—	*	*	310	—	—
SOLID WHITE TUNA										
OIL PACK, 2 oz	140	14	10	<1	—	*	*	310	—	—
SPRING WATER PACK, 2 oz	100	14	5	<1	—	*	*	310	—	—
USDA										
ABALONE										
cnd, 3.5 oz, 100 gm	80	16	<1	2	0	14	2.40	255	396	47
raw, 3.5 oz, 100 gm	98	19	<1	3	0	37	2.40	255	396	55
ALBACORE, raw, 3.5 oz, 100 gm	177	25	8	0	0	26	1.60	40	293	55
ALEWIFE										
cnd, s & l, 3.5 oz, 100 gm	141	16	8	0	0	50	.90	50	286	46
raw, 3.5 oz, 100 gm	127	19	5	0	0	50	.90	50	286	55
ANCHOVY, 5 anchovies, 20 gm	35	4	2	<1	0	34	.58	165	118	11
BARRACUDA, PACIFIC, raw, 3.5 oz, 100 gm	113	21	3	0	0	16	1.60	40	293	55
BASS										
BLACK SEA, raw, 3.5 oz, 100 gm	93	19	1	0	0	20	1.00	68	256	55
SMALL & LARGE MOUTH, raw, 3.5 oz, 100 gm	104	19	3	0	0	20	1.00	68	256	55
STRIPED										
oven fried, 3.5 oz, 100 gm	196	22	9	7	0	20	1.00	68	256	63
raw, 3.5 oz, 100 gm	105	19	3	0	0	20	1.00	68	256	55

FOOD & DESCRIPTION MEASURE OR QUANTITY	CALORIES	PROTEIN (GM)	FAT (GM)	CARBO- HYDRATE (GM)	FIBER (GM)	CALCIUM (MG)	IRON (MG)	SODIUM (MG)	POTASSIUM (MG)	CHOLES- TEROL (MG)
WHITE, raw, 3.5 oz, 100 gm	98	18	2	0	0	20	1.00	68	256	55
BLUEFISH										
baked or broiled, with butter										
or margarine, 3.5 oz,										
100 gm	159	26	5	0	0	29	.70	104	420	70
fried, 3.5 oz, 100 gm	205	23	10	5	0	35	.90	146	420	61
raw, 3.5 oz, 100 gm	117	21	3	0	0	23	.60	74	420	55
BONITO, ATLANTIC, PACIFIC										
& STRIPED, raw, 3.5 oz,										
100 gm	168	24	7	0	0	26	1.60	40	293	55
BUFFALOFISH, raw, 3.5 oz,										
100 gm	113	18	4	0	0	50	.90	52	293	55
BULLHEAD, BLACK, raw, 3.5										
oz, 100 gm	84	16	2	0	0	23	.40	60	330	55
BURBOT										
fried, 3.5 oz, 100 gm	165	37	6	0	0	40	1.20	177	348	117
raw, 3.5 oz, 100 gm	82	17	<1	0	0	23	.70	61	304	55
BUTTERFISH										
GULF WATERS, raw, 3.5 oz,										
100 gm	95	16	3	0	0	20	.50	54	330	55
NORTHERN WATERS, raw,										
3.5 oz, 100 gm	169	18	10	0	0	20	.50	54	330	55
CARP, raw, 3.5 oz, 100 gm	115	18	4	0	0	50	.90	50	286	55
CATFISH, FRESHWATER, raw,										
3.5 oz, 100 gm	103	18	3	0	0	23	.40	60	330	55
CAVIAR, STURGEON, granular										
1 tbsp, 16 gm	42	4	2	<1	0	44	1.90	352	29	48
1 oz, 28 gm	74	8	4	<1	0	78	3.30	624	51	85
CAVIAR, STURGEON, pressed,										
1 tbsp, 17 gm	54	6	3	<1	0	47	2.01	374	31	65
1 oz, 28 gm	90	10	5	1	0	78	3.35	624	51	109
CLAMS										
cnd, dr, solids, chopped or										
minced, 7.5–8 oz can,										
3.9–4.2 oz, 114 gm										
drained weight	112	18	3	2	0	63	4.67	137	160	72
1 c, 160 gm	157	25	4	3	0	88	6.56	192	224	101
cnd, s & l										
7.5–8 oz can, 220 gm	114	17	2	6	0	121	9.00	1254	308	70
1 pound, 454 gm	236	36	3	13	0	249	18.60	2588	635	145
raw, meat only										
soft, 38 large, 38–62										
medium, 62+ small, 1										
pint, 1 lb, 454 gm	372	64	9	6	0	313	15.44	163	1067	227
hard, 14 or fewer chowders,										
14–22 medium, 22–31										
cherrystone, 31+										
littlenecks, 1 pint, 1 lg,										
454 gm	363	50	4	27	0	313	34.00	930	1411	227
4 cherrystone or 5										
littlenecks, 70 gm	56	8	<1	4	0	48	5.30	144	218	35
CLAM LIQUOR, bouillon,										
nectar										
1 c, 240 gm	46	6	<1	5	0	0	0	960	0	22
1 oz, 30 gm	6	<1	<1	<1	0	0	0	120	0	3
COD										
cnd, dr, solids, flaked, 1 c,										
140 gm	119	27	<1	0	0	43	1.40	154	570	77
1 lb, 454 gm	386	87	1	0	0	141	4.54	499	1848	250
dehyd, lightly salted,										
shredded, 1 oz, 28 gm	106	23	<1	0	0	26	1.00	2296	45	66
dried, salted, 1 oz, 28 gm	37	8	<1	0	0	64	1.02	2296	45	23
raw, 3.5 oz, 100 gm	78	18	<1	0	0	10	.40	70	382	50
steak or fillet, broiled with										

FOOD & DESCRIPTION MEASURE OR QUANTITY	CALORIES	PROTEIN (GM)	FAT (GM)	CARBO-HYDRATE (GM)	FIBER (GM)	CALCIUM (MG)	IRON (MG)	SODIUM (MG)	POTASSIUM (MG)	CHOLES-TEROL (MG)
butter or margarine, 3.5 oz, 100 gm	170	29	5	0	0	31	1.00	110	407	81
CRAB										
cnd										
BLUE CRAB, dr, solids, 6.5 oz can, 125 gm	126	22	3	1	0	56	1.00	1250	138	126
KING CRAB, dr, solids, 7.5 oz can, 180 gm	182	31	5	2	0	81	1.40	1800	198	182
not packed, solids, claw, 1 c, 115 gm	116	20	3	1	0	52	.90	1150	127	116
white or king, 1 c, 135 gm	136	24	3	2	0	61	1.10	1350	149	136
packed, solids, 1 c, 160 gm	162	28	4	2	0	72	1.30	1600	176	162
DEVILED, 1 c, 240 gm	451	27	23	32	0	113	2.90	2081	398	245
3.5 oz, 100 gm	188	11	9	13	0	47	1.20	867	166	102
STEAMED										
flakes, not packed, 1 c, 125 gm	116	22	2	<1	0	54	1.00	263	225	125
pieces										
not packed, 1 c, 155 gm	144	27	3	<1	0	67	1.20	326	279	155
packed, 1 c, 210 gm	195	36	4	1	0	90	1.70	441	378	210
CRAPPIE, WHITE, raw, 3.5 oz, 100 gm	79	17	<1	0	0	12	.60	68	230	55
CRAYFISH, FRESHWATER or SPINY LOBSTER, raw, 3.5 oz, 100 gm	72	15	<1	1	0	77	1.50	210	180	66
CROAKER										
ATLANTIC, raw, 3.5 oz, 100 gm	96	18	2	0	0	10	.40	87	234	55
bkd, 3.5 oz, 100 gm	133	24	3	0	0	31	1.00	120	323	75
WHITE, raw, 3.5 oz, 100 gm	84	18	<1	0	0	10	.40	87	234	55
YELLOWFIN, raw, 3.5 oz, 100 gm	89	19	<1	0	0	10	.40	87	234	55
DOGFISH, SPINY, GRAYFISH, raw, 3.5 oz, 100 gm	156	18	9	0	0	20	.50	54	330	55
DRUM										
FRESHWATER, raw, 3.5 oz, 100 gm	121	17	5	0	0	50	.90	70	286	55
RED, REDFISH, raw, 3.5 oz, 100 gm	80	18	<1	0	0	10	.40	55	273	55
EEL, AMERICAN, raw, 3.5 oz, 100 gm	233	16	18	0	0	18	.70	74	420	55
smoked, 3.5 oz, 100 gm	330	19	28	0	0	18	.70	6231	157	64
EULACHON, SMELT, raw, 3.5 oz, 100 gm	118	15	6	0	0	50	.90	50	286	55
FINNAN HADDIE, SMOKED HADDOCK, 3.5 oz, 100 gm	103	23	<1	0	0	18	.70	6231	157	76
FISH CAKES										
fried, 1 regular or 5 bite-size pieces, 60 gm	103	9	5	6	—	7	.24	106	209	25
fz, fried, reheated, 1 regular or 5 bite-size pieces, 60 gm	162	6	11	10	—	7	.24	106	209	16
FISH FLAKES, cnd, s & l										
7 oz can, 198 gm	220	49	1	0	0	97	1.60	81	552	139
1 c, 165 gm	183	41	1	0	0	81	1.30	68	460	116
FISH STICKS, fz, breaded, ckd, 4 × 1 × ½″, 1 oz, 28 gm	50	5	3	2	0	3	.10	50	99	13
FLATFISH, FLOUNDER, SOLE, SANDDABS, raw, 3.5 oz, 100 gm	79	17	<1	0	0	12	.80	78	342	50
FLOUNDER, bkd with butter or margarine, 3.5 oz, 100										

FOOD & DESCRIPTION MEASURE OR QUANTITY	CALORIES	PROTEIN (GM)	FAT (GM)	CARBO-HYDRATE (GM)	FIBER (GM)	CALCIUM (MG)	IRON (MG)	SODIUM (MG)	POTASSIUM (MG)	CHOLES-TEROL (MG)
gm	202	30	8	0	0	23	1.40	237	587	90
FROG'S LEGS, 3.5 oz, 100 gm	73	16	<1	0	0	18	1.50	58	285	50
GROUPER, RED, BLACK, SPECKLED HIND, raw, 3.5 oz, 100 gm	87	19	<1	0	0	23	.70	61	304	55
HADDOCK										
fried, pan or oven, 3.5 oz, 100 gm	165	20	6	6	0	40	1.20	177	348	64
smoked, canned or uncanned, 3.5 oz, 100 gm	103	23	<1	0	0	23	.70	6231	157	76
raw, 3.5 oz, 100 gm	79	18	<1	0	0	23	.70	61	304	60
HAKE or WHITING, raw, 3.5 oz, 100 gm	74	17	<1	0	0	41	.70	74	363	55
HALIBUT										
ATLANTIC & PACIFIC, raw, 3.5 oz, 100 gm	100	21	1	0	0	13	.70	54	449	50
broiled with butter or margarine, 3.5 oz, 100 gm	171	25	7	0	0	16	.80	134	525	60
CALIFORNIA, raw, 3.5 oz, 100 gm	97	20	1	0	0	13	.70	54	449	50
GREENLAND, raw, 3.5 oz, 100 gm	146	16	8	0	0	13	.70	54	449	50
smoked, 3.5 oz, 100 gm	224	21	15	0	0	13	.70	6231	157	50
HERRING										
in tomato sauce, 1 herring with 1 tbsp sauce, 55 gm	97	9	6	2	—	81	.99	41	231	43
BISMARCK, pickled										
1 herring, 50 gm	112	10	8	0	0	33	.70	3116	79	50
1 oz, 28 gm	63	6	4	0	0	19	.40	1766	45	28
plain, cnd, s & l, 15 oz, 425 gm	884	85	58	0	0	625	7.70	315	1785	412
smoked, kippered, cnd, dr solids, fillet 7 × 2¼ × ¼", 1 fillet, 65 gm	137	14	8	0	0	43	.90	4050	102	71
contents from 3.25 oz can, dr, 80 gm	169	18	10	0	0	53	1.10	4985	126	87
fillet, 4⅜ × 1¾ × ¼", 40 gm	84	9	5	0	0	26	.60	2492	63	44
JACK MACKEREL, raw, 3.5 oz, 100 gm	143	22	6	0	0	8	2.10	74	420	55
KINGFISH, NORTHERN & SOUTHERN GULF, WHITING, 3.5 oz, 100 gm	105	18	3	0	0	12	.60	83	250	55
LAKE HERRING, CISCO, raw, 3.5 oz, 100 gm	96	18	2	0	0	12	.50	47	319	55
LAKE TROUT										
raw, 3.5 oz, 100 gm	168	18	10	0	0	26	.80	81	292	55
SISCOWET, raw										
less than 6.5 lbs round weight, 3.5 oz, 100 gm	241	14	20	0	0	26	.80	81	292	55
over 6.5 lbs round weight, 3.5 oz, 100 gm	524	8	54	0	0	26	.80	81	292	55
LINGCOD, raw, 3.5 oz, 100 gm	84	18	<1	0	0	13	.70	59	433	55
LOBSTER, NORTHERN										
cnd or ckd, 3.5 oz, 100 gm	95	19	2	<1	0	65	.80	210	180	85
raw, whole, 3.5 oz, 100 gm	91	17	2	0	0	29	.60	210	180	77
MACKEREL										
ATLANTIC										
broiled with butter or										

FOOD & DESCRIPTION MEASURE OR QUANTITY	CALORIES	PROTEIN (GM)	FAT (GM)	CARBO-HYDRATE (GM)	FIBER (GM)	CALCIUM (MG)	IRON (MG)	SODIUM (MG)	POTASSIUM (MG)	CHOLES-TEROL (MG)
margarine, 3.5 oz, 100 gm	236	22	16	0	0	6	1.20	74	420	101
cnd, s & l, 3.5 oz, 100 gm	183	19	11	0	0	185	2.10	74	420	94
raw, 3.5 oz, 100 gm	191	19	12	0	0	5	1.00	74	420	95
PACIFIC										
cnd, s & l, 15 oz, 425 gm	765	90	43	0	0	1105	9.35	315	1785	400
3.5 oz, 100 gm	180	21	10	0	0	260	2.20	74	420	94
raw, 3.5 oz, 100 gm	159	22	7	0	0	8	2.10	74	420	95
SALTED										
1 fillet, 112 gm	342	21	28	0	0	74	1.57	6979	176	106
1 oz, 28 gm	86	5	7	0	0	19	.40	1766	45	27
3.5 oz, 100 gm	305	19	25	0	0	66	1.40	6231	157	95
smoked, 3.5 oz, 100 gm	219	24	13	0	0	66	1.40	6231	157	95
MENHADEN, ATLANTIC, cnd, s & l, 3.5 oz, 100 gm	172	19	10	0	0	147	1.30	74	420	55
MUSKELLUNGE, raw, 3.5 oz, 100 gm	109	20	3	0	0	28	.60	111	753	55
MUSSELS										
ATLANTIC & PACIFIC										
raw, s & l, 3.5 oz, 100 gm	66	10	1	3	0	88	3.40	289	315	50
raw, meat only, 3.5 oz, 100 gm	95	14	2	3	0	88	3.40	289	315	50
PACIFIC										
cnd, dr solids, 3.5 oz, 100 gm	114	18	3	2	0	88	3.40	289	315	45
OCEAN PERCH										
ATLANTIC, REDFISH										
fried, 3.5 oz, 100 gm	227	19	13	7	0	33	1.30	153	284	58
raw, 3.5 oz, 100 gm	88	18	1	0	0	20	1.00	79	269	55
PACIFIC, raw, 3.5 oz, 100 gm	95	19	2	0	0	20	1.00	63	390	55
fried, fz, breaded, fillet, 88 gm	281	17	17	15	0	29	1.14	135	250	51
OCTOPUS, raw, 3.5 oz, 100 gm	73	15	<1	0	0	29	.70	74	363	55
OYSTERS										
fried, 2.5 select, 1 oz, 28 gm	68	2	4	5	—	43	2.30	58	58	13
raw										
EASTERN, dr, 18–27 select or 27–44 standard, 12 oz, 340 gm	224	29	6	12	0	320	18.70	248	411	170
1 c, 240 gm	158	20	4	8	0	226	13.20	175	290	120
2 select or 3 standard, 1 oz, 28 gm	19	2	<1	1	0	27	1.60	21	34	14
PACIFIC & WESTERN, dr, 6–9 medium, 9–13 small, 12 oz, 340 gm	309	36	8	22	0	289	24.50	248	411	170
4–6 medium, 6–9 small, 1 c, 240 gm	218	25	5	15	0	204	17.30	175	290	120
PERCH										
WHITE, raw, 3.5 oz, 100 gm	118	19	4	0	0	50	.90	50	286	55
YELLOW, raw, 3.5 oz, 100 gm	91	20	<1	0	0	12	.60	68	230	55
PICKEREL, CHAIN, raw, 3.5 oz, 100 gm	84	19	<1	0	0	50	.70	68	230	55
PIKE										
BLUE, raw, 3.5 oz, 100 gm	90	19	<1	0	0	13	.40	51	319	55
NORTHERN, raw, 3.5 oz, 100 gm	88	18	1	0	0	13	.40	51	319	55
WALLEYE, raw, 3.5 oz, 100 gm	93	19	1	0	0	13	.40	51	319	55
POLLOCK, raw, 3.5 oz, 100 gm	95	20	<1	0	0	13	.70	48	350	55
POMPANO, raw, 3.5 oz, 100										

FOOD & DESCRIPTION MEASURE OR QUANTITY	CALORIES	PROTEIN (GM)	FAT (GM)	CARBO-HYDRATE (GM)	FIBER (GM)	CALCIUM (MG)	IRON (MG)	SODIUM (MG)	POTASSIUM (MG)	CHOLES-TEROL (MG)
gm	166	19	10	0	0	45	1.10	47	191	55
RED & GRAY SNAPPER, raw, 3.5 oz, 100 gm	93	20	<1	0	0	16	.80	67	323	55
REDHORSE, SILVER, raw, 3.5 oz, 100 gm	98	18	2	0	0	13	.70	54	449	55
ROCKFISH, BLACK, CANARY, YELLOWTAIL, RASPHEAD & BOCACCIO oven-steamed fillets, 3.5 oz, 100 gm	107	18	3	2	0	16	.80	68	446	53
raw, 3.5 oz, 100 gm	97	19	2	0	0	13	.70	60	388	55
ROE										
CARP, COD, HADDOCK, HERRING, PIKE, SHAD, 3.5 oz, 100 gm	130	24	2	2	0	30	.60	73	132	360
COD & SHAD										
ckd, 3.5 oz, 100 gm	126	22	3	2	0	13	2.30	73	132	325
cnd, 3.5 oz, 100 gm	118	22	3	<1	0	15	1.20	73	132	317
HERRING, cnd, s & l, 8 oz, 227 gm	268	49	6	<1	0	34	2.72	166	300	720
SALMON, STURGEON, TURBOT, 3.5 oz, 100 gm	207	25	10	1	0	13	.60	73	132	360
SABLEFISH, raw, 3.5 oz, 100 gm	190	13	15	0	0	79	.90	56	358	55
SALMON										
broiled or baked with butter or margarine, 3.5 oz, 100 gm	182	27	7	0	0	127	1.20	116	443	47
cnd, s & l										
ATLANTIC, 1 can, 7.75 oz, 220 gm	447	48	27	0	0	339	1.98	163	924	81
CHINOOK, KING, salt-free, 1 can, 7.75 oz, 220 gm	462	43	31	0	0	339	2.00	105	805	75
CHUM, salt-free, 1 can, 7.75 oz, 220 gm	306	47	11	0	0	548	1.50	105	739	81
COHO, 1 can, 7.75 oz, 220 gm	337	46	16	0	0	537	2.00	772	746	79
HUMPBACK (pink), 1 can, 7.75 oz, 220 gm	310	45	13	0	0	431	1.80	851	794	77
SOCKEYE (red), 1 can, 7.75 oz, 220 gm	376	45	21	0	0	570	2.60	1148	757	77
raw										
ATLANTIC, 3.5 oz, 100 gm	217	23	13	0	0	79	.90	74	420	39
CHINOOK, KING, 3.5 oz, 100 gm	222	19	16	0	0	79	.90	45	399	33
CHUM, 3.5 oz, 100 gm	186	21	11	0	0	127	.70	53	429	33
COHO, 3.5 oz, 100 gm	186	21	11	0	0	175	.90	48	421	33
HUMPBACK (pink), 3.5 oz, 100 gm	119	20	4	0	0	127	.80	64	306	35
SOCKEYE, 3.5 oz, 100 gm	186	21	11	0	0	127	1.20	48	391	35
smoked, 1 oz, 28 gm	50	6	3	0	0	4	.40	1766	45	11
SARDINES										
ATLANTIC										
cnd, in oil, dr, solids, 1 oz, 28 gm	58	7	3	—	0	124	.80	233	167	40
s & l, 1 oz, 28 gm	88	6	7	<1	0	100	1	145	159	34
PACIFIC										
cnd										
in brine or mustard, s & l, 3.5 oz, 100 gm	196	19	12	2	0	303	5.20	760	260	110
in oil, dr, solids, 3.5 oz, 100 gm	203	24	11	0	0	437	2.90	823	590	120
in tomato sauce, s & l, 3.5										

FOOD & DESCRIPTION MEASURE OR QUANTITY	CALORIES	PROTEIN (GM)	FAT (GM)	CARBO-HYDRATE (GM)	FIBER (GM)	CALCIUM (MG)	IRON (MG)	SODIUM (MG)	POTASSIUM (MG)	CHOLES-TEROL (MG)
oz, 100 gm	197	19	12	2	0	449	4.10	400	320	110
raw, 3.5 oz, 100 gm	160	19	9	0	0	33	1.80	74	420	112
SCALLOPS										
fried, fz, SEA, 1 scallop, 10 gm	19	2	<1	1	0	8	.35	12	15	4
3.5 oz, 100 gm	194	18	8	11	0	76	3.50	120	147	41
raw, BAY or SEA, 3.5 oz	81	15	<1	3	0	26	1.80	255	396	35
steamed, BAY or SEA, 3.5 oz, 100 gm	112	23	1	3	0	115	3.00	265	476	53
SEA BASS, WHITE, raw, 3.5 oz, 100 gm	96	21	<1	0	0	41	.70	74	363	55
SHAD, AMERICAN										
cnd, s & l, 3.5 oz, 100 gm	152	17	9	0	0	24	.70	79	377	50
raw, 3.5 oz, 100 gm	170	19	10	0	0	20	.50	54	330	55
bkd, 3.5 oz, 100 gm	201	23	11	0	0	24	.60	79	377	69
SHEEPSHEAD, ATLANTIC, raw, 3.5 oz, 100 gm	113	21	3	0	0	50	.90	101	234	55
SHRIMP										
dr solids, 1 c, 128 gm	148	31	1	<1	0	147	4.00	179	156	192
large, 3¼", 10 shrimp, 58 gm	67	14	<1	<1	0	67	1.80	81	71	87
medium, 2½", 10 shrimp, 32 gm	37	8	<1	<1	0	37	1.00	45	39	48
small, 2", 10 shrimp, 17 gm	20	4	<1	<1	0	20	.50	24	21	26
1 oz, 28 gm	33	7	<1	<1	0	33	.90	40	35	43
french-fried, 1 oz, 28 gm	64	6	3	3	0	20	.60	53	65	43
3.5 oz, 100 gm	225	20	11	10	0	72	2.00	186	229	150
fz, breaded, raw, 3.5 oz, 100 gm	139	12	<1	20	.10	38	1.00	140	122	102
raw, 3.5 oz, 100 gm	91	18	<1	2	0	63	1.60	140	220	150
SHRIMP or LOBSTER PASTE, cnd, 3.5 oz, 100 gm	180	21	9	2	0	115	3.10	140	122	172
SKATE or RAJAFISH, raw, 3.5 oz, 100 gm	98	22	<1	0	0	10	.40	70	382	55
SMELT, ATLANTIC, JACK & BAY										
cnd, s & l, 3.5 oz, 100 gm	200	18	14	0	0	358	1.70	70	382	54
raw, 3.5 oz, 100 gm	98	19	2	0	0	10	.40	70	382	55
SNAIL, raw, 3.5 oz, 100 gm	90	16	1	2	0	10	3.50	70	382	50
GIANT AFRICAN, raw, 3.5 oz, 100 gm	73	10	1	4	0	10	3.50	70	382	50
SQUID, raw, 3.5 oz, 100 gm	84	16	<1	2	0	12	.50	74	363	55
STURGEON										
steamed, 3.5 oz, 100 gm	160	25	6	0	0	40	2.00	108	235	77
raw, 3.5 oz, 100 gm	94	18	2	0	0	13	.70	54	449	55
smoked, 3.5 oz, 100 gm	149	31	2	0	0	13	.70	6231	157	95
SUCKERS										
CARP, raw, 3.5 oz, 100 gm	111	19	3	0	0	13	.70	56	336	55
WHITE & MULLET, raw, 3.5 oz, 100 gm	104	21	2	0	0	13	.70	56	336	55
SWORDFISH										
broiled with butter, 3.5 oz, 100 gm	174	28	6	0	0	27	1.30	134	525	80
cnd, s & l, 3.5 oz, 100 gm	102	18	3	0	0	27	1.30	134	525	50
raw, 3.5 oz, 100 gm	118	19	4	0	0	19	.90	54	449	55
TAUTOG, BLACKFISH, raw, 3.5 oz, 100 gm	89	19	1	0	0	13	.70	54	449	55
TERRAPIN, DIAMOND BACK, raw, 3.5 oz, 100 gm	111	19	4	0	0	50	3.20	50	286	50
TILEFISH										
baked, 3.5 oz, 100 gm	138	25	4	0	0	16	.80	134	525	77
raw, 3.5 oz, 100 gm	79	18	<1	0	0	13	.70	54	449	55
TROUT										
BROOK, raw, 3.5 oz, 100 gm	101	19	2	0	0	12	.50	47	319	49

FOOD & DESCRIPTION MEASURE OR QUANTITY	CALORIES	PROTEIN (GM)	FAT (GM)	CARBO- HYDRATE (GM)	FIBER (GM)	CALCIUM (MG)	IRON (MG)	SODIUM (MG)	POTASSIUM (MG)	CHOLES- TEROL (MG)
RAINBOW & STEELHEAD										
cnd, 3.5 oz, 100 gm	209	21	13	0	0	26	.80	81	292	53
raw, 3.5 oz, 100 gm	195	22	11	0	0	26	.80	81	292	55
TUNA										
cnd in oil										
s & l, 3.5 oz, 100 gm	288	24	21	0	0	6	1.10	800	301	55
dr, solids, 3.5 oz, 100 gm	197	29	8	0	0	8	1.90	800	301	65
cnd in water										
s & l, 3.5 oz, 100 gm	127	28	<1	0	0	16	1.60	875	279	63
salt-free, 3.5 oz, 100 gm	127	28	<1	0	0	16	1.60	41	279	63
raw										
BLUEFIN, 3.5 oz, 100 gm	145	25	4	0	0	16	1.30	37	279	57
YELLOWFIN, 3.5 oz, 100 gm	133	25	3	0	0	16	1.30	37	279	56
TURTLE, GREEN										
cnd, 3.5 oz, 100 gm	106	23	<1	0	0	118	1.40	68	230	50
raw, 3.5 oz, 100 gm	89	20	<1	0	0	118	1.40	68	230	50
WEAKFISH										
broiled with butter or margarine, 3.5 oz, 100 gm	208	25	11	0	0	29	.70	560	465	82
raw, 3.5 oz, 100 gm	121	17	6	0	0	23	.60	75	317	55
WHITEFISH, LAKE, flesh only										
raw, 3.5 oz, 100 gm	155	19	8	0	0	26	.40	52	299	55
smoked, 3.5 oz, 100 gm	155	21	7	0	0	22	1.40	6231	157	61
WRECKFISH, raw, 3.5 oz, 100 gm	114	18	4	0	0	47	3.20	74	282	55
YELLOWTAIL, PACIFIC COAST, raw, 3.5 oz, 100 gm	138	21	5	0	0	23	.60	74	420	55
Van De Camp										
BATTER-DIPPED										
FISH STICKS, 4 oz	220	9	14	15	—	20	1.08	330	—	—
FISH FILLETS, 3 oz	180	8	10	15	—	20	.72	230	—	—
FISH & CHIPS, half fish & half chips, 7 oz	440	18	25	36	—	40	1.80	640	—	—
FISH KABOBS, 4 oz	240	12	15	15	—	20	1.44	430	—	—
HADDOCK, 4 oz	240	13	12	18	—	—	—	430	—	—
HALIBUT, 4 oz	260	12	16	17	—	20	1.44	440	—	—
PERCH, 4 oz	270	12	15	21	—	—	—	510	—	—
SOLE, 4 oz	280	14	14	24	—	40	1.44	578	—	—
COUNTRY SEASONED FISH										
FILLETS, 2 oz	200	7	13	12	—	20	.90	335	—	—
LIGHT & CRISPY										
FISH STICKS, 3.75 oz	270	8	19	16	—	—	.72	300	—	—
FISH FILLETS, 2 oz	180	6	14	9	—	—	.54	175	—	—
FISH NUGGETS, 2 oz	130	7	8	9	—	—	.54	160	—	—
HADDOCK FILLETS, 2 oz	180	5	13	10	—	—	.72	160	—	—
PERCH FILLETS, 2 oz	170	6	12	10	—	—	1.26	115	—	—
LIGHTLY BREADED										
COD, 5 oz	290	17	19	11	—	—	.72	371	—	—
FLOUNDER, 5 oz	300	16	18	17	—	30	.72	412	—	—
SOLE, 5 oz	300	16	18	17	—	30	.72	412	—	—
TODAY'S CATCH										
COD, 4 oz	80	18	0	0	—	—	.36	150	—	—
FISH FILLETS, 4 oz	90	20	0	0	—	—	1.80	80	—	—
FLOUNDER, 4 oz	90	18	0	2	—	—	.72	130	—	—
HADDOCK, 4 oz	90	19	0	0	—	—	1.44	70	—	—
PERCH, 4 oz	110	20	3	0	—	20	.72	180	—	—
SOLE, BABY, 4 oz	80	17	0	0	—	20	1.08	220	—	—

13

FRUITS

FOOD & DESCRIPTION MEASURE OR QUANTITY	CALORIES	PROTEIN (GM)	FAT (GM)	CARBO-HYDRATE (GM)	FIBER (GM)	CALCIUM (MG)	IRON (MG)	SODIUM (MG)	POTASSIUM (MG)	CHOLES-TEROL (MG)
Birds Eye–										
General Foods										
AWAKE, 6 oz	80	0	0	21	tr	*	*	15	60	—
MIXED FRUIT, QUICK THAW,										
light syrup, 5 oz	100	1	0	27	.6	*	.36	0	190	—
ORANGE PLUS, 6 oz	100	0	0	24	tr	20	*	10	170	—
RED RASPBERRIES, LITE										
SYRUP, QUICK THAW,										
5 oz	100	1	0	26	3.1	20	1.08	0	160	—
STRAWBERRIES										
HALVED, LITE SYRUP,										
QUICK THAW, 5 oz	60	1	0	16	.6	*	.72	5	135	—
HALVED IN SYRUP, QUICK										
THAW, 5 oz	120	1	0	30	.6	*	1.08	5	135	—
WHOLE, LITE SYRUP, 4 oz	60	1	0	14	.5	*	.72	0	125	—
Del Monte										
APPLES, dried, sliced, 2 oz,										
57 gm	140	0	0	37	—	*	.72	<50	255	—
APPLESAUCE, cnd, ½ c,										
113.5 gm	90	0	0	24	—	0	.36	<5	75	—
LITE, ½ c, 113.5 gm	50	0	0	13	—	0	*	<10	85	—
APRICOTS, cnd, halved,										
unpeeled, ½ c, 120.5										
gm	100	0	0	26	—	*	.36	<10	165	—
LITE, halved, ½ c, 120.5 gm	60	0	0	16	—	*	*	<10	165	—
cnd, whole, peeled, ½ c,										
120.5 gm	100	0	0	27	—	*	.36	<10	150	—
APRICOTS, DRIED, 2 oz, 57										
gm	140	2	0	35	—	20	2.70	<10	825	—
APRICOT NECTAR, 6 oz, 188										
gm	100	1	0	26	—	*	.72	<10	215	—
BANANA, 1 medium, 175 gm	101	1	<1	26	—	10	.72	1	440	—
CHERRIES, cnd										
DARK, SWEET, pitted, ½ c,										
117 gm	90	0	0	24	—	*	.36	<10	180	—
with pits, ½ c, 117 gm	90	0	0	23	—	*	.36	<10	170	—
LIGHT, SWEET, with pits, ½										
c, 120.5 gm	100	0	0	26	—	*	.36	<10	165	—
CHUNKY MIXED FRUIT, cnd,										
½ c, 120.5 gm	80	0	0	23	—	0	.36	<10	90	—
LITE, ½ c, 120.5 gm	50	0	0	14	—	0	*	<10	105	—
CURRANTS, ZANTE, DRIED,										
½ c, 67 gm	200	2	0	53	—	60	1.80	<10	700	—

FOOD & DESCRIPTION MEASURE OR QUANTITY	CALORIES	PROTEIN (GM)	FAT (GM)	CARBO-HYDRATE (GM)	FIBER (GM)	CALCIUM (MG)	IRON (MG)	SODIUM (MG)	POTASSIUM (MG)	CHOLES-TEROL (MG)
FIGS, cnd, whole, ½ c, 120.5 gm	100	0	0	28	—	20	*	<10	150	—
FRUIT COCKTAIL, cnd, ½ c, 120.5 gm	80	0	0	23	—	0	.36	<10	105	—
LITE, ½ c, 120.5 gm	50	0	0	15	—	0	*	<10	105	—
FRUIT FOR SALAD, cnd, ½ c, 120.5 gm	90	0	0	22	—	0	*	<10	90	—
GRAPEFRUIT JUICE, cnd, unsw, 6 oz, 184 gm	70	1	0	17	—	*	.36	<10	255	—
MANDARIN ORANGES, cnd, 5.5 oz, 156 gm	100	0	0	25	—	*	.36	<10	120	—
MIXED FRUIT CUP, cnd, single serving, 5 oz, 142 gm	100	0	0	27	—	*	.36	<10	110	—
MIXED FRUIT, DRIED, diced, .9 oz, 25 gm	80	0	0	18	—	*	.72	25	260	—
2 oz, 57 gm	130	1	0	34	—	20	1.44	10	470	—
ORANGE JUICE, cnd, unsw, 6 oz, 185 gm	80	1	0	19	—	*	.72	<10	300	—
PAPAYA, fresh, ⅓ medium fruit, 100 gm	60	0	0	15	—	*	.36	<5	160	—
PEACHES, FREESTONE, cnd, halved or sliced ½ c, 113.5 gm	90	0	0	23	—	0	*	<10	105	—
LITE, ½ c, 113.5 gm	60	0	0	13	—	0	*	<10	100	—
CLING, diced, single serving, 5 oz, 113.5 gm	110	0	0	28	—	*	.36	<10	110	—
halved or sliced, ½ c, 113.5 gm	80	0	0	22	—	0	*	<10	100	—
LITE, ½ c, 113.5 gm	50	0	0	13	—	0	*	<10	100	—
SPICED, with pits, 3.5 oz, 103 gm	80	0	0	20	—	0	*	<10	80	—
PEACHES, DRIED, uncooked, 2 oz, 57 gm	140	2	0	35	—	*	1.80	<10	595	—
PEARS, BARTLETT, cnd, halved or sliced, ½ c, 113.5 gm	80	0	0	22	—	0	*	<10	70	—
LITE, ½ c, 113.5 gm	50	0	0	14	—	0	*	<10	50	—
PINEAPPLE, fresh, 2 sl, 168 gm	90	1	0	24	—	20	.36	<5	180	—
PINEAPPLE, cnd chunks, tidbits, slices, juice pack, ½ c, 113.5 gm	70	0	0	18	—	*	*	<10	95	—
crushed, chunks, slices, syrup pack, ½ c, 113.5 gm	90	0	0	23	—	*	*	<10	160	—
spears, juice pack, 2 spears, 89 gm	50	0	0	14	—	20	.36	10	75	—
PINEAPPLE JUICE, cnd, unsw, 6 oz, 188 gm	100	0	0	25	—	20	.72	<10	240	—
PRUNES, dried, pitted, uncooked, 2 oz, 57 gm	140	1	0	35	—	20	1.08	<10	455	—
with pits, 2 oz, 57 gm	120	1	0	31	—	20	1.08	<10	390	—
moist pack, 2 oz, 57 gm	120	1	0	30	—	20	1.80	<10	325	—
PRUNE JUICE, cnd, unsw, 6 oz, 191 gm	120	1	0	33	—	*	1.44	<10	500	—
RAISINS GOLDEN, 3 oz, 85 gm	260	3	0	68	—	40	1.44	<10	655	—
NATURAL, 3 oz, 85 gm	250	3	0	68	—	40	1.80	15	665	—
TROPICAL FRUIT SALAD, cnd, ½ c, 113.5 gm	90	0	0	26	—	*	.36	<10	150	—

FOOD & DESCRIPTION MEASURE OR QUANTITY	CALORIES	PROTEIN (GM)	FAT (GM)	CARBO- HYDRATE (GM)	FIBER (GM)	CALCIUM (MG)	IRON (MG)	SODIUM (MG)	POTASSIUM (MG)	CHOLES- TEROL (MG)
Dole										
BANANA, fresh, 1 medium, 8¾", 175 gm	101	1	<1	26	—	10	.80	1	440	—
GRAPES, THOMPSON SEEDLESS, fresh, ½ c, 80 gm	54	<1	<1	14	—	10	.30	3	138	—
MANDARIN ORANGES, cnd, light syrup, ½ c, 126 gm	76	<1	<1	20	—	9	.46	8	99	—
ORANGE, NAVEL, fresh, with skin, 1 medium, 206 gm	71	2	<1	18	—	56	.60	1	272	—
PINEAPPLE, cnd, all cuts juice pack, ½ c, 114 gm	70	<1	<1	18	—	10	.36	1	139	—
syrup pack, ½ c, 128 gm	95	<1	<1	25	—	14	.40	2	123	—
PINEAPPLE, fresh, ½ c, 78 gm	41	<1	<1	11	—	13	.40	1	113	—
PINEAPPLE JUICE, 6 oz	103	<1	<1	25	—	28	.60	2	280	—
Dromedary—Nabisco										
DATES, chopped, ¼ c	130	1	0	31	—	20	.72	0	190	—
pitted, 5 fruits	100	1	0	23	—	20	.72	0	190	—
Duffy—Mott										
APPLE JUICE, 6 oz	78	0	0	19	—	—	—	—	—	—
blended, west coast, 6 oz	86	0	0	21	—	—	—	—	—	—
blended with concentrate, 6 oz	81	0	0	20	—	—	—	—	—	—
concentrate, shelf stable, diluted, 6 oz	86	0	0	21	—	—	—	—	—	—
from concentrate, 6 oz	83	0	0	20	—	—	—	—	—	—
natural style, 6 oz	83	0	0	20	—	—	—	—	—	—
southern, from concentrate, 6 oz	83	0	0	20	—	—	—	—	—	—
APPLE CRANBERRY CURRANT JUICE, shelf stable, from concentrate, diluted, 6 oz	98	0	0	24	—	—	—	—	—	—
APPLE CRANBERRY JUICE, 6 oz	79	0	0	19	—	—	—	—	—	—
APPLE GRAPE JUICE, 6 oz	84	0	0	20	—	—	—	—	—	—
shelf stable, concentrate, diluted, 6 oz	93	0	0	22	—	—	—	—	—	—
APPLE RASPBERRY JUICE, 10 oz	130	0	0	31	—	—	—	—	—	—
APPLESAUCE, cnd, with sugar, 4 oz	119	0	0	29	—	—	—	—	—	—
CHUNKY, 4 oz	119	0	0	29	—	—	—	—	—	—
CINNAMON, 4 oz	119	0	0	29	—	—	—	—	—	—
NATURAL STYLE, 4 oz	53	0	0	12	—	—	—	—	—	—
GRAPEFRUIT JUICE, 10 oz	115	1	0	26	—	—	—	—	—	—
ORANGE BLEND JUICE, 10 oz	130	1	0	30	—	—	—	—	—	—
PRUNE JUICE WITH PULP, 6 oz	129	1	0	31	—	—	—	—	—	—
SUPER MOTT'S PRUNE JUICE, 6 oz	143	1	0	34	—	—	—	—	—	—
Featherweight										
APPLESAUCE, cnd, water pack, ½ c	50	0	0	12	—	—	—	<3	8	—
APRICOTS, cnd, juice pack, ½ c	50	1	0	12	—	—	—	<10	210	—
water pack, ½ c	35	0	0	9	—	—	—	<3	200	—

FOOD & DESCRIPTION MEASURE OR QUANTITY	CALORIES	PROTEIN (GM)	FAT (GM)	CARBO-HYDRATE (GM)	FIBER (GM)	CALCIUM (MG)	IRON (MG)	SODIUM (MG)	POTASSIUM (MG)	CHOLES-TEROL (MG)
CHERRIES, cnd, DARK, water										
pack, ½ c	60	1	0	13	—	—	—	<3	162	—
LIGHT, water pack, ½ c	50	1	0	11	—	—	—	<3	159	—
FRUIT COCKTAIL, cnd, juice										
pack, ½ c	50	1	0	12	—	—	—	<10	100	—
water pack, ½ c	40	0	0	10	—	—	—	<3	115	—
FRUIT FOR SALAD, cnd, juice										
pack, ½ c	50	1	0	12	—	—	—	<10	171	—
GRAPEFRUIT SEGMENTS,										
cnd, juice pack, ½ c	40	0	0	9	—	—	—	<10	200	—
MANDARIN ORANGES, cnd,										
water pack, ½ c	35	0	0	8	—	—	—	<10	146	—
PEACHES, cnd, halved or										
sliced, juice pack, ½ c	50	1	0	12	—	—	—	<10	220	—
water pack, ½ c	30	0	0	8	—	—	—	<3	120	—
PEARS, cnd, juice pack,										
halved, ½ c	60	0	0	15	—	—	—	<10	150	—
water pack, ½ c	40	0	0	10	—	—	—	<3	60	—
PINEAPPLE, cnd, slices or										
chunks, juice pack, ½ c	70	0	0	18	—	—	—	<10	113	—
water pack, ½ c	60	0	0	15	—	—	—	<10	113	—
PRUNES, STEWED, water										
pack, ½ c	130	1	1	35	—	—	—	<3	348	—
PURPLE PLUMS, cnd, whole,										
juice pack, ½ c	80	1	0	18	—	—	—	<10	184	—

Libby

FOOD & DESCRIPTION	CALORIES	PROTEIN	FAT	CARBO-HYDRATE	FIBER	CALCIUM	IRON	SODIUM	POTASSIUM	CHOLES-TEROL
APRICOT NECTAR, cnd, 6 oz	110	1	0	27	—	20	.36	5	285	—
BANANA NECTAR, cnd, 6 oz	60	0	0	14	—	*	.36	5	—	—
GRAPEFRUIT JUICE, cnd,										
unsw, 6 oz	75	1	0	18	—	20	.72	5	300	—
GUAVA NECTAR, cnd, 6 oz	70	0	0	17	—	*	.72	5	—	—
MANGO NECTAR, cnd, 6 oz	60	0	0	14	—	*	.36	5	—	—
ORANGE JUICE, cnd										
sweetened, 6 oz	100	1	0	23	—	20	.72	5	370	—
unsw, 6 oz	90	2	0	20	—	20	.72	5	370	—
ORANGE AND GRAPEFRUIT										
JUICE, cnd, unsw, 6 oz	80	1	0	19	—	20	.72	5	340	—
PEACH NECTAR, cnd, 6 oz	90	0	0	23	—	*	.36	5	145	—
PEAR NECTAR, cnd, 6 oz	100	0	0	25	—	*	*	5	75	—
PEAR/PASSION FRUIT										
NECTAR, cnd, 6 oz	60	0	0	14	—	*	.36	5	—	—
STRAWBERRY NECTAR, cnd,										
6 oz	60	0	0	14	—	*	.36	5	—	—

USDA
[All weights are edible portions]

FOOD & DESCRIPTION	CALORIES	PROTEIN	FAT	CARBO-HYDRATE	FIBER	CALCIUM	IRON	SODIUM	POTASSIUM	CHOLES-TEROL
ACEROLA, raw, 1 fruit, 4.8 gm	2	<1	<1	<1	.02	1	.01	0	7	0
1 c, 98 gm	31	<1	<1	8	.39	12	.20	7	143	0
ACEROLA JUICE, raw, 1 c,										
242 gm	51	<1	<1	12	.73	24	1.21	7	235	0
APPLE, raw, with skin, 1 fruit,										
138 gm	81	<1	<1	21	1.06	10	.25	1	159	0
slices, 1 c, 110 gm	64	<1	<1	17	.84	8	.20	0	126	0
APPLE, peeled, 1 fruit,										
128 gm	72	<1	<1	19	.69	5	.09	0	144	0
slices, 1 c, 110 gm	62	<1	<1	16	.59	4	.08	0	124	0
ckd, boiled, ½ c, 86 gm	46	<1	<1	12	1.64d	4	.16	1	76	0
microwaved, ½ c, 85 gm	48	<1	<1	12	2.01d	4	.14	1	79	0
APPLE, cnd, sweetened,										
sliced, unheated, ½ c,										
102 gm	68	<1	<1	17	1.85d	4	.23	3	69	0

FOOD & DESCRIPTION MEASURE OR QUANTITY	CALORIES	PROTEIN (GM)	FAT (GM)	CARBO-HYDRATE (GM)	FIBER (GM)	CALCIUM (MG)	IRON (MG)	SODIUM (MG)	POTASSIUM (MG)	CHOLES-TEROL (MG)
APPLE, dehyd, low moisture, sulfured, unheated, ½ c, 30 gm	104	<1	<1	28	1.23	6	.60	37	192	0
ckd, ½ c, 97 gm	71	<1	<1	19	.84	4	.41	25	132	0
APPLE, dried, sulfured uncooked, 10 rings, 64 gm	155	<1	<1	42	1.84	9	.90	56	288	0
1 c, 86 gm	209	<1	<1	57	2.47	12	1.21	75	387	0
ckd, sweetened, ½ c, 140 gm	116	<1	<1	29	.88	4	.44	27	137	0
ckd, unsw, ½ c, 128 gm	72	<1	<1	20	.86	4	.42	26	134	0
APPLE, fz, unsw, sliced, unheated, ½ c, 86 gm	41	<1	<1	11	1.75d	4	.16	3	67	0
heated, ½ c, 103 gm	48	<1	<1	12	1.96d	5	.19	3	78	0
APPLE JUICE, cnd, 1 c, 248 gm	116	<1	<1	29	.52	16	.92	7	296	0
fz concentrate, 6 oz, 211 gm	349	1	<1	87	—	43	1.92	54	945	0
fz concentrate, diluted, 1 c, 239 gm	111	<1	<1	28	—	14	.61	17	301	0
APPLESAUCE cnd, sweetened, ½ c, 128 gm	97	<1	<1	25	1.42d	5	.45	4	78	0
cnd, unsw, ½ c, 122 gm	53	<1	<1	14	.95d	4	.15	2	91	0
APRICOT, raw, 3 whole, 106 gm	51	1	<1	12	1.42d	15	.58	1	313	0
halves, 1 c, 155 gm	74	2	<1	17	2.05d	22	.84	1	458	0
APRICOT, cnd, s & l extra-heavy syrup, without skin 2 fruits, 90 gm	87	<1	<1	22	.31	7	.56	12	113	0
1 c, 246 gm	236	1	<1	61	.85	19	1.53	32	310	0
extra-light syrup, 3 halves, 84 gm	41	<1	<1	11	.35	8	.25	2	118	0
halves, 1 c, 247 gm	121	1	<1	31	1.03	25	.74	5	346	0
heavy syrup, 3 halves, 85 gm	70	<1	<1	18	.34	7	.26	3	119	0
halves, 1 c, 258 gm	214	1	<1	55	1.04	22	.77	10	361	0
heavy syrup, without skin, 2 halves, 90 gm	75	<1	<1	19	.32	8	.38	9	120	0
whole, 1 c, 258 gm	214	1	<1	55	.90	22	1.10	27	345	0
juice pack, 3 halves, 84 gm	40	<1	<1	10	.39d	10	.25	3	139	0
halves, 1 c, 248 gm	119	2	<1	31	1.17d	30	.74	9	409	0
light syrup, 3 halves, 85 gm	54	<1	<1	14	.35	10	.33	3	117	0
halves, 1 c, 253 gm	160	1	<1	42	1.04	28	.99	10	349	0
water pack, 3 halves, 84 gm	22	<1	<1	5	.36	7	.26	2	161	0
halves, 1 c, 243 gm	65	2	<1	16	1.03	19	.77	7	465	0
water pack, without skin, 1 c, 227 gm	51	2	<1	12	.84	19	1.23	25	350	0
2 whole, 90 gm	20	<1	<1	5	.33	8	.49	10	139	0
APRICOT, dehyd, sulfured, low moisture uncooked, ½ c, 60 gm	192	3	<1	50	2.37	37	3.79	8	1110	0
ckd, ½ c, 124 gm	156	2	<1	40	1.93	30	3.08	6	902	0
APRICOT, dried, sulfured, 10 halves, 35 gm	83	1	<1	22	1.03	16	1.65	3	482	0
1 c, 130 gm	310	5	<1	80	3.83	59	6.11	13	1791	0
ckd, sweetened, ½ c, 135 gm	153	2	<1	39	1.28	20	2.05	4	598	0
ckd, unsw, ½ c, 125 gm	106	2	<1	27	1.31	20	2.08	4	611	0
APRICOT, fz, sweetened, ½ c, 121 gm	119	<1	<1	30	.73	12	1.09	5	277	0
APRICOT NECTAR, cnd, 1 c, 251 gm	141	<1	<1	36	.75d	17	.96	9	286	0
BANANA, raw, 1 fruit, 114 gm	105	1	<1	27	1.60d	7	.35	1	451	0
mashed, 1 c, 225 gm	207	2	1	53	3.15d	13	.69	2	890	0
BANANA, dehyd, 1 tbsp, 6.2 gm	21	<1	<1	5	.12	1	.07	0	92	0
1 c, 100 gm	346	4	2	88	1.88	22	1.15	3	1491	0
BLACKBERRIES, raw, ½ c, 72										

FOOD & DESCRIPTION MEASURE OR QUANTITY	CALORIES	PROTEIN (GM)	FAT (GM)	CARBO-HYDRATE (GM)	FIBER (GM)	CALCIUM (MG)	IRON (MG)	SODIUM (MG)	POTASSIUM (MG)	CHOLES-TEROL (MG)
gm	37	<1	<1	9	3.26d	23	.41	0	141	0
BLACKBERRIES, cnd, heavy syrup, ½ c, 128 gm	118	2	<1	30	3.33	27	.83	3	127	0
BLACKBERRIES, fz, unsw, 1 c, 151 gm	97	2	<1	24	4.08	44	1.21	2	211	0
18 oz pkg, 510 gm	326	6	2	80	13.77	150	4.08	7	714	0
BLUEBERRIES, raw, 1 c, 145 gm	82	<1	<1	20	4.35d	9	.24	9	129	0
BLUEBERRIES, cnd, heavy syrup, ½ c, 128 gm	112	<1	<1	28	1.15	7	.42	4	51	0
BLUEBERRIES, fz, sweetened, 1 c, 230 gm	187	<1	<1	50	2.07	13	.90	3	137	0
sweetened, 10 oz pkg, 284 gm	231	1	<1	62	2.56	16	1.11	4	169	0
unsw, 1 c, 155 gm	78	<1	<1	19	4.94d	12	.28	1	83	0
20 oz pkg, 567 gm	287	2	4	69	18.08d	43	1.02	5	304	0
BOYSENBERRIES, cnd, heavy syrup, ½ c, 128 gm	113	1	<1	29	2.43	23	.55	4	115	0
BOYSENBERRIES, fz, unsw, 1 c, 132 gm	66	1	<1	16	3.56	36	1.12	2	183	0
10 oz pkg, 284 gm	141	3	<1	35	7.67	78	2.41	4	395	0
BREADFRUIT, raw, ¼ small fruit, 96 gm	99	1	<1	26	1.42	17	.52	2	470	0
1 c, 220 gm	227	2	<1	60	3.25	38	1.19	4	1077	0
CARAMBOLA, raw, 1 fruit, 127 gm	42	<1	<1	10	2.61d	6	.33	2	207	0
cubes, 1 c, 137 gm	45	<1	<1	11	1.52d	6	.35	2	223	0
CARISSA, raw, 1 fruit, 20 gm	12	<1	<1	3	.18	2	.26	1	52	0
sliced, 1 c, 150 gm	92	<1	2	20	1.35	17	1.97	4	390	0
CHERIMOYA, raw, 1 fruit, 547 gm	515	7	2	131	12.03	126	2.74	—	—	0
CHERRIES, SOUR, red, raw, with pits, 1 c, 103 gm	51	1	<1	13	.21	16	.33	3	178	0
pitted, 1 c, 155 gm	77	2	<1	19	.31	24	.50	5	268	0
CHERRIES, SOUR, cnd, red extra-heavy syrup, ½ c, 130 gm	148	<1	<1	38	.13	13	1.64	9	118	0
heavy syrup, ½ c, 128 gm	116	<1	<1	30	.13	13	1.66	9	119	0
light syrup, ½ c, 126 gm	94	<1	<1	24	.13	13	1.66	9	119	0
water pack, ½ c, 122 gm	43	<1	<1	11	.12	13	1.67	9	120	0
CHERRIES, SOUR, fz, red, unsw, 1 c, 155 gm	72	1	<1	17	.46	20	.82	1	192	0
18 oz pkg, 510 gm	237	5	2	56	1.53	65	2.70	4	632	0
CHERRIES, SWEET, raw, pitted, 10 fruits, 68 gm	49	<1	<1	11	1.05d	10	.26	0	152	0
1 c, 145 gm	104	2	1	24	2.23d	21	.56	1	325	0
CHERRIES, SWEET, cnd, s & l extra-heavy syrup, ½ c, 130 gm	133	<1	<1	34	.40	11	.45	3	185	0
heavy syrup, ½ c, 129 gm	107	<1	<1	27	.40	12	.46	3	187	0
juice pack, ½ c, 125 gm	68	1	<1	17	.31d	17	.73	3	163	0
light syrup, ½ c, 126 gm	85	<1	<1	22	.40	12	.45	3	186	0
water pack, ½ c, 124 gm	57	<1	<1	15	.25	13	.45	2	162	0
CHERRIES, SWEET, fz, 1 c, 259 gm	232	3	<1	58	1.04	31	.90	3	514	0
10 oz pkg, 284 gm	254	3	<1	63	1.14	34	.99	3	564	0
CRABAPPLES, raw, sliced, 1 c, 110 gm	83	<1	<1	22	.66	20	.39	1	213	0
CRANBERRIES, raw, whole, 1 c, 95 gm	46	<1	<1	12	1.14	7	.19	1	67	0
chopped, 1 c, 110 gm	54	<1	<1	14	1.32	8	.22	1	78	0
CRANBERRY JUICE COCKTAIL, bottled, 1 c, 253 gm	147	<1	<1	38	—	8	.40	10	61	0

FOOD & DESCRIPTION MEASURE OR QUANTITY	CALORIES	PROTEIN (GM)	FAT (GM)	CARBO-HYDRATE (GM)	FIBER (GM)	CALCIUM (MG)	IRON (MG)	SODIUM (MG)	POTASSIUM (MG)	CHOLES-TEROL (MG)
CRANBERRY SAUCE, cnd, sweetened, ½ c, 138 gm	209	<1	<1	54	.41	5	.30	40	35	0
CRANBERRY-ORANGE RELISH, cnd, ½ c, 138 gm	246	<1	<1	64	.83	15	.28	44	53	0
CURRANTS, EUROPEAN BLACK, raw, ½ c, 56 gm	36	<1	<1	9	3.04d	31	.86	1	180	0
CURRANTS, RED & WHITE, ½ c, 56 gm	31	<1	<1	8	1.9	18	.56	1	154	0
CURRANTS, ZANTE, dried, ½ c, 72 gm	204	3	<1	53	1.13	62	2.34	6	642	0
CUSTARD-APPLE, raw, 100 gm	101	2	<1	25	3.4	30	.71	4	382	0
DATES, dried, 10 fruits, 83 gm	228	2	<1	61	4.23d	27	.96	2	541	0
chopped, 1 c, 178 gm	489	4	<1	131	9.08d	58	2.05	5	1161	0
ELDERBERRIES, raw, 1 c, 145 gm	105	<1	<1	27	10.15	55	2.32	—	406	0
FIGS, raw, 1 medium, 50 gm	37	<1	<1	10	.60	18	.18	1	116	0
1 large, 64 gm	47	<1	<1	12	.77	22	.23	1	148	0
FIGS, cnd, s & l extra-heavy syrup, 3 fruits, 85 gm	91	<1	<1	24	.46	22	.24	1	83	0
1 c, 261 gm	280	<1	<1	73	1.41	68	.72	3	254	0
heavy syrup, 3 fruits, 85 gm	75	<1	<1	19	.47	23	.24	1	85	0
1 c, 259 gm	228	<1	<1	59	1.42	69	.73	3	258	0
light syrup, 3 fruits, 85 gm	58	<1	<1	15	.48	23	.25	1	86	0
1 c, 252 gm	173	<1	<1	45	1.41	69	.73	3	256	0
water pack, 3 fruits, 80 gm	42	<1	<1	11	.46	22	.24	1	83	0
1 c, 248 gm	130	<1	<1	35	1.42	69	.73	3	256	0
FIGS, dried, uncooked, 10 fruits, 187 gm	477	6	2	122	8.97	269	4.18	20	1332	0
1 c, 199 gm	508	6	2	130	9.54	286	4.45	22	1418	0
ckd, ½ c, 130 gm	140	2	<1	36	2.63	79	1.23	6	391	0
FRUIT COCKTAIL, cnd, s & l extra-heavy syrup, ½ c, 130 gm	115	<1	<1	30	.57	8	.36	7	112	0
extra-light syrup, ½ c, 123 gm	55	<1	<1	14	.57	10	.37	5	128	0
juice pack, ½ c, 124 gm	56	<1	<1	15	.76d	10	.26	4	118	0
light syrup, ½ c, 126 gm	72	<1	<1	19	.57	8	.37	7	112	0
heavy syrup, ½ c, 128 gm	93	<1	<1	24	.57	8	.36	7	112	0
water pack, ½ c, 122 gm	40	<1	<1	10	.57	6	.31	5	115	0
FRUIT SALAD, cnd, s & l extra-heavy syrup, ½ c, 130 gm	114	<1	<1	30	.77	8	.36	7	104	0
heavy syrup, ½ c, 128 gm	94	<1	<1	24	.77	8	.36	7	103	0
juice pack, ½ c, 124 gm	62	<1	<1	16	.82d	14	.31	7	144	0
light syrup, ½ c, 126 gm	73	<1	<1	19	.77	8	.37	7	104	0
water pack, ½ c, 122 gm	37	<1	<1	10	.76	8	.36	4	95	0
FRUIT SALAD, TROPICAL, cnd, heavy syrup, ½ c, 128 gm	110	<1	<1	29	.57	17	.66	3	168	0
GOOSEBERRIES, raw, 1 c, 150 gm	67	1	<1	15	2.85	38	.47	1	297	0
GOOSEBERRIES, cnd, light syrup, ½ c, 126 gm	93	<1	<1	24	1.51	20	.42	3	97	0
GRAPEFRUIT, raw, ½ fruit, 120 gm	38	<1	<1	10	.24	14	.10	0	167	0
segments, s & l, 1 c, 230 gm	74	1	<1	19	.46	27	.20	1	321	0
PINK & RED, ARIZONA, CALIFORNIA, raw, ½ fruit, 123 gm	46	<1	<1	12	.25	13	.09	1	181	0
segments, s & l, 1 c, 230 gm	86	1	<1	22	.46	25	.17	1	338	0
PINK & RED, FLORIDA, raw,										

FOOD & DESCRIPTION MEASURE OR QUANTITY	CALORIES	PROTEIN (GM)	FAT (GM)	CARBO-HYDRATE (GM)	FIBER (GM)	CALCIUM (MG)	IRON (MG)	SODIUM (MG)	POTASSIUM (MG)	CHOLES-TEROL (MG)
½ fruit, 123 gm	37	<1	<1	9	.25	18	.15	0	156	0
segments, s & l, 1 c, 230 gm	68	1	<1	17	.46	35	.28	1	292	0
WHITE, raw, all areas										
½ fruit, 118 gm	39	<1	<1	10	.24	14	.07	0	175	0
segments, s & l, 1 c, 230 gm	76	2	<1	19	.46	28	.14	0	340	0
WHITE, CALIFORNIA, raw										
½ fruit, 118 gm	43	1	<1	11	.24	14	.09	0	169	0
segments, s & l, 1 c, 230 gm	84	2	<1	21	.46	27	.17	1	330	0
WHITE, FLORIDA, ½ fruit, 118 gm	38	<1	<1	10	.20d	18	.06	0	177	0
segments, s & l, 1 c, 230 gm	75	1	<1	19	.39d	35	.12	1	345	0
GRAPEFRUIT, cnd, s & l										
juice pack, ½ c, 124 gm	46	<1	<1	11	.22	19	.26	9	209	0
light syrup, s & l, ½ c, 127 gm	76	<1	<1	20	.41	18	.51	2	164	0
water pack, s & l, ½ c, 122 gm	44	<1	<1	11	.40	18	.50	2	161	0
GRAPEFRUIT JUICE, fresh, 1 fruit, 196 gm	76	<1	<1	18	—	18	.39	2	318	0
1 c, 247 gm	96	1	<1	23	—	22	.49	2	400	0
cnd, sweetened, 1 c, 250 gm	116	1	<1	28	.00	20	.89	4	405	0
cnd, unsw, 1 c, 247 gm	93	1	<1	22	.00	18	.50	3	378	0
fz concentrate, 6 oz, 207 gm	302	4	<1	72	—	56	1.02	6	1002	0
diluted, 1 c, 247 gm	102	1	<1	24	—	19	.34	2	337	0
GRAPES, American type, slip skin										
10 fruits, 24 gm	15	<1	<1	4	.18	3	.07	0	46	0
1 c, 92 gm	58	<1	<1	16	.70	13	.27	2	176	0
GRAPES, European type, adherent skin										
10 fruits, 50 gm	36	<1	<1	9	.83d	5	.13	1	93	0
1 c, 160 gm	114	1	<1	28	2.64d	17	.41	3	296	0
GRAPES, Thompson seedless, cnd, s&l										
heavy syrup, ½ c, 128 gm	94	<1	<1	25	.25	13	1.20	7	132	0
water pack, ½ c, 122 gm	48	<1	<1	13	.25	13	1.19	7	131	0
GRAPE JUICE, cnd, 1 c, 253 gm	155	1	<1	38	—	22	.60	7	334	0
fz concentrate, sweetened, 6 oz, 216 gm	386	1	<1	96	—	28	.77	15	159	0
diluted, 1 c, 250 gm	128	<1	<1	32	—	9	.26	5	53	0
GROUNDCHERRIES, raw, ½ c, 70 gm	37	1	<1	8	1.96	6	.70	—	—	0
GUAVAS, raw, 1 fruit, 90 gm	45	<1	<1	11	5.04	18	.28	2	256	0
1 c, 165 gm	83	1	<1	20	9.24	33	.51	·4	469	0
GUAVAS, STRAWBERRY, raw, 1 fruit, 6 gm	4	<1	<1	1	.38	1	.01	2	18	0
1 c, 244 gm	169	1	1	42	15.62	52	.53	89	713	0
GUAVA SAUCE, ckd, ½ c, 119 gm	43	<1	<1	11	2.37	8	.21	4	268	0
JACKFRUIT, raw, 100 gm	94	1	<1	24	1.00	34	.60	3	303	0
JAVA-PLUM, raw, 3 fruits, 9 gm	5	<1	<1	1	.02	2	.02	1	7	0
1 c, 135 gm	82	<1	<1	21	.37	25	.25	18	106	0
JUJUBE, raw, 100 gm	79	1	<1	20	1.40	21	.48	3	250	0
dried, 100 gm	287	4	1	74	3.00	79	1.80	9	531	0
KIWIFRUIT, raw, 1 medium, 76 gm	46	<1	<1	11	.84	20	.31	4	252	0
1 large, 91 gm	55	<1	<1	14	1.00	24	.37	4	302	0
KUMQUATS, raw, 1 fruit, 19										

FOOD & DESCRIPTION MEASURE OR QUANTITY	CALORIES	PROTEIN (GM)	FAT (GM)	CARBO- HYDRATE (GM)	FIBER (GM)	CALCIUM (MG)	IRON (MG)	SODIUM (MG)	POTASSIUM (MG)	CHOLES- TEROL (MG)
gm	12	<1	<1	3	.70	8	.07	1	37	0
LEMON, peeled, raw,										
1 medium, 58 gm	17	<1	<1	5	.23	15	.35	1	80	0
1 large, 84 gm	25	<1	<1	8	.34	22	.50	2	116	0
LEMON, unpeeled, raw,										
1 medium, 108 gm	22	1	<1	12	—	66	.76	3	157	0
1 wedge, 27 gm	5	<1	<1	3	—	16	.19	1	39	0
LEMON JUICE, fresh, 1 tbsp,										
15.2 gm	4	<1	0	1	—	1	0	0	19	0
1 c, 244 gm	60	<1	0	21	—	18	.08	2	303	0
cnd, 1 tbsp, 15.2 gm	3	<1	<1	<1	—	2	.02	3	15	0
1 c, 244 gm	52	<1	<1	16	—	26	.31	50	248	0
fz, single strength, 1 tbsp,										
15.2 gm	3	<1	<1	<1	—	1	.02	0	14	0
1 c, 244 gm	53	1	<1	16	—	19	.30	2	218	0
LEMON PEEL, raw, 1 tsp, 2										
gm	0	<1	<1	<1	—	3	.02	0	3	0
1 tbsp, 6 gm	0	<1	<1	<1	—	8	.05	0	10	0
LIME, raw, 1 fruit, 67 gm	20	<1	<1	7	.34	22	.40	1	68	0
LIME JUICE, raw, 1 tbsp, 15.4										
gm	4	<1	<1	1	—	1	0	0	17	0
1 c, 246 gm	66	1	<1	22	—	22	.08	2	268	0
LIME JUICE, cnd, 1 tbsp, 15.4										
gm	3	<1	<1	1	—	2	.03	2	12	0
1 c, 246 gm	51	<1	<1	16	—	30	.56	39	185	0
LOGANBERRIES, fz, 1 c, 147										
gm	80	2	<1	19	—	38	.94	1	213	0
LOGANBERRIES, raw, 1 fruit,										
3.2 gm	2	<1	0	<1	.01	0	0	0	9	0
dried, 100 gm	286	5	<1	74	2.00	45	5.40	48	658	0
LOQUATS, raw, 1 fruit, 9.9 gm	5	<1	<1	1	.05	2	.03	0	26	0
LYCHEES, raw, 1 fruit, 9.6 gm	6	<1	<1	2	.02	0	.03	0	16	0
1 c, 190 gm	125	2	<1	31	.39	10	.59	1	325	0
LYCHEES, dried, 100 gm	277	4	1	71	1.40	33	1.70	3	1110	0
MAMMY-APPLE, raw, 1 fruit,										
846 gm	431	4	4	106	8.46	93	5.92	127	398	0
MANGOS, raw, 1 fruit, 207 gm	135	1	<1	35	2.24d	21	.26	4	322	0
sliced, 1 c, 165 gm	108	<1	<1	28	1.78d	17	.21	3	257	0
MELON, CANTALOUPE, raw,										
½ fruit, 267 gm	94	2	<1	22	.85d	28	.57	23	825	0
cubed, 1 c, 160 gm	57	1	<1	13	.51d	17	.34	14	494	0
CASABA, raw, 1/10 fruit, 164										
gm	43	1	<1	10	.82	8	.66	20	344	0
cubed, 1 c, 170 gm	45	2	<1	11	.85	9	.68	20	357	0
HONEYDEW, raw, 1/10 fruit,										
129 gm	46	<1	<1	12	.77	8	.09	13	350	0
cubed, 1 c, 170 gm	60	<1	<1	16	1.02	10	.12	17	461	0
MELON BALLS, fz, cantaloupe										
& honeydew, 1 c, 173										
gm	55	1	<1	14	—	17	.50	53	484	0
MIXED FRUIT, cnd, heavy										
syrup, ½ c, 128 gm	92	<1	<1	24	.51	1	.46	5	108	0
MIXED FRUIT, dried, 11 oz										
pkg, 293 gm	712	7	1	188	8.48	110	7.93	52	2332	0
MIXED FRUIT, fz, sweetened,										
1 c, 250 gm	245	4	<1	61	—	18	.70	8	327	0
10 oz pkg, 284 gm	278	4	<1	69	—	20	.80	9	372	0
MULBERRIES, raw, 10 fruits,										
15 gm	7	<1	<1	1	.14	6	.28	2	29	0
1 c, 140 gm	61	2	<1	14	1.34	55	2.59	14	271	0
NECTARINES, raw, 1 fruit, 136										
gm	67	1	<1	16	.54	6	.21	0	288	0
sliced, 1 c, 138 gm	68	1	<1	16	.55	6	.21	0	292	0
OHELOBERRIES, raw, 10										

FOOD & DESCRIPTION MEASURE OR QUANTITY	CALORIES	PROTEIN (GM)	FAT (GM)	CARBO-HYDRATE (GM)	FIBER (GM)	CALCIUM (MG)	IRON (MG)	SODIUM (MG)	POTASSIUM (MG)	CHOLES-TEROL (MG)
fruits, 11 gm	3	<1	<1	<1	.15	1	.01	0	4	0
1 c, 140 gm	39	<1	<1	10	1.85	10	.13	2	54	0
ORANGE, peeled, raw, all varieties										
1 fruit, 131 gm	62	1	<1	15	.56	52	.13	0	237	0
sections, without										
membrane, 1 c, 180 gm	85	2	<1	21	.77	72	.18	0	326	0
FLORIDA, raw, 1 fruit, 151 gm	69	1	<1	17	.52	65	.13	1	254	0
sections, without										
membrane, 1 c, 185 gm	84	1	<1	21	.64	80	.16	1	312	0
NAVEL, CALIFORNIA, raw, 1 fruit, 140 gm	65	1	<1	16	.64	56	.17	1	250	0
sections, without										
membrane, 1 c, 165 gm	76	2	<1	19	.76	66	.20	1	294	0
VALENCIA, CALIFORNIA, raw, 1 fruit, 121 gm	59	1	<1	14	.61	48	.11	0	217	0
sections, without										
membrane, 1 c, 180 gm	88	2	<1	21	.90	72	.16	0	322	0
with peel, raw, 1 fruit, 159 gm	64	2	<1	25	—	111	1.27	3	312	0
1 c, 170 gm	68	2	<1	26	—	119	1.36	3	333	0
ORANGE-GRAPEFRUIT JUICE, cnd, 1 c, 247 gm	107	1	<1	25	—	21	1.15	8	390	0
ORANGE JUICE, fresh, 1 fruit, 86 gm	39	<1	<1	9	.09	9	.17	1	172	0
1 c, 248 gm	111	2	<1	26	.25	27	.50	2	496	0
cnd, 1 c, 249 gm	104	1	<1	25	.25	21	1.10	6	436	0
chilled, 1 c, 249 gm	110	2	<1	25	—	24	.41	2	473	0
fz concentrate, 6 oz, 213 gm	339	5	<1	81	.39	67	.74	7	1435	0
diluted, 1 c, 249 gm	112	2	<1	27	.13	22	.24	2	474	0
ORANGE PEEL, raw, 1 tsp, 2 gm	—	<1	0	<1	—	3	.02	0	4	0
1 tbsp, 6 gm	—	<1	<1	2	—	10	.05	0	13	0
PAPAYA, raw, 1 fruit, 304 gm	117	2	<1	30	2.77d	72	.30	8	780	0
cubed, 1 c, 140 gm	54	<1	<1	14	1.27d	33	.14	4	359	0
PAPAYA NECTAR, cnd, 1 c, 250 gm	142	<1	<1	36	—	24	.86	14	78	0
PASSION FRUIT, purple, raw, 1 fruit, 18 gm	18	<1	<1	4	1.97	2	.29	5	63	0
PASSION FRUIT JUICE										
purple, 1 c, 247 gm	126	<1	<1	34	.10	9	.59	—	—	0
yellow, 1 c, 247 gm	149	2	<1	36	.42	9	.89	15	687	0
PEACH, raw, 1 fruit, 87 gm	37	<1	<1	10	.54d	5	.10	0	171	0
sliced, 1 c, 170 gm	73	1	<1	19	1.05d	9	.19	1	334	0
PEACH, cnd, s & l										
extra-heavy syrup, 1 half, 81 gm	77	<1	<1	21	.23	3	.24	6	67	0
sliced or halved, 1 c, 262 gm	251	1	<1	68	.75	9	.77	21	217	0
extra-light syrup, 1 half, 77 gm	32	<1	<1	9	.15	4	.23	4	57	0
sliced or halved, 1 c, 247 gm	104	<1	<1	27	.49	12	.74	12	183	0
heavy syrup, 1 half, 81 gm	60	<1	<1	16	.24	2	.22	5	74	0
sliced or halved, 1 c, 256 gm	190	1	<1	51	.74	8	.69	16	235	0
juice pack, 1 half, 77 gm	34	<1	<1	9	.35d	5	.21	3	98	0
sliced or halved, 1 c, 248 gm	109	2	<1	29	1.12d	15	.66	11	317	0
light syrup, 1 half, 81 gm	44	<1	<1	12	.24	3	.29	4	79	0
sliced or halved, 1 c, 251 gm	136	1	<1	37	.75	9	.90	13	244	0
water pack, 1 half, 77 gm	18	<1	<1	5	.24	2	.24	3	76	0

FOOD & DESCRIPTION MEASURE OR QUANTITY	CALORIES	PROTEIN (GM)	FAT (GM)	CARBO- HYDRATE (GM)	FIBER (GM)	CALCIUM (MG)	IRON (MG)	SODIUM (MG)	POTASSIUM (MG)	CHOLES- TEROL (MG)
sliced or halved, 1 c, 244 gm	58	1	<1	15	.75	6	.77	8	241	0
PEACH, dehyd, sulfured, low moisture										
uncooked, ½ c, 58 gm	188	3	<1	48	2.30	22	3.20	6	783	0
ckd, ½ c, 121 gm	161	2	<1	41	1.97	19	2.74	5	671	0
PEACH, dried, sulfured, 10 halves, 130 gm	311	5	<1	80	3.81	37	5.28	9	1295	0
1 c, 160 gm	383	6	1	98	4.68	45	6.50	12	1594	0
ckd, sweetened, ½ c, 135 gm	139	1	<1	36	1.16	11	1.62	3	395	0
ckd, unsw, ½ c, 129 gm	99	1	<1	25	1.21	12	1.68	3	413	0
PEACH, fz, sweetened, sliced, 1 c, 250 gm	235	2	<1	60	1.00	6	.93	16	325	0
10 oz pkg, 284 gm	267	2	<1	68	1.14	7	1.06	18	370	0
PEACH, SPICED, cnd, heavy syrup, s & l										
1 fruit, 88 gm	66	<1	<1	18	.22	5	.25	3	75	0
whole fruits, 1 c, 242 gm	180	<1	<1	49	.61	15	.69	9	206	0
PEACH NECTAR, cnd, 1 c, 249 gm	134	<1	<1	35	.40d	13	.47	17	101	0
PEAR, raw, 1 fruit, 166 gm	98	<1	<1	25	4.08d	19	.41	1	208	0
halves, 1 c, 165 gm	97	<1	<1	25	4.06d	19	.41	1	207	0
PEAR, cnd, s & l										
extra-light syrup, 1 half, 77 gm	36	<1	<1	9	.46	5	.15	2	34	0
halved, 1 c, 247 gm	116	<1	<1	30	1.49	17	.49	5	110	0
extra-heavy syrup, 1 half, 79 gm	77	<1	<1	20	.45	4	.17	4	50	0
halved, 1 c, 261 gm	254	<1	<1	66	1.50	12	.57	13	166	0
heavy syrup, 1 half, 79 gm	58	<1	<1	15	.46	4	.17	4	51	0
halved, 1 c, 255 gm	188	<1	<1	49	1.49	12	.56	13	165	0
juice pack, 1 half, 77 gm	38	<1	<1	10	.71d	7	.22	3	74	0
halved, 1 c, 248 gm	123	<1	<1	32	2.28d	21	.71	10	238	0
light syrup, 1 half, 79 gm	45	<1	<1	12	.47	4	.22	4	52	0
halved, 1 c, 251 gm	144	<1	<1	38	1.49	13	.70	13	165	0
water pack, 1 half, 77 gm	22	<1	<1	6	.47	3	.16	2	41	0
halved, 1 c, 244 gm	71	<1	<1	19	1.49	9	.52	5	130	0
PEAR, dried, sulfured, 10 halves, 175 gm	459	3	1	122	9.95	59	3.68	10	932	0
1 c, 180 gm	472	3	1	125	10.24	60	3.78	10	959	0
ckd, sweetened, 1 c, 280 gm	392	2	<1	104	7.33	43	2.72	8	687	0
ckd, unsw, 1 c, 255 gm	325	2	<1	86	7.04	41	2.60	7	659	0
PEAR NECTAR, cnd, 1 c, 250 gm	149	<1	<1	39	1.63d	11	.65	9	33	0
PERSIMMON, Japanese, raw, 1 fruit, 168 gm	118	<1	<1	31	2.49	13	.26	3	270	0
dried, 1 fruit, 34 gm	93	<1	<1	25	1.23	8	.25	1	273	0
PERSIMMON, native, raw, 1 fruit, 25 gm	32	<1	<1	8	.38	7	.63	0	78	0
PINEAPPLE, raw, 1 sl, 84 gm	42	<1	<1	10	1.29d	6	.31	1	95	0
diced, 1 c, 155 gm	77	<1	<1	19	2.39d	11	.57	1	175	0
PINEAPPLE, cnd, s & l										
extra-heavy syrup, 1 sl, 58 gm	48	<1	<1	12	.25	8	.22	1	59	0
chunked or crushed, 1 c, 260 gm	217	<1	<1	56	1.12	35	.98	3	265	0
heavy syrup, 1 sl, 58 gm	45	<1	<1	12	.25	8	.22	1	60	0
chunked or crushed, 1 c, 255 gm	199	<1	<1	52	1.11	35	.98	3	264	0
juice pack, 1 sl, 58 gm	35	<1	<1	9	.44d	8	.16	1	70	0
chunked or tidbits, 1 c, 250 gm	150	1	<1	39	1.88d	34	.70	4	304	0
light syrup, 1 sl, 58 gm	30	<1	<1	8	.26	8	.23	1	61	0
1 c, 252 gm	131	<1	<1	34	1.12	36	.98	3	266	0

FOOD & DESCRIPTION MEASURE OR QUANTITY	CALORIES	PROTEIN (GM)	FAT (GM)	CARBO-HYDRATE (GM)	FIBER (GM)	CALCIUM (MG)	IRON (MG)	SODIUM (MG)	POTASSIUM (MG)	CHOLES-TEROL (MG)
water pack, 1 sl, 58 gm	19	<1	<1	5	.26	9	.23	1	74	0
tidbits, 1 c, 246 gm	79	1	<1	20	1.11	37	.98	3	313	0
PINEAPPLE, fz, chunked, sweetened, 1 c, 245 gm	208	<1	<1	54	.74	22	.98	5	245	0
PINEAPPLE JUICE, cnd, 1 c, 250 gm	139	<1	<1	34	.25	42	.65	2	334	0
fz concentrate, 6 oz, 216 gm	387	3	<1	96	.65	84	1.94	6	1020	0
fz, diluted, 1 c, 250 gm	129	1	<1	32	.25	28	.75	3	340	0
PITANGA, raw, 1 fruit, 7 gm	2	<1	<1	<1	.04	1	.01	0	7	0
1 c, 173 gm	57	1	<1	13	1.04	16	.35	5	178	0
PLANTAIN, raw, 1 fruit, 179 gm	218	2	<1	57	.90	5	1.07	7	893	0
sliced, 1 c, 148 gm	181	2	<1	47	.74	4	.89	6	739	0
ckd, sliced, 1 c, 154 gm	179	1	<1	48	—	3	.89	8	716	0
PLUM, raw, 1 fruit, 66 gm	36	<1	<1	9	.40	2	.07	0	113	0
sliced, 1 c, 165 gm	91	1	1	21	.99	6	.17	1	284	0
PLUM, purple, cnd, s & l extra-heavy syrup, 3 fruits, 133 gm	135	<1	<1	35	.43	12	1.09	25	118	0
1 c, 261 gm	265	<1	<1	69	.84	24	2.15	50	232	0
heavy syrup, 3 fruits, 133 gm	119	<1	<1	31	.44	12	1.12	26	121	0
1 c, 258 gm	230	<1	<1	60	.85	24	2.17	50	234	0
juice pack, 3 fruits, 95 gm	55	<1	<1	14	.37d	9	.32	1	147	0
1 c, 252 gm	146	1	<1	38	.98d	25	.84	3	389	0
light syrup, 3 fruits, 133 gm	83	<1	<1	22	.45	13	1.14	26	123	0
1 c, 252 gm	158	<1	<1	41	.85	24	2.16	50	233	0
water pack, 3 fruits, 95 gm	39	<1	<1	10	.24	6	.15	1	120	0
1 c, 249 gm	102	<1	<1	27	.62	17	.40	2	314	0
POMEGRANATE, raw, 1 fruit, 154 gm	104	1	<1	26	.31	5	.46	5	399	0
PRICKLY PEAR, raw, 1 fruit, 103 gm	42	<1	<1	10	1.87	58	.31	6	226	0
PRUNE, cnd, heavy syrup, s & l, 5 fruits, 86 gm	90	<1	<1	24	.60	15	.35	2	194	0
1 c, 234 gm	245	2	<1	65	1.63	40	.95	5	528	0
PRUNE, dehyd, low moisture uncooked, ½ c, 66 gm	224	2	<1	59	1.91	48	2.32	4	699	0
ckd, ½ c, 140 gm	158	2	<1	42	1.35	34	1.64	3	494	0
PRUNE, dried, uncooked, 10 fruits, 84 gm	201	2	<1	53	1.72	43	2.08	3	626	0
1 c, 161 gm	385	4	<1	101	3.29	82	3.99	6	1200	0
ckd, sweetened, ½ c, 119 gm	147	1	<1	39	1.02	25	1.24	2	371	0
ckd, unsw, ½ c, 106 gm	113	1	<1	30	.97	24	1.18	2	354	0
PRUNE JUICE, cnd, 1 c, 256 gm	181	2	<1	45	.03	30	3.03	11	706	0
PUMMELO, raw, 1 fruit, 609 gm	228	5	<1	59	1.10	23	.69	7	1317	0
sliced, 1 c, 190 gm	71	1	<1	18	.34	7	.22	2	411	0
QUINCE, raw, 1 fruit, 92 gm	53	<1	<1	14	1.56	10	.64	4	181	0
RAISINS GOLDEN, seedless, not packed, 1 c, 145 gm	437	5	<1	115	2.08	76	2.59	17	1082	0
packed, 1 c, 165 gm	498	6	<1	131	2.36	87	2.95	20	1232	0
SEEDED, 1 c, 145 gm	428	4	<1	114	.97	41	3.75	41	1197	0
packed, 1 c, 165 gm	488	4	<1	129	1.11	46	4.27	47	1362	0
SEEDLESS, 1 c, 145 gm	434	5	<1	115	1.85	71	3.02	17	1089	0
packed, 1 c, 165 gm	494	5	<1	131	2.11	81	3.43	19	1239	0
RASPBERRIES, raw, 1 c, 123 gm	61	1	<1	14	5.79d	27	.70	0	187	0
RASPBERRIES, red, cnd, heavy syrup, ½ c, 128 gm	117	1	<1	30	—	14	.54	4	120	0
1 c, 250 gm	256	2	<1	65	5.53	38	1.62	1	285	0
RASPBERRIES, red, fz,										

FOOD & DESCRIPTION MEASURE OR QUANTITY	CALORIES	PROTEIN (GM)	FAT (GM)	CARBO-HYDRATE (GM)	FIBER (GM)	CALCIUM (MG)	IRON (MG)	SODIUM (MG)	POTASSIUM (MG)	CHOLES-TEROL (MG)
sweetened, 10 oz pkg, 284 gm	291	2	<1	74	6.28	43	1.84	1	324	0
RHUBARB, raw, diced, ½ c, 61 gm	13	<1	<1	3	.43	52	.14	2	175	0
fz, uncooked, ½ c, 68 gm	14	<1	<1	3	—	132	.20	1	73	0
fz, ckd, sweetened, ½ c, 120 gm	139	<1	<1	37	.96	174	.25	2	115	0
ROSE-APPLE, raw, 100 gm	25	<1	<1	6	1.10	29	.07	0	123	0
ROSELLE, raw, 1 c, 57 gm	28	<1	<1	6	.65	123	.84	3	118	0
SAPODILLA, raw, 1 fruit, 170 gm	140	<1	2	34	9.01d	36	1.36	20	328	0
pulp, 1 c, 241 gm	199	1	3	48	12.77d	51	1.93	29	465	0
SAPOTE, raw, 1 fruit, 225 gm	301	5	1	76	4.28	88	2.25	21	773	0
SOURSOP, raw,										
1 fruit, 625 gm	416	6	2	105	6.88	88	3.75	87	1739	0
pulp, 1 c, 225 gm	150	2	<1	38	2.48	32	1.35	31	626	0
STRAWBERRIES, raw, 1 c, 149 gm	45	<1	<1	10	2.83d	21	.57	2	247	0
STRAWBERRIES, cnd, heavy syrup, ½ c, 127 gm	117	<1	<1	30	—	16	.62	5	109	0
STRAWBERRIES, fz sweetened, sliced, 1 c, 255 gm	245	1	<1	66	1.57	28	1.49	8	249	0
10 oz pkg, 284 gm	273	2	<1	74	1.75	31	1.66	9	277	0
whole, sweetened, 1 c, 255 gm	200	1	<1	54	1.50	29	1.21	3	249	0
10 oz pkg, 284 gm	223	1	<1	60	1.68	32	1.34	3	277	0
unsw, 1 c, 149 gm	52	<1	<1	14	1.18	23	1.12	3	220	0
20 oz pkg, 567 gm	200	2	<1	52	4.5	88	4.25	11	838	0
SUGAR-APPLE, raw, 1 fruit, 155 gm	146	3	<1	37	2.28	37	.93	15	384	0
pulp, 1 c, 250 gm	236	5	<1	59	3.68	59	1.50	24	619	0
TAMARIND, raw, 1 fruit, 2 gm	5	<1	<1	1	.10	1	.06	1	13	0
pulp, 1 c, 120 gm	287	3	<1	75	6.12	89	3.36	33	753	0
TANGERINE, raw, 1 fruit, 84 gm	37	<1	<1	9	.28	12	.09	1	132	0
sections, without membrane, 1 c, 195 gm	86	1	<1	22	.65	27	.20	3	305	0
TANGERINE, cnd, s & l, juice pack, ½ c, 124 gm	46	<1	<1	12	.13	14	.33	7	165	0
light syrup, ½ c, 126 gm	76	<1	<1	20	.16	9	.46	8	99	0
TANGERINE JUICE, fresh, 1 c, 247 gm	106	1	<1	25	.25	44	.49	2	440	0
cnd, sweetened, 1 c, 249 gm	125	1	<1	30	.25	45	.50	2	443	0
fz concentrate, sweetened, 6 oz, 214 gm	344	3	<1	83	—	57	.72	7	850	0
diluted, 1 c, 241 gm	110	1	<1	27	—	18	.23	2	273	0
WATERMELON, raw, 1/16 fruit, 482 gm	152	3	2	35	.96d	38	.83	10	560	0
diced, 1 c, 160 gm	50	<1	<1	11	.32d	13	.28	3	186	0

14

MEATS

FOOD & DESCRIPTION MEASURE OR QUANTITY	CALORIES	PROTEIN (GM)	FAT (GM)	CARBO-HYDRATE (GM)	FIBER (GM)	CALCIUM (MG)	IRON (MG)	SODIUM (MG)	POTASSIUM (MG)	CHOLES-TEROL (MG)
Beef										
Armour–Dial, Inc.										
BEEF TRIPE, 6 oz	210	28	9	1	—	40	.72	280	—	—
DRIED BEEF, sliced, 1 oz	45	5	1	1	—	*	1.08	1220	—	—
USDA										
BRAIN										
pan-fried, 3 oz, 85 gm	167	11	13	0	0	8	1.89	134	301	1696
yield from 1 lb raw with refuse, 351 gm	690	44	56	0	0	32	7.79	555	1243	7003
simmered, 3 oz, 85 gm	136	9	11	0	0	8	1.88	102	204	1746
yield from 1 lb raw with refuse, 391 gm	627	43	49	0	0	36	8.64	469	938	8030
BRISKET, FLAT HALF										
braised, lean & fat, 3 oz, 85 gm	347	19	30	0	0	8	1.85	55	187	78
yield from 1 lb raw with refuse, 321 gm	1311	71	112	0	0	29	7.00	207	704	296
braised, lean only, 3 oz, 85 gm	223	24	13	0	0	5	2.37	66	232	77
yield from 1 lb raw with refuse, 209 gm	549	59	33	0	0	13	5.82	161	571	190
BRISKET, POINT HALF										
braised, lean & fat, 3 oz, 85 gm	311	21	25	0	0	7	1.92	47	203	81
yield from 1 lb raw with refuse, 320 gm	1172	79	93	0	0	26	7.21	179	764	304
braised, lean only, 3 oz, 85 gm	181	27	7	0	0	4	2.42	54	253	81
yield from 1 lb raw with refuse, 217 gm	461	68	19	0	0	11	6.17	137	646	206
BRISKET, WHOLE										
braised, lean & fat, 3 oz, 85 gm	332	20	28	0	0	7	1.86	52	195	79
yield from 1 lb raw with refuse, 322 gm	1258	74	104	0	0	28	7.04	198	739	301
braised, lean only, 3 oz, 85 gm	205	25	11	0	0	5	2.36	61	244	79
yield from 1 lb raw with refuse, 213 gm	513	63	27	0	0	12	5.90	153	610	197
CHUCK, ARM POT ROAST ALL GRADES										
braised, lean & fat, 3 oz, 85 gm	297	23	22	0	0	9	2.61	51	207	84

FOOD & DESCRIPTION MEASURE OR QUANTITY	CALORIES	PROTEIN (GM)	FAT (GM)	CARBO-HYDRATE (GM)	FIBER (GM)	CALCIUM (MG)	IRON (MG)	SODIUM (MG)	POTASSIUM (MG)	CHOLES-TEROL (MG)
yield from 1 lb raw with refuse, 275 gm	962	75	71	0	0	28	8.43	164	671	273
braised, lean only, 3 oz, 85 gm	196	28	8	0	0	7	3.22	56	246	85
yield from 1 lb raw with refuse, 202 gm	467	67	20	0	0	18	7.66	134	584	203
CHOICE GRADE										
braised, lean & fat, 3 oz, 85 gm	301	23	23	0	0	9	2.59	50	207	84
yield from 1 lb raw with refuse, 277 gm	982	75	73	0	0	28	8.45	165	674	274
braised, lean only, 3 oz, 85 gm	199	28	9	0	0	7	3.22	56	246	85
yield from 1 lb raw with refuse, 202 gm	473	67	21	0	0	18	7.66	134	584	203
GOOD GRADE										
braised, lean & fat, 3 oz, 85 gm	287	23	21	0	0	9	2.64	51	209	84
yield from 1 lb raw with refuse, 265 gm	894	73	65	0	0	27	8.22	159	653	263
braised, lean only, 3 oz, 85 gm	189	28	8	0	0	7	3.22	5 6	246	85
yield from 1 lb raw with refuse, 198 gm	439	65	18	0	0	17	7.5	131	573	199
PRIME GRADE										
braised, lean & fat, 3 oz, 85 gm	332	22	26	0	0	9	2.5	201	177	84
yield from 1 lb raw with refuse, 277 gm	1082	72	86	0	0	29	8.15	655	577	274
braised, lean only, 3 oz, 85 gm	222	28	11	0	0	7	3.22	56	246	85
yield from 1 lb raw with refuse, 191 gm	499	63	26	0	0	17	7.24	126	552	192
CHUCK BLADE ROAST										
ALL GRADES										
braised, lean & fat, 3 oz, 85 gm	325	22	26	0	0	11	2.52	53	190	87
yield from 1 lb raw with refuse, 251 gm	961	64	76	0	0	32	7.43	158	560	258
braised, lean only, 3 oz, 85 gm	230	26	13	0	0	11	3.13	60	223	90
yield from 1 lb raw with refuse, 182 gm	492	57	28	0	0	23	6.7	129	478	192
CHOICE GRADE										
braised, lean & fat, 3 oz, 85 gm	330	22	26	0	0	11	2.51	53	189	87
yield from 1 lb raw with refuse, 253 gm	982	64	78	0	0	33	7.46	159	563	260
braised, lean only, 3 oz, 85 gm	234	26	13	0	0	11	3.13	60	223	90
yield from 1 lb raw with refuse, 183 gm	503	57	29	0	0	23	6.74	130	481	193
GOOD GRADE										
braised, lean & fat, 3 oz, 85 gm	311	22	24	0	0	11	2.55	54	192	88
yield from 1 lb raw with refuse, 241 gm	882	62	68	0	0	31	7.24	153	543	248
braised, lean only, 3 oz, 85 gm	218	26	12	0	0	11	3.13	60	223	90
yield from 1 lb raw with refuse, 178 gm	456	55	24	0	0	22	6.56	127	467	188
PRIME GRADE										
braised, lean & fat, 3 oz, 85 gm	354	22	29	0	0	11	2.52	53	190	87

FOOD & DESCRIPTION MEASURE OR QUANTITY	CALORIES	PROTEIN (GM)	FAT (GM)	CARBO-HYDRATE (GM)	FIBER (GM)	CALCIUM (MG)	IRON (MG)	SODIUM (MG)	POTASSIUM (MG)	CHOLES-TEROL (MG)
yield from 1 lb raw with refuse, 247 gm	1029	63	84	0	0	32	7.33	155	552	254
braised, lean only, 3 oz, 85 gm	270	26	17	0	0	11	3.13	60	223	90
yield from 1 lb raw wih refuse, 179 gm	569	56	37	0	0	22	6.59	127	470	189
CORNED BEEF BRISKET										
ckd, 3 oz, 85 gm	213	15	16	<1	0	7	1.58	964	123	83
yield from 1 lb raw with refuse, 320 gm	802	58	61	2	0	25	5.94	3628	464	314
cnd, 3 oz, 85 gm	213	23	13	0	0	—	1.77	856	116	73
jelled loaf, 1 oz, 28 gm	43	6	2	0	0	3	.58	270	29	13
CURED THIN-SLICED BEEF, 1 oz, 28 gm	50	8	1	2	0	3	.76	408	122	12
DRIED BEEF, 1 oz, 28 gm	47	8	1	<1	0	2	1.28	984	126	—
FLANK										
CHOICE GRADE										
braised, lean & fat, 3 oz, 85 gm	218	23	13	0	0	6	2.89	61	293	61
yield from 1 lb raw with refuse, 268 gm	689	74	41	0	0	18	9.11	191	922	193
braised, lean only, 3 oz, 85 gm	208	24	12	0	0	6	2.95	61	298	60
yield from 1 lb raw with refuse, 260 gm	635	73	36	0	0	17	9.02	188	912	185
broiled, lean & fat, 3 oz, 85 gm	216	21	14	0	0	5	2.12	70	338	60
yield from 1 lb raw with refuse, 340 gm	863	85	55	0	0	21	8.49	278	1353	241
broiled, lean only, 3 oz, 85 gm	207	22	13	0	0	5	2.15	70	344	60
yield from 1 lb raw with refuse, 332 gm	808	84	50	0	0	20	8.41	274	1344	233
GROUND BEEF, EXTRA LEAN (17 percent fat raw)										
Baked, medium, 3 oz, 85 gm	213	21	14	0	0	6	1.94	42	190	70
yield from 1 lb raw with refuse, 345 gm	863	84	56	0	0	23	7.87	170	772	283
baked, well done, 3 oz, 85 gm	232	26	14	0	0	7	2.52	54	247	91
yield from 1 lb raw with refuse, 268 gm	733	81	43	0	0	23	7.93	172	780	286
broiled, medium, 3 oz, 85 gm	217	22	14	0	0	6	2.00	59	266	71
yield from 1 lb raw with refuse, 336 gm	859	85	55	0	0	25	7.90	234	1052	281
broiled, well done, 3 oz, 85 gm	225	24	13	0	0	7	2.35	70	314	84
yield from 1 lb raw with refuse, 281 gm	744	80	44	0	0	24	7.78	230	1037	277
pan-fried, medium, 3 oz, 85 gm	216	21	14	0	0	6	2.01	59	265	69
yield from 1 lb raw with refuse, 340 gm	866	85	56	0	0	24	8.02	238	1060	274
pan-fried, well done, 3 oz, 85 gm	224	24	14	0	0	7	2.32	69	306	79
yield from 1 lb raw with refuse, 295 gm	777	83	47	0	0	24	8.05	238	1063	275
GROUND BEEF, LEAN (21 percent fat raw)										
baked, medium, 3 oz, 85 gm	227	20	16	0	0	8	1.78	47	190	66
yield from 1 lb raw with refuse, 336 gm	899	80	62	0	0	32	7.02	187	752	262
baked, well done, 3 oz, 85										

FOOD & DESCRIPTION MEASURE OR QUANTITY	CALORIES	PROTEIN (GM)	FAT (GM)	CARBO-HYDRATE (GM)	FIBER (GM)	CALCIUM (MG)	IRON (MG)	SODIUM (MG)	POTASSIUM (MG)	CHOLES-TEROL (MG)
gm	248	25	16	0	0	10	2.26	61	243	84
yield from 1 lb raw with refuse, 263 gm	768	78	48	0	0	32	7.00	187	751	261
broiled, medium, 3 oz, 85 gm	231	21	16	0	0	9	1.79	65	256	74
yield from 1 lb raw with refuse, 322 gm	876	80	59	0	0	34	6.79	248	970	280
broiled, well done, 3 oz, 85 gm	238	24	15	0	0	10	2.08	76	296	86
yield from 1 lb raw with refuse, 281 gm	785	79	50	0	0	34	6.88	250	980	283
pan-fried, medium, 3 oz, 85 gm	234	21	16	0	0	8	1.85	65	254	71
yield from 1 lb raw with refuse, 327 gm	901	79	62	0	0	32	7.13	251	978	275
pan-fried, well done, 3 oz, 85 gm	235	23	15	0	0	9	2.11	74	289	81
yield from 1 lb raw with refuse, 286 gm	791	79	51	0	0	31	7.09	249	973	273
GROUND BEEF, REGULAR (27 percent fat raw)										
baked, medium, 3 oz, 85 gm	244	20	18	0	0	8	2.05	51	188	74
yield from 1 lb raw with refuse, 318 gm	913	73	67	0	0	31	7.66	191	703	276
baked, well done, 3 oz, 85 gm	269	24	18	0	0	10	2.54	63	233	92
yield from 1 lb raw with refuse, 254 gm	804	73	55	0	0	31	7.59	189	696	274
broiled, medium, 3 oz, 85 gm	246	20	18	0	0	9	2.07	70	248	76
yield from 1 lb raw with refuse, 304 gm	880	73	63	0	0	33	7.42	251	887	273
broiled, well done, 3 oz, 85 gm	248	23	17	0	0	10	2.33	79	278	86
yield from 1 lb raw with refuse, 272 gm	793	74	53	0	0	33	7.45	252	891	274
pan-fried, medium, 3 oz, 85 gm	260	20	19	0	0	10	2.08	71	255	75
yield from 1 lb raw with refuse, 308 gm	941	74	69	0	0	34	7.55	258	924	273
pan-fried, well done, 3 oz, 85 gm	243	23	16	0	0	11	2.30	79	283	83
yield from 1 lb raw with refuse, 277 gm	792	75	52	0	0	35	7.51	257	921	272
GROUND BEEF PATTIES, fz, broiled, medium, 3 oz, 85 gm	240	21	17	0	0	9	1.79	66	250	80
yield from 1 lb raw with refuse, 313 gm	882	77	62	0	0	33	6.57	242	919	294
HEART, simmered, 3 oz, 85 gm	148	24	5	<1	0	5	6.38	54	198	164
yield from 1 lb raw with refuse, 257 gm	450	74	14	1	0	16	19.30	162	599	496
KIDNEYS, simmered, 3 oz, 85 gm	122	22	3	<1	0	15	6.21	114	152	329
yield from 1 lb raw with refuse. 197 am	283	50	7	2	0	34	14.40	264	353	762
LIVER, braised, 3 oz, 85 gm	137	21	4	3	0	6	5.75	60	200	331
yield from 1 lb raw with refuse, 336 gm	542	82	16	11	0	23	22.74	235	789	1308
pan-fried, 3 oz, 85 gm	184	23	7	7	0	9	5.34	90	309	410
yield from 1 lb raw with refuse, 295 gm	639	79	24	23	0	31	18.53	313	1074	1423
LUNGS, braised, 3 oz, 85 gm	102	17	3	0	0	9	4.59	86	147	236
yield from 1 lb raw with refuse, 303 gm	365	62	11	0	0	33	16.37	306	525	840

195

FOOD & DESCRIPTION MEASURE OR QUANTITY	CALORIES	PROTEIN (GM)	FAT (GM)	CARBO-HYDRATE (GM)	FIBER (GM)	CALCIUM (MG)	IRON (MG)	SODIUM (MG)	POTASSIUM (MG)	CHOLES-TEROL (MG)
PANCREAS, braised, 3 oz, 85 gm	230	23	15	0	0	14	2.22	51	209	—
yield from 1 lb raw with refuse, 222 gm	601	60	38	0	0	36	5.79	133	546	—
RIB, EYE, SMALL END, 10–12 ribs										
CHOICE GRADE										
broiled, lean & fat, 3 oz, 85 gm	250	22	18	0	0	11	1.98	55	299	70
yield from 1 lb raw with refuse, 328 gm	966	83	68	0	0	43	7.66	211	1156	271
broiled, lean only, 3 oz, 85 gm	191	24	10	0	0	11	2.18	58	335	68
yield from 1 lb raw with refuse, 277 gm	623	78	32	0	0	36	7.11	190	1093	223
RIB, LARGE END, 6–9 ribs										
ALL GRADES										
broiled, lean & fat, 3 oz, 85 gm	321	17	27	0	0	9	1.72	51	245	74
yield from 1 lb raw with refuse, 287 gm	1083	58	93	0	0	29	5.79	173	827	248
broiled, lean only, 3 oz, 85 gm	198	21	12	0	0	7	2.11	59	314	70
yield from 1 lb raw with refuse, 194 gm	453	48	28	0	0	16	4.81	135	716	160
roasted, lean & fat, 3 oz, 85 gm	313	19	26	0	0	8	1.97	54	246	72
yield from 1 lb raw with refuse, 280 gm	1030	64	84	0	0	27	6.49	179	809	237
roasted, lean only, 3 oz, 85 gm	207	23	12	0	0	7	2.40	62	303	68
yield from 1 lb raw with refuse, 200 gm	487	55	28	0	0	16	5.64	146	713	161
CHOICE GRADE										
broiled, lean & fat, 3 oz, 85 gm	327	17	28	0	0	9	1.71	51	244	74
yield from 1 lb raw with refuse, 288 gm	1107	58	95	0	0	30	5.79	173	826	249
broiled, lean only, 3 oz, 85 gm	203	21	13	0	0	7	2.11	59	314	70
yield from 1 lb raw with refuse, 194 gm	464	48	29	0	0	16	4.81	135	716	160
roasted, lean & fat, 3 oz, 85 gm	316	19	26	0	0	8	1.97	54	245	72
yield from 1 lb raw with refuse, 280 gm	1040	64	85	0	0	27	6.48	179	808	237
roasted, lean only, 3 oz, 85 gm	210	23	12	0	0	7	2.40	62	303	68
yield from 1 lb raw with refuse, 200 gm	495	55	29	0	0	16	5.64	146	713	161
GOOD GRADE										
broiled, lean & fat, 3 oz, 85 gm	301	17	25	0	0	9	1.75	52	250	73
yield from 1 lb raw with refuse, 285 gm	1009	58	84	0	0	29	5.85	174	839	246
broiled, lean only, 3 oz, 85 gm	183	21	10	0	0	7	2.11	59	314	70
yield from 1 lb raw with refuse, 199 gm	428	49	24	0	0	17	4.94	139	734	164
roasted, lean & fat, 3 oz, 85 gm	304	19	24	0	0	8	1.98	54	247	72
yield from 1 lb raw with refuse, 280 gm	1000	64	81	0	0	27	6.51	179	812	237
roasted, lean only, 3 oz, 85										

FOOD & DESCRIPTION MEASURE OR QUANTITY	CALORIES	PROTEIN (GM)	FAT (GM)	CARBO-HYDRATE (GM)	FIBER (GM)	CALCIUM (MG)	IRON (MG)	SODIUM (MG)	POTASSIUM (MG)	CHOLES-TEROL (MG)
gm	197	23	11	0	0	7	2.40	62	303	68
yield from 1 lb raw with refuse, 202 gm	468	56	26	0	0	16	5.70	148	720	163
PRIME GRADE										
broiled, lean & fat, 3 oz, 85										
gm	361	17	32	0	0	9	1.69	51	241	74
yield from 1 lb raw with refuse, 298 gm	1267	59	112	0	0	31	5.94	178	846	259
broiled, lean only, 3 oz, 85										
gm	250	21	18	0	0	7	2.11	59	314	70
yield from 1 lb raw with refuse, 196 gm	575	48	41	0	0	17	4.86	136	723	162
roasted, lean & fat, 3 oz, 85										
gm	346	19	29	0	0	8	1.93	54	240	72
yield from 1 lb raw with refuse, 279 gm	1136	62	97	0	0	27	6.33	176	787	238
roasted, lean only, 3 oz, 85										
gm	241	23	16	0	0	7	2.40	62	303	68
yield from 1 lb raw with refuse, 192 gm	543	53	35	0	0	15	5.42	140	685	155
RIB, SMALL END, 10–12 ribs										
ALL GRADES										
broiled, lean & fat, 3 oz, 85										
gm	277	20	21	0	0	11	1.89	53	281	71
yield from 1 lb raw with refuse, 291 gm	950	70	72	0	0	39	6.46	181	964	244
broiled, lean only, 3 oz, 85										
gm	188	24	10	0	0	11	2.18	58	335	68
yield from 1 lb raw with refuse, 223 gm	492	63	25	0	0	29	5.72	153	880	179
roasted, lean & fat, 3 oz, 85										
gm	305	19	25	0	0	11	1.66	56	276	72
yield from 1 lb raw with refuse, 273 gm	981	61	80	0	0	36	5.33	179	887	231
roasted, lean only, 3 oz, 85										
gm	201	23	11	0	0	11	1.96	64	344	68
yield from 1 lb raw with refuse, 197 gm	465	53	27	0	0	26	4.53	148	796	159
CHOICE GRADE										
broiled, lean & fat, 3 oz, 85										
gm	282	20	22	0	0	11	1.88	53	280	71
yield from 1 lb raw with refuse, 291 gm	965	70	74	0	0	39	6.43	181	960	244
broiled, lean only, 3 oz, 85										
gm	191	24	10	0	0	11	2.18	58	335	68
yield from 1 lb raw with refuse, 222 gm	499	62	26	0	0	29	5.70	152	876	178
roasted, lean & fat, 3 oz, 85										
gm	312	19	26	0	0	11	1.65	55	275	72
yield from 1 lb raw with refuse, 273 gm	1002	61	82	0	0	36	5.31	178	882	231
roasted, lean only, 3 oz, 85										
gm	206	23	12	0	0	11	1.96	64	344	68
yield from 1 lb raw with refuse, 196 gm	476	52	28	0	0	26	4.51	147	792	158
GOOD GRADE										
broiled, lean & fat, 3 oz, 85										
gm	263	21	19	0	0	11	1.91	53	285	71
yield from 1 lb raw with refuse, 287 gm	889	70	66	0	0	38	6.44	180	963	240
broiled, lean only, 3 oz, 85										
gm	178	24	8	0	0	11	2.18	58	335	68
yield from 1 lb raw with refuse, 226 gm	473	63	22	0	0	29	5.80	155	892	182

FOOD & DESCRIPTION MEASURE OR QUANTITY	CALORIES	PROTEIN (GM)	FAT (GM)	CARBO-HYDRATE (GM)	FIBER (GM)	CALCIUM (MG)	IRON (MG)	SODIUM (MG)	POTASSIUM (MG)	CHOLES-TEROL (MG)
roasted, lean & fat, 3 oz, 85 gm	283	19	22	0	0	11	1.69	56	282	72
yield from 1 lb raw with refuse, 270 gm	900	61	71	0	0	36	5.35	179	896	227
roasted, lean only, 3 oz, 85 gm	183	23	10	0	0	11	1.96	344	186	68
yield from 1 lb raw with refuse, 201 gm	433	54	23	0	0	26	4.62	813	439	162
PRIME GRADE										
broiled, lean & fat, 3 oz 85 gm	309	20	25	0	0	11	1.86	52	277	71
yield from 1 lb raw with refuse, 286 gm	1041	68	83	0	0	38	6.27	176	933	240
broiled, lean only, 3 oz, 85 gm	221	24	13	0	0	11	2.18	58	335	68
yield from 1 lb raw with refuse, 215 gm	559	60	33	0	0	28	5.52	147	848	173
roasted, lean & fat, 3 oz, 85 gm	357	19	31	0	0	11	1.63	55	269	72
yield from 1 lb raw with refuse, 272 gm	1142	59	99	0	0	36	5.21	175	861	231
roasted, lean only, 3 oz, 85 gm	259	23	18	0	0	11	1.96	64	344	68
yield from 1 lb raw with refuse, 188 gm	572	50	40	0	0	25	4.32	141	760	151
RIB, WHOLE, 6–12 ribs										
ALL GRADES										
broiled, lean & fat, 3 oz, 85 gm	308	18	25	0	0	10	1.77	52	257	73
yield from 1 lb raw with refuse, 287 gm	1039	62	86	0	0	33	5.98	175	868	245
broiled, lean only, 3 oz, 85 gm	194	22	11	0	0	9	2.14	59	323	69
yield from 1 lb raw with refuse, 202 gm	461	53	26	0	0	21	5.08	140	766	165
roasted, lean & fat, 3 oz, 85 gm	324	19	27	0	0	10	1.80	54	250	72
yield from 1 lb raw with refuse, 274 gm	1042	60	87	0	0	30	5.78	173	805	233
roasted, lean only, 3 oz, 85 gm	204	23	12	0	0	9	2.22	63	320	68
yield from 1 lb raw with refuse, 187 gm	449	51	26	0	0	18	4.88	138	708	150
CHOICE GRADE										
broiled, lean & fat, 3 oz 85 gm	313	18	26	0	0	10	1.76	52	256	73
yield from 1 lb raw with refuse, 288 gm	1060	62	88	0	0	33	5.97	175	866	247
broiled, lean only, 3 oz, 85 gm	198	22	12	0	0	9	2.14	59	323	69
yield from 1 lb raw refuse, 201 gm	469	52	27	0	0	21	5.06	139	763	164
roasted, lean & fat, 3 oz, 85 gm	328	19	28	0	0	10	1.79	54	249	72
yield from 1 lb raw with refuse, 275 gm	1062	60	89	0	0	31	5.78	173	805	234
roasted, lean only, 3 oz, 85 gm	209	23	12	0	0	9	2.22	63	320	68
yield from 1 lb raw with refuse, 186 gm	456	51	27	0	0	18	4.85	137	699	149
GOOD GRADE										
broiled, lean & fat, 3 oz, 85 gm	289	19	23	0	0	9	1.80	52	262	72
yield from 1 lb raw with										

FOOD & DESCRIPTION MEASURE OR QUANTITY	CALORIES	PROTEIN (GM)	FAT (GM)	CARBO-HYDRATE (GM)	FIBER (GM)	CALCIUM (MG)	IRON (MG)	SODIUM (MG)	POTASSIUM (MG)	CHOLES-TEROL (MG)
refuse, 285 gm	969	62	78	0	0	31	6.04	174	878	242
broiled, lean only, 3 oz, 85 gm	181	22	10	0	0	9	2.14	59	323	69
yield from 1 lb raw with refuse, 207 gm	440	54	23	0	0	21	5.21	143	785	169
roasted, lean & fat, 3 oz, 85 gm	306	19	25	0	0	10	1.83	54	255	72
yield from 1 lb raw with refuse, 272 gm	978	61	80	0	0	30	5.84	174	815	230
roasted, lean only, 3 oz, 85 gm	191	23	10	0	0	9	2.22	63	320	68
yield from 1 lb raw with refuse, 191 gm	430	52	23	0	0	19	4.98	140	718	153
PRIME GRADE										
broiled, lean & fat, 3 oz, 85 gm	347	18	30	0	0	10	1.74	51	252	73
yield from 1 lb raw with refuse, 294 gm	1199	62	104	0	0	34	6.02	177	870	253
broiled, lean only, 3 oz, 85 gm	238	22	16	0	0	9	2.14	59	323	69
yield from 1 lb raw with refuse, 201 gm	562	52	38	0	0	21	5.06	139	763	164
roasted, lean only, 3 oz, 85 gm	248	23	17	0	0	9	2.22	63	320	68
yield from 1 lb raw with refuse, 184 gm	536	50	36	0	0	18	4.79	135	691	148
roasted, lean only, 3 oz, 85 gm	248	23	17	0	0	9	2.22	63	320	68
yield from 1 lb raw with refuse, 184 gm	536	50	36	0	0	18	4.79	135	691	148
SHORTRIBS, CHOICE GRADE										
braised, lean & fat, 3 oz, 85 gm	400	18	36	0	0	10	1.96	43	191	80
yield from 1 lb raw with refuse, 226 gm	1064	49	95	0	0	28	5.21	114	507	212
braised, lean only, 3 oz, 85 gm	251	26	15	0	0	9	2.86	50	266	79
yield from 1 lb raw with refuse, 123 gm	363	38	22	0	0	13	4.13	72	385	114
ROUND, BOTTOM										
ALL GRADES										
braised, lean & fat, 3 oz, 85 gm	222	25	13	0	0	5	2.76	43	248	81
yield from 1 lb raw with refuse, 278 gm	725	83	41	0	0	16	9.04	140	812	266
braised, lean only, 3 oz, 85 gm	189	27	8	0	0	4	2.94	44	262	81
yield from 1 lb raw with refuse, 254 gm	564	80	25	0	0	12	8.78	131	783	243
CHOICE GRADE										
braised, lean & fat, 3 oz, 85 gm	224	25	13	0	0	5	2.76	43	248	81
yield from 1 lb raw with refuse, 278 gm	734	83	42	0	0	16	9.04	140	812	266
braised, lean only, 3 oz, 85 gm	191	27	8	0	0	4	2.94	44	262	81
yield from 1 lb raw with refuse, 254 gm	571	80	25	0	0	12	8.78	131	783	243
GOOD GRADE										
braised, lean & fat, 3 oz, 85 gm	215	25	12	0	0	5	2.77	43	249	81
yield from 1 lb raw with refuse, 277 gm	700	83	38	0	0	16	9.02	140	810	265
braised, lean only, 3 oz, 85										

FOOD & DESCRIPTION MEASURE OR QUANTITY	CALORIES	PROTEIN (GM)	FAT (GM)	CARBO-HYDRATE (GM)	FIBER (GM)	CALCIUM (MG)	IRON (MG)	SODIUM (MG)	POTASSIUM (MG)	CHOLES-TEROL (MG)
gm	182	27	7	0	0	4	2.94	44	262	81
yield from 1 lb raw with refuse, 254 gm	543	80	22	0	0	12	8.78	131	783	243
PRIME GRADE										
braised, lean & fat, 3 oz, 85 gm	253	25	16	0	0	5	2.71	43	244	81
yield from 1 lb raw with refuse, 287 gm	853	84	55	0	0	17	9.15	144	824	275
braised, lean only, 3 oz, 85 gm	212	27	11	0	0	4	2.94	44	262	81
yield from 1 lb raw with refuse, 250 gm	622	79	32	0	0	12	8.64	128	771	239
ROUND EYE OF										
ALL GRADES										
roasted, lean & fat, 3 oz, 85 gm	206	23	12	0	0	5	1.56	50	308	62
yield from 1 lb raw with refuse, 358 gm	869	96	51	0	0	20	6.58	212	1296	260
roasted, lean only, 3 oz, 85 gm	155	25	6	0	0	4	1.65	52	336	59
yield from 1 lb raw with refuse, 315 gm	575	91	21	0	0	14	6.13	194	1245	219
CHOICE GRADE										
roasted, lean & fat, 3 oz, 85 gm	207	23	12	0	0	5	1.56	50	308	62
yield from 1 lb raw with refuse, 357 gm	871	96	51	0	0	20	6.56	211	1292	259
roasted, lean only, 3 oz, 85 gm	156	25	6	0	0	4	1.65	52	336	59
yield from 1 lb raw with refuse, 314 gm	578	91	21	0	0	14	6.11	194	1241	218
GOOD GRADE										
roasted, lean & fat, 3 oz, 85 gm	201	23	12	0	0	5	1.56	50	308	62
yield from 1 lb raw with refuse, 359 gm	851	96	49	0	0	20	6.60	213	1302	260
roasted, lean only, 3 oz, 85 gm	151	25	5	0	0	4	1.65	52	336	59
yield from 1 lb raw with refuse, 316 gm	562	92	19	0	0	14	6.15	195	1249	219
PRIME GRADE										
roasted, lean & fat, 3 oz, 85 gm	213	23	13	0	0	5	1.57	51	311	61
yield from 1 lb raw with refuse, 355 gm	888	96	53	0	0	20	6.56	211	1298	256
roasted, lean only, 3 oz, 85 gm	168	25	7	0	0	4	1.65	52	336	59
yield from 1 lb raw with refuse, 317 gm	628	92	26	0	0	14	6.17	196	1253	220
ROUND, FULL CUT										
CHOICE GRADE										
broiled, lean & fat, 3 oz, 85 gm	233	22	16	0	0	6	2.05	51	311	71
yield from 1 lb raw with refuse, 304 gm	832	78	55	0	0	21	7.34	183	1113	255
broiled, lean only, 3 oz, 85 gm	165	24	7	0	0	5	2.28	54	352	70
yield from 1 lb raw with refuse, 254 gm	493	72	20	0	0	14	6.81	162	1053	208
GOOD GRADE										
broiled, lean & fat, 3 oz, 85 gm	222	22	14	0	0	6	2.07	51	313	71
yield from 1 lb raw with refuse, 302 gm	790	78	51	0	0	20	7.34	182	1113	253

FOOD & DESCRIPTION MEASURE OR QUANTITY	CALORIES	PROTEIN (GM)	FAT (GM)	CARBO-HYDRATE (GM)	FIBER (GM)	CALCIUM (MG)	IRON (MG)	SODIUM (MG)	POTASSIUM (MG)	CHOLES-TEROL (MG)
broiled, lean only, 3 oz, 85 gm	157	24	6	0	0	5	2.28	54	352	70
yield from 1 lb raw with refuse, 255 gm	470	73	18	0	0	14	6.85	163	1057	209
ROUND, TIP										
ALL GRADES										
roasted, lean & fat, 3 oz, 85 gm	213	23	13	0	0	6	2.30	53	300	70
yield from 1 lb raw with refuse, 328 gm	823	87	50	0	0	21	8.88	203	1158	272
roasted, lean only, 3 oz, 85 gm	162	24	6	0	0	5	2.50	55	328	69
yield from 1 lb raw with refuse, 287 gm	546	82	22	0	0	16	8.44	186	1109	233
CHOICE GRADE										
roasted, lean & fat, 3 oz, 85 gm	216	22	13	0	0	6	2.3	53	300	70
yield from 1 lb raw with refuse, 329 gm	837	87	52	0	0	21	8.88	204	1159	273
roasted, lean only, 3 oz, 85 gm	164	24	7	0	0	5	2.50	55	328	69
yield from 1 lb raw with refuse, 287 gm	552	82	22	0	0	16	8.44	186	1109	233
GOOD GRADE										
roasted, lean & fat, 3 oz, 85 gm	205	23	12	0	0	5	2.31	53	302	70
yield from 1 lb raw with refuse, 324 gm	780	86	46	0	0	21	8.82	201	1151	268
roasted, lean only, 3 oz, 85 gm	156	24	6	0	0	5	2.50	55	328	69
yield from 1 lb raw with refuse, 286 gm	524	82	19	0	0	16	8.41	186	1105	232
PRIME GRADE										
roasted, lean & fat, 3 oz, 85 gm	242	22	16	0	0	6	2.26	52	294	71
yield from 1 lb raw with refuse, 328 gm	932	85	63	0	0	22	8.70	201	1134	273
roasted, lean only, 3 oz, 85 gm	181	24	9	0	0	5	2.50	55	328	69
yield from 1 lb raw with refuse, 278 gm	593	80	28	0	0	15	8.17	181	1074	225
ROUND, TOP										
ALL GRADES										
broiled, lean & fat, 3 oz, 85 gm	179	26	7	0	0	5	2.39	51	365	72
yield from 1 lb raw with refuse, 332 gm	701	102	29	0	0	21	9.32	199	1424	281
broiled, lean only, 3 oz, 85 gm	162	27	5	0	0	5	2.45	52	376	72
yield from 1 lb raw with refuse, 319 gm	610	101	20	0	0	19	9.19	194	1411	269
CHOICE GRADE										
broiled, lean & fat, 3 oz, 85 gm	181	26	8	0	0	5	2.39	51	365	72
yield from 1 lb raw with refuse, 333 gm	709	103	30	0	0	21	9.35	200	1429	282
broiled, lean only, 3 oz, 85 gm	165	27	5	0	0	5	2.45	52	376	72
yield from 1 lb raw with refuse, 319 gm	617	101	21	0	0	19	9.19	194	1411	269
pan-fried, lean & fat, 3 oz, 85 gm	246	27	15	0	0	5	2.43	57	390	82
yield from 1 lb raw with refuse, 283 gm	819	90	48	0	0	18	8.09	188	1298	274

FOOD & DESCRIPTION MEASURE OR QUANTITY	CALORIES	PROTEIN (GM)	FAT (GM)	CARBO-HYDRATE (GM)	FIBER (GM)	CALCIUM (MG)	IRON (MG)	SODIUM (MG)	POTASSIUM (MG)	CHOLES-TEROL (MG)
pan-fried, lean only, 3 oz, 85 gm	193	30	7	0	0	4	2.68	60	436	83
yield from 1 lb raw with refuse, 245 gm	556	86	21	0	0	12	7.71	173	1257	238
GOOD GRADE										
broiled, lean & fat, 3 oz, 85 gm	176	26	7	0	0	5	2.38	51	363	72
yield from 1 lb raw with refuse, 332 gm	686	102	28	0	0	21	9.29	199	1419	281
broiled, lean only, 3 oz, 85 gm	156	27	5	0	0	5	2.45	52	376	72
yield from 1 lb raw with refuse, 317 gm	583	100	17	0	0	19	9.14	192	1402	267
PRIME GRADE										
broiled, lean & fat, 3 oz, 85 gm	201	26	10	0	0	5	2.38	51	363	72
yield from 1 lb raw with refuse, 331 gm	738	102	39	0	0	21	9.26	198	1414	281
broiled, lean only, 3 oz, 85 gm	183	27	8	0	0	5	2.45	52	376	72
yield from 1 lb raw with refuse, 315 gm	678	100	28	0	0	19	9.08	191	1393	265
SHANK, CROSS CUTS, CHOICE GRADE										
simmered, lean & fat, 3 oz, 85 gm	208	27	10	0	0	26	3.06	52	355	67
yield from 1 lb raw with refuse, 208 gm	508	66	25	0	0	63	7.5	128	868	165
simmered, lean only, 3 oz, 85 gm	171	29	5	0	0	27	3.28	54	380	66
yield from 1 lb raw with refuse, 189 gm	380	64	12	0	0	60	7.29	120	845	147
SHORT LOIN, PORTERHOUSE STEAK, CHOICE GRADE										
broiled, lean & fat, 3 oz, 85 gm	254	21	18	0	0	7	2.26	52	303	70
yield from 1 lb raw with refuse, 269 gm	803	68	57	0	0	23	7.15	165	959	222
broiled, lean only, 3 oz, 85 gm	185	24	9	0	0	6	2.55	56	346	68
yield from 1 lb raw with refuse, 222 gm	483	63	24	0	0	16	6.66	145	903	178
SMOKED CHOPPED BEEF, 1 oz, 28 gm	50	8	1	2	0	3	.76	408	122	12
SPLEEN, braised, 3 oz, 85 gm	123	21	4	0	0	10	33.46	48	242	295
yield from 1 lb raw with refuse, 308 gm	447	77	13	0	0	37	121.23	176	875	1069
T-BONE STEAK, CHOICE GRADE										
broiled, lean & fat, 3 oz, 85 gm	276	20	21	0	0	8	2.16	51	288	71
yield from 1 lb raw with refuse, 274 gm	888	66	67	0	0	24	6.95	164	928	229
broiled, lean only, 3 oz, 85 gm	182	24	9	0	0	6	2.55	56	346	68
yield from 1 lb raw with refuse, 209 gm	447	59	22	0	0	15	6.27	137	850	167
TENDERLOIN										
ALL GRADES										
broiled, lean & fat, 3 oz, 85 gm	226	22	15	0	0	7	2.76	52	323	72
yield from 1 lb raw with refuse, 322 gm	857	84	55	0	0	26	10.47	196	1224	274
broiled, lean only, 3 oz, 85										

FOOD & DESCRIPTION MEASURE OR QUANTITY	CALORIES	PROTEIN (GM)	FAT (GM)	CARBO-HYDRATE (GM)	FIBER (GM)	CALCIUM (MG)	IRON (MG)	SODIUM (MG)	POTASSIUM (MG)	CHOLES-TEROL (MG)
gm	174	24	8	0	0	6	3.05	54	356	72
yield from 1 lb raw with refuse, 283 gm	577	80	26	0	0	20	10.13	178	1186	238
roasted, lean & fat, 3 oz, 85 gm	258	21	19	0	0	7	2.71	47	291	74
yield from 1 lb raw refuse, 336 gm	1018	82	74	0	0	27	10.72	188	1152	292
roasted, lean only, 3 oz, 85 gm	186	23	10	0	0	6	3.11	50	334	73
yield from 1 lb raw with refuse, 275 gm	602	76	31	0	0	19	10.07	162	1081	237
CHOICE GRADE										
broiled, lean & fat, 3 oz, 85 gm	230	22	15	0	0 ·	6	2.76	51	322	73
yield from 1 lb raw with refuse, 325 gm	881	84	58	0	0	26	10.53	195	1232	280
broiled, lean only, 3 oz, 85 gm	176	24	8	0	0	6	3.05	54	356	72
yield from 1 lb raw with refuse, 283 gm	586	80	27	0	0	20	10.13	178	1186	238
roasted, lean & fat, 3 oz, 85 gm	262	21	19	0	0	7	2.70	47	290	74
yield from 1 lb raw with refuse, 336 gm	1035	82	76	0	0	27	10.65	188	1146	292
roasted, lean only, 3 oz, 85 gm	189	23	10	0	0	6	3.11	50	334	73
yield from 1 lb raw with refuse, 272 gm	607	75	32	0	0	19	9.96	160	1069	234
GOOD GRADE										
broiled, lean & fat, 3 oz, 85 gm	216	22	13	0	0	6	2.79	52	326	73
yield from 1 lb raw with refuse, 317 gm	805	83	50	0	0	25	10.40	193	1214	273
broiled, lean only, 3 oz, 85 gm	167	24	7	0	0	6	3.05	5	356	72
yield from 1 lb raw with refuse, 280 gm	549	79	23	0	0	20	10.02	176	1173	235
roasted, lean & fat, 3 oz, 85 gm	245	21	17	0	0	7	2.73	48	294	74
yield from 1 lb raw with refuse, 334 gm	962	82	68	0	0	27	10.75	187	1156	291
roasted, lean only, 3 oz, 85 gm	177	23	9	0	0	6	3.11	50	334	73
yield from 1 lb raw with refuse, 277 gm	576	76	28	0	0	19	10.14	163	1089	238
PRIME GRADE										
broiled, lean & fat, 3 oz, 85 gm	270	21	20	0	0	7	2.64	50	307	73
yield from 1 lb raw with refuse, 319 gm	1014	79	75	0	0	26	9.89	188	1155	274
broiled, lean only, 3 oz, 85 gm	197	24	11	0	0	6	3.05	54	356	72
yield from 1 lb raw with refuse, 258 gm	599	73	32	0	0	18	9.24	163	1081	217
roasted, lean & fat, 3 oz, 85 gm	305	20	24	0	0	7	2.57	47	277	75
yield from 1 lb raw with refuse, 325 gm	1164	76	93	0	0	29	9.85	179	1060	286
roasted, lean only, 3 oz, 85 gm	217	23	13	0	0	6	3.11	50	334	73
yield from 1 lb raw with refuse, 247 gm	630	68	38	0	0	17	9.04	146	971	212
THYMUS, braised, 3 oz, 85 gm	271	19	21	0	0	—	1.27	99	368	250

FOOD & DESCRIPTION MEASURE OR QUANTITY	CALORIES	PROTEIN (GM)	FAT (GM)	CARBO-HYDRATE (GM)	FIBER (GM)	CALCIUM (MG)	IRON (MG)	SODIUM (MG)	POTASSIUM (MG)	CHOLES-TEROL (MG)
yield from 1 lb raw with refuse, 381 gm	1214	83	95	0	0	—	5.69	442	1650	1119
TOP LOIN										
ALL GRADES										
broiled, lean & fat, 3 oz, 85 gm	238	22	16	0	0	7	1.91	54	299	67
yield from 1 lb raw with refuse, 332 gm	930	85	62	0	0	30	7.44	209	1165	262
broiled, lean only, 3 oz, 85 gm	172	24	8	0	0	7	2.10	57	336	65
yield from 1 lb raw with refuse, 278 gm	564	80	25	0	0	22	6.87	189	1101	211
CHOICE GRADE										
broiled, lean & fat, 3 oz, 85 gm	243	22	17	0	0	8	1.90	54	297	68
yield from 1 lb raw with refuse, 333 gm	952	85	65	0	0	30	7.46	210	1166	263
broiled, lean only, 3 oz, 85 gm	176	24	8	0	0	7	2.10	57	336	65
yield from 1 lb raw with refuse, 278 gm	575	80	26	0	0	22	6.87	189	1101	211
GOOD GRADE										
broiled, lean & fat, 3 oz, 85 gm	223	22	14	0	0	7	1.92	54	302	67
yield from 1 lb raw with refuse, 326 gm	854	85	55	0	0	29	7.37	209	1157	258
broiled, lean only, 3 oz, 85 gm	162	24	6	0	0	7	2.10	57	336	65
yield from 1 lb raw with refuse, 278 gm	528	80	21	0	0	22	6.87	189	1101	211
PRIME GRADE										
broiled, lean & fat, 3 oz, 85 gm	288	21	22	0	0	8	1.84	53	285	68
yield from 1 lb raw with refuse, 323 gm	1095	80	84	0	0	29	7.01	200	1085	258
broiled, lean only, 3 oz, 85 gm	208	24	12	0	0	7	2.10	57	336	65
yield from 1 lb raw with refuse, 254 gm	622	73	35	0	0	20	6.27	173	1006	193
TONGUE, simmered, 3 oz, 85 gm	241	19	18	<1	0	6	2.88	51	153	91
yield from 1 lb raw with refuse, 259 gm	732	57	54	<1	0	19	8.78	155	466	278
WEDGE-BONE SIRLOIN										
ALL GRADES										
broiled, lean & fat, 3 oz, 85 gm	238	23	15	0	0	9	2.56	53	306	77
yield from 1 lb raw with refuse, 285 gm	797	78	51	0	0	31	8.57	178	1025	257
broiled, lean only, 3 oz, 85 gm	177	26	7	0	0	9	2.85	56	342	76
yield from 1 lb raw with refuse, 242 gm	504	73	21	0	0	25	8.12	161	974	216
CHOICE GRADE										
broiled, lean & fat, 3 oz, 85 gm	240	23	16	0	0	9	2.55	53	305	77
yield from 1 lb raw with refuse, 284 gm	804	78	52	0	0	31	8.53	177	1020	256
broiled, lean only, 3 oz, 85 gm	180	26	8	0	0	9	2.85	56	342	76
yield from 1 lb raw with refuse, 241 gm	509	73	22	0	0	25	8.09	160	970	215
pan-fried, lean & fat, 3 oz, 85 gm	288	23	21	0	0	10	2.76	58	328	84

FOOD & DESCRIPTION MEASURE OR QUANTITY	CALORIES	PROTEIN (GM)	FAT (GM)	CARBO-HYDRATE (GM)	FIBER (GM)	CALCIUM (MG)	IRON (MG)	SODIUM (MG)	POTASSIUM (MG)	CHOLES-TEROL (MG)
yield from 1 lb raw with refuse, 269 gm	913	74	66	0	0	31	8.74	184	1037	265
pan-fried, lean only, 3 oz, 85 gm	202	28	9	0	0	9	3.32	65	395	85
yield from 1 lb raw with refuse, 207 gm	492	67	23	0	0	22	8.08	159	963	206
GOOD GRADE										
broiled, lean & fat, 3 oz, 85 gm	232	23	15	0	0	9	2.55	53	305	77
yield from 1 lb raw with refuse, 284 gm	777	78	49	0	0	31	8.53	177	1020	256
broiled, lean only, 3 oz, 85 gm	170	26	7	0	0	9	2.85	56	342	76
yield from 1 lb raw with refuse, 241 gm	482	73	19	0	0	25	8.09	160	970	215
PRIME GRADE										
broiled, lean & fat, 3 oz, 85 gm	271	23	19	0	0	9	2.49	52	297	77
yield from 1 lb raw with refuse, 275 gm	878	73	63	0	0	31	8.04	169	961	248
broiled, lean only, 3 oz, 85 gm	201	26	10	0	0	9	2.85	56	342	76
yield from 1 lb raw with refuse, 223 gm	527	68	26	0	0	23	7.48	148	898	199

Game

USDA

FOOD & DESCRIPTION MEASURE OR QUANTITY	CALORIES	PROTEIN (GM)	FAT (GM)	CARBO-HYDRATE (GM)	FIBER (GM)	CALCIUM (MG)	IRON (MG)	SODIUM (MG)	POTASSIUM (MG)	CHOLES-TEROL (MG)
BEAVER, roasted, 3.5 oz, 100 gm	248	29	14	0	0	21	1.50	41	368	100
MUSKRAT, roasted, 3.5 oz, 100 gm	153	27	4	0	0	21	1.50	41	368	100
OPOSSUM, 3.5 oz, 100 gm	221	30	10	0	0	21	1.50	41	368	100
RABBIT, DOMESTICATED, stewed										
yield from 1 lb with bones, ready-to-cook, 8.6 oz, 245 gm	529	72	25	0	0	51	3.70	100	902	223
chopped or diced, 1 c, 140 gm	302	41	14	0	0	29	2.10	57	515	127
ground, 1 c, 110 gm	238	32	11	0	0	23	1.70	45	405	100
3.5 oz, 100 gm	216	29	10	0	0	21	1.50	41	368	91
RACCOON, roasted, 3.5 oz, 100 gm	255	29	15	0	0	21	1.50	41	368	100
REINDEER										
lean only, 3.5 oz, 100 gm	127	22	4	0	0	12	5.30	90	320	65
lean & fat										
forequarter, 3.5 oz, 100 gm	178	22	9	0	0	11	3.00	90	320	68
hindquarter, 3.5 oz, 100 gm	256	19	19	0	0	11	2.70	90	320	68
side, 3.5 oz, 100 gm	217	21	14	0	0	11	2.80	90	320	68
VENISON, lean only, 3.5 oz, 100 gm	126	21	4	0	0	10	1.50	90	320	65

Lamb

USDA

FOOD & DESCRIPTION MEASURE OR QUANTITY	CALORIES	PROTEIN (GM)	FAT (GM)	CARBO-HYDRATE (GM)	FIBER (GM)	CALCIUM (MG)	IRON (MG)	SODIUM (MG)	POTASSIUM (MG)	CHOLES-TEROL (MG)
LEG, roasted										
lean & fat										
yield from 1 lb with bone, 267 gm	745	68	51	0	0	29	4.50	166	757	262
yield from 1 lb without bone, 318 gm	887	81	60	0	0	35	5.40	197	902	312

FOOD & DESCRIPTION MEASURE OR QUANTITY	CALORIES	PROTEIN (GM)	FAT (GM)	CARBO-HYDRATE (GM)	FIBER (GM)	CALCIUM (MG)	IRON (MG)	SODIUM (MG)	POTASSIUM (MG)	CHOLES-TEROL (MG)
l c, 140 gm	391	35	27	0	0	15	2.40	87	396	137
1 piece, 3 oz, 85 gm	237	22	16	0	0	9	1.40	53	241	83
lean only										
yield from 1 lb with bone, 221 gm	411	63	16	0	0	29	4.90	155	710	221
yield from 1 lb without bone, 264 gm	491	76	19	0	0	34	5.80	186	849	264
1 c, 140 gm	260	40	10	0	0	18	3.10	98	450	140
1 piece, 3 oz, 85 gm	158	24	6	0	0	11	1.90	60	273	85
LOIN CHOP, broiled										
lean & fat										
yield from 1 lb with bone, 285 gm	1023	63	84	0	0	26	3.70	154	702	279
yield from 1 chop, ⅓ lb raw weight, 95 gm	341	21	28	0	0	9	1.20	51	234	93
yield from 1 chop, ¼ lb raw weight, 71 gm	255	16	21	0	0	6	.90	38	175	70
1 piece, 3 oz, 85 gm	305	19	25	0	0	8	1.11	46	209	83
lean only										
yield from 1 lb with bone, 196 gm	368	55	15	0	0	24	3.90	135	619	196
yield from 1 chop, ⅓ lb raw weight, 65 gm	122	18	5	0	0	8	1.30	45	205	65
yield from 1 chop, ¼ lb raw weight, 49 gm	92	14	4	0	0	6	1.00	34	155	49
1 piece, 3 oz, 85 gm	160	24	6	0	0	10	1.70	59	269	85
RIB CHOPS										
Lean & fat										
yield from 1 lb with bone, 268 gm	1091	54	95	0	0	24	2.90	132	604	263
yield from 1 chop, ⅓ lb raw weight, 89 gm	362	18	32	0	0	8	1.00	44	200	87
yield from 1 chop, ¼ lb raw weight, 67 gm	273	14	24	0	0	6	.70	33	151	66
1 piece, 3 oz, 85 gm	346	17	30	0	0	8	.94	42	191	83
lean only										
yield from 1 lb with bone, 171 gm	361	47	18	0	0	19	3.20	114	521	171
yield from 1 chop, ⅓ lb raw weight, 57 gm	120	16	6	0	0	6	1.10	38	174	57
yield from 1 chop, ¼ lb raw weight, 43 gm	91	12	5	0	0	5	.80	29	131	43
1 piece, 3 oz, 85 gm	179	23	9	0	0	9	1.61	57	259	85
SHOULDER										
lean & fat										
yield from 1 lb with bone, 270 gm	913	59	73	0	0	27	3.20	144	656	265
yield from 1 lb without bone, 318 gm	1075	69	87	0	0	32	3.80	169	773	312
1 c, 140 gm	473	30	38	0	0	14	1.70	74	340	137
1 piece, 3 oz, 85 gm	287	18	23	0	0	9	1.02	45	207	83
lean only										
yield from 1 lb with bone, 200 gm	410	54	20	0	0	24	3.80	131	600	200
yield from 1 lb without bone, 235 gm	482	63	24	0	0	28	4.50	154	706	235
1 c, 140 gm	287	38	14	0	0	17	2.70	92	420	140
1 piece, 3 oz, 85 gm	174	23	9	0	0	10	1.62	56	255	85

FOOD & DESCRIPTION MEASURE OR QUANTITY	CALORIES	PROTEIN (GM)	FAT (GM)	CARBO-HYDRATE (GM)	FIBER (GM)	CALCIUM (MG)	IRON (MG)	SODIUM (MG)	POTASSIUM (MG)	CHOLES-TEROL (MG)
Pork & Pork Products										
Hormel										
BLACK LABEL										
BACON, ckd, sliced, 2 sl	60	4	5	0	—	—	—	298	—	—
HAM, cnd										
1.5 pound ham, 4 oz, 113 gm	150	21	7	0	—	—	—	1324	—	—
3 pound ham, 4 oz, 113 gm	140	20	7	0	—	—	—	1315	—	—
5 pound ham, 4 oz, 113 gm	140	20	7	0	—	—	—	1245	—	—
BREADED PORK STEAKS, 3 oz, 85 gm	220	12	15	11	—	—	—	—	—	—
CURE 81 HAM, 4 oz, 113 gm	160	22	8	0	—	—	—	1322	—	—
CURE MASTER HAM, 4 oz, 113 gm	140	22	5	1	—	—	—	1361	—	—
EXL CANNED HAM, 4 oz, 113 gm	120	22	4	0	—	—	—	1382	—	—
HAM										
BONE-IN, 4 oz, 113 gm	210	17	15	1	—	—	—	—	—	—
CHOPPED, 8 lb can, 3 oz, 85 gm	240	12	21	1	—	—	—	1062	—	—
CHUNK, 6.75 gm, 191 gm	310	32	20	0	—	—	—	2241	—	—
HAM PATTY, 1 patty	180	7	16	0	—	—	—	456	—	—
HAM AND CHEESE PATTY, 1 patty	190	7	18	0	—	—	—	468	—	—
HAM ROLL, 4 oz, 113 gm	170	21	10	0	—	—	—	1338	—	—
HOLIDAY GLAZE HAM, 4 oz, 113 gm	130	21	4	2	—	—	—	—	—	—
LIGHT & LEAN HAM, boneless, 2 oz, 57 gm	60	10	2	0	—	—	—	574	—	—
PORK, CHOPPED, 8 lb can, 3 oz, 85 gm	200	12	16	2	—	—	—	1073	—	—
PORK TONGUE, CURED, 3 oz, 85 gm	190	17	13	0	—	—	—	966	—	—
RANGE BRAND SLICED BACON, ckd, 2 sl	110	6	9	0	—	—	—	392	—	—
RED LABEL BACON, ckd, 3 sl	110	6	10	0	—	—	—	—	—	—
USDA										
BACKFAT, fresh, raw, 1 oz, 28 gm	230	<1	25	0	0	1	.05	3	18	16
BACON										
ckd, 3 medium sl, 19 gm	109	6	9	<1	0	2	.31	303	92	16
yield from 1 lb raw, 4.48 oz, 127 gm	732	39	63	<1	0	15	2.05	2026	617	107
raw, 3 medium sl, 20/lb, 68 gm	378	6	39	<1	0	5	.41	466	95	46
1 thick sl, 12/lb, 38 gm	211	3	22	<1	0	3	.23	260	53	26
BELLY, fresh, raw, 1 oz, 28 gm	147	3	15	0	0	1	.15	9	52	20
BRAINS, braised, 3 oz, 85 gm	117	10	8	0	0	8	1.55	77	166	2169
yield from 1 lb with refuse, 382 gm	526	46	36	0	0	34	6.95	348	745	9749
CHITTERLINGS, ckd, simmered, 3 oz, 85 gm	258	9	24	0	0	23	3.15	33	7	122
yield from 1 lb with refuse, 171 gm	518	18	49	0	0	47	6.33	66	13	245
EARS, ckd, simmered, 1 ear, 111 gm, from 1 raw ear	183	18	12	0	0	20	1.65	183	44	99
yield from 1 lb raw with refuse, 422 gm	700	67	46	0	0	78	6.33	703	170	380

FOOD & DESCRIPTION MEASURE OR QUANTITY	CALORIES	PROTEIN (GM)	FAT (GM)	CARBO-HYDRATE (GM)	FIBER (GM)	CALCIUM (MG)	IRON (MG)	SODIUM (MG)	POTASSIUM (MG)	CHOLES-TEROL (MG)
FAT										
cooked, 1 oz, 28 gm	200	2	21	0	0	1	.09	9	23	26
raw, 1 oz, 28 gm	202	1	22	0	0	1	.08	5	27	26
FEET, fresh, simmered										
1 foot, yield from 8 oz raw, 71 gm	138	14	9	0	0	32	—	—	—	71
pickled, 1 oz, 28 gm	58	4	5	<1	0	9	—	—	—	26
HAM, boneless										
extra lean & regular										
roasted, 3 oz, 85 gm	140	19	7	<1	0	7	1.19	1177	308	48
1 c, 140 gm	231	31	11	<1	0	11	1.95	1938	507	80
unheated, 1 oz, 28 gm	46	5	2	<1	0	2	.26	362	84	15
1 c, 140 gm	227	26	12	3	0	10	1.26	1789	415	74
extra lean										
roasted, 3 oz, 85 gm	123	18	5	1	0	7	1.26	1023	244	45
1 c, 140 gm	203	29	8	2	0	11	2.07	1684	402	74
unheated, 1 oz, 28 gm	37	5	1	<1	0	2	.22	405	99	13
1 c, 140 gm	183	27	7	1	0	10	1.07	2000	489	66
regular, 11% fat										
roasted, 3 oz, 85 gm	151	19	8	0	0	7	1.14	1275	348	50
1 c, 140 gm	249	32	13	0	0	12	1.88	2100	573	83
unheated, 1 oz, 28 gm	52	5	3	<1	0	2	.28	373	94	16
1 c, 140 gm	255	25	15	4	0	10	1.39	1844	465	80
HAM, cnd										
extra lean & regular										
roasted, 3 oz, 85 gm	142	18	7	<1	0	6	.91	908	298	34
1 c, 140 gm	234	29	12	<1	0	10	1.50	1495	491	57
unheated, 1 oz, 28 gm	41	5	2	0	0	2	.26	362	95	11
l c, 140 gm	202	25	10	0	0	8	1.26	1787	468	54
extra lean, 4% fat										
roasted, 3 oz, 85 gm	116	18	4	<1	0	5	.78	965	296	25
1 c, 140 gm	191	30	7	<1	0	8	1.29	1589	487	41
unheated, 1 oz, 28 gm	34	5	1	0	0	2	.27	356	103	11
1 c, 140 gm	168	26	6	0	0	8	1.32	1757	510	53
regular										
roasted, 3 oz, 85 gm	192	17	13	<1	0	7	1.16	800	304	52
1 c, 140 gm	317	29	21	<1	0	12	1.92	1317	500	86
unheated, 3 oz, 85 gm	162	14	11	<1	0	5	.71	1055	269	33
1 c, 140 gm	266	24	18	<1	0	8	1.16	1736	442	55
HAM, COUNTRY-STYLE, lean only, raw, 1 oz, 28 gm	55	8	2	<1	0	—	—	—	—	—
HAM, CENTER SLICE, lean & fat, unheated, 1 oz, 28 gm	57	6	4	<1	0	2	.21	393	95	15
HAM LEG, fresh										
RUMP HALF, lean & fat, roasted, 3 oz, 85 gm	233	23	15	0	0	6	.89	52	303	81
1 c, 140 gm	384	37	25	0	0	10	1.46	85	499	133
RUMP HALF, lean only, roasted, 3 oz, 85 gm	187	25	9	0	0	6	.96	55	332	81
1 c, 140 gm	309	41	15	0	0	10	1.59	90	547	134
SHANK HALF, lean & fat, roasted, 3 oz, 85 gm	258	21	19	0	0	5	.83	50	263	78
1 c, 140 gm	425	34	31	0	0	9	1.36	82	434	129
SHANK HALF, lean only, roasted, 3 oz, 85 gm	183	24	9	0	0	6	.95	54	306	78
1 c, 140 gm	301	39	15	0	0	10	1.56	90	504	129
WHOLE, lean & fat, roasted, 3 oz, 85 gm	250	21	18	0	0	5	.85	51	280	79
1 c, 140 gm	411	35	29	0	0	9	1.4	83	461	131
WHOLE, lean only, roasted, 3 oz, 85 gm	187	24	9	0	0	6	.95	55	317	80
1 c, 140 gm	309	40	15	0	0	10	1.57	90	523	131

FOOD & DESCRIPTION MEASURE OR QUANTITY	CALORIES	PROTEIN (GM)	FAT (GM)	CARBO-HYDRATE (GM)	FIBER (GM)	CALCIUM (MG)	IRON (MG)	SODIUM (MG)	POTASSIUM (MG)	CHOLES-TEROL (MG)
HAM STEAK, boneless, extra lean, unheated, 1 oz, 28 gm	35	6	1	0	0	1	.28	360	92	13
HAM, WHOLE, lean & fat										
roasted, 3 oz, 85 gm	207	18	14	0	0	6	.74	1009	243	52
1 c, 140 gm	341	30	23	0	0	10	1.22	1661	400	86
unheated, 3 oz, 85 gm	209	16	16	<1	0	6	.60	1092	264	48
1 c, 140 gm	345	26	26	<1	0	10	1.00	1797	434	78
WHOLE, lean only										
roasted, 3 oz, 85 gm	133	21	5	0	0	6	.79	1128	269	47
1 c, 140 gm	219	35	8	0	0	10	1.31	1858	443	78
unheated, 3 oz, 85 gm	125	19	5	<1	0	6	.69	1289	316	44
1 c. 140 gm	206	31	8	<1	0	10	1.13	2122	519	73
HEART, braised, yield from 1 raw heart, 226 gm raw, 129 gm ckd	191	30	7	<1	0	9	7.52	46	266	285
1 c, 145 gm	214	34	7	<1	0	10	8.45	51	299	320
JOWL, raw, 1 oz, 28 gm	186	2	20	0	0	1	.12	7	42	25
KIDNEYS, braised, 3 oz, 85 gm	128	22	4	0	0	11	4.50	68	121	408
1 c, 140 gm	211	36	7	0	0	18	7.41	111	200	673
LIVER, braised, 3 oz, 85 gm	141	22	4	3	0	9	15.23	42	128	302
yield from 1 lb, 354 gm	585	92	16	13	0	37	63.44	173	532	1257
LOIN										
BLADE, lean & fat										
braised, 3 oz, 85	348	20	29	0	0	12	1.10	59	284	92
1 chop, 67 gm, 89 gm with refuse	275	16	23	0	0	9	.87	46	224	72
broiled, 3 oz, 85 gm	334	18	29	0	0	9	.77	57	283	83
1 chop, 59 gm, 104 gm with refuse	303	16	26	0	0	8	.70	52	256	75
pan-fried, 3 oz, 85 gm	352	16	31	0	0	8	.70	52	253	81
1 chop, 89 gm, 121 gm with refuse	368	17	33	0	0	9	.73	55	265	85
roasted, 3 oz, 85 gm	310	18	26	0	0	10	.91	52	249	76
1 chop, 88 gm, 118 gm with refuse	321	19	27	0	0	11	.94	54	258	79
BLADE, lean only										
braised, 3 oz, 85 gm	266	25	18	0	0	14	1.38	69	354	96
1 chop, 50 gm, 89 with refuse	156	15	10	0	0	9	.81	41	209	57
broiled, 3 oz, 85 gm	255	21	18	0	0	11	.92	65	347	85
1 chop, 59 gm, 104 gm with refuse	177	15	13	0	0	8	.64	45	241	59
pan-fried, 3 oz, 85 gm	240	21	17	0	0	11	.89	63	335	82
1 chop, 62 gm, 121 gm with refuse	175	15	12	0	0	8	.65	46	245	60
roasted, 3 oz, 85 gm	238	21	16	0	0	12	1.07	58	294	76
1 chop, 71 gm, 118 gm with refuse	198	18	14	0	0	10	.89	48	246	63
CENTER, lean & fat										
braised, 3 oz, 85 gm	301	25	22	0	0	5	.71	43	269	91
1 chop, 75 gm, 91 gm with refuse	266	22	19	0	0	4	.62	38	238	81
broiled, 3 oz, 85 gm	269	23	19	0	0	4	.69	59	305	82
1 chop, 87 gm, 106 gm with refuse	275	24	19	0	0	4	.71	61	312	84
pan-fried, 3 oz, 85 gm	318	20	26	0	0	4	.71	61	308	87
1 chop, 89 gm, 112 gm with refuse	333	21	27	0	0	4	.74	64	323	92
roasted, 3 oz, 85 gm	259	22	18	0	0	5	.84	54	274	78
1 chop, 88 gm, 109 gm with refuse	268	22	19	0	0	5	.87	56	284	80

209

FOOD & DESCRIPTION MEASURE OR QUANTITY	CALORIES	PROTEIN (GM)	FAT (GM)	CARBO-HYDRATE (GM)	FIBER (GM)	CALCIUM (MG)	IRON (MG)	SODIUM (MG)	POTASSIUM (MG)	CHOLES-TEROL (MG)
CENTER, lean only										
braised, 3 oz, 85 gm	231	30	12	0	0	5	.81	46	316	95
1 chop, 61 gm, 91 gm with refuse	166	21	8	0	0	4	.58	33	227	68
broiled, 3 oz, 85 gm	196	27	9	0	0	4	.78	66	357	83
1 chop, 72 gm, 106 gm with refuse	166	23	8	0	0	3	.66	56	302	71
pan-fried, 3 oz, 85 gm	226	24	14	0	0	4	.85	72	387	91
1 chop, 67 gm, 112 gm with refuse	178	19	11	0	0	3	.67	57	305	71
roasted, 3 oz, 85 gm	204	24	11	0	0	5	.93	59	307	78
1 chop, 72 gm, 109 gm with refuse	180	21	10	0	0	4	.82	52	271	68
RIB, CENTER, lean & fat										
braised, 3 oz, 85 gm	312	24	23	0	0	9	.91	41	351	81
1 chop, 67 gm, 89 gm with refuse	246	19	18	0	0	7	.71	32	277	64
broiled, 3 oz, 85 gm	291	21	22	0	0	11	.61	52	315	79
1 chop, 77 gm, 104 gm with refuse	264	19	20	0	0	10	.56	47	285	72
pan-fried, 3 oz, 85 gm	331	18	28	0	0	6	.56	38	299	71
1 chop, 88 gm, 119 gm with refuse	343	19	29	0	0	6	.58	40	309	74
roasted, 3 oz, 85 gm	271	21	20	0	0	8	.76	37	313	69
1 chop, 79 gm, 109 gm with refuse	252	20	19	0	0	8	.71	35	291	64
RIB, CENTER, lean only										
braised, 3 oz, 85 gm	236	29	12	0	0	10	1.07	44	426	82
1 chop, 53 gm, 89 gm with refuse	147	18	8	0	0	6	.67	28	266	51
broiled, 3 oz, 85 gm	219	25	13	0	0	13	.69	57	373	80
1 chop, 63 gm, 104 with refuse	162	18	9	0	0	9	.51	42	276	59
pan-fried, 3 oz, 85 gm	219	24	13	0	0	7	.68	43	396	69
1 chop, 62 gm, 119 gm with refuse	160	17	9	0	0	5	.49	31	288	50
roasted, 3 oz, 85 gm	208	24	12	0	0	9	.85	39	359	67
1 chop, 66 gm, 109 gm with refuse	162	19	9	0	0	7	.66	30	279	52
SIRLOIN, lean & fat										
braised, 3 oz, 85 gm	299	24	22	0	0	5	.96	45	314	90
1 chop, 71 gm, 89 gm with refuse	250	20	18	0	0	5	.80	38	262	75
broiled, 3 oz, 85 gm	281	21	21	0	0	4	.66	46	312	82
1 chop, 84 gm, 106 gm with refuse	278	20	21	0	0	4	.66	46	308	81
roasted, 3 oz, 85 gm	247	21	17	0	0	8	.85	50	286	77
1 chop, 84 gm, 109 gm with refuse	244	21	17	0	0	8	.84	49	283	76
SIRLOIN, lean only										
braised, 3 oz, 85 gm	221	28	11	0	0	6	1.13	50	377	94
1 chop, 57 gm, 89 gm with refuse	149	19	7	0	0	4	.76	34	253	63
broiled, 3 oz, 85 gm	207	24	12	0	0	5	.75	51	369	83
1 chop, 68 gm, 106 gm with refuse	165	19	9	0	0	4	.6	41	295	67
roasted, 3 oz, 85 gm	201	23	11	0	0	8	.92	53	315	77
1 chop, 74 gm, 109 gm with refuse	175	20	10	0	0	7	.8	46	274	67
TENDERLOIN, lean only										
roasted, 3 oz, 85 gm	141	24	4	0	0	7	1.31	57	457	79
yield from 1 lb raw, 358 gm	596	103	17	0	0	31	5.52	238	1928	333
TOP LOIN, lean & fat										

FOOD & DESCRIPTION MEASURE OR QUANTITY	CALORIES	PROTEIN (GM)	FAT (GM)	CARBO-HYDRATE (GM)	FIBER (GM)	CALCIUM (MG)	IRON (MG)	SODIUM (MG)	POTASSIUM (MG)	CHOLES-TEROL (MG)
braised, 3 oz, 85 gm	324	24	25	0	0	9	.88	40	339	81
1 chop, 70 gm, 89 gm with refuse	267	19	20	0	0	7	.72	33	279	67
broiled, 3 oz, 85 gm	306	20	24	0	0	10	.60	51	303	79
1 chop, 82 gm, 104 gm with refuse	295	19	23	0	0	10	.58	49	293	76
pan-fried, 3 oz, 85 gm	333	18	28	0	0	6	.56	38	298	71
1 chop, 86 gm, 115 gm with refuse	337	19	29	0	0	6	.57	39	301	72
roasted, 3 oz, 85 gm	280	21	21	0	0	8	.74	37	305	69
1 chop, 83 gm, 107 gm with refuse	274	20	21	0	0	8	.73	36	298	68
TOP LOIN, lean only										
braised, 3 oz, 85 gm	236	29	12	0	0	10	1.07	44	426	82
1 chop, 53 gm, 89 gm with refuse	147	18	8	0	0	6	.67	28	265	51
broiled, 3 oz, 85 gm	219	25	13	0	0	13	.69	57	373	80
1 chop, 64 gm, 104 gm with refuse	165	18	10	0	0	9	.52	43	281	60
pan-fried, 3 oz, 85 gm	219	24	13	0	0	7	.68	43	396	69
1 chop, 61 gm, 115 gm with refuse	157	17	9	0	0	5	.49	31	284	49
roasted, 3 oz, 85 gm	208	24	12	0	0	9	.85	39	359	67
1 chop, 68 gm, 107 gm with refuse	167	19	9	0	0	7	.68	31	287	54
WHOLE, lean & fat										
braised, 3 oz, 85 gm	312	23	24	0	0	7	.99	56	293	87
1 chop, 71 gm, 89 gm with refuse	261	19	20	0	0	6	.82	46	245	73
broiled, 3 oz, 85 gm	294	20	23	0	0	6	.69	56	298	80
1 chop, 82 gm, 104 gm with refuse	284	19	22	0	0	5	.66	54	287	77
roasted, 3 oz, 85 gm	271	20	21	0	0	7	.86	53	271	77
1 chop, 82 gm, 106 gm with refuse	262	19	20	0	0	7	.83	52	261	74
WHOLE, lean only										
braised, 3 oz, 85 gm	232	28	12	0	0	8	1.19	63	356	90
1 chop, 55 gm, 89 gm with refuse	150	18	8	0	0	5	.77	41	230	58
broiled, 3 oz, 85 gm	218	24	13	0	0	6	.79	64	355	81
1 chop, 66 gm, 104 gm with refuse	169	18	10	0	0	5	.61	49	276	63
roasted, 3 oz, 85 gm	204	23	12	0	0	7	.98	59	312	77
1 chop, 69 gm, 106 gm with refuse	166	19	10	0	0	6	.79	48	253	62
LUNG										
braised, 3 oz, 85 gm	84	14	34	0	0	7	13.95	68	129	329
yield from 1 lb raw with refuse, 300 gm	297	50	9	0	0	25	49.23	242	454	1161
PANCREAS										
braised, 3 oz, 85 gm	186	24	9	0	0	13	2.29	35	143	268
yield from 1 lb raw, 245 gm	537	70	26	0	0	38	6.59	102	412	772
SALT PORK, raw, 1 oz, 28 gm	212	1	23	0	0	2	.12	404	19	25
SHOULDER										
ARM PICNIC, lean & fat										
braised, 3 oz, 85 gm	293	23	22	0	0	6	1.37	74	286	93
1 c, 140 gm	483	38	36	0	0	10	2.25	123	470	153
roasted, 3 oz, 85 gm	281	19	22	0	0	6	1.01	59	249	80
1 c, 140 gm	463	31	37	0	0	11	1.66	97	410	132
ARM PICNIC, lean only										
braised, 3 oz, 85 gm	211	27	10	0	0	7	1.66	87	344	97
1 c, 140 gm	347	45	17	0	0	12	2.73	143	566	160
roasted, 3 oz, 85 gm	194	23	11	0	0	7	1.21	68	299	81
1 c, 140 gm	319	37	18	0	0	12	1.99	112	492	133

FOOD & DESCRIPTION MEASURE OR QUANTITY	CALORIES	PROTEIN (GM)	FAT (GM)	CARBO-HYDRATE (GM)	FIBER (GM)	CALCIUM (MG)	IRON (MG)	SODIUM (MG)	POTASSIUM (MG)	CHOLES-TEROL (MG)
ARM PICNIC, CURED, lean & fat										
3 oz, 85 gm	238	17	18	0	0	9	.81	912	220	49
1 c, 140 gm	392	29	30	0	0	14	1.33	1501	362	82
ARM PICNIC, CURED, lean only										
roasted, 3 oz, 85 gm	145	21	6	0	0	9	.91	1046	248	41
1 c, 140 gm	238	35	10	0	0	15	1.51	1723	409	68
BLADE ROLL, CURED, lean & fat										
roasted, 3 oz, 85 gm	244	15	20	<1	0	6	.75	827	165	57
unheated, 1 oz, 28 gm	76	5	6	0	0	2	.23	354	84	15
BOSTON BLADE, lean & fat										
braised, 3 oz, 85 gm	316	22	24	0	0	6	1.46	57	296	95
1 steak, 160 gm, 180 gm with refuse	594	42	46	0	0	11	2.75	107	557	178
broiled, 3 oz, 85 gm	297	19	24	0	0	5	.99	63	298	87
1 steak, 185 gm, 210 gm with refuse	647	40	53	0	0	10	2.16	138	649	190
roasted, 3 oz, 85 gm	273	19	21	0	0	6	1.2	57	266	82
1 steak, 185 gm, 213 gm with refuse	594	40	47	0	0	12	2.62	125	579	179
BOSTON BLADE, lean only										
braised, 3 oz, 85 gm	250	26	15	0	0	6	1.74	64	350	99
1 steak, 130 gm, 180 gm with refuse	382	41	23	0	0	10	2.67	98	536	151
broiled, 3 oz, 85 gm	233	21	16	0	0	5	1.15	71	348	89
1 steak, 151 gm, 210 gm with refuse	413	38	28	0	0	9	2.04	126	618	159
roasted, 3 oz, 85 gm	218	21	14	0	0	6	1.36	62	300	83
1 steak, 158 gm, 213 gm with refuse	404	38	27	0	0	11	2.53	116	557	155
WHOLE, lean & fat										
roasted, 3 oz, 85 gm	277	19	22	0	0	6	1.11	58	258	81
1 c, 140 gm	456	31	36	0	0	10	1.83	96	425	134
WHOLE, lean only										
roasted, 3 oz, 85 gm	207	22	13	0	0	6	1.29	65	299	82
1 c, 140 gm	341	36	21	0	0	11	2.13	107	493	135
SPARERIBS, lean & fat										
braised, 3 oz, 85 gm	338	25	26	0	0	40	1.58	79	272	103
yield from 1 lb raw with refuse, 6.25 oz, 177 gm	703	51	54	0	0	83	3.28	165	566	214
SPLEEN										
braised, 3 oz, 85 gm	127	24	3	0	0	11	18.9	—	193	428
yield from 1 lb raw, 10.55 oz, 299 gm	446	84	10	0	0	38	66.47	—	679	1506
STOMACH, raw, 1 oz, 28 gm	44	5	3	0	0	3	.62	15	57	55
TAIL										
simmered, 3 oz, 85 gm	336	14	30	0	0	12	—	—	—	110
yield from 1 lb raw, 9.7 oz, 275 gm	1088	47	98	0	0	39	—	—	—	355
TONGUE										
braised, 3 oz, 85 gm	230	20	16	0	0	16	4.24	93	201	124
yield from 1 lb with refuse, 8.15 oz, 231 gm	690	61	47	0	0	49	12.72	279	604	371

Sausages & Luncheon Meats

Armour

FOOD & DESCRIPTION MEASURE OR QUANTITY	CALORIES	PROTEIN (GM)	FAT (GM)	CARBO-HYDRATE (GM)	FIBER (GM)	CALCIUM (MG)	IRON (MG)	SODIUM (MG)	POTASSIUM (MG)	CHOLES-TEROL (MG)
LOWER SALT ALL BEEF BOLOGNA, 1 oz, 28 gm	90	3	8	1	—	—	—	190	200	15
LOWER SALT ALL BEEF HOT										

FOOD & DESCRIPTION MEASURE OR QUANTITY	CALORIES	PROTEIN (GM)	FAT (GM)	CARBO-HYDRATE (GM)	FIBER (GM)	CALCIUM (MG)	IRON (MG)	SODIUM (MG)	POTASSIUM (MG)	CHOLES-TEROL (MG)
DOGS, 2 oz, 56 gm	170	7	15	2	—	—	—	390	400	30
LOWER SALT ALL MEAT BOLOGNA, 1 oz, 28 gm	90	3	8	1	—	—	—	200	200	15
LOWER SALT ALL MEAT HOT DOGS, 2 oz, 56 gm	170	7	15	2	—	—	—	380	390	30
LOWER SALT BACON, .3 oz, 9 gm	38	3	3	<1	—	—	—	127	80	6
LOWER SALT HAM, 1 oz, 28 gm	35	5	1	<1	—	—	—	221	146	14
LOWER SALT SALAMI, 1 oz, 28 gm	80	3	7	2	—	—	—	200	200	20

Armour–Dial

BANNER SAUSAGE, 2.67 oz, 76 gm	160	10	12	2	—	*	1.08	560	—	—
CHOPPED BEEF, 3 oz, 85 gm	280	11	24	3	—	*	1.44	1250	—	—
CHOPPED HAM, 3 oz, 85 gm	240	13	20	2	—	*	.36	1280	—	—
DEVILED HAM, 1.5 oz, 43 gm	120	6	9	0	—	*	*	380	—	—
DEVILED TREET, 1.5 oz, 43 gm	120	6	10	1	—	*	.36	390	—	—
LUNCH TONGUE, 3 oz, 85 gm	200	15	14	1	—	20	2.7	1400	—	—
POTTED MEAT, 1.5 oz, 43 gm	80	5	6	0	—	*	1.08	460	—	—
HOT 'N SPICY, 1.5 oz, 43 gm	80	5	6	0	—	—	—	490	—	—
TREET, 3 oz, 85 gm	290	9	26	4	—	*	.72	1190	—	—
VIENNA SAUSAGE IN BARBEQUE SAUCE, 2.5 oz, 71 gm	200	6	18	4	—	*	.72	580	—	—
IN BEEF STOCK, 2 oz, 57 gm	180	5	17	1	—	*	.36	390	—	—
HOT 'N SPICY, 2 oz, 57 gm	190	6	17	2	—	—	—	750	—	—
SMOKED, 2 oz, 57 gm	180	5	17	1	—	*	1.08	400	—	—

Ball Park

BOLOGNA, 35 gm	107	4	10	0	—	—	—	363	—	—
FRANK, 2 oz, 57 gm	174	7	17	0	—	—	—	545	—	—
BEEF, 2 oz, 57 gm	167	7	16	0	—	—	—	545	—	—
KNOCKWURST, 4 oz, 113 gm	349	13	33	0	—	—	—	1090	—	—
BEEF, 4 oz, 113 gm	335	13	31	0	—	—	—	1090	—	—

Buddig

BEEF, 1 oz, 28 gm	38	5	2	<1	—	3	.91	425	75	16
CHICKEN, 1 oz, 28 gm	50	5	3	<1	—	4	.48	340	55	12
CORNED BEEF, 1 oz, 28 gm	38	5	2	<1	—	3	.91	380	75	16
HAM, 1 oz, 28 gm	48	5	3	<1	—	11	.62	400	80	20
PASTRAMI, 1 oz, 28 gm	38	5	2	<1	—	3	.91	320	75	16
TURKEY, 1 oz, 28 gm	50	5	3	<1	—	4	.51	400	55	6
TURKEY HAM, 1 oz, 28 gm	37	5	2	<1	—	3	.48	425	85	19
TURKEY SALAMI, 1 oz, 28 gm	37	5	2	<1	—	3	.48	340	85	19

Dietz and Watson

BOLOGNA, 1 oz, 28 gm	85	4	7	<1	—	—	—	255	—	—
30% LOWER SALT, 1 oz, 28 gm	78	4	7	<1	—	—	—	196	—	—
FRANKFURTER, 1 oz, 28 gm	85	4	8	<1	—	—	—	249	—	—
GOURMET LITE, 1 oz, 28 gm	75	4	6	<1	—	—	—	160	155	—
BEEF, 1 oz, 28 gm	79	4	7	<1	—	—	—	249	—	—
GOURMET LITE, 1 oz, 28 gm	75	4	6	<1	—	—	—	160	155	—
SALAMI, 1 oz, 28 gm	71	4	6	<1	—	—	—	255	—	—
30% LOWER SALT, 1 oz, 28 gm	72	4	6	<1	—	—	—	196	—	—

FOOD & DESCRIPTION MEASURE OR QUANTITY	CALORIES	PROTEIN (GM)	FAT (GM)	CARBO- HYDRATE (GM)	FIBER (GM)	CALCIUM (MG)	IRON (MG)	SODIUM (MG)	POTASSIUM (MG)	CHOLES- TEROL (MG)
TURKEY BREAST, NO SALT ADDED, 1 oz, 28 gm	33	7	<1	<1	—	—	—	27	—	—
Grillmaster										
BOLOGNA 1 sl, 35 gm	89	5	7	1	—	—	—	454	—	—
CHICKEN CHEESE FRANK, 1 frank, 2 oz, 57 gm	146	8	12	2	—	—	—	683	—	—
CHICKEN FRANK, 1 frank, 2 oz, 57 gm	130	7	11	2	—	—	—	641	—	—
COTTO SALAMI, 1 sl, 32 gm	81	5	7	<1	—	—	—	404	—	—
MAC & CHEESE LOAF, 1 sl, 32 gm	85	4	7	2	—	—	—	482	—	—
P & P LOAF, 1 sl, 32 gm	80	4	7	2	—	—	—	421	—	—
RED HOTS, 1 link, 76 gm	183	9	15	1	—	—	—	797	—	—
SMOKED SAUSAGE, 1 link, 2 oz, 57 gm	157	8	14	<1	—	—	—	584	—	—
ROPE STYLE, 4 oz, 113 gm	306	15	26	4	—	—	—	1142	—	—
SPICED LUNCHEON LOAF, 1 sl, 32 gm	83	5	7	<1	—	—	—	404	—	—
Hillshire Farm										
BEEF POLSKA KIELBASA, 1 oz, 28 gm	95	4	9	<1	—	2	.49	283	53	8
BEEF SMOKED SAUSGAGE, 1 oz, 28 gm	95	4	8	<1	—	2	.54	281	49	8
BRATWURST, FULLY COOKED, 1 oz, 28 gm	87	3	8	1	—	1	.29	195	43	8
CHEDDARWURST, 1 oz, 28 gm	98	4	9	<1	—	19	.29	259	60	9
ITALIAN SAUSAGE (before cooking)										
HOT, 1 oz, 28 gm	91	4	8	<1	—	1	.31	236	68	11
MILD, 1 oz, 28 gm	91	4	8	<1	—	1	.34	206	66	7
KNOCKWURST, 1 oz, 28 gm	93	3	8	1	—	2	.45	276	51	12
METTWURST, 1 oz, 28 gm	97	4	9	1	—	2	.6	272	63	7
OUR OLD FASHIONED BEEF FRANKS, 1 oz, 28 gm	89	3	8	1	—	2	.46	249	45	7
POLSKA KIELBASA, ENDLESS, 1 oz, 28 gm	96	4	9	1	—	2	.57	258	54	7
SMOKED SAUSAGE, ENDLESS, 1 oz, 28 gm	95	4	9	<1	—	1	.54	259	55	6
SMOKED SAUSAGE LINKS, 1 oz, 28 gm	96	4	9	1	—	1	.54	259	55	6
Hormel										
BEEF BOLOGNA, 2 sl	170	6	16	1	—	—	—	592	—	—
BEEF SALAMI, 2 sl	50	3	5	0	—	—	—	219	—	—
BEEFY SUMMER SAUSAGE, 1 oz, 28 gm	100	5	9	0	—	—	—	313	—	—
BOLOGNA COARSE GROUND										
BEEF, 2 oz, 57 gm	160	8	14	1	—	—	—	576	—	—
REGULAR, 2 oz, 57 gm	160	8	14	1	—	—	—	578	—	—
FINE GROUND, 2 oz, 57 gm	170	7	16	1	—	—	—	596	—	—
BRAUNSCHWEIGER (liverwurst), 1 oz, 28 gm	80	4	7	0	—	—	—	322	—	—
BREAST OF TURKEY, 2 sl	60	9	2	0	—	—	—	484	—	—
BROWN 'N SERVE SAUSAGE ckd, 2 sausages	140	6	13	0	—	—	—	430	—	—
uncooked, 2 sausages	180	7	17	0	—	—	—	411	—	—
CAPOCOLLO, 1 oz, 28 gm	80	5	6	0	—	—	—	273	—	—
CHICKEN LUNCHEON LOAF,										

FOOD & DESCRIPTION MEASURE OR QUANTITY	CALORIES	PROTEIN (GM)	FAT (GM)	CARBO- HYDRATE (GM)	FIBER (GM)	CALCIUM (MG)	IRON (MG)	SODIUM (MG)	POTASSIUM (MG)	CHOLES- TEROL (MG)
2 oz, 57 gm	130	7	10	0	—	—	—	608	—	—
CHICKEN SANDWICH MAKIN'S ½ oz, 14 gm	25	1	2	1	—	—	—	126	—	—
CHICKEN SPREAD, ½ oz, 14 gm	30	2	2	0	—	—	—	—	—	—
CHICKEN VIENNA SAUSAGE, 4 sausages	180	8	16	1	—	—	—	—	—	—
CHOPPED HAM, 8 lb can, 3 oz, 85 gm	240	12	21	1	—	—	—	1062	—	—
SLICED, 2 sl	88	11	5	0	—	—	—	685	—	—
CHOPPED PORK, 8 lb can, 3 oz, 85 gm	200	12	16	2	—	—	—	1073	—	—
CHUNK HAM, 6.75 oz, 191 gm	310	32	20	0	—	—	—	2241	—	—
CHUNK PEPPERONI, chub, 1 oz, 28 gm	140	6	12	0	—	—	—	423	—	—
CORNED BEEF SPREAD, ½ oz, 14 gm	35	2	3	0	—	—	—	—	—	—
CORN DOGS BATTER WRAPPED WIENERS, 1 wiener	220	7	12	21	—	—	—	656	—	—
COTTO SALAMI, 2 sl	105	9	7	1	—	—	—	750	—	—
chub, 1 oz, 28 gm	100	5	9	0	—	—	—	385	—	—
DEVILED HAM, 1 tbsp	35	2	3	0	—	—	—	108	—	—
DEVILED SPAM, luncheon meat, 1 tbsp	35	2	3	0	—	—	—	125	—	—
DI LUSSO GENOA SALAMI, 1 oz, 28 gm	100	6	8	0	—	—	—	443	—	—
DINTY MOORE CORNED BEEF, 2 oz, 57 gm	130	15	8	0	—	—	—	—	—	—
EXL DELI HAM, 4 oz, 112 gm	130	20	6	0	—	—	—	1368	—	—
FRANK 'N STUFF CHILI FRANKS, 1 frank	165	7	15	2	—	—	—	517	—	—
GENOA SALAMI, 1 oz, 28 gm	110	6	10	0	—	—	—	456	—	—
GRAN VALORE GENOA SALAMI, 1 oz, 28 gm	110	6	10	0	—	—	—	453	—	—
HAM & CHEESE LOAF, 3 oz, 85 gm	260	13	22	1	—	—	—	1135	—	—
SLICES, 2 sl	110	11	7	0	—	—	—	668	—	—
HARD SALAMI, PERMA-FRESH, 2 sl	80	4	7	0	—	—	—	339	—	—
HARD SALAMI, 1 oz, 28 gm	110	7	10	0	—	—	—	468	—	—
SLICED, 1 oz, 28 gm	110	6	10	0	—	—	—	483	—	—
HONEY LOAF, 2 sl	90	0	5	1	—	—	—	584	—	—
IOWA BRAND LOAF, 2 sl	90	10	6	0	—	—	—	607	—	—
JELLIED BEEF LOAF, 2 sl	90	14	4	0	—	—	—	900	—	—
KOLBASE POLISH SAUSAGE, 3 oz, 85 gm	220	12	19	1	—	—	—	904	—	—
LEONI BRAND PEPPERONI, 1 oz, 28 gm	130	6	12	0	—	—	—	508	—	—
LITTLE SIZZLERS PORK SAUSAGE, ckd, 2 sausages	103	6	9	0	—	—	—	172	—	—
LIVER LOAF, 2 sl	160	9	13	1	—	—	—	704	—	—
LIVERWURST SPREAD, ½ oz, 14 gm	35	2	3	0	—	—	—	—	—	—
LUMBERJACK BEEF ROLL, 2 oz, 28 gm	101	5	9	0	—	—	—	304	—	—
MEAT BOLOGNA, 2 sl	180	7	16	0	—	—	—	599	—	—
MEXICAL DOGS, 5 oz, 140 gm	400	14	21	41	—	—	—	952	—	—
MIDGET LINKS PORK SAUSAGE, ckd, 2 sausages	143	7	13	0	—	—	—	327	—	—
NATIONAL BRAND HARD										

FOOD & DESCRIPTION MEASURE OR QUANTITY	CALORIES	PROTEIN (GM)	FAT (GM)	CARBO-HYDRATE (GM)	FIBER (GM)	CALCIUM (MG)	IRON (MG)	SODIUM (MG)	POTASSIUM (MG)	CHOLES-TEROL (MG)
SALAMI, 1 oz, 28 gm	120	6	11	0	—	—	—	463	—	—
OLD SMOKEHOUSE, THURINGER, 1 oz, 28 gm	90	4	8	1	—	—	—	328	—	—
11 oz chub, 1 oz, 28 gm	100	5	9	0	—	—	—	332	—	—
SLICED, 1 oz, 28 gm	100	5	9	0	—	—	—	321	—	—
OLIVE LOAF, 2 sl	110	7	7	5	—	—	—	810	—	—
PARTY SALAMI, 1 oz, 28 gm	90	5	8	0	—	—	—	399	—	—
PEPPERONI, 1 oz, 28 gm	140	6	13	0	—	—	—	462	—	—
PERMA-FRESH, 2 sl	80	3	7	0	—	—	—	281	—	—
PICCOLO SALAMI, from 10 oz stick, 1 oz	120	6	11	0	—	—	—	512	—	—
PICKLE LOAF, 2 sl	102	8	7	3	—	—	—	752	—	—
POLISH SAUSAGE, 2 sausages	170	9	14	0	—	—	—	574	—	—
PORK LUNCHEON MEAT, 3 oz, 85 gm	240	11	21	2	—	—	—	1056	—	—
POTTED MEAT FOOD PRODUCT, 1 tbsp	30	2	2	0	—	—	—	145	—	—
PROSCIUTTO HAM, BONELESS, 1 oz, 28 gm	90	7	7	0	—	—	—	502	—	—
ROAST BEEF SPREAD, ½ oz, 14 gm	31	2	2	0	—	—	—	—	—	—
ROSA GRANDE PEPPERONI, 1 oz, 28 gm	140	6	13	0	—	—	—	512	—	—
ROSA PEPPERONI, 1 oz, 28 gm	140	6	13	0	—	—	—	626	—	—
SAN REMO BRAND GENOA SALAMI, 1 oz, 28 gm	118	7	10	0	—	—	—	544	—	—
SAUSAGE PATTIES, HOT, 1 patty	150	7	13	0	—	—	—	549	—	—
MILD, 1 patty	150	7	13	0	—	—	—	541	—	—
SKINLESS KIELBASA, POLISH SAUSAGE, ½ link	180	12	14	1	—	—	—	826	—	—
SLICED CANADIAN BACON, 1 oz, 28 gm	45	6	2	0	—	—	—	315	—	—
SMOKED BREAST OF TURKEY, 2 sl	60	10	2	0	—	—	—	540	—	—
SMOKED PORK SAUSAGE, 3 oz, 85 gm	290	12	27	1	—	—	—	—	—	—
SMOKIE CHEEZERS, 2 sausages	168	9	15	1	—	—	—	623	—	—
SMOKIES SMOKED SAUSAGE, 2 sausages	160	9	14	2	—	—	—	597	—	—
SPAM LUNCHEON MEAT, 2 oz, 57 gm	170	8	15	0	—	—	—	862	—	—
SMOKE FLAVORED LUNCHEON MEAT, 2 oz, 57 gm	170	8	15	0	—	—	—	774	—	—
SPAM WITH CHEESE CHUNKS, 2 oz, 57 gm	170	8	16	0	—	—	—	811	—	—
SPICED HAM, 3 oz, 85 gm	240	13	21	1	—	—	—	1093	—	—
SPICED LUNCHEON MEAT, 3 oz, 85 gm	280	11	26	2	—	—	—	1110	—	—
SLICED, 2 sl	118	9	9	1	—	—	—	702	—	—
SUMMER SAUSAGE, 2 sl	140	10	11	0	—	—	—	706	—	—
TANGY SUMMER SAUSAGE, chub, 1 oz, 28 gm	90	5	7	0	—	—	—	317	—	—
TATER DOGS BATTER WRAPPED WIENERS, 1 wiener	210	6	14	15	—	—	—	170	—	—
THURINGER SUMMER SAUSAGE, 1 oz, 28 gm	90	4	9	0	—	—	—	332	—	—
VIENNA SAUSAGE, no broth, 4 sausages	200	7	18	1	—	—	—	479	—	—

FOOD & DESCRIPTION MEASURE OR QUANTITY	CALORIES	PROTEIN (GM)	FAT (GM)	CARBO-HYDRATE (GM)	FIBER (GM)	CALCIUM (MG)	IRON (MG)	SODIUM (MG)	POTASSIUM (MG)	CHOLES-TEROL (MG)
VIKING CERVELAT, chub,										
1 oz, 28 gm	90	5	8	0	—	—	—	325	—	—
WEINER, BEEF,										
12 oz pkg, 1 weiner	100	4	10	1	—	—	—	362	—	—
1 lb pkg, 1 weiner	140	5	13	1	—	—	—	463	—	—
WEINER, MEAT,										
12 oz pkg, 1 weiner	110	4	10	1	—	—	—	378	—	—
1 lb pkg, 1 weiner	140	5	13	1	—	—	—	486	—	—
BEEF, 1 weiner	170	7	15	2	—	—	—	619	—	—
WRANGLERS										
SMOKED FRANK, RANGE										
BR., 1 frank	170	7	16	1	—	—	—	600	—	—
SMOKED FRANK WITH										
CHEESE, 1 frank	180	8	16	1	—	—	—	546	—	—

Kahn's

FOOD & DESCRIPTION MEASURE OR QUANTITY	CALORIES	PROTEIN (GM)	FAT (GM)	CARBO-HYDRATE (GM)	FIBER (GM)	CALCIUM (MG)	IRON (MG)	SODIUM (MG)	POTASSIUM (MG)	CHOLES-TEROL (MG)
BEEF BOLOGNA, 3.5 oz, 100										
gm	309	11	29	5	—	13	1.64	1090	111	—
BEEF, ENDLESS, 3.5 oz, 100										
gm	320	13	29	2	—	—	1.15	1070	150	51
BEEF FRANKS, 1 link, 1.5 oz,										
43 gm	148	5	14	2	—	5	.64	495	50	—
JUMBO, 2 oz, 57 gm	185	6	17	3	—	6	.79	619	63	—
BIG RED SMOKEY, 1 link, 2										
oz, 57 gm	175	7	16	2	—	6	.63	590	96	—
BRATWURST, 1 link, 2 oz, 57										
gm	180	6	17	2	—	22	.64	—	—	—
LAUDERDALE JUMBO, 2 oz,										
57 gm	178	6	16	3	—	7	.89	619	63	—
DELUXE JUMBO BOLOGNA,										
3.5 oz, 100 gm	308	11	29	3	—	35	1.24	1113	90	—
L'L REDS ROOKIE, 2 links, 2										
oz, 57 gm	171	7	15	2	—	6	.61	579	95	—
POLSKA KIELBASA, 100 gm	324	13	29	3	—	—	1.5	1050	170	57
WEINERS, 1 weiner, 1.5 oz,										
45 gm	150	5	14	2	—	3	.44	505	41	—
JUMBO, 1 weiner, 2 oz, 57										
gm	187	6	18	2	—	4	.55	631	51	—
LAUDERDALE JUMBO, 1										
weiner, 2 oz, 57 gm	184	6	17	2	—	6	.65	631	51	—

Land O'Frost

FOOD & DESCRIPTION MEASURE OR QUANTITY	CALORIES	PROTEIN (GM)	FAT (GM)	CARBO-HYDRATE (GM)	FIBER (GM)	CALCIUM (MG)	IRON (MG)	SODIUM (MG)	POTASSIUM (MG)	CHOLES-TEROL (MG)
BEEF, SMOKED, 1 oz, 28 gm	40	6	2	1	—	—	—	430	—	12
BEEF, SPICY, 1 oz, 28 gm	40	6	2	1	—	—	—	400	—	12
CHICKEN, SMOKED, 1 oz, 28										
gm	60	5	4	1	—	—	—	400	—	38
CORNED BEEF, 1 oz, 28 gm	40	6	2	1	—	—	—	370	—	12
HAM, 1 oz, 28 gm	50	5	3	1	—	—	—	430	—	16
PASTRAMI, 1 oz, 28 gm	40	6	2	1	—	—	—	370	—	12
REDI-EAT										
BEEF, SMOKED, 1 oz, 28 gm	50	5	3	1	—	—	—	430	—	12
CHICKEN, SMOKED, 1 oz, 28										
gm	60	5	4	1	—	—	—	400	—	38
HAM, SMOKED, 1 oz, 28 gm	60	5	5	1	—	—	—	430	—	17
TURKEY, SMOKED, 1 oz, 28										
gm	50	5	3	1	—	—	—	430	—	11
SMOKEY CANYON										
BEEF, 1 oz, 28 gm	40	6	2	1	—	—	—	430	—	12
CHICKEN, 1 oz, 28 gm	60	5	4	1	—	—	—	400	—	38
CORNED BEEF, 1 oz, 28 gm	40	6	2	1	—	—	—	370	—	12
HAM, 1 oz, 28 gm	50	5	3	1	—	—	—	430	—	16
PASTRAMI, 1 oz, 28 gm	40	6	2	1	—	—	—	370	—	12
TURKEY, 1 oz, 28 gm	50	5	3	1	—	—	—	430	—	11

FOOD & DESCRIPTION MEASURE OR QUANTITY	CALORIES	PROTEIN (GM)	FAT (GM)	CARBO-HYDRATE (GM)	FIBER (GM)	CALCIUM (MG)	IRON (MG)	SODIUM (MG)	POTASSIUM (MG)	CHOLES-TEROL (MG)
TURKEY, SMOKED, 1 oz, 28 gm	50	5	3	1	—	—	—	430	—	11
TURKEY HAM, 1 oz, 28 gm	35	5	2	0	—	—	—	400	—	11
TURKEY HAM, chub, 1 oz, 28 gm	36	5	2	1	—	—	—	340	—	11
Land O'Lakes										
TURKEY HAM, 3 oz, 85 gm	100	18	2	2	—	*	1.08	845	225	55
Libby										
CORNED BEEF, 2.3 oz, 65 gm	160	17	9	2	—	*	1.44	720	85	—
2.4 oz, 68 gm	160	17	9	2	—	*	1.44	750	90	—
DEVILED HAM, 1.5 oz, 43 gm	130	7	11	0	—	*	.36	—	—	—
POTTED MEAT, 1.83 oz, 52 gm	100	7	9	0	—	*	.72	320	70	—
VIENNA SAUSAGE IN BARBECUE SAUCE, 2.5 oz, 71 gm	180	8	15	2	—	20	1.08	—	—	—
IN BEEF BROTH, 3½ links, 57 gm	160	6	15	1	—	20	.72	330	40	—
Light & Lean—Hormel										
BBQ HAM, 2 sl	50	8	2	0	—	—	—	—	—	—
BLACK PEPPERED HAM, 2 sl	50	9	2	0	—	—	—	—	—	—
BOLOGNA, 2 sl	140	6	12	2	—	—	—	—	—	—
THIN SLICES, 2 sl	70	3	6	1	—	—	—	—	—	—
BREAST OF TURKEY, 2 sl	60	8	2	0	—	—	—	—	—	—
CANADIAN STYLE BACON, 2 sl	35	6	1	0	—	—	—	—	—	—
CHOPPED HAM, 2 sl	70	8	4	0	—	—	—	—	—	—
COOKED HAM, 2 sl	50	9	2	0	—	—	—	—	—	—
COTTO SALAMI, 2 sl	80	6	6	0	—	—	—	—	—	—
GLAZED HAM, 2 sl	50	9	2	0	—	—	—	—	—	—
HAM AND CHEESE LOAF, 2 sl	90	8	6	0	—	—	—	—	—	—
NEW ENGLAND BRAND LUNCHEON MEAT, 2 sl	90	10	6	0	—	—	—	—	—	—
PICKLE LOAF, 2 sl	100	8	6	3	—	—	—	—	—	—
RED PEPPERED HAM, 2 sl	50	9	2	0	—	—	—	—	—	—
SMOKED COOKED HAM, 2 sl	50	9	2	0	—	—	—	—	—	—
SPICED LUNCHEON MEAT, 2 sl	120	8	9	1	—	—	—	—	—	—
SUMMER SAUSAGE, 2 sl	100	6	8	0	—	—	—	—	—	—
Louis Rich										
TURKEY BOLOGNA, 1 sl, 28 gm	60	4	5	<1	—	32	.41	214	45	20
BREAKFAST SAUSAGES, ckd, 1 oz, 28 gm	65	6	4	0	—	5	.52	191	76	23
COTTO SALAMI, 1 sl, 28 gm	50	4	4	<1	—	5	.48	251	56	23
FRANK, 1 link, 45 gm	100	5	9	1	—	58	.71	454	89	39
HAM, thigh, 1 sl, 28 gm	35	5	1	<1	—	2	.35	262	70	17
CHOPPED, 1 sl, 28 gm	40	5	2	<1	—	2	.32	250	67	17
LUNCHEON LOAF, 1 sl, 28 gm	40	5	3	<1	—	2	.14	287	56	13
PASTRAMI, 1 sl, 28 gm	35	5	1	<1	—	2	.40	272	81	15
SMOKED SAUSAGE, 1 sl, 28 gm	55	5	4	<1	—	5	.41	219	59	19
SUMMER SAUSAGE, 1 sl, 28 gm	50	5	3	<1	—	4	.53	304	65	22
Morningstar Farms										
BREAKFAST										

FOOD & DESCRIPTION MEASURE OR QUANTITY	CALORIES	PROTEIN (GM)	FAT (GM)	CARBO-HYDRATE (GM)	FIBER (GM)	CALCIUM (MG)	IRON (MG)	SODIUM (MG)	POTASSIUM (MG)	CHOLES-TEROL (MG)
LINKS, 3 links, 68 gm	200	13	14	5	—	20	2.70	675	75	0
PATTIES, 2 patties, 76 gm	220	16	14	7	—	40	2.70	870	115	0
STRIPS, 3 strips, 25 gm	80	3	5	6	—	—	.36	330	25	0
GRILLERS, 1 patty, 64 gm	190	14	13	5	—	40	2.70	345	284	0

Oscar Mayer

FOOD & DESCRIPTION MEASURE OR QUANTITY	CALORIES	PROTEIN (GM)	FAT (GM)	CARBO-HYDRATE (GM)	FIBER (GM)	CALCIUM (MG)	IRON (MG)	SODIUM (MG)	POTASSIUM (MG)	CHOLES-TEROL (MG)
BACON, cooked, 1 sl, 6 gm	35	2	3	<1	—	0	.11	115	24	5
CENTER CUT, cooked, 1 sl, 4 gm	21	1	2	<1	—	0	.06	83	21	4
THICK SLICE, cooked, 1 sl, 11 gm	64	3	6	<1	—	1	.20	208	45	10
BACON & CHEDDAR CHEESE HOT DOG, 1 link, 45 gm	143	6	13	1	—	17	.42	515	85	30
BACON BITS, ¼ oz, 7 gm	21	3	1	<1	—	1	.14	181	38	6
BAR-B-Q LOAF, 1 oz, 28 gm	47	5	3	2	—	16	.34	353	93	13
BEEF BOLOGNA, 1 sl, 23 gm	74	3	7	<1	—	2	.31	253	38	12
BEEF COTTO SALAMI, 1 sl, 23 gm	45	4	3	<1	—	2	.63	274	47	15
BEEF FRANK, 1 link, 45 gm	144	5	13	1	—	6	.61	460	70	27
BEEF LEBANON BOLOGNA, 1 link, 45 gm	50	5	3	<1	—	3	.59	296	70	16
BEEF SALAMI FOR BEER, 1 sl, 23 gm	67	3	6	<1	—	2	.37	273	41	21
BEEF SMOKIES, 1 link, 43 gm	122	5	11	<1	—	4	.71	425	74	27
BEEF SUMMER SAUSAGES, THURINGER, CERVELAT, 1 sl, 23 gm	73	4	6	<1	—	2	.54	316	53	17
BOLOGNA, 1 sl, 23 gm	74	3	7	<1	—	2	.24	243	38	13
WITH CHEESE, 1 sl, 23 gm	74	3	7	<1	—	13	.28	242	40	14
BRAUNSCHWEIGER, LIVER SAUSAGE, sliced 1 sl, 28 gm	95	4	9	<1	—	2	2.63	321	56	50
TUBE, 1 oz, 28 gm	96	4	9	<1	—	2	2.68	319	50	41
CANADIAN BACON, 1 oz, 28 gm	35	6	1	<1	—	2	.19	391	83	12
CHEESE HOT DOGS, 1 link, 45 gm	145	6	13	1	—	28	.36	484	74	30
CHEESE SMOKIES, 1 link, 43 gm	127	6	11	<1	—	17	.48	448	80	28
CHOPPED HAM, sliced with natural juices, 1 oz, 28 gm	61	5	4	<1	—	2	.26	355	81	14
CHILI CON CARNE CONCENTRATE, 1 oz, 28 gm	78	4	6	3	—	6	.81	426	98	14
CRACKED BLACK PEPPER HAM, 1 sl, 21 gm	24	4	<1	<1	—	1	.23	269	61	11
CORNED BEEF, 1 sl, 21 gm	20	4	<1	0	—	1	.60	248	65	8
COTTO SALAMI, 1 sl, 23 gm	54	3	4	<1	—	1	.48	275	47	15
GARLIC BEEF BOLOGNA, 1 link, 45 gm	73	3	7	<1	—	3	.29	235	36	13
GENOA SALAMI, 1 sl, 9 gm	35	2	3	<1	—	2	.14	157	29	8
GERMAN BRAND BRAUNSCHWEIGER, 1 oz, 28 gm	94	4	8	<1	—	3	2.79	341	60	46
HAM AND CHEESE LOAF, 1 oz, 28 gm	76	5	6	<1	—	17	.24	351	75	17
HAM AND CHEESE SPREAD, 1 oz, 28 gm	66	5	5	<1	—	51	.18	329	47	16
HAM SALAD SPREAD, 1 oz, 28 gm	62	3	4	4	—	2	.17	265	39	11
HARD SALAMI, 1 sl, 9 gm	34	2	3	<1	—	1	.15	163	31	7
HEAD CHEESE, 1 oz, 28 gm	55	5	4	0	—	4	.38	338	9	21

FOOD & DESCRIPTION MEASURE OR QUANTITY	CALORIES	PROTEIN (GM)	FAT (GM)	CARBO-HYDRATE (GM)	FIBER (GM)	CALCIUM (MG)	IRON (MG)	SODIUM (MG)	POTASSIUM (MG)	CHOLES-TEROL (MG)
HONEY HAM, 1 sl, 21 gm	27	4	1	<1	—	1	.25	272	60	11
HONEY LOAF, 1 oz, 28 gm	35	5	1	1	—	6	.33	364	100	12
ITALIAN STYLE BEEF, 1 sl, 21 gm	22	4	<1	<1	—	2	.59	259	66	9
ITALIAN STYLE COOKED HAM, 1 sl, 21 gm	24	4	<1	<1	—	1	.28	264	58	9
JUBILEE HAM, BONELESS, 1 oz, 28 gm	47	5	3	<1	—	2	.25	375	91	15
CANNED, 1 oz, 28 gm	31	5	1	0	—	1	.27	283	88	13
SLICED, 1 oz, 28 gm	29	5	1	0	—	1	.33	349	77	13
STEAKS, 1 sl, 57 gm	59	10	2	<1	—	2	.67	711	157	27
LEAN 'N TASTY BEEF BREAKFAST STRIPS, heated, 1 strip, 12 gm	46	3	4	<1	—	1	.23	182	36	13
PORK BREAKFAST STRIPS, heated, 1 strip, 12 gm	52	3	5	<1	—	1	.15	196	43	14
LIVER CHEESE, pork fat–wrapped, 1 sl, 38 gm	116	6	10	<1	—	3	4.31	436	83	75
LITTLE FRIERS PORK SAUSAGE, ckd, 1 link, 20 gm	77	3	7	<1	—	5	.22	206	48	16
LITTLE SMOKIES SAUSAGE, 1 link, 9 gm	28	1	3	<1	—	1	.11	92	17	6
LITTLE WIENERS, 1 link, 9 gm	28	1	3	<1	—	1	.10	91	14	5
LUNCHEON MEAT, 1 oz, 28 gm	99	4	9	<1	—	3	.29	346	53	16
LUXURY LOAF, 1 sl, 28 gm	38	5	1	1	—	11	.32	302	105	13
NACHO STYLE CHEESE HOT DOGS, 1 link, 45 gm	138	5	13	1	—	23	.34	558	75	30
NEW ENGLAND BRAND SAUSAGE, 1 sl, 23 gm	31	4	2	<1	—	1	.28	292	69	13
OLD FASHIONED LOAF, 1 oz, 28 gm	64	4	4	3	—	28	.29	321	94	14
OLIVE LOAF, 1 oz, 28 gm	63	3	4	3	—	31	.17	375	80	10
PASTRAMI, 1 sl, 21 gm	21	4	<1	<1	—	1	.53	266	64	8
PEPPERED LOAF, 1 oz, 28 gm	43	5	2	1	—	13	.36	366	97	13
PICKLE AND PIMIENTO LOAF, 1 oz, 28 gm	64	4	4	3	—	35	.19	376	87	10
PICNIC LOAF, 1 oz, 28 gm	62	4	4	1	—	12	.31	315	73	12
SALAMI FOR BEER, 1 sl, 23 gm	55	3	5	<1	—	2	.25	264	50	15
SANDWICH SPREAD, 1 oz, 28 gm	67	2	5	4	—	3	.25	261	29	10
SMOKED CHICKEN BREAST, 1 oz, 28 gm	27	5	<1	<1	—	2	.19	385	75	11
SMOKED COOKED HAM, 1 sl, 21 gm	23	4	<1	<1	—	1	.19	265	65	10
SMOKED TURKEY BREAST, 1 sl, 21 gm	20	4	<1	<1	—	2	.15	294	68	7
SMOKIE LINKS SAUSAGE, 1 link, 43 gm	124	5	11	<1	—	3	.47	432	82	27
SUMMER SAUSAGE, THURINGER, CERVELAT, 1 sl, 23 gm	73	4	7	<1	—	2	.48	327	51	17
WIENERS, 1 link, 45 gm	144	5	13	1	—	5	.48	456	74	27

Purnell's "Old Folks"

DIETER'S DELIGHT WHOLE BEEF SAUSAGE, 2 patties, 85 gm	210	14	17	1	—	—	—	50	—	—

FOOD & DESCRIPTION MEASURE OR QUANTITY	CALORIES	PROTEIN (GM)	FAT (GM)	CARBO-HYDRATE (GM)	FIBER (GM)	CALCIUM (MG)	IRON (MG)	SODIUM (MG)	POTASSIUM (MG)	CHOLES-TEROL (MG)
Russer Foods										
LIL' SALT										
BOLOGNA, 1 oz, 28 gm	81	4	7	2	—	—	—	200	—	—
COOKED HAM, 1 oz, 28 gm	27	5	<1	<1	—	—	—	220	—	—
COOKED SALAMI, 1 oz, 28 gm	63	4	4	2	—	—	—	200	—	—
OLD FASHIONED LOAF, 1 oz, 28 gm	74	4	5	1	—	—	—	200	—	—
P & P LOAF, 1 oz, 28 gm	67	4	5	1	—	—	—	200	—	—
SMOKED HAM, 1 oz, 28 gm	27	5	<1	<1	—	—	—	—	—	—
Swanson–Campbell										
CHICKEN SPREAD, 1 oz, 28 gm	60	4	4	2	—	60	.36	140	—	—
USDA										
BARBECUE LOAF, PORK, BEEF, 1 oz, 28 gm	49	4	3	2	—	15	.33	378	93	11
BEERWURST, BEER SALAMI										
BEEF, 1 oz, 28 gm	92	3	8	<1	0	3	.39	264	52	16
PORK, 1 oz, 28 gm	67	4	5	<1	0	2	.22	352	72	17
BERLINER, PORK, BEEF, 1 oz, 28 gm	65	4	5	<1	0	3	.33	368	80	13
BLOOD SAUSAGE, 1 oz, 28 gm	107	4	10	<1	—	—	—	—	—	34
BOCKWURST, pork, veal, milk, eggs, raw, 1 oz, 28 gm	87	4	8	<1	—	—	—	—	—	—
BOLOGNA, BEEF, 1 oz, 28 gm	89	3	8	<1	0	3	.40	284	44	16
BEEF & PORK, 1 oz, 28 gm	89	3	8	<1	0	3	.43	289	51	16
PORK, 1 oz, 28 gm	70	4	6	<1	0	3	.22	336	80	17
TURKEY, 1 oz, 28 gm	57	4	4	<1	—	24	.43	249	56	28
BRATWURST, PORK, cooked, 1 oz, 28 gm	85	4	7	<1	—	13	.36	158	60	17
BRAUNSCHWEIGER (liver sausage), PORK, 1 oz, 28 gm	102	4	9	<1	0	2	2.65	324	57	44
BROTWURST, pork & beef, non-fat dry milk added, 1 oz, 28 gm	92	4	8	<1	—	14	.29	315	80	18
BREAKFAST STRIPS, cured, ckd										
from 15 slice per–12 oz pkg, 3 sl, 34 gm	156	10	12	<1	0	5	.67	714	158	36
from 12 oz raw, 6 oz, 170 gm	780	49	62	2	0	24	3.34	3568	791	179
CANADIAN BACON										
unheated, 2 sl, 2 oz, 57 gm	89	12	4	<1	0	5	.38	799	195	28
grilled, 2 sl, 57 gm raw, 47 gm	86	11	4	<1	0	5	.38	719	181	27
CHEESEFURTER, CHEESE SMOKIE, pork & beef, 1 oz, 28 gm	93	4	8	<1	—	16	.30	307	58	19
CHICKEN ROLL, light meat, 1 oz, 28 gm	45	6	2	<1	—	12	.27	166	65	14
CHICKEN SPREAD, cnd, 1 oz, 28 gm	55	4	3	2	—	35	.66	—	—	—
CORNED BEEF LOAF, JELLIED, 1 oz, 28 gm	46	7	2	0	—	3	.58	294	25	12
DUTCH BRAND LOAF, pork & beef, 1 oz, 28 gm	68	4	5	2	—	24	.35	354	107	13
FRANKFURTER										
BEEF, 8 per lb, 1 frank, 57 gm	184	6	17	1	0	7	.76	584	90	27

221

FOOD & DESCRIPTION MEASURE OR QUANTITY	CALORIES	PROTEIN (GM)	FAT (GM)	CARBO- HYDRATE (GM)	FIBER (GM)	CALCIUM (MG)	IRON (MG)	SODIUM (MG)	POTASSIUM (MG)	CHOLES- TEROL (MG)
10 per lb, 1 frank, 45 gm	145	5	13	1	0	6	.60	461	71	22
BEEF & PORK, 8 per lb, 1 frank, 57 gm	183	6	17	1	0	6	.66	639	95	29
10 per lb, 1 frank, 45 gm	144	5	13	1	0	5	.52	504	75	22
CHICKEN, 10 per lb, 1 frank, 45 gm	116	6	9	3	—	43	.90	617	—	45
TURKEY, 10 per lb, 1 frank, 45 gm	102	6	8	<1	—	48	.83	642	80	48
HAM										
chopped, cnd, cured, 1 oz, 28 gm	68	5	5	<1	0	2	.27	387	81	14
minced, cured, 1 oz, 28 gm	75	5	6	<1	0	3	.22	353	88	20
sliced										
extra lean, 5% fat, 1 oz, 28 gm	37	5	1	<1	0	2	.22	405	99	13
regular, 11% fat, 1 oz, 28 gm	52	5	3	<1	0	2	.28	373	94	16
HAM & CHEESE LOAF or ROLL, 1 oz, 28 gm	73	5	6	<1	—	16	.26	381	83	16
HAM & CHEESE SPREAD, 1 oz, 28 gm	69	5	5	<1	—	62	.22	339	46	17
HAM PATTIES, cured										
grilled, 1 patty, 59.5 gm	203	8	18	1	0	5	.96	632	145	43
1 oz, 28 gm	97	4	9	<1	0	3	.46	301	69	20
unheated										
1 patty, 65 gm	206	8	18	1	0	5	.69	709	156	46
1 oz, 28 gm	89	4	8	<1	0	2	.30	308	68	20
HAM SALAD SPREAD, 1 oz, 28 gm	61	2	4	3	—	2	.17	259	42	10
1 tbsp, 15 gm	32	1	2	2	—	1	.09	137	22	6
HEADCHEESE, PORK, 1 oz, 28 gm	60	5	4	<1	0	4	.33	356	9	23
HONEY LOAF, PORK, BEEF, 1 oz, 28 gm	36	4	1	2	—	5	.38	374	97	10
HONEY ROLL, SAUSAGE, BEEF, 1 oz, 28 gm	52	5	3	<1	0	3	.62	375	83	14
ITALIAN SAUSAGE, PORK										
ckd										
1 link, from 5 per lb raw, 67 gm	216	13	17	1	0	16	1.00	618	204	52
1 link, from 2 per lb raw, 83 gm	268	17	21	1	0	20	1.24	765	253	65
1 oz, 28 gm	92	6	7	<1	0	7	.43	261	86	22
raw										
1 link, 5 per lb, 91 gm	315	13	29	<1	0	16	1.07	665	230	69
1 link, 4 per lb, 113 gm	391	16	35	<1	0	20	1.33	826	286	86
1 oz, 28 gm	98	4	9	<1	0	5	.33	207	72	22
KIELBASA, KOLBASSY, pork, beef, non-fat milk added, 1 oz, 28 gm	88	4	8	<1	0	12	.41	305	77	19
KNACKWURST, KNOCKWURST, PORK, BEEF, 1 oz, 28 gm	87	3	8	<1	0	3	.26	286	57	16
LEBANON BOLOGNA, BEEF, 1 oz, 28 gm	64	6	4	<1	0	4	.67	359	87	19
LIVER CHEESE, PORK, 1 oz, 28 gm	86	4	7	<1	—	2	3.07	347	64	49
LIVER SAUSAGE, LIVERWURST, PORK, 1 oz, 28 gm	93	4	8	<1	—	7	1.81	—	—	45
LUNCHEON MEAT, BEEF LOAF, 1 oz, 28 gm	87	4	7	<1	0	3	.66	377	59	18
thin-sliced, 1 oz, 28 gm	35	6	<1	<1	0	—	.60	470	116	12
PORK & BEEF, 1 oz, 28 gm	100	4	9	<1	0	3	.24	367	57	15

FOOD & DESCRIPTION MEASURE OR QUANTITY	CALORIES	PROTEIN (GM)	FAT (GM)	CARBO-HYDRATE (GM)	FIBER (GM)	CALCIUM (MG)	IRON (MG)	SODIUM (MG)	POTASSIUM (MG)	CHOLES-TEROL (MG)
PORK, cnd, 1 oz, 28 gm	95	4	9	<1	0	2	.20	365	61	18
LUNCHEON SAUSAGE, PORK, BEEF, 1 oz, 28 gm	74	4	6	<1	0	4	.40	335	70	18
LUXURY LOAF, PORK, 1 oz, 28 gm	40	5	1	1	—	10	.30	347	107	10
MORTADELLA, BEEF, PORK, 1 oz, 28 gm	88	5	7	<1	—	5	.40	353	46	16
MOTHER'S LOAF, PORK, 1 oz, 28 gm	80	3	6	2	—	12	.38	320	64	13
NEW ENGLAND BRAND SAUSAGE, PORK, BEEF, 1 oz, 28 gm	46	5	2	1	0	2	.27	346	91	14
OLIVE LOAF, PORK, 1 oz, 28 gm	67	3	5	3	—	31	.15	421	84	11
PATE										
CHICKEN LIVER, cnd, 1 oz, 28 gm	57	4	4	2	—	3	2.60	—	—	—
1 tbsp, 13 gm	26	2	2	<1	—	1	1.19	—	—	—
GOOSE LIVER, smoked, cnd, 1 oz, 28 gm	131	3	12	1	0	—	—	—	—	43
1 tbsp, 13 gm	60	1	6	<1	0	—	—	—	—	20
PEPPERED LOAF, PORK, BEEF, 1 oz, 28 gm	42	5	2	1	—	15	.30	432	112	13
PEPPERONI, PORK, BEEF, 1 oz, 28 gm	141	6	12	<1	0	3	.40	578	98	—
PICKLE & PIMIENTO LOAF, PORK, 1 oz, 28 gm	74	3	6	2	—	27	.29	394	96	10
PICNIC LOAF, PORK, BEEF, 1 oz, 28 gm	66	4	5	1	—	13	.29	330	76	11
POLISH SAUSAGE, PORK, 1 oz, 28 gm	92	4	8	<1	0	3	.41	248	67	20
PORK & BEEF SAUSAGE, fresh ckd										
from approximately 8 per lb, 1 patty, 27 gm	107	4	10	<1	0	—	.31	217	—	—
from approximately 16 per lb, 1 link, 13 gm	52	2	5	<1	0	—	.15	105	—	—
PORK SAUSAGE, fresh, raw, 1 oz, 28 gm	118	3	11	<1	0	5	.26	228	58	19
ckd, from approximately 8 per lb										
1 patty, 27 gm	100	5	8	<1	0	9	.34	349	97	22
from approximately 16 per lb, 1 link, 13 gm	48	3	4	<1	0	4	.16	168	47	11
POULTRY SALAD SANDWICH SPREAD, 1 oz, 28 gm	57	3	4	2	—	3	.17	107	52	9
SALAMI										
BEEF, cooked, 2 oz, 28 gm	72	4	6	<1	0	2	.57	328	64	17
BEEF & PORK, 1 oz, 28 gm	71	4	6	<1	0	4	.76	302	56	18
TURKEY, 1 oz, 28 gm	56	5	4	<1	—	6	.46	285	69	23
DRY or HARD										
PORK, 1 oz, 28 gm	115	6	10	<1	0	4	.37	641	—	22
PORK & BEEF, 1 oz, 28 gm	119	6	10	<1	0	2	.43	527	107	22
SANDWICH SPREAD, PORK, BEEF, 1 oz, 28 gm	67	2	5	3	—	3	.22	287	31	11
SMOKED LINK SAUSAGE										
PORK										
1 link, 4 × 1⅛″, 68 gm	265	15	22	1	0	20	.79	1020	228	46
1 small link, 2 × ¾″, 16 gm	62	4	5	<1	0	5	.19	240	54	11
1 oz, 28 gm	110	6	9	<1	0	9	.33	425	95	19
PORK, BEEF										
1 link, 4 × 1⅛″, 68 gm	229	9	21	<1	0	7	.99	642	129	48
1 small link, 2 × ¾″, 16 gm	54	2	5	<1	0	2	.23	151	30	11
1 oz, 28 gm	95	4	9	<1	0	3	.41	268	54	20

FOOD & DESCRIPTION MEASURE OR QUANTITY	CALORIES	PROTEIN (GM)	FAT (GM)	CARBO-HYDRATE (GM)	FIBER (GM)	CALCIUM (MG)	IRON (MG)	SODIUM (MG)	POTASSIUM (MG)	CHOLES-TEROL (MG)
PORK, BEEF, with flour, non-fat milk										
1 link, 4 × 1⅛", 68 gm	182	10	15	3	—	12	1.05	741	105	59
1 small link, 2 × ¾", 16 gm	43	2	3	<1	—	3	.25	174	25	14
1 oz, 28 gm	76	4	6	1	—	5	.44	309	44	25
PORK, BEEF, with non-fat milk										
1 link, 4 × 1⅛", 68 gm	213	9	19	1	0	28	1.00	798	194	44
1 small link, 2 × ¾", 16 gm	50	2	4	<1	0	6	.23	188	46	10
1 oz, 28 gm	89	4	8	<1	0	12	.42	333	81	18
THURINGER, CERVELAT, SUMMER SAUSAGES, BEEF, PORK										
1 oz, 28 gm	98	5	8	<1	0	2	.58	412	65	19
TURKEY BOLOGNA, 1 oz, 28 gm	57	4	4	<1	—	24	.43	249	56	28
TURKEY BREAST MEAT, TURKEY LOAF, salt added, 1 oz, 28 gm	31	6	<1	0	0	2	.11	406	79	12
TURKEY HAM, cured turkey thigh meat, 1 oz, 28 gm	36	5	1	<1	—	3	.78	282	92	—
TURKEY PASTRAMI, 1 oz, 28 gm	40	5	2	<1	—	3	.47	296	74	—
TURKEY ROLL										
light and dark meat, 1 oz, 28 gm	42	5	2	<1	—	9	.38	166	77	16
light meat, 1 oz, 28 gm	42	5	2	<1	—	11	.36	139	71	12
TURKEY SALAMI, 1 oz, 28 gm	56	5	4	<1	—	6	.46	285	69	23
VIENNA SAUSAGE, cnd, beef, pork										
1 sausage, 1 oz, 28 gm	79	3	7	<1	0	3	.25	270	29	15
1 sausage, 16 gm	45	2	4	<1	0	2	.14	152	16	8

Veal

Hormel

BREADED VEAL STEAK, 4 oz	240	17	13	13	—	—	—	—	—	—
VEAL STEAK, 4 oz	130	22	4	2	—	—	—	—	—	—

USDA

BRAIN, CALF, raw, 3.5 oz, 100 gm	125	10	9	<1	0	10	2.40	125	219	2000
CHUCK CUTS & BONELESS FOR STEW										
braised, pot roasted, stewed										
yield from 1 lb with bone, 8.4 oz, 240 gm	564	67	31	0	0	29	8.40	117	536	242
yield from 1 lb without bone, 10.6 oz, 299 gm	703	83	38	0	0	36	10.50	146	667	302
1 c chopped or diced, not packed, 140 gm	329	39	18	0	0	17	4.90	68	313	141
3 oz, 85 gm	200	24	11	0	0	10	3.00	41	190	86
LIVER, CALF										
raw, 3.5 oz, 100 gm	140	19	5	4	0	8	8.80	73	281	300
fried, 3.5 oz, 100 gm	261	30	13	4	0	13	14.20	118	453	438
LOIN, braised or broiled										
yield from 1 lb with bone, 9.53 oz, 269 gm	629	71	36	0	0	30	8.60	174	795	272
yield from 1 lb without bone, 11.4 oz, 324 gm	758	86	43	0	0	36	10.40	209	958	327
1 c chopped or diced, not packed, 140 gm	328	37	19	0	0	15	4.50	91	414	141

FOOD & DESCRIPTION MEASURE OR QUANTITY	CALORIES	PROTEIN (GM)	FAT (GM)	CARBO-HYDRATE (GM)	FIBER (GM)	CALCIUM (MG)	IRON (MG)	SODIUM (MG)	POTASSIUM (MG)	CHOLES-TEROL (MG)
3 oz, 85 gm	199	22	11	0	0	9	2.72	55	251	86
LUNGS, CALF, raw, 3.5 oz, 100 gm	106	17	4	0	0	5	4.00	86	193	150
PANCREAS, raw, 3.5 oz, 100 gm	161	19	9	0	0	8	2.80	67	276	250
PLATE, BREAST OF VEAL BRAISED OR STEWED										
yield from 1 lb with bone, 8.3 oz, 237 gm	718	62	50	0	0	28	7.80	108	495	239
yield from 1 lb without bone, 10.6 oz, 299 gm	906	78	63	0	0	36	9.90	137	624	302
3 oz, 85 gm	258	22	18	0	0	10	2.81	39	178	86
RIB ROAST										
yield from 1 lb with bone, 8.5 oz, 241 gm	648	66	41	0	0	29	8.20	161	735	243
yield from 1 lb without bone, 11 oz, 313 gm	842	85	53	0	0	38	10.60	208	953	316
1 c chopped or diced, 140 gm	377	38	24	0	0	17	4.80	93	427	141
1 c ground, 110 gm	296	30	19	0	0	13	3.70	73	335	111
3 oz, 85 gm	229	23	14	0	0	10	2.90	57	259	86
ROUND WITH RUMP (ROASTS AND LEG CUTLETS)										
braised or broiled										
yield from 1 lb with bone, 8.7 oz, 247 gm	534	67	27	0	0	27	7.90	164	749	249
yield from 1 lb without bone, 11.3 oz, 321 gm	693	87	36	0	0	35	10.30	213	974	324
1 c chopped or diced, not packed, 140 gm	302	38	16	0	0	15	4.50	93	424	141
3 oz, 85 gm	184	23	9	0	0	9	2.70	56	258	86
SWEETBREAD, THYMUS, CALF										
braised, 3.5 oz, 100 gm	168	33	3	0	0	10	1.60	116	433	466
raw, 3.5 oz, 100 gm	94	18	2	0	0	10	1.60	96	360	250

15

NUTS AND SEEDS

FOOD & DESCRIPTION MEASURE OR QUANTITY	CALORIES	PROTEIN (GM)	FAT (GM)	CARBO-HYDRATE (GM)	FIBER (GM)	CALCIUM (MG)	IRON (MG)	SODIUM (MG)	POTASSIUM (MG)	CHOLES-TEROL (MG)
Arrowhead Mills										
FLAX SEED, 1 oz, 28 gm	140	5	10	11	—	—	—	1	—	—
PEANUT BUTTER										
CREAMY, 2 tbsp	190	9	16	6	—	—	—	2	—	—
CRUNCHY, 2 tbsp	190	9	16	6	—	—	—	2	—	—
PEANUTS, 2 oz, 56 gm	320	15	27	11	—	—	—	3	—	—
SESAME SEEDS, 1 oz, 28 gm	160	5	14	6	—	—	—	15	—	—
SUNFLOWER SEEDS, 1 oz, 28 gm	160	7	13	6	—	—	—	9	—	—
Bama–Borden										
PEANUT BUTTER										
CREAMY, 2 tbsp	200	8	16	7	—	*	.36	160	190	—
CRUNCHY, 2 tbsp	200	8	16	6	—	20	.36	135	215	—
Blue Diamond										
ALMONDS										
BARBEQUE, 1 oz, 28 gm	150	7	15	6	—	100	1.08	170	125	—
BLANCHED, SLICED, 1 oz, 28 gm	150	7	13	5	—	80	1.08	5	205	—
BLANCHED, WHOLE, 1 oz, 28 gm	150	7	13	5	—	80	1.08	5	175	—
CHEESE, 1 oz, 28 gm	140	7	12	8	—	100	1.08	90	110	—
DRY ROASTED, UNSALTED, 1 oz, 28 gm	150	7	14	5	—	100	1.44	5	215	—
HICKORY SMOKE, DRY ROASTED, 1 oz, 28 gm	150	7	13	5	—	100	1.44	120	195	—
ONION GARLIC, 1 oz, 28 gm	140	7	13	7	—	100	1.08	155	135	—
ROASTED, SALTED, 1 oz, 28 gm	150	7	15	4	—	80	.72	110	90	—
BLANCHED, 1 oz, 28 gm	150	7	14	4	—	60	.72	80	180	—
SLICED, 1 oz, 28 gm	150	7	13	5	—	80	1.08	5	195	—
SMOKEHOUSE, 1 oz, 28 gm	150	7	14	5	—	60	1.08	115	100	—
WHOLE, 1 oz, 28 gm	150	7	13	5	—	80	1.44	5	220	—
HAZELNUTS										
ROASTED, SALTED, Oregon, 1 oz, 28 gm	160	5	16	4	—	60	1.08	115	160	—
SLICED, Oregon, 1 oz, 28 gm	140	6	14	6	—	40	1.08	5	225	—
WHOLE, Oregon, 1 oz, 28 gm	150	5	14	5	—	40	1.08	5	150	—
MACADAMIA NUTS, DRY ROASTED, Hawaiian, 1 oz, 28 gm	170	2	19	4	—	20	.36	115	90	—
PISTACHIOS, DRY ROASTED, California, 1 oz, 28 gm	140	7	13	6	—	40	1.08	160	270	—

FOOD & DESCRIPTION MEASURE OR QUANTITY	CALORIES	PROTEIN (GM)	FAT (GM)	CARBO- HYDRATE (GM)	FIBER (GM)	CALCIUM (MG)	IRON (MG)	SODIUM (MG)	POTASSIUM (MG)	CHOLES- TEROL (MG)
RED PISTACHIOS, DRY										
ROASTED, California, 1 oz, 28 gm	130	6	12	7	—	40	108	230	235	—
Dia-Mel										
PEANUT BUTTER, 2 tbsp	200	8	17	5	—	—	—	2	—	0
Featherweight										
PEANUT BUTTER, ls, 1 oz, 28 gm	180	8	15	4			—	<3	191	—
Hammons Products										
BLACK WALNUTS, 1 oz, 28 gm	180	8	15	3	—	20	1.44	—	—	0
Jif—Procter & Gamble										
PEANUT BUTTER										
CREAMY, 2 tbsp	190	9	16	6	—	*	.36	155	—	0
CRUNCHY, 2 tbsp	190	9	16	6	—	*	.36	130	—	0
Planters—Nabisco										
ALMONDS										
BLANCHED, WHOLE, SLICED, 1 oz, 28 gm	170	6	15	6	—	60	1.08	0	225	0
DRY ROASTED, 1 oz, 28 gm	170	6	15	6	—	80	1.08	200	200	0
SMOKED, 1 oz, 28 gm	170	5	15	6	—	60	1.08	160	200	0
CASHEWS										
DRY ROASTED										
SALT FREE, 1 oz, 28 gm	160	5	13	9	—	*	1.08	0	190	0
SALTED, 1 oz, 28 gm	160	5	13	9	—	*	1.08	230	190	0
HONEY ROAST, 1 oz, 28 gm,	170	4	12	11	—	*	1.44	170	135	0
OIL ROASTED, halves										
SALT FREE, 1 oz, 28 gm	170	5	14	8	—	*	1.08	0	170	0
SALTED, 1 oz, 28 gm	170	5	14	8	—	*	1.08	135	170	0
CASHEWS & PEANUTS, HONEY ROAST, 1 oz, 28 gm	170	5	12	9	—	*	1.08	170	150	0
MIXED NUTS										
DRY ROASTED										
SALT FREE, 1 oz, 28 gm	170	6	15	7	—	20	1.08	0	160	0
SALTED, 1 oz, 28 gm	160	5	14	7	—	20	1.08	270	140	0
OIL ROASTED										
DELUXE, 1 oz, 28 gm	180	4	17	6	—	20	1.08	135	180	0
SALT FREE, 1 oz, 28 gm	180	5	16	6	—	20	.72	0	130	0
SALTED, 1 oz, 28 gm	180	5	16	6	—	20	.72	130	130	0
PEANUTS										
COCKTAIL										
OIL ROASTED										
SALT FREE, 1 oz, 28 gm	170	7	15	5	—	*	.36	0	90	0
SALTED, 1 oz, 28 gm	170	7	15	5	—	*	.36	160	90	0
DRY ROASTED										
Lite, ⅔ oz, 19 gm	90	6	6	5	—	*	.36	180	160	0
SALT FREE, 1 oz, 28 gm	170	7	15	5	—	*	.36	0	190	0
SALTED, 1 oz, 28 gm	160	7	14	6	—	*	.36	250	200	0
HONEY ROASTED, 1 oz, 28 gm	170	6	13	8	—	*	.36	180	160	0
OIL ROASTED, SALTED, 1 oz, 28 gm	170	7	15	5	—	*	.36	160	200	0
REDSKIN, oil roasted, 1 oz, 28 gm	170	7	15	5	—	*	.36	150	190	0
ROASTED-IN-SHELL										

FOOD & DESCRIPTION MEASURE OR QUANTITY	CALORIES	PROTEIN (GM)	FAT (GM)	CARBO-HYDRATE (GM)	FIBER (GM)	CALCIUM (MG)	IRON (MG)	SODIUM (MG)	POTASSIUM (MG)	CHOLES-TEROL (MG)
SALT FREE, 1 oz, 28 gm	160	7	14	6	—	20	.72	0	190	0
SALTED, 1 oz, 28 gm	160	7	14	6	—	20	.72	160	190	0
SPANISH										
DRY ROASTED, 1 oz, 28 gm	160	7	14	6	—	*	.72	200	190	0
OIL ROASTED, 1 oz, 28 gm	170	7	15	5	—	*	.36	150	190	0
RAW, 1 oz, 28 gm	150	7	12	7	—	*	.72	0	190	0
SWEET 'N CRUNCHY, 1 oz, 28 gm	140	4	8	15	—	20	.36	20	105	0
TAVERN NUTS, 1 oz, 28 gm	170	7	15	6	—	*	.36	65	190	0
PECANS, chips, halves, pieces, 1 oz, 28 gm	190	2	20	5	—	20	.36	0	170	0
PISTACHIOS										
DRY ROASTED, 1 oz, 28 gm	170	5	15	6	—	20	1.08	250	280	0
RED, 1 oz, 28 gm	170	5	15	6	—	20	1.08	250	280	0
SALTED, 1 oz, 28 gm	170	5	15	6	—	20	1.08	250	280	0
SESAME NUT MIX										
DRY ROASTED, 1 oz, 28 gm	160	5	12	8	—	*	.36	330	140	0
OIL ROASTED, 1 oz, 28 gm	160	5	13	8	—	20	.72	220	110	0
SUNFLOWER NUTS										
DRY ROASTED										
SALT FREE, 1 oz, 28 gm	170	7	15	5	—	20	1.08	0	240	0
SALTED, 1 oz, 28 gm	160	7	14	5	—	20	1.08	260	240	0
OIL ROASTED, 1 oz, 28 gm	170	6	15	5	—	20	.72	190	190	0
SUNFLOWER SEEDS, 1 oz, 28 gm	160	7	14	5	—	20	1.08	30	200	0
WALNUTS										
BLACK, 1 oz, 28 gm	180	7	17	3	—	20	.72	0	160	0
ENGLISH, whole, halves or pieces, 1 oz, 28 gm	190	4	20	3	—	20	.72	0	115	0

Sahadi–Lipton

SESAME TAHINI, 2 tbsp, 1 oz	190	6	17	4	—	20	1.44	75	—	—

Skippy–Best Foods

PEANUT BUTTER										
CREAMY, 1 tbsp, 16 gm	95	5	8	2	.3	5	.30	75	105	0
CRUNCHY, 1 tbsp, 16 gm	95	5	8	2	.3	5	.30	65	100	0

Smucker's

GOOBER GRAPE PEANUT BUTTER, 1 tbsp	180	5	10	18	—	0	.36	120	—	0
PEANUT BUTTER										
NATURAL, 2 tbsp, 32 gm	200	8	16	6	—	0	.72	125	—	0
NO SALT, 2 tbsp, 32 gm	200	8	17	6	—	0	.72	0	—	0

USDA

NUTS										
ACORNS										
dried, 1 oz, 28 gm	145	2	9	15	.96	15	.30	0	201	0
flour, 1 oz, 28 gm	142	2	9	16	.80	12	.34	—	202	0
raw, 1 oz, 28 gm,	105	2	7	12	.73	12	.22	0	153	0
ALMONDS										
dried, unblanched, 1 oz, 28 gm	167	6	15	6	1.34d	75	1.04	3	208	0
chopped, 1 c, 130 gm	766	26	68	27	6.14d	346	4.76	14	952	0
sliced or diced, 1 c, 94 gm	554	19	49	19	4.44d	250	3.44	10	688	0
slivered, 1 c, 135 gm	795	27	70	28	6.37d	359	4.94	15	988	0
whole kernel, 1 c, 142 gm	837	28	74	29	6.70d	377	5.19	15	1039	0
dried, blanched, 1 oz, 28 gm	166	6	15	5	.65	70	1.03	3	213	0
whole kernel, 1 c, 145 gm	850	30	76	27	3.32	358	5.26	15	1088	0
dry-roasted, unblanched salt-free, 1 oz, 28 gm	167	5	15	7	1.40	80	1.08	3	219	0

FOOD & DESCRIPTION MEASURE OR QUANTITY	CALORIES	PROTEIN (GM)	FAT (GM)	CARBO-HYDRATE (GM)	FIBER (GM)	CALCIUM (MG)	IRON (MG)	SODIUM (MG)	POTASSIUM (MG)	CHOLES-TEROL (MG)
1 c, 138 gm	810	23	71	33	6.81	389	5.25	15	1063	0
salted, 1 oz, 28 gm	167	5	15	7	1.40	80	1.08	222	219	0
1 c, 138 gm	810	23	71	33	6.81	389	5.25	1076	1063	0
oil-roasted, blanched										
salt-free, 1 oz, 28 gm	174	5	16	5	.89	55	1.51	3	197	0
1 c, 142 gm	870	27	80	26	4.43	276	7.53	17	984	0
salted, 1 oz, 28 gm	174	5	16	5	.89	55	1.51	220	197	0
1 c, 142 gm	870	27	80	26	4.43	276	7.53	1102	984	0
oil-roasted, unblanched										
salt-free, 1 oz, 28 gm	176	6	16	5	1.40	66	1.09	3	194	0
1 c, 157 gm	970	32	91	25	7.74	367	6.02	16	1073	0
salted, 1 oz, 28 gm	176	6	16	5	1.40	66	1.09	221	194	0
1 c, 157 gm	970	32	91	25	7.74	367	6.02	1223	1073	0
toasted, unblanched, 1 oz, 28 gm	167	6	14	7	1.41	80	1.4	3	220	0
ALMOND BUTTER										
salt-free, 1 tbsp, 16 gm	101	2	9	3	.24	43	.59	2	121	0
salted, 1 tbsp, 16 gm	101	2	9	3	.24	43	.59	72	121	0
with honey & cinnamon										
salt-free, 1 tbsp, 16 gm	96	3	8	4	.24	43	.59	2	120	0
salted, 1 tbsp, 16 gm	96	3	8	4	.24	43	.59	27	120	0
ALMOND MEAL, partially defatted										
salt-free, 1 oz, 28 gm	116	11	5	8	.65	120	2.41	2	398	0
salted, 1 oz, 28 gm	116	11	5	8	.65	120	2.41	211	398	0
ALMOND PASTE										
1 oz, 28 gm	127	3	8	12	1.70	65	.90	3	184	0
firmly packed, 1 c, 227 gm	1012	27	62	99	13.62	523	7.16	21	1468	0
ALMOND POWDER										
full fat, 1 oz, 28 gm	168	6	15	6	.54	62	.80	2	201	0
not packed, 1 c, 65 gm	385	13	34	15	1.24	142	1.82	4	461	0
partially defatted, 1 oz, 28 gm	112	11	5	9	.80	67	.99	3	204	0
not packed, 1 c, 65 gm	255	24	10	21	1.82	154	2.26	6	467	0
BEECHNUTS, dried, 1 oz, 28 gm	164	2	14	10	1.05	0	—	—	—	0
BRAZIL NUTS, dried, unblanched, 1 oz, 28 gm	186	4	19	4	.65	50	.97	0	170	0
1 c, 140 gm	919	20	93	18	3.20	246	4.76	2	840	0
BUTTERNUTS, dried, 1 oz, 28 gm	174	7	16	3	.53	15	1.14	0	119	0
CASHEWS										
dry-roasted										
salt-free, 1 oz, 28 gm	163	4	13	9	.20	13	1.70	4	160	0
1 c, 137 gm	787	21	64	45	.96	62	8.22	21	774	0
salted, 1 oz, 28 gm	163	4	13	9	.20	13	1.70	181	160	0
1 c, 137 gm	787	21	64	45	.96	62	8.22	877	774	0
oil-roasted										
salt-free, 1 oz, 28 gm	163	5	14	8	.36	12	1.16	5	151	0
1 c, 130 gm	748	21	63	37	1.65	53	5.33	22	689	0
salted, 1 oz, 28 gm	163	5	14	8	.36	12	1.16	177	151	0
1 c, 130 gm	748	21	63	37	1.65	53	5.33	814	689	0
CASHEW BUTTER										
salt-free, 1 oz, 28 gm	167	5	14	8	.22	12	1.43	4	155	0
1 tbsp, 16 gm	94	3	8	4	.12	7	.80	2	87	0
salted, 1 oz, 28 gm	167	5	14	8	.22	12	1.43	174	155	0
1 tbsp, 16 gm	94	3	8	4	.12	7	.80	98	87	0
CHESTNUTS, CHINESE										
boiled, steamed, 1 oz, 28 gm	44	<1	<1	10	.32	3	.27	1	87	0
dried, 1 oz, 28 gm	103	2	<1	23	.76	8	.65	2	206	0
raw, 1 oz, 28 gm	64	1	<1	14	.47	5	.40	1	127	0
roasted, 1 oz, 28 gm	68	1	<1	15	.50	5	.43	1	135	0
CHESTNUTS, EUROPEAN										
boiled, steamed, 1 oz, 28 gm	37	<1	<1	8	.20	13	.49	8	203	0

FOOD & DESCRIPTION MEASURE OR QUANTITY	CALORIES	PROTEIN (GM)	FAT (GM)	CARBO-HYDRATE (GM)	FIBER (GM)	CALCIUM (MG)	IRON (MG)	SODIUM (MG)	POTASSIUM (MG)	CHOLES-TEROL (MG)
dried										
peeled, 1 oz, 28 gm	105	1	1	22	1.42	18	.68	11	281	0
with peel, 1 oz, 28 gm	106	2	1	22	1.55	19	.68	11	280	0
raw										
peeled, 1 oz, 28 gm	56	<1	<1	13	.27	5	.27	1	137	0
with peel, 1 oz, 28 gm	60	<1	<1	13	2.82d	8	.29	1	147	0
1 c, 145 gm	308	4	3	66	14.40d	40	1.46	4	751	0
roasted, 1 oz, 28 gm	70	<1	<1	15	3.32d	8	.26	1	168	0
1 c, 143 gm	350	5	3	76	16.73d	42	1.30	3	846	0
CHESTNUTS, JAPANESE										
boiled, steamed, 1 oz, 28 gm	16	<1	<1	4	.10	3	.15	1	34	0
dried, 1 oz, 28 gm	102	1	<1	23	.64	20	.96	10	218	0
1 c, 155 gm	558	8	2	126	3.51	111	5.24	52	1191	0
raw, 1 oz, 28 gm	44	<1	<1	10	.28	9	.41	4	94	0
roasted, 1 oz, 28 gm	57	<1	<1	13	.31	10	.60	—	—	0
COCONUT										
dried, creamed, 1 oz, 28 gm	194	2	20	6	1.12	7	.95	11	156	0
dried, sweetened										
cnd, flaked, 1 oz, 28 gm	126	<1	9	12	.61	4	.53	6	92	0
1 c, 77 gm	341	3	24	32	1.65	11	1.42	15	249	0
packaged, flaked, 1 oz, 28 gm	135	<1	9	14	.60	4	.51	73	90	0
1 c, 74 gm	351	2	24	35	1.55	10	1.33	189	234	0
shredded, 1 oz, 28 gm	142	<1	10	14	.62	4	.54	75	96	0
1 c, 93 gm	466	3	33	44	2.02	14	1.78	244	313	0
dried, toasted, 1 oz, 28 gm	168	2	13	13	.68	8	.96	11	157	0
dried, unsw, 1 oz, 28 gm	187	2	18	7	1.51	7	.94	11	154	0
raw, 1 piece 2 × 2 × ½″, 45 gm	159	2	15	7	1.92	6	1.09	9	160	0
shredded, grated, not packed, 1 c, 80 gm	283	3	27	12	3.41	12	1.94	16	285	0
COCONUT CREAM, sweetened										
cnd, 1 tbsp, 19 gm	36	<1	3	2	—	0	.10	10	19	0
1 c, 296 gm	568	8	52	25	—	4	1.50	149	299	0
raw, 1 tbsp, 15 gm	49	<1	5	1	—	2	.34	1	49	0
1 c, 240 gm	792	9	83	16	—	26	5.47	10	781	0
COCONUT MILK										
cnd, 1 tbsp, 15 gm	30	<1	3	<1	—	3	.50	2	33	0
1 c, 226 gm	445	5	48	6	—	40	7.46	29	497	0
fz, 1 tbsp, 15 gm	30	<1	3	<1	—	1	.12	2	35	0
1 c, 240 gm	486	4	50	13	—	11	1.94	29	556	0
raw, 1 tbsp, 15 gm	35	<1	4	<1	—	2	.25	2	39	0
1 c, 240 gm	552	6	57	13	—	39	3.94	37	630	0
COCONUT WATER										
1 tbsp, 15 gm	3	<1	<1	<1	0	4	.04	16	38	0
1 c, 240 gm	46	2	<1	9	.05	58	.69	252	600	0
FILBERTS/HAZELNUTS										
dried, blanched, 1 oz, 28 gm	191	4	19	5	.51	55	.96	1	131	0
dried, unblanched, 1 oz, 28 gm	179	4	18	4	1.08	53	.93	1	126	0
chopped, 1 c, 115 gm	727	15	72	18	4.37	216	3.76	3	512	0
ground, 1 c, 75 gm	474	10	47	11	2.85	141	2.45	2	334	0
whole, 1 c, 135 gm	853	18	85	21	5.13	254	4.41	4	601	0
dry-roasted, unblanched										
salt-free, 1 oz, 28 gm	188	3	19	5	1.12	55	.96	1	131	0
salted, 1 oz, 28 gm	188	3	19	5	1.12	55	.96	221	131	0
oil-roasted, unblanched										
salt-free, 1 oz, 28 gm	187	4	18	5	.71	56	.97	1	132	0
salted, 1 oz, 28 gm	187	4	18	5	.71	56	.97	223	132	0
GINKGO NUTS										
cnd, 1 oz, 28 gm	32	<1	<1	6	.46	1	.08	87	51	0
1 c, 155 gm	173	4	3	34	2.51	6	.45	476	278	0
dried, 1 oz, 28 gm	99	3	<1	21	.28	6	.45	4	283	0
raw, 1 oz, 28 gm	52	1	<1	11	.14	1	.28	2	145	0

FOOD & DESCRIPTION MEASURE OR QUANTITY	CALORIES	PROTEIN (GM)	FAT (GM)	CARBO-HYDRATE (GM)	FIBER (GM)	CALCIUM (MG)	IRON (MG)	SODIUM (MG)	POTASSIUM (MG)	CHOLES-TEROL (MG)
HICKORY NUTS, dried, 1 oz, 28 gm	187	4	18	5	.92	17	.60	0	124	0
MACADAMIA NUTS										
dried, 1 oz, 28 gm	199	2	21	4	1.50	20	.68	1	104	0
1 c, 134 gm	940	11	99	18	7.08	94	3.23	6	493	0
oil-roasted										
salt-free, 1 oz, 28 gm	204	2	22	4	.49	13	.51	2	94	0
whole or halves, 1 c, 134 gm	962	10	103	17	2.32	60	2.41	9	441	0
salted, 1 oz, 28 gm	204	2	22	4	.49	13	.51	74	94	0
whole or halves, 1 c, 134 gm	962	10	103	17	2.32	60	2.41	348	441	0
MIXED NUTS (WITHOUT PEANUTS)										
oil-roasted										
salt-free, 1 oz, 28 gm	175	4	16	6	.63	30	.73	3	154	0
1 c, 144 gm	886	22	81	32	3.18	153	3.70	16	783	0
salted, 1 oz, 28 gm	175	4	16	6	.63	30	.73	198	154	0
1 c, 144 gm	886	22	81	32	3.18	153	3.70	1008	783	0
MIXED NUTS (WITH PEANUTS)										
dry-roasted										
salt-free, 1 oz, 28 gm	169	5	15	7	.26	20	1.05	3	169	0
1 c, 137 gm	814	24	70	35	1.23	96	5.07	16	817	0
salted, 1 oz, 28 gm	169	5	15	7	.26	20	1.05	190	169	0
1 c, 137 gm	814	24	70	35	1.23	96	5.07	917	817	0
oil-roasted										
salt-free, 1 oz, 28 gm	175	5	16	6	.61	31	.91	3	165	0
1 c, 142 gm	876	24	80	30	3.06	153	4.56	16	825	0
salted, 1 oz, 28 gm	175	5	16	6	.61	31	.91	185	165	0
1 c, 142 gm	876	24	80	30	3.06	153	4.56	926	825	0
NUTS, ARTIFICIAL, wheat-based										
macadamia flavor, 1 oz, 28 gm	176	3	16	8	.17	6	.57	13	74	0
other flavors, 1 oz, 28 gm	184	4	18	6	.28	6	.74	26	91	0
unflavored, no color, 1 oz, 28 gm	177	4	16	7	.23	7	.68	143	90	0
PEANUT KERNELS										
dried, 1 oz, 28 gm	161	7	14	5	1.39	17	.92	5	204	0
1 c, 146 gm	827	37	72	24	7.14	85	4.71	23	1047	0
oil-roasted										
salt-free, 1 oz, 28 gm	165	8	14	5	.68	24	.54	4	200	0
1 c, 145 gm	841	39	71	27	3.47	125	2.78	22	1020	0
salted, 1 oz, 28 gm	165	8	14	5	.68	24	.54	122	200	0
1 c, 145 gm	841	39	71	27	3.47	125	2.78	626	1020	0
PEANUT BUTTER, SMOOTH										
salt-free, 1 tbsp, 16 gm	95	5	8	3	.53	5	.29	3	110	0
1 c, 258 gm	1526	73	132	41	8.57	85	4.67	44	1767	0
salted, 1 tbsp, 16 gm	95	5	8	3	.53	5	.29	75	110	0
1 c, 158 gm	1526	73	132	41	8.57	85	4.67	1210	1767	0
PEANUT FLOUR, defatted										
salt-free, 1 tbsp, 4 gm	13	2	<1	1	.16	6	.08	1	52	0
1 c, 60 gm	196	31	<1	21	2.43	84	1.26	9	774	0
salted, 1 tbsp, 4 gm	13	2	<1	1	.16	6	.08	7	52	0
1 c, 60 gm	196	31	<1	21	2.43	84	1.26	108	774	0
PECANS										
dried, 1 oz, 28 gm	190	2	19	5	.45	10	.60	0	111	0
chopped, 1 c, 119 gm	794	9	80	22	1.90	43	2.53	1	466	0
ground, 1 c, 95 gm	634	7	64	17	1.52	34	2.02	<1	372	0
halves, 1 c, 108 gm	721	8	73	20	1.72	39	2.30	1	423	0
dry-roasted										
salt-free, 1 oz, 28 gm	187	2	18	6	.47	10	.62	0	105	0
salted, 1 oz, 28 gm	187	2	18	6	.47	10	.62	221	105	0

FOOD & DESCRIPTION MEASURE OR QUANTITY	CALORIES	PROTEIN (GM)	FAT (GM)	CARBO-HYDRATE (GM)	FIBER (GM)	CALCIUM (MG)	IRON (MG)	SODIUM (MG)	POTASSIUM (MG)	CHOLES-TEROL (MG)
oil-roasted										
salt-free, 1 oz, 28 gm	195	2	20	5	.46	10	.60	0	102	0
1 c, 110 gm	754	8	78	18	1.77	37	2.33	1	395	0
salted, 1 oz, 28 gm	195	2	20	5	.46	10	.60	214	102	0
1 c, 110 gm	754	8	78	18	1.77	37	2.33	832	395	0
PECAN FLOUR, 1 oz, 28 gm	93	9	<1	14	.43	9	.56	0	95	0
PILINUTS/CANARYTREE,										
dried, 1 oz, 28 gm	204	3	23	1	.80	41	1.00	1	144	0
1 c, 120 gm	863	13	95	5	3.36	174	4.23	4	609	0
PINE NUTS/PIGNOLIAS, dried,										
1 oz, 28 gm	146	7	14	4	.23	7	2.61	1	170	0
1 tbsp, 10 gm	51	2	5	1	.08	3	.92	0	60	0
PINE NUTS/PINYON, dried, 1										
oz, 28 gm	161	3	17	5	1.34	2	.87	20	178	0
10 kernels, 1 gm	6	<1	<1	<1	.05	0	.03	1	6	0
PISTACHIOS										
dried, 1 oz, 28 gm	164	6	14	7	.53	38	1.92	2	310	0
1 c, 128 gm	739	26	62	32	2.40	173	8.67	7	1399	0
dry-roasted										
salt-free, 1 oz, 28 gm	172	4	15	8	.51	20	.90	2	275	0
1 c, 128 gm	776	19	68	35	2.31	90	4.06	8	1242	0
salted, 1 oz, 28 gm	172	4	15	8	.51	20	.90	221	275	0
1 c, 128 gm	776	19	68	35	2.31	90	4.06	998	1242	0
SOYBEAN NUTS										
roasted and toasted, salt-										
free, 1 oz, 28 gm	129	11	7	9	1.01	39	1.26	1	417	0
whole kernels, 1 c, 108 gm	490	40	26	33	3.83	149	4.81	4	1588	0
salted, 1 oz, 28 gm	129	11	7	9	1.01	39	1.26	46	417	0
whole kernels, 1 c, 108 gm	490	40	26	33	3.83	149	4.81	176	1588	0
WALNUTS										
BLACK, dried, 1 oz, 28 gm	172	7	16	3	1.83	16	.87	0	149	0
chopped, 1 c, 125 gm	759	30	71	15	8.08	72	3.84	2	655	0
ground, 1 c, 80 gm	486	19	45	10	5.17	46	2.46	<1	419	0
ENGLISH/PERSIAN, dried,										
1 oz, 28 gm	182	4	18	5	1.31	27	.69	3	142	0
halves, 1 c, 100 gm	642	14	62	18	4.60	94	2.44	10	502	0
pieces, 1 c, 120 gm	770	17	74	22	5.52	113	2.93	12	602	0
SEEDS										
BREADFRUIT SEEDS										
boiled, 1 oz, 28 gm	48	2	<1	9	.51	17	.17	—	—	0
raw, 1 oz, 28 gm	54	2	2	8	.48	10	1.04	—	—	0
roasted, 1 oz, 28 gm	59	2	<1	11	.62	24	.26	—	—	0
BREADNUT TREE SEEDS										
dried, 1 oz, 28 gm	104	2	<1	23	1.59	27	1.31	—	—	0
raw, 1 oz, 28 gm	62	2	<1	13	.72	28	.59	—	—	0
CHIA SEEDS, dried, 1 oz, 28										
gm	134	5	7	14	7.19	150	2.84	—	—	0
COTTONSEED KERNELS,										
roasted, 1 tbsp, 10 gm	51	3	4	2	.20	10	.54	3	135	0
1 c, 149 gm	754	49	54	33	2.98	149	8.05	37	2012	0
COTTONSEED FLOUR, partially										
defatted										
1 tbsp, 5 gm	18	2	<1	2	.10	24	.63	2	89	0
1 c, 94 gm	337	39	6	38	1.88	449	11.90	33	1666	0
low-fat, 1 oz, 28 gm	94	14	<1	10	.69	135	3.57	10	500	0
COTTONSEED MEAL, 1 oz, 28										
gm	104	14	1	11	.69	143	3.79	10	531	0
LOTUS SEEDS										
dried, 1 oz, 28 gm	94	4	<1	18	.69	46	1.00	1	389	0
1 c, 32 gm	106	5	<1	21	.77	52	1.13	1	438	0
raw, 1 oz, 28 gm	25	1	<1	5	.18	12	.27	0	104	0
PUMPKIN, SQUASH SEEDS										
kernels, dried										

FOOD & DESCRIPTION MEASURE OR QUANTITY	CALORIES	PROTEIN (GM)	FAT (GM)	CARBO- HYDRATE (GM)	FIBER (GM)	CALCIUM (MG)	IRON (MG)	SODIUM (MG)	POTASSIUM (MG)	CHOLES- TEROL (MG)
1 oz, 28 gm	154	7	13	5	.63	12	4.25	5	229	0
1 c, 138 gm	747	34	63	25	3.07	59	20.66	24	1114	0
kernels, roasted										
salt-free, 1 oz, 28 gm	148	9	12	4	.51	12	4.24	5	229	0
1 c, 227 gm	1184	75	96	31	4.11	97	33.92	40	1829	0
salted, 1 oz, 28 gm	148	9	12	4	.51	12	4.24	163	229	0
1 c, 227 gm	1184	75	96	31	4.11	97	33.92	1305	1829	0
whole, roasted										
salt-free, 1 oz, 28 gm	127	5	6	15	10.2	16	.94	5	261	0
1 c, 64 gm	285	12	12	34	22.98	35	2.12	12	588	0
salted, 1 oz, 28 gm	127	5	6	15	10.2	16	.94	163	261	0
1 c, 64 gm	285	12	12	34	22.98	35	2.12	368	588	0
SAFFLOWER SEEDS, dried 1 oz, 28 gm	147	5	11	10	.70	22	—	—	—	0
SAFFLOWER SEED MEAL, partially defatted, 1 oz, 28 gm	97	10	<1	14	2.16	22	—	—	—	0
SESAME SEEDS										
kernels, dried										
1 tbsp, 8 gm	47	2	4	<1	.24	10	.62	3	33	0
1 c, 150 gm	882	40	82	14	4.44	197	11.70	59	610	0
kernels, toasted, 1 oz, 28 gm	161	5	14	7	1.42	37	2.21	11	115	0
whole, dried										
1 tbsp, 9 gm	52	2	4	2	.41	88	1.31	1	42	0
1 c, 144 gm	825	26	72	34	6.62	1404	20.95	16	674	0
whole, roasted & toasted, 1 oz, 28 gm	161	5	14	7	2.41	281	4.19	3	135	0
SESAME SEED BUTTER										
paste from whole seeds										
1 oz, 28 gm	169	5	14	7	1.55	273	5.45	3	165	0
1 tbsp, 16 gm	95	3	8	4	.87	154	3.07	2	93	0
tahini, raw, stone-ground kernels										
1 oz, 28 gm	162	5	14	7	1.42	119	.71	21	118	0
1 tbsp, 15 gm	86	3	7	4	.75	63	.38	11	62	0
tahini, roasted & toasted kernels										
1 oz, 28 gm	169	5	15	6	1.42	121	2.54	33	118	0
1 tbsp, 15 gm	89	3	8	3	.75	64	1.34	17	62	0
tahini, unroasted kernels										
1 oz, 28 gm	173	5	16	5	.86	40	1.80	0	130	0
1 tbsp, 14 gm	85	3	8	3	.42	20	.89	0	64	0
SESAME FLOUR										
high-fat, 1 oz, 28 gm	149	9	11	8	1.81	45	4.31	12	120	0
low-fat, 1 oz, 28 gm	95	14	<1	10	1.42	42	4.04	11	113	0
partially defatted, 1 oz, 28 gm	109	11	3	10	1.71	43	4.06	12	121	0
SESAME MEAL, partially defatted, 1 oz, 28 gm	161	5	14	7	1.14	43	4.13	11	115	0
SISYMBRIUM SEEDS, whole, dried, 1 oz, 28 gm	90	3	1	17	8.43	464	.03	26	605	0
1 c, 74 gm	235	9	3	43	21.98	1208	.08	68	1576	0
SUNFLOWER SEED kernels, dried										
1 oz, 28 gm	162	6	14	5	1.18	33	1.92	1	196	0
1 c, 144 gm	821	33	71	27	5.99	168	9.75	4	992	0
dry-roasted										
salt-free, 1 oz, 28 gm	165	5	14	7	.51	20	1.08	1	221	0
1 c, 128 gm	745	25	64	31	2.32	90	4.87	4	1088	0
salted, 1 oz, 28 gm	165	5	14	7	.51	20	1.08	241	241	0
1 c, 128 gm	745	25	64	31	2.32	90	4.87	998	1088	0
oil-roasted										
salt-free, 1 oz, 28 gm	175	6	16	4	.51	16	1.90	1	137	0
1 c, 135 gm	830	29	78	20	2.41	76	9.05	4	652	0

FOOD & DESCRIPTION MEASURE OR QUANTITY	CALORIES	PROTEIN (GM)	FAT (GM)	CARBO-HYDRATE (GM)	FIBER (GM)	CALCIUM (MG)	IRON (MG)	SODIUM (MG)	POTASSIUM (MG)	CHOLES-TEROL (MG)
salted, 1 oz, 28 gm	175	6	16	4	.51	16	1.90	171	137	0
1 c, 135 gm	830	29	78	20	2.41	76	9.05	814	652	0
toasted										
salt-free, 1 oz, 28 gm	176	5	16	6	.52	16	1.93	1	139	0
1 c, 134 gm	829	23	76	28	2.43	76	9.13	4	658	0
salted, 1 oz, 28 gm	176	5	16	6	.52	16	1.93	174	139	0
1 c, 134 gm	829	23	76	28	2.43	76	9.13	821	658	0
SUNFLOWER SEED BUTTER										
salt-free, 1 oz, 28 gm	165	6	14	8	1.39d	35	1.35	1	20	0
1 tbsp, 16 gm	93	3	8	4	.79d	19	.76	1	12	0
salted, 1 oz, 28 gm	165	6	14	8	1.39d	35	1.35	147	20	0
1 tbsp, 16 gm	93	3	8	4	.79d	19	.76	83	12	0
SUNFLOWER SEED FLOUR, partially defatted, 1 tbsp, 5 gm	16	2	<1	2	.26	6	.33	0	3	0
1 c, 80 gm	261	38	1	29	4.15	91	5.3	2	54	0
WATERMELON SEEDS, dried, 1 oz, 28 gm	158	8	13	4	.86	15	2.07	28	184	0
1 c, 108 gm	602	31	51	17	3.29	59	7.86	107	700	0

234

16

PANTRY STAPLES

FOOD & DESCRIPTION MEASURE OR QUANTITY	CALORIES	PROTEIN (GM)	FAT (GM)	CARBO-HYDRATE (GM)	FIBER (GM)	CALCIUM (MG)	IRON (MG)	SODIUM (MG)	POTASSIUM (MG)	CHOLES-TEROL (MG)
Flour										
Arrowhead Mills										
BARLEY, 2 oz	200	7	1	43	—	—	—	2	—	—
BROWN RICE, 2 oz	200	4	1	44	—	—	—	5	—	—
CAROB POWDER, 2 oz	100	3	1	46	—	—	—	—	—	—
CORNMEAL, 1 oz	210	4	2	43	—	—	—	1	—	—
HI-LYSINE, 2 oz	210	4	2	43	—	—	—	1	—	—
MILLET, 2 oz	185	6	2	41	—	—	—	2	—	—
OAT, 2 oz	200	7	1	43	—	—	—	1	—	—
RYE, 2 oz	190	9	1	39	—	—	—	1	—	—
SOY, 2 oz	250	20	11	18	—	—	—	1	—	—
TRITICALE, 2 oz	190	7	1	41	—	—	—	1	—	—
WHEAT										
BUCKWHEAT, 2 oz	190	7	1	41	—	—	—	0	—	—
DURUM, 2 oz	190	7	1	40	—	—	—	2	—	—
GRAHAM, 2 oz	200	8	1	40	—	—	—	2	—	—
PASTRY, 2 oz	180	6	1	41	—	—	—	2	—	—
UNBLEACHED, 2 oz	200	7	1	53	—	—	—	1	—	—
WHEAT GERM, 2 oz	210	15	6	26	—	—	—	2	—	—
WHOLE WHEAT, 2 oz	200	8	1	40	—	—	—	2	—	—
Aunt Jemima—Quaker										
FLOUR, SELF RISING, ¼ c	109	3	<1	24	.10	60	1.25	368	32	—
Featherweight										
RICE FLOUR, 1 c	500	11	1	113	—	—	—	7	184	—
Five Roses—Catelli										
DARK RYE, 1 c, 84 gm	294	10	1	63	.84	23	2.18	<1	171	—
WHEAT										
ALL PURPOSE, 1 c, 116 gm	418	14	1	84	.35	32	3.36	2	110	—
GRAHAM, 1 c, 127 gm	423	18	2	86	2.92	43	6.35	4	470	—
UNBLEACHED, 1 c, 116 gm	418	14	1	84	.35	32	3.36	2	110	—
WHOLE WHEAT, 1 c, 127 gm	423	18	2	86	2.92	43	6.35	4	470	—
General Mills										
BISQUICK, 2 oz	240	4	8	37	—	80	1.08	700	80	—
WHEAT										
DRIFTED SNOW, 1 c, 4 oz	400	11	1	87	—	200	4.50	0	130	—
GOLD MEDAL										
ALL-PURPOSE, 1 c, 4 oz	400	11	1	87	—	200	4.50	0	130	—
BETTER FOR BREAD—HIGH										

FOOD & DESCRIPTION MEASURE OR QUANTITY	CALORIES	PROTEIN (GM)	FAT (GM)	CARBO-HYDRATE (GM)	FIBER (GM)	CALCIUM (MG)	IRON (MG)	SODIUM (MG)	POTASSIUM (MG)	CHOLES-TEROL (MG)
PROTEIN, 1 c, 4 oz	400	14	1	83	—	20	4.50	0	120	—
SELF-RISING, 1 c, 4 oz	380	10	1	83	—	350	4.50	1520	130	—
UNBLEACHED, 1 c, 4 oz	400	11	1	87	—	20	4.50	0	140	—
WHOLE WHEAT, 1 c, 4 oz	390	16	2	78	—	20	4.50	0	410	—
WHOLE WHEAT BLEND, 1 c, 4 oz	370	14	2	84	—	20	4.50	0	340	—
LA PINA, 1 c, 4 oz	400	10	1	87	—	20	4.50	0	180	—
RED BAND										
PLAIN, ALL-PURPOSE, 1 c, 4 oz	400	11	1	87	—	200	4.50	0	120	—
SELF-RISING, 1 c, 4 oz	380	9	1	83	—	350	4.50	1520	140	—
WHOLE WHEAT BLEND, 1 c, 4 oz	400	13	2	82	—	20	3.60	0	—	—
SOFTASILK, 1 c, 4 oz	100	2	0	23	—	*	1.08	0	110	—
WHITE DEER, ALL-PURPOSE, 1 c, 4 oz	400	11	1	87	—	200	4.50	0	140	—
WONDRA, 1 c, 4 oz	400	11	1	87	—	20	4.50	0	130	—

Pillsbury

BALLARD										
ALL PURPOSE, 1 c	400	10	1	87	—	0	4.50	<5	110	—
SELF RISING, BLEACHED or UNBLEACHED, 1 c	380	9	1	84	—	300	4.50	1290	100	—
PILLSBURY BEST										
ALL PURPOSE, 1 c	400	11	1	87	—	0	4.50	<5	110	—
BOHEMIAN STYLE RYE AND WHEAT, 1 c	400	11	1	86	—	20	3.60	<5	170	—
BREAD, 1 c	400	14	2	83	—	0	4.50	<5	90	—
MEDIUM RYE, 1 c	400	12	2	83	—	20	2.70	<5	230	—
SAUCE 'N GRAVY, 2 tbsp	50	1	0	11	—	0	.36	<5	15	—
SELF RISING, BLEACHED or UNBLEACHED, 1 c	380	9	1	84	—	300	4.50	1290	100	—
UNBLEACHED, ALL PURPOSE, 1 c	400	12	1	86	—	0	4.50	<5	140	—
WHOLE WHEAT, 1 c	400	15	2	80	—	20	3.60	10	420	—

USDA

CAROB (St.-John's-bread), 1 c, 140 gm	252	6	2	113	—	493	—	—	—	—
1 tbsp, 8 gm	14	<1	<1	7	—	28	—	—	—	—
RYE										
DARK, spooned into cup, 1 c, 128 gm	419	21	3	87	—	69	5.80	1	1101	—
LIGHT										
sifted, 1 c, 88 gm	314	8	<1	69	—	19	1.00	1	137	—
unsifted, 1 c, 102 gm	364	10	1	80	—	22	1.10	1	159	—
MEDIUM, sifted, 1 c, 88 gm	308	10	2	66	—	24	2.30	1	179	—
SOYBEAN										
DEFATTED, stirred, 1 c, 100 gm	326	47	1	38	—	265	11.10	1	1820	—
FULL FAT										
stirred, 1 c, 70 gm	295	26	14	21	—	139	5.90	1	1162	—
unstirred, 1 c, 85 gm	358	31	17	26	—	169	7.10	1	1411	—
LOW-FAT, stirred, 1 c, 88 gm	313	38	6	32	—	231	8.00	1	1636	—
WHEAT										
ALL-PURPOSE										
sifted, spooned into cup, 1 c, 115 gm	419	12	1	88	—	18	3.30	2	109	—
unsifted, dipped with cup, 1 c, 137 gm	499	14	1	104	—	22	4.00	3	130	—
unsifted, spooned into cup, 1 c, 125 gm	455	13	1	95	—	20	3.60	3	119	—
BREAD										

FOOD & DESCRIPTION MEASURE OR QUANTITY	CALORIES	PROTEIN (GM)	FAT (GM)	CARBO-HYDRATE (GM)	FIBER (GM)	CALCIUM (MG)	IRON (MG)	SODIUM (MG)	POTASSIUM (MG)	CHOLES-TEROL (MG)
sifted, 1 c, 115 gm	420	14	1	86	—	18	3.30	2	109	—
unsifted, dipped with cup, 1 c, 137 gm	500	16	2	102	—	22	4.00	3	130	—
BUCKWHEAT										
DARK, sifted, 1 c, 98 gm	326	12	3	71	—	32	2.70	—	—	—
LIGHT, sifted, 1 c, 98 gm	340	6	1	78	—	11	1.00	—	314	—
CAKE or PASTRY										
sifted, spooned into cup, 1 c, 96 gm	349	7	<1	76	—	16	.50	2	91	—
unsifted, dipped with cup, 1 c, 118 gm	430	9	<1	94	—	20	.60	2	112	—
unsifted, spooned into cup, 1 c, 109 gm	397	8	<1	87	—	19	.50	2	104	—
CORN, 1 c, 117 gm	431	9	3	90	—	7	2.10	1	—	—
GLUTEN, 45% gluten, 55% patent flour										
unsifted, dipped with cup, 1 c, 140 gm	529	58	3	66	—	56	—	3	84	—
unsifted or sifted, spooned into cup, 1 c, 135 gm	510	56	3	64	—	54	—	3	81	—
INSTANT BLENDING, unsifted, spooned into cup, 1 c, 129 gm	470	14	1	98	—	21	3.70	3	123	—
SELF-RISING										
sifted, 1 c, 115 gm	405	11	1	85	—	305	3.30	1241	—	—
unsifted, 1 c, 125 gm	440	12	1	93	—	331	3.60	1349	—	—
WHOLE-WHEAT, stirred, 1 c, 120 gm	400	16	2	85	—	49	4.00	4	444	—

Grains

Arrowhead Mills

AMARANTH, 2 oz	200	8	3	35	—	—	—	2	—	—
BARLEY										
HULLED, 2 oz	200	5	1	34	—	—	—	2	—	—
PEARLED, 2 oz	200	5	1	45	—	—	—	2	—	—
BUCKWHEAT GROATS										
BROWN, 2 oz	190	7	1	41	—	—	—	2	—	—
WHITE , 2 oz	190	7	1	41	—	—	—	2	—	—
CORN, 2 oz	210	4	2	43	—	—	—	—	—	—
MILLET, 2 oz	90	3	1	21	—	—	—	1	—	—
OAT										
BRAN, 1 oz	110	6	2	17	—	—	—	2	—	—
GROATS, 2 oz	220	8	4	38	—	—	—	1	—	—
RYE, 2 oz	190	7	1	42	—	—	—	1	—	—
TRITICALE, 2 oz	190	7	1	41	—	—	—	—	—	—
WHEAT										
BRAN, 2 oz	200	10	2	30	—	—	—	5	—	—
HARD RED WINTER or SOFT PASTRY, 2 oz	190	8	1	41	—	—	—	2	—	—

Aunt Jemima–Quaker

CORNMEAL										
WHITE or YELLOW, enriched, 3 tbsp	102	2	<1	22	.20	1	.81	1	51	—
SELF-RISING, WHITE, 1/6 c	98	2	<1	21	.20	109	.81	381	44	—
CORNMEAL MIX										
BOLTED, WHITE, 1/6 c	99	2	<1	21	.20	60	1.08	337	68	—
BOLTED, YELLOW, 1/6 c	97	2	<1	21	.10	60	1.08	369	40	—
BUTTERMILK, self-rising, white, 3 tbsp	101	3	1	20	.30	60	1.08	439	87	—

FOOD & DESCRIPTION MEASURE OR QUANTITY	CALORIES	PROTEIN (GM)	FAT (GM)	CARBO-HYDRATE (GM)	FIBER (GM)	CALCIUM (MG)	IRON (MG)	SODIUM (MG)	POTASSIUM (MG)	CHOLES-TEROL (MG)
Ogilvie–Catelli										
WHEAT GERM, 1 tbsp, 9 gm	32	3	<1	5	.18	6	.99	<1	85	—
Quaker										
BARLEY, SCOTCH										
PEARLED, ¼ c dry	172	6	<1	36	.40	11	1.24	5	130	—
QUICK PEARLED, ¼ c dry	172	6	<1	36	.40	11	1.24	5	130	—
MASA HARINA DE MAIZ, ⅓ c	137	4	2	27	.70	77	2.93	2	115	—
MASA TRIGO, ⅓ C	149	4	4	25	.10	66	2.60	794	36	—
USDA										
CORNMEAL, WHITE or YELLOW										
BOLTED, dry, 1 c, 122 gm	442	11	4	91	—	21	2.20	1	303	—
DEGERMED, enriched, dry, 1 c, 138 gm	502	11	2	108	—	8	4.00	1	166	—
SELF RISING										
DEGERMED, 1 c, 141 gm	491	11	2	106	—	409	1.40	1946	159	—
WITH FLOUR added, 1 c, 141 gm	491	11	2	106	—	412	1.40	1946	154	—
WHOLE GROUND, 1 c, 134 gm	465	11	4	96	—	402	2.30	1849	314	—
with flour added, 1 c, 134 gm	465	12	4	96	—	403	2.10	1849	284	—
UNBOLTED, dry, 1 c, 122 gm	433	11	5	90	—	24	2.90	1	346	—

Jams & Jellies

Dia-Mel

PRESERVES, JELLY, 1 tsp	2	0	0	0	—	—	—	<1	—	0

Featherweight

JELLY										
LOW CALORIE										
GRAPE, 1 tbsp	6	0	0	1	—	—	—	16	14	—
REDUCED CALORIE										
APPLE, 1 tbsp	16	0	0	4	—	—	—	12	14	—
BLACKBERRY, 1 tbsp	16	0	0	4	—	—	—	10	14	—
CHERRY, 1 tbsp	16	0	0	4	—	—	—	50	14	—
GRAPE, 1 tbsp	16	0	0	4	—	—	—	21	14	—
PLUM, 1 tbsp	16	0	0	4	—	—	—	9	14	—
STRAWBERRY, 1 tbsp	16	0	0	4	—	—	—	11	14	—
PRESERVES										
LOW CALORIE										
STRAWBERRY, 1 tbsp	6	0	0	1	—	—	—	7	18	—
REDUCED CALORIE										
APRICOT, 1 tbsp	16	0	0	4	—	—	—	6	18	—
BLACKBERRY, 1 tbsp	16	0	0	4	—	—	—	8	18	—
ORANGE MARMALADE, 1 tbsp	16	0	0	4	—	—	—	11	18	—
PEACH, 1 tbsp	16	0	0	4	—	—	—	7	18	—
RED RASPBERRY, 1 tbsp	16	0	0	4	—	—	—	6	18	—
STRAWBERRY, 1 tbsp	16	0	0	4	—	—	—	10	18	—

Habitant–Catelli

JAM										
APPLE AND RASPBERRY, 1 tbsp, 20 gm	43	<1	<1	11	.08	<1	.03	<1	4	—
APPLE AND STRAWBERRY, 1										

FOOD & DESCRIPTION MEASURE OR QUANTITY	CALORIES	PROTEIN (GM)	FAT (GM)	CARBO-HYDRATE (GM)	FIBER (GM)	CALCIUM (MG)	IRON (MG)	SODIUM (MG)	POTASSIUM (MG)	CHOLES-TEROL (MG)
tbsp, 20 gm	43	<1	<1	11	.05	<1	.03	<1	4	—
RASPBERRY, 1 tbsp, 20 gm	45	<1	<1	12	.12	<1	.04	<1	5	—
STRAWBERRY, 1 tbsp, 20 gm	44	<1	<1	11	.07	<1	.04	<1	6	—

Laura Secord–Catelli

JAM										
RASPBERRY, 1 tbsp, 20 gm	42	<1	<1	11	.16	<1	.05	<1	7	—
STRAWBERRY, 1 tbsp, 20 gm	42	<1	<1	11	.06	<1	.05	<1	8	—
MARMALADE										
ORANGE, 1 tbsp, 20 gm	44	<1	<1	12	.06	4	.04	<1	11	—
SEVILLE ORANGE, 1 tbsp, 20 gm	38	<1	<1	11	.03	8	.05	<1	10	—
3-FRUIT, 1 tbsp, 20 gm	45	<1	tr	12	.07	4	.03	<1	10	—

Smucker's

BUTTER										
APPLE, NATURAL & CIDER, 2 tsp	25	0	0	6	—	*	*	0	—	—
PEACH, 2 tsp	30	0	0	8	—	*	*	0	—	—
JAM AND PRESERVES										
IMITATION STRAWBERRY, artificially sweetened, 2 tsp	4	0	0	1	—	*	*	0	—	—
single service, .5 oz	38	0	0	9	—	*	*	0	—	—
SLENDERELLA, 2 tsp	16	0	0	4	—	*	*	0	—	—
SWEETENED with sugar, 2 tsp	35	0	0	9	—	*	*	0	—	—
JELLY										
IMITATION GRAPE, artificially sweetened, 2 tsp	4	0	0	1	—	*	*	0	—	—
single service, .5 oz	38	0	0	9	—	*	*	0	—	—
artificially sweetened, imitation, .38 oz	2	0	0	<1	—	*	*	<10	—	—
SLENDERELLA, 2 tsp	16	0	0	4	—	*	*	0	—	—
SWEETENED with sugar, 2 tsp	35	0	0	9	—	*	*	0	—	—
LOW SUGAR SPREADS, 8 flavors, 2 tsp	16	0	0	4	—	*	*	0	—	—
MARMALADE, ORANGE, 2 tsp	35	0	0	9	—	*	*	0	—	—

USDA

JAM & PRESERVES, sweetened with sugar, 1 tbsp, 20 gm	54	<1	tr	14	—	4	.20	2	18	—
JELLIES, sweetened with sugar, 1 tbsp, 18 gm	49	tr	tr	13	—	4	.30	3	14	—
MARMALADE, sweetened with sugar, 1 tbsp, 20 gm	51	<1	tr	14	—	7	.10	3	7	—

Welch

JAMS, JELLIES & PRESERVES, 2 tsp	35	0	0	9	—	*	*	5	5	—

Miscellaneous

Argo and Kingsford–Best Foods

CORNSTARCH, 1 tbsp, 8 gm	30	tr	tr	7	tr	*	*	tr	—	—

FOOD & DESCRIPTION MEASURE OR QUANTITY	CALORIES	PROTEIN (GM)	FAT (GM)	CARBO-HYDRATE (GM)	FIBER (GM)	CALCIUM (MG)	IRON (MG)	SODIUM (MG)	POTASSIUM (MG)	CHOLES-TEROL (MG)
Featherweight										
BAKING POWDER, LOW SODIUM, no cereal, 1 tsp	8	0	0	2	—	—	—	2	530	—
STARCH										
POTATO, 1 c	620	0	1	154	—	—	—	51	107	—
WHEAT STARCH, 1 c	410	0	0	100	—	—	—	27	7	—
Fleischmann–Nabisco										
YEAST										
ACTIVE DRY, 1 pkt	20	3	0	3	—	*	1.08	10	150	—
COMPRESSED, 1 cube	15	2	0	2	—	*	.72	5	100	—
RAPID RISE, 1 pkt	20	3	0	3	—	*	1.08	10	150	—
Kellogg										
CORN FLAKE CRUMBS, 1 oz, ¼ c	110	2	0	25	tr	1	1.80	285	25	0
Nabisco										
COMET CUPS, 1 cone	20	0	0	4	—	*	*	5	5	—
CHOCOLATE FLAVORED, 1 cone	25	0	0	5	—	*	*	5	10	—
SUGAR CONES, 1 cone	40	1	0	9	—	*	.36	35	15	—
Nestlé										
CHOCO-BAKE, 1 oz	180	4	15	8	—	*	*	—	—	—
MORSELS										
BUTTERSCOTCH FLAVORED, 1 oz	150	1	7	19	—	40	*	15	50	0
MILK CHOCOLATE, 1 oz	150	2	9	17	—	60	*	20	120	5
PEANUT BUTTER, 1 oz	160	5	10	12	—	*	.36	60	205	—
TOLL HOUSE SEMI-SWEET, 1 oz	150	2	8	18	—	*	.72	0	100	—
USDA										
BAKING POWDER										
SODIUM ALUMINUM SULFATE										
MONOCALCIUM PHOSPHATE MONOHYDRATE, 1 tsp, 3 gm	4	tr	tr	<1	—	58	—	329	5	—
MONOCALCIUM PHOSPHATE MONOHYDRATE & CALCIUM CARBONATE, 1 tsp, 3 gm	2	tr	tr	<1	—	173	—	349	—	—
MONOCALCIUM PHOSPHATE MONOHYDRATE & CALCIUM SULFATE, 1 tsp, 3 gm	3	tr	tr	<1	—	183	—	290	—	—
SPECIAL LOW SODIUM, commercial, 1 tsp, 4 gm	7	tr	tr	2	—	207	—	tr	471	—
STRAIGHT PHOSPHATE, 1 tsp, 4 gm	5	tr	tr	1	—	239	—	312	6	—
TARTRATE, 1 tsp, 3 gm	2	tr	tr	<1	—	0	0	204	106	—
CHOCOLATE, bitter or baking, 1 oz, 28 gm	143	3	15	8	—	22	1.90	1	235	—
grated, 1 c, 132 gm	667	14	70	38	—	103	8.80	5	1096	—
COCOA, dry powder										

FOOD & DESCRIPTION MEASURE OR QUANTITY	CALORIES	PROTEIN (GM)	FAT (GM)	CARBO-HYDRATE (GM)	FIBER (GM)	CALCIUM (MG)	IRON (MG)	SODIUM (MG)	POTASSIUM (MG)	CHOLES-TEROL (MG)
HIGH–MEDIUM FAT										
PLAIN, 1 tbsp, 5 gm	14	<1	1	3	—	7	.60	tr	82	—
PROCESSED WITH ALKALI, 1 tbsp, 5 gm	14	<1	1	3	—	7	.60	39	35	—
LOW–MEDIUM FAT										
PLAIN, 1 tbsp, 5 gm	12	1	<1	3	—	8	.60	tr	82	—
PROCESSED WITH ALKALI, 1 tbsp, 5 gm	12	1	<1	3	—	8	.60	39	35	—
CORNSTARCH, stirred, 1 tbsp, 8 gm	29	tr	tr	7	—	0	0	tr	tr	—
GELATIN										
capsule, 1, .6 gm	2	<1	tr	0	—	—	—	—	—	—
dry, 1 env, 7 gm	23	6	tr	0	—	—	—	—	—	—
MALT, dry, 1 oz, 28 gm	104	<1	<1	22	—	—	1.10	—	—	—
MALT EXTRACT, dried, 1 oz,										
28 gm	104	2	tr	25	—	14	2.50	23	65	—
SALT, TABLE, 1 tsp, 5.5 gm	0	0	0	0	—	14	tr	2132	tr	—
TAPIOCA, PEARL or QUICK-COOKING, dry										
1 c, 152 gm	535	<1	<1	131	—	15	.60	5	27	—
1 tbsp, 8 gm	30	<1	tr	7	—	1	tr	tr	2	—
YEAST										
BAKER'S										
COMPRESSED										
1 pkg, .6 oz, 18 gm	15	2	<1	2	—	2	.90	3	110	—
1 oz, 28 gm	24	3	<1	3	—	4	1.40	5	173	—
DRY										
1 pkg, ¼ oz, 7 gm	20	3	<1	3	—	3	1.10	4	140	—
1 oz, 28 gm	80	11	<1	11	—	12	4.60	15	566	—
BREWER'S, debittered										
1 tbsp, 8 gm	23	3	<1	3	—	17	1.40	10	152	—
1 oz, 28 gm	80	11	<1	11	—	60	4.90	34	537	—
TORULA, 1 oz, 28 gm	79	11	<1	11	—	120	5.50	4	580	—

Sugars & Sweeteners

Dia-Mel–Estee

FRUCTOSE, 1 tsp	12	0	0	3	—	—	—	0	—	0
SWEET'N IT, 6 drops	0	0	0	0	—	—	—	1	—	0

Featherweight

ARTIFICIAL SWEETENER										
LIQUID, 3 drops	0	0	0	0	—	—	—	1	<1	—
SACCHARIN, ¼ grain tablet	0	0	0	0	—	—	—	2	0	—

Pillsbury

ARTIFICIAL SWEETENER										
SPRINKLE SWEET, 1 tsp	2	0	0	<1	—	0	0	1	0	—
SWEET* 10, ⅛ tsp	0	0	0	0	—	0	0	2	0	—

USDA

HONEY, strained or extracted										
1 c, 339 gm	1031	1	0	279	—	17	1.70	17	173	—
1 tbsp, 21 gm	64	<1	0	17	—	1	.10	1	11	—
SUGAR										
BROWN										
packed into cup, 1 c, 220 gm	821	0	0	212	—	187	7.50	66	757	—
not packed, 1 c, 145 gm	541	0	0	140	—	123	4.90	44	499	—
GRANULATED										

FOOD & DESCRIPTION MEASURE OR QUANTITY	CALORIES	PROTEIN (GM)	FAT (GM)	CARBO-HYDRATE (GM)	FIBER (GM)	CALCIUM (MG)	IRON (MG)	SODIUM (MG)	POTASSIUM (MG)	CHOLES-TEROL (MG)
1 c, 200 gm	770	0	0	199	—	0	.20	2	6	—
1 tbsp, 12 gm	46	0	0	12	—	0	tr	tr	tr	—
cubes, ½" cube, 2 cubes, 5 gm	19	0	0	5	—	0	tr	tr	tr	—
tablets, ⅛ × ¾ × 5⁄16" tablet, 1 tablet, 5 gm	19	0	0	5	—	0	tr	tr	tr	—
MAPLE, 1 oz, 28 gm	99	—	—	26	—	41	.40	4	69	—
POWDERED sifted, spooned into cup, 1 c, 100 gm	385	0	0	100	—	0	.10	1	3	—
unsifted, 1 c, 120 gm	462	0	0	119	—	0	.10	1	4	—
1 tbsp, 8 gm	31	0	0	8	—	0	tr	tr	tr	—

Weight Watchers

SWEETENER, sugar substitute, granulated, 1 pkt, 1 gm	4	0	0	1	—	—	—	16	1	—

Syrups & Toppings

Aunt Jemima–Quaker

BUTTER LITE, 2 tbsp	52	0	0	13	—	0	0	67	0	—
LITE, 2 tbsp	60	0	0	15	—	0	0	66	1	—
REGULAR, 2 tbsp	103	0	0	26	—	0	0	21	3	—

Estee–Dia-Mel

BLUEBERRY, 1 tbsp	1	0	0	<1	—	—	—	15	—	0
CHOCOLATE, 1 tbsp	6	0	0	1	—	—	—	3	—	0
PANCAKE, 1 tbsp	1	0	0	<1	—	—	—	10	—	0

Featherweight

BLUEBERRY, 1 tbsp	14	0	0	3	—	—	—	20	10	—
PANCAKE, 1 tbsp	12	0	0	3	—	—	—	20	9	—

Golden Griddle–Best Foods

GOLDEN GRIDDLE SYRUP, 1 tbsp, 20 gm	50	0	0	13	0	*	*	20	—	—

Habitant–Catelli

BUTTER PECAN FLAVORED, 1 tbsp, 21 gm	60	0	0	15	0	0	.01	<1	<1	—
TABLE SYRUP, 1 tbsp, 21 gm	50	0	0	13	0	2	.11	<1	10	—

Karo–Best Foods

DARK CORN SYRUP, 1 tbsp, 20.5 gm	60	0	0	15	0	*	*	40	—	—
LIGHT CORN SYRUP, 1 tbsp, 20.5 gm	60	0	0	15	0	*	*	30	—	—
PANCAKE SYRUP, 1 tbsp, 20.5 gm	60	0	0	15	0	*	*	35	—	—

Lever Brothers

MRS. BUTTERWORTH'S SYRUP, 3 tbsp, 59 gm	165	0	<1	40	—	22	*	77	2	—

Nestlé

QUIK SYRUP, 1 oz, 28 gm	80	<1	0	18	—	*	*	35	115	—

FOOD & DESCRIPTION MEASURE OR QUANTITY	CALORIES	PROTEIN (GM)	FAT (GM)	CARBO-HYDRATE (GM)	FIBER (GM)	CALCIUM (MG)	IRON (MG)	SODIUM (MG)	POTASSIUM (MG)	CHOLES-TEROL (MG)
Smucker's										
SYRUP, FRUIT, 2 tbsp	100	0	0	26	—	*	*	0	—	—
TOPPING										
BUTTERSCOTCH FLAVORED, 2 tbsp	140	0	1	33	—	20	*	75	—	—
CARAMEL FLAVORED, 2 tbsp	140	1	1	33	—	20	*	110	—	—
HOT CARAMEL, 2 tbsp	150	1	4	28	—	*	*	75	—	—
CHOCOLATE FLAVORED SYRUP, 2 tbsp	130	1	0	27	—	*	.36	35	—	—
CHOCOLATE FUDGE, 2 tbsp	130	1	1	31	—	20	*	45	—	—
HOT FUDGE, 2 tbsp	110	1	4	18	—	*	*	55	—	—
MAGIC SHELL, 2 tbsp, 34 gm	190	1	15	16	—	*	*	25-50	—	—
PEANUT BUTTER CARAMEL, 2 tbsp	150	3	2	29	—	*	*	105	—	—
PECANS IN SYRUP, 2 tbsp	130	2	1	28	—	*	.36	0	—	—
PINEAPPLE, 2 tbsp	130	0	0	32	—	*	*	0	—	—
STRAWBERRY, 2 tbsp	120	0	0	30	—	*	*	0	—	—
SWISS MILK CHOCOLATE FUDGE, 2 tbsp	140	3	1	31	—	40	*	70	—	—
WALNUTS IN SYRUP, 2 tbsp	130	2	1	27	—	*	3.96	0	—	—
USDA										
CHOCOLATE SYRUP, cnd										
THICK FUDGE, 2 tbsp, 1 oz, 38 gm	124	2	5	20	—	48	.50	33	107	—
THIN, 2 tbsp, 1 oz, 38 gm	92	<1	<1	24	—	6	.60	20	106	—
TABLE										
CANE & MAPLE BLEND, 1 tbsp, 20 gm	50	0	0	13	—	3	tr	tr	5	—
MAPLE, 1 tbsp, 20 gm	50	—	—	13	—	20	.20	2	35	—
SORGHUM, 1 tbsp, 21 gm	53	—	—	14	—	35	2.60	—	—	—
TABLE BLENDS (chiefly corn), 1 tbsp, 21 gm	59	0	0	15	—	9	.80	14	1	—

17

POULTRY

FOOD & DESCRIPTION MEASURE OR QUANTITY	CALORIES	PROTEIN (GM)	FAT (GM)	CARBO- HYDRATE (GM)	FIBER (GM)	CALCIUM (MG)	IRON (MG)	SODIUM (MG)	POTASSIUM (MG)	CHOLES- TEROL (MG)
Fresh Poultry										
Note: Weights given are for edible portion.										
USDA										
CAPON [Figures are for a 6½-pound capon, approximately.]										
FLESH WITH SKIN, roasted,										
3.5 oz, 100 gm	229	29	12	0	0	14	1.49	49	255	86
½ capon, 637 gm	1457	184	74	0	0	91	9.47	313	1626	549
CHICKEN, BROILER-FRYER [All analyses are based on a 3½-pound raw chicken, including the weight of the giblets and neck.]										
FLESH & SKIN										
batter-dipped, fried, 3.5 oz, 100 gm	289	23	17	9	.04	21	1.37	292	185	87
½ chicken, 466 gm	1347	105	81	44	.17	97	6.37	1360	863	404
flour-coated, fried, 3.5 oz, 100 gm	269	29	15	3	.01	17	1.38	84	234	90
½ chicken, 314 gm	844	90	47	10	.04	52	4.33	264	735	283
roasted, 3.5 oz, 100 gm	239	27	14	0	0	15	1.26	82	223	88
½ chicken, 299 gm	715	82	41	0	0	45	3.78	244	667	263
stewed, 3.5 oz, 100 gm	219	25	13	0	0	13	1.16	67	166	78
½ chicken, 334 gm	730	82	42	0	0	44	3.87	224	556	262
FLESH ONLY										
fried, 3.5 oz, 100 gm	219	31	9	2	.01	17	1.35	91	257	94
½ chicken, 258 gm	565	79	24	4	.03	44	3.48	235	663	243
1 c, 140 gm	307	43	13	2	.01	24	1.89	127	360	131
roasted, 3.5 oz, 100 gm	190	29	7	0	0	15	1.21	86	243	89
½ chicken, 243 gm	462	70	18	0	0	36	2.94	209	590	216
1 c, 140 gm	266	41	10	0	0	21	1.69	120	340	125
stewed, 3.5 oz, 100 gm	177	27	7	0	0	14	1.17	70	180	83
½ chicken, 262 gm	464	71	18	0	0	37	3.07	183	472	217
1 c, 140 gm	248	38	9	0	0	19	1.63	98	252	116
GIBLETS, 1 each of GIZZARD, HEART & LIVER										
raw, 75 gm	93	13	3	1	0	7	4.39	58	171	196
flour-coated, fried, 44 gm	122	14	6	2	.01	8	4.54	50	145	196
simmered, 45 gm	71	12	2	<1	0	5	2.90	26	71	177

244

FOOD & DESCRIPTION MEASURE OR QUANTITY	CALORIES	PROTEIN (GM)	FAT (GM)	CARBO-HYDRATE (GM)	FIBER (GM)	CALCIUM (MG)	IRON (MG)	SODIUM (MG)	POTASSIUM (MG)	CHOLES-TEROL (MG)
GIZZARD, raw, 3.5 oz, 100 gm	118	18	4	<1	0	8	3.51	76	236	130
1 gizzard, 37 gm	44	7	2	<1	0	3	1.3	28	87	48
simmered, 3.5 oz, 100 gm	153	27	4	1	0	10	4.15	67	179	194
1 c, 145 gm	222	39	5	2	0	14	6.02	97	259	281
1 gizzard, 22 gm	34	6	<1	<1	0	2	.91	15	39	43
HEART, raw, 3.5 oz, 100 gm	153	16	9	<1	0	12	5.96	74	176	136
1 heart, 6.1 gm	9	<1	<1	<1	0	1	.36	5	11	8
simmered, 3.5 oz, 100 gm	185	26	8	<1	0	19	9.03	48	132	242
1 c, 145 gm	268	38	11	<1	0	27	13.09	69	192	350
1 heart, 3.3 gm	6	<1	<1	<1	0	<1	.30	2	4	8
LIVER, raw, 3.5 oz, 100 gm	125	18	4	3	0	11	8.56	79	228	439
1 liver, 32 gm	40	6	1	1	0	3	2.74	25	73	140
simmered, 3.5 oz, 100 gm	157	24	5	<1	0	14	8.47	51	140	631
1 c, 140 gm	219	34	8	1	0	20	11.86	71	196	883
1 liver, 20 gm	31	5	1	<1	0	3	1.69	10	28	126
LIGHT FLESH WITH SKIN										
batter-dipped, fried, 3.5 oz, 100 gm	277	24	15	10	.04	20	1.26	287	185	84
½ chicken, 188 gm	520	44	29	18	.07	37	2.37	539	348	157
flour-coated, fried, 3.5 oz, 100 gm	246	30	12	2	.01	16	1.21	77	239	87
½ chicken, 130 gm	320	40	16	2	.01	20	1.57	100	311	113
roasted, 3.5 oz, 100 gm	222	29	11	0	0	15	1.14	75	227	84
½ chicken, 132 gm	293	38	14	0	0	19	1.51	99	299	111
stewed, 3.5 oz, 100 gm	201	26	10	0	0	13	.98	63	167	74
½ chicken, 150 gm	302	39	15	0	0	19	1.46	95	251	111
DARK FLESH WITH SKIN										
batter-dipped, fried, 3.5 oz, 100 gm	298	22	19	9	.04	21	1.44	295	185	89
½ chicken, 278 gm	828	61	52	26	.1	59	4	821	515	247
flour-coated, fried, 3.5 oz, 100 gm	285	27	17	4	.02	17	1.5	89	230	92
½ chicken, 184 gm	523	50	31	8	.03	32	2.76	164	424	169
roasted, 3.5 oz, 100 gm	253	26	16	0	0	15	1.36	87	220	91
½ chicken, 167 gm	423	43	26	0	0	25	2.27	145	367	152
stewed, 3.5 oz, 100 gm	233	24	15	0	0	14	1.31	70	166	82
½ chicken, 184 gm	428	43	27	0	0	25	2.4	129	305	151
LIGHT FLESH WITHOUT SKIN										
fried, 3.5 oz, 100 gm	192	33	6	<1	0	16	1.14	81	263	90
1 c, 140 gm	268	46	8	<1	0	22	1.59	114	368	125
½ chicken, 106 gm	204	35	6	<1	0	17	1.21	86	279	95
roasted, 3.5 oz, 100 gm	173	31	5	0	0	15	1.06	77	247	85
1 c, 140 gm	242	43	6	0	0	21	1.49	108	345	118
½ chicken, 107 gm	185	33	5	0	0	16	1.13	82	264	91
stewed, 3.5 oz, 100 gm	159	29	4	0	0	13	.93	65	180	77
1 c, 140 gm	223	40	6	0	0	18	1.31	91	252	107
½ chicken, 119 gm	189	34	5	0	0	15	1.11	77	214	92
DARK FLESH WITHOUT SKIN										
fried, 3.5 oz, 100 gm	239	29	12	3	.01	18	1.49	97	253	96
1 c, 140 gm	334	41	16	4	.01	25	2.09	136	354	135
½ chicken, 152 gm	363	44	18	4	.02	27	2.26	147	385	146
roasted, 3.5 oz, 100 gm	205	27	10	0	0	15	1.33	93	240	93
1 c, 140 gm	286	38	14	0	0	21	1.86	130	336	130
½ chicken, 136 gm	279	37	13	0	0	20	1.81	126	326	126
stewed, 3.5 oz, 100 gm	192	26	9	0	0	14	1.36	74	181	88
1 c, 140 gm	269	36	13	0	0	20	1.90	104	253	123
½ chicken, 143 gm	275	37	13	0	0	20	1.94	106	259	126
BACK, FLESH WITH SKIN										
batter-dipped, fried, 3.5 oz, 100 gm	331	22	22	10	.04	26	1.49	317	180	88
½ back, 120 gm	397	26	26	12	.05	31	1.79	380	216	105
flour-coated, fried, 3.5 oz,										

FOOD & DESCRIPTION MEASURE OR QUANTITY	CALORIES	PROTEIN (GM)	FAT (GM)	CARBO-HYDRATE (GM)	FIBER (GM)	CALCIUM (MG)	IRON (MG)	SODIUM (MG)	POTASSIUM (MG)	CHOLES-TEROL (MG)
100 gm	331	28	21	7	.03	24	1.62	90	226	89
½ back, 72 gm	238	20	15	5	.02	17	1.17	65	163	64
roasted, 3.5 oz, 100 gm	300	26	21	0	0	21	1.42	87	210	88
½ back, 53 gm	159	14	11	0	0	11	.75	46	111	46
stewed, 3.5 oz, 100 gm	258	22	18	0	0	18	1.22	64	145	78
½ back, 61 gm	158	14	11	0	0	11	.74	39	89	48
BACK, FLESH ONLY										
fried, 3.5 oz, 100 gm	288	30	15	6	.02	26	1.65	99	251	93
½ back, 58 gm	167	17	9	3	.01	15	.96	58	146	54
roasted, 3.5 oz, 100 gm	239	28	13	0	0	24	1.39	96	237	90
½ back, 40 gm	96	11	5	0	0	10	.56	38	95	36
stewed, 3.5 oz, 100 gm	209	25	11	0	0	21	1.27	67	158	85
½ back, 42 gm	88	11	5	0	0	9	.53	28	66	36
BREAST, FLESH WITH SKIN										
batter-dipped, fried, 3.5 oz, 100 gm	260	25	13	9	.04	20	1.25	275	201	85
½ breast, 140 gm	364	35	18	13	.05	28	1.75	385	282	119
flour-coated, fried, 3.5 oz, 100 gm	222	32	9	2	.01	16	1.19	76	259	89
½ breast, 98 gm	218	31	9	2	.01	16	1.17	75	253	88
roasted, 3.5 oz, 100 gm	197	30	8	0	0	14	1.07	71	245	84
½ breast, 98 gm	193	29	8	0	0	14	1.04	69	240	83
stewed, 3.5 oz, 100 gm	184	27	7	0	0	13	.92	62	178	75
½ breast, 110 gm	202	30	8	0	0	14	1.01	68	195	83
BREAST, FLESH WITHOUT SKIN										
fried, 3.5 oz, 100 gm	187	33	5	<1	0	16	1.14	79	276	91
½ breast, 86 gm	161	29	4	<1	0	14	.98	68	237	78
roasted, 3.5 oz, 100 gm	165	31	4	0	0	15	1.04	74	256	85
½ breast, 86 gm	142	27	3	0	0	13	.89	63	220	73
stewed, 3.5 oz, 100 gm	151	29	3	0	0	13	.88	63	187	77
½ breast, 95 gm	144	28	3	0	0	12	.84	59	178	73
DRUMSTICK, FLESH WITH SKIN										
batter-dipped, fried, 3.5 oz, 100 gm	268	22	16	8	.03	17	1.35	269	186	86
1 drumstick, 72 gm	193	16	11	6	.02	12	.97	194	134	62
flour-coated, fried, 3.5 oz, 100 gm	245	27	14	2	.01	12	1.34	89	229	90
1 drumstick, 49 gm	120	13	7	<1	0	6	.66	44	112	44
roasted, 3.5 oz, 100 gm	216	27	11	0	0	12	1.33	90	229	91
1 drumstick, 52 gm	112	14	6	0	0	6	.69	47	119	48
stewed, 3.5 oz, 100 gm	204	25	11	0	0	11	1.33	76	184	83
1 drumstick, 57 gm	116	14	6	0	0	7	.76	43	105	48
DRUMSTICK, FLESH WITHOUT SKIN										
fried, 3.5 oz, 100 gm	195	29	8	0	0	12	1.32	96	249	94
1 drumstick, 42 gm	82	12	3	0	0	5	.55	40	105	40
roasted, 3.5 oz, 100 gm	172	28	6	0	0	12	1.30	95	246	93
1 drumstick, 44 gm	76	12	2	0	0	5	.57	42	108	41
stewed, 3.5 oz, 100 gm	169	28	6	0	0	11	1.37	80	199	88
1 drumstick, 46 gm	78	13	3	0	0	5	.63	37	92	40
LEG, FLESH WITH SKIN										
batter-dipped, fried, 3.5 oz, 100 gm	273	22	16	9	.03	18	1.40	279	189	90
1 leg, 158 gm	431	34	26	14	.05	28	2.21	442	299	142
flour-coated, fried, 3.5 oz, 100 gm	254	27	14	3	.01	13	1.43	88	233	94
1 leg, 112 gm	285	30	16	3	.01	15	1.60	99	261	105
roasted, 3.5 oz, 100 gm	232	26	13	0	0	12	1.33	87	225	92
1 leg, 114 gm	265	30	15	0	0	14	1.52	99	256	105
stewed, 3.5 oz, 100 gm	220	24	13	0	0	11	1.35	73	176	84
1 leg, 125 gm	275	30	16	0	0	14	1.69	92	220	105
LEG, FLESH WITHOUT SKIN										

FOOD & DESCRIPTION MEASURE OR QUANTITY	CALORIES	PROTEIN (GM)	FAT (GM)	CARBO-HYDRATE (GM)	FIBER (GM)	CALCIUM (MG)	IRON (MG)	SODIUM (MG)	POTASSIUM (MG)	CHOLES-TEROL (MG)
fried, 3.5 oz, 100 gm	208	28	9	<1	0	13	1.40	96	254	99
1 leg, 94 gm	195	27	9	<1	0	12	1.31	90	239	93
roasted, 3.5 oz, 100 gm	191	27	8	0	0	12	1.31	91	242	94
1 leg, 95 gm	182	26	8	0	0	12	1.24	87	230	89
stewed, 3.5 oz	185	26	8	0	0	11	1.40	78	190	89
1 leg, 101 gm	187	27	8	0	0	11	1.41	78	192	90
NECK, FLESH WITH SKIN										
batter-dipped, fried, 3.5 oz, 100 gm	330	20	24	9	.03	31	2.15	276	151	91
1 neck, 52 gm	172	10	12	5	.02	16	1.12	143	78	47
flour-coated, fried, 3.5 oz, 100 gm	332	24	24	4	.02	31	2.42	82	180	94
1 neck, 36 gm	119	9	9	2	.01	11	.87	29	65	34
simmered, 3.5 oz, 100 gm	247	20	18	0	0	27	2.30	52	108	70
1 neck, 38 gm	94	7	7	0	0	10	.87	20	41	27
NECK, FLESH WITHOUT SKIN										
fried, 3.5 oz, 100 gm	229	27	12	2	.01	41	2.98	99	213	105
1 neck, 22 gm	50	6	3	<1	0	9	.66	22	47	23
simmered, 3.5 oz, 100 gm	179	25	8	0	0	44	2.63	64	140	79
1 neck, 18 gm	32	4	1	0	0	8	.47	12	25	14
THIGH, FLESH WITH SKIN										
batter-dipped, fried, 3.5 oz, 100 gm	277	22	17	9	.04	18	1.45	288	192	93
1 thigh, 86 gm	238	19	14	8	.03	16	1.24	248	165	80
flour-coated, fried, 3.5 oz, 100 gm	262	27	15	3	.01	14	1.49	88	237	97
1 thigh, 62 gm	162	17	9	2	.01	8	.93	55	147	60
roasted, 3.5 oz, 100 gm	247	25	15	0	0	12	1.34	84	222	93
1 thigh, 62 gm	153	16	10	0	0	8	.83	52	137	58
stewed, 3.5 oz, 100 gm	232	23	15	0	0	11	1.37	71	170	84
1 thigh, 68 gm	158	16	10	0	0	8	.93	49	115	57
THIGH, FLESH WITHOUT SKIN										
fried, 3.5 oz, 100 gm	218	28	10	1	.01	13	1.46	95	259	102
1 thigh, 52 gm	113	15	5	<1	0	7	.76	49	134	53
roasted, 3.5 oz, 100 gm	209	26	11	0	0	12	1.31	88	238	95
1 thigh, 52 gm	109	13	6	0	0	6	.68	46	124	49
stewed, 3.5 oz, 100 gm	195	25	10	0	0	11	1.42	75	183	90
1 thigh, 55 gm	107	14	5	0	0	6	.78	41	101	49
WING, FLESH WITH SKIN										
batter-dipped, fried, 3.5 oz, 100 gm	324	20	22	11	.04	20	1.29	320	138	79
1 wing, 49 gm	159	10	11	5	.02	10	.63	157	68	39
flour-coated, fried, 3.5 oz, 100 gm	321	26	22	2	.01	15	1.25	77	177	81
1 wing, 32 gm	103	8	7	<1	0	5	.40	25	57	26
roasted, 3.5 oz, 100 gm	290	27	19	0	0	15	1.27	82	184	84
1 wing, 34 gm	99	9	7	0	0	5	.43	28	62	29
stewed, 3.5 oz, 100 gm	249	23	17	0	0	12	1.13	67	139	70
1 wing, 40 gm	100	9	7	0	0	5	.45	27	56	28
WING, FLESH WITHOUT SKIN										
fried, 3.5 oz, 100 gm	211	30	9	0	0	15	1.14	91	208	84
1 wing, 20 gm	42	6	2	0	0	3	.23	18	42	17
roasted, 3.5 oz, 100 gm	203	30	8	0	0	16	1.16	92	210	85
1 wing, 21 gm	43	6	2	0	0	3	.24	19	44	18
stewed, 3.5 oz, 100 gm	181	27	7	0	0	13	1.12	73	153	74
1 wing, 24 gm	43	7	2	0	0	3	.27	18	37	18
CHICKEN, ROASTING [Figures are for a 4½-pound chicken, approximately.]										
FLESH WITH SKIN										
roasted, 3.5 oz, 100 gm	223	24	13	0	0	12	1.26	73	211	76
½ chicken, 480 gm	1071	115	64	0	0	58	6.05	349	1014	365
FLESH WITHOUT SKIN										

FOOD & DESCRIPTION MEASURE OR QUANTITY	CALORIES	PROTEIN (GM)	FAT (GM)	CARBO-HYDRATE (GM)	FIBER (GM)	CALCIUM (MG)	IRON (MG)	SODIUM (MG)	POTASSIUM (MG)	CHOLES-TEROL (MG)
roasted, 3.5 oz, 100 gm	167	25	7	0	0	12	.1.21	75	229	75
1 c, 140 gm	233	35	9	0	0	16	1.70	105	321	104
½ chicken, 390 gm	651	98	26	0	0	47	4.72	293	893	293
GIBLETS, 1 each of GIZZARD, HEART & LIVER, simmered, 68 gm	112	18	4	<1	0	8	4.14	41	109	243
1 c, 145 gm	239	39	8	1	0	18	8.83	86	232	517
LIGHT FLESH										
roasted, 3.5 oz, 100 gm	153	27	4	0	0	13	1.08	51	236	75
1 c, 140 gm	214	38	6	0	0	18	1.51	71	330	105
½ chicken, 177 gm	271	48	7	0	0	23	1.91	90	418	133
DARK FLESH										
roasted, 3.5 oz, 100 gm	178	23	9	0	0	11	1.33	95	224	75
1 c, 140 gm	250	33	12	0	0	15	1.86	133	313	104
½ chicken, 214 gm	381	50	19	0	0	24	2.85	203	479	161
CHICKEN, STEWING [Figures are for a 2.9-pound chicken, approximately.]										
FLESH WITH SKIN										
stewed, 3.5 oz, 100 gm	285	27	19	0	0	13	1.37	73	182	79
½ chicken, 261 gm	744	70	49	0	0	33	3.56	190	476	205
FLESH WITHOUT SKIN										
STEWED, 3.5 oz, 100 gm	237	30	12	0	0	13	1.43	78	202	83
1 c, 140 gm	332	43	17	0	0	18	2.01	109	282	117
½ chicken, 201 gm	476	61	24	0	0	26	2.87	157	406	167
GIBLETS, 1 EACH OF GIZZARD, HEART & LIVER, simmered, 50 gm	97	13	5	<1	0	7	3.22	28	77	178
1 c, 145 gm	281	37	13	<1	0	19	9.33	81	224	515
LIGHT FLESH, stewed, 3.5 oz, 100 gm	213	33	8	0	0	14	1.19	58	199	70
1 c, 140 gm	298	46	11	0	0	19	1.67	81	279	98
½ chicken, 94 gm	200	31	8	0	0	13	1.12	55	187	66
DARK FLESH, stewed, 3.5 oz, 100 gm	258	28	15	0	0	12	1.64	95	204	95
1 c, 140 gm	361	39	21	0	0	17	2.30	133	285	132
½ chicken, 108 gm	279	30	17	0	0	13	1.77	103	220	103
DUCK, DOMESTICATED [Figures are for a 1.94-pound duck, approximately.]										
FLESH WITH SKIN, roasted, 3.5 oz, 100 gm	337	19	28	0	0	11	2.70	59	204	84
½ duck, 382 gm	1287	73	108	0	0	43	10.31	227	780	320
FLESH WITHOUT SKIN, roasted, 3.5 oz, 100 gm	201	23	11	0	0	12	2.7	65	252	89
½ duck, 221 gm	445	52	25	0	0	26	5.97	143	557	198
GOOSE, DOMESTICATED, [Figures are for a 3.59-pound goose, approximately.]										
FLESH WITH SKIN, roasted, 3.5 oz, 100 gm	305	25	22	0	0	13	2.83	70	329	91
½ goose, 774 gm	2362	195	170	0	0	104	21.90	543	2546	708
FLESH WITHOUT SKIN, roasted, 3.5 oz, 100 gm	238	29	13	0	0	14	2.87	76	388	96
½ goose, 591 gm	1406	171	75	0	0	84	16.96	447	2291	569
TURKEY, all classes [Figures are for a 15.45-pound turkey, approximately.]										
FLESH WITH SKIN, roasted, 3.5 oz, 100 gm	208	28	10	0	0	26	1.79	68	280	82

FOOD & DESCRIPTION MEASURE OR QUANTITY	CALORIES	PROTEIN (GM)	FAT (GM)	CARBO-HYDRATE (GM)	FIBER (GM)	CALCIUM (MG)	IRON (MG)	SODIUM (MG)	POTASSIUM (MG)	CHOLES-TEROL (MG)
FLESH WITHOUT SKIN,										
roasted, 3.5 oz, 100 gm	170	29	5	0	0	25	1.78	70	298	76
1 c, 140 gm	238	41	7	0	0	35	2.49	99	418	107
GIBLETS, 1 each of										
GIZZARD, HEART &										
LIVER										
SIMMERED										
1 of each, 158 gm	264	42	8	3	0	21	10.60	93	316	660
1 c, 145 gm	243	39	7	3	0	18	9.72	85	291	606
GIZZARD, simmered										
1 c, 145 gm	236	43	6	<1	0	22	7.88	79	306	336
1 gizzard, 67 gm	109	20	3	<1	0	10	3.64	36	141	155
HEART, simmered										
1 c, 145 gm	257	39	9	3	0	19	9.98	79	265	327
1 heart, 16 gm	28	4	<1	<1	0	2	1.10	9	29	36
LIVER, simmered										
1 c, 140 gm	237	34	8	5	0	15	10.92	89	272	876
1 liver, 75 gm	127	18	4	3	0	8	5.85	48	146	470
NECK, FLESH WITHOUT										
SKIN, 1 neck, 152 gm	274	41	11	0	0	56	3.49	84	226	186
LIGHT FLESH WITH SKIN,										
roasted, 3.5 oz, 100 gm	197	29	8	0	0	21	1.41	63	285	76
½ turkey, 1050 gm	2069	300	87	0	0	225	14.84	658	2996	794
DARK FLESH WITH SKIN,										
roasted, 3.5 oz, 100 gm	221	27	12	0	0	33	2.27	76	274	89
½ turkey, 808 gm	1789	222	93	0	0	263	18.37	612	2214	720
LIGHT FLESH WITHOUT										
SKIN, roasted, 3.5 oz,										
100 gm	157	30	3	0	0	19	1.35	64	305	69
1 c, 140 gm	219	42	5	0	0	27	1.88	89	426	97
½ turkey, 906 gm	1422	271	29	0	0	172	12.23	580	2763	625
DARK FLESH WITHOUT SKIN,										
roasted, 3.5 oz, 100 gm	187	29	7	0	0	32	2.33	79	290	85
1 c, 140 gm	262	40	10	0	0	45	3.27	110	406	119
½ turkey, 704 gm	1316	201	51	0	0	225	16.40	556	2042	598
BACK, FLESH WITH SKIN,										
roasted, 3.5 oz, 100 gm	243	27	14	0	0	33	2.19	73	260	91
½ back, 262 gm	637	70	38	0	0	87	5.74	191	682	238
BREAST, FLESH WITH SKIN,										
roasted, 3.5 oz, 100 gm	189	29	7	0	0	21	1.40	63	288	74
½ breast, 864 gm	1637	248	64	0	0	182	12.05	541	2491	643
LEG, FLESH WITH SKIN,										
roasted, 3.5 oz, 100 gm	208	28	10	0	0	32	2.30	77	280	85
1 leg, 546 gm	1133	152	54	0	0	176	12.56	420	1530	466
WING, FLESH WITH SKIN,										
roasted, 3.5 oz, 100 gm	229	27	12	0	0	24	1.46	61	266	81
1 wing, 186 gm	426	51	23	0	0	44	2.72	114	494	150
FRYER-ROASTER TURKEY										
[Figures are for a										
7-pound turkey,										
approximately.]										
FLESH WITH SKIN, roasted,										
3.5 oz, 100 gm	172	28	6	0	0	22	1.95	66	250	105
½ turkey, 808 gm	1392	228	46	0	0	180	15.72	532	2023	849
FLESH WITHOUT SKIN,										
roasted, 3.5 oz, 100 gm	150	30	3	0	0	20	1.96	67	263	98
1 c, 140 gm	210	41	4	0	0	28	2.75	94	368	138
½ turkey, 687 gm	1031	203	18	0	0	137	13.00	460	1807	673
LIGHT FLESH WITH SKIN,										
roasted, 3.5 oz, 100 gm	164	29	5	0	0	18	1.61	57	262	95
½ turkey, 433 gm	711	125	20	0	0	77	6.98	247	1135	413
DARK FLESH WITH SKIN,										
roasted, 3.5 oz, 100 gm	182	28	7	0	0	27	2.33	76	237	117
½ turkey, 374 gm	680	104	26	0	0	103	8.73	285	885	436

FOOD & DESCRIPTION MEASURE OR QUANTITY	CALORIES	PROTEIN (GM)	FAT (GM)	CARBO-HYDRATE (GM)	FIBER (GM)	CALCIUM (MG)	IRON (MG)	SODIUM (MG)	POTASSIUM (MG)	CHOLES-TEROL (MG)
LIGHT FLESH WITHOUT SKIN, roasted, 3.5 oz, 100 gm	140	30	1	0	0	15	1.57	56	277	86
1 c, 140 gm	195	42	2	0	0	20	2.20	79	388	121
½ turkey, 367 gm	514	111	4	0	0	55	5.76	206	1017	316
DARK FLESH WITHOUT SKIN, roasted, 3.5 oz, 100 gm	162	29	4	0	0	26	2.41	79	246	112
1 c, 140 gm	227	40	6	0	0	37	3.38	110	345	157
½ turkey, 320 gm	518	92	14	0	0	83	7.71	253	787	358
BACK, FLESH WITH SKIN, roasted, 3.5 oz, 100 gm	204	26	10	0	0	36	1.85	70	208	108
½ back, 130 gm	265	34	13	0	0	47	2.41	90	270	140
BACK, FLESH WITHOUT SKIN, roasted, 3.5 oz, 100 gm	170	28	6	0	0	36	1.85	73	217	95
½ back, 96 gm	164	27	5	0	0	35	1.77	70	209	91
BREAST, FLESH WITH SKIN, roasted, 3.5 oz, 100 gm	153	29	3	0	0	15	1.57	53	279	90
½ breast, 344 gm	526	100	11	0	0	51	5.38	182	961	310
BREAST, FLESH WITHOUT SKIN, roasted, 3.5 oz, 100 gm	135	30	<1	0	0	12	1.53	52	292	83
½ breast, 306 gm	413	92	2	0	0	38	4.68	159	892	255
LEG, FLESH WITH SKIN, roasted, 3.5 oz, 100 gm	170	28	5	0	0	23	2.59	80	252	70
1 leg, 245 gm	418	70	13	0	0	56	6.35	195	617	171
LEG, FLESH WITHOUT SKIN, roasted, 3.5 oz, 100 gm	159	29	4	0	0	22	2.66	81	258	119
1 leg, 224 gm	355	65	8	0	0	49	5.95	182	579	267
WING, FLESH WITH SKIN, roasted, 3.5 oz, 100 gm	207	28	10	0	0	29	1.81	73	196	115
1 wing, 90 gm	186	25	9	0	0	26	1.62	65	177	104
WING, FLESH WITHOUT SKIN, roasted, 3.5 oz, 100 gm	163	31	3	0	0	26	1.78	78	204	102
1 wing, 60 gm	98	19	2	0	0	15	1.07	47	122	61
TURKEY, YOUNG HEN [Figures are for a 12½-pound turkey, approximately.]										
FLESH WITH SKIN, roasted, 3.5 oz, 100 gm	218	28	11	0	0	26	1.78	64	282	78
½ turkey, 1524 gm	3323	428	166	0	0	399	27.16	977	4291	1190
FLESH WITHOUT SKIN, roasted, 3.5 oz, 100 gm	175	29	6	0	0	25	1.76	67	299	73
1 c, 140 gm	244	41	8	0	0	35	2.46	93	418	102
½ turkey, 1328 gm	2324	388	73	0	0	332	23.37	890	3971	969
LIGHT FLESH WITH SKIN, roasted, 3.5 oz, 100 gm	207	29	9	0	0	23	1.39	58	286	74
½ turkey, 859 gm	1778	246	81	0	0	195	11.96	501	2454	633
DARK FLESH WITH SKIN, roasted, 3.5 oz, 100 gm	232	27	13	0	0	31	2.28	72	276	84
½ turkey, 665 gm	1544	182	85	0	0	204	15.18	476	1836	557
LIGHT FLESH WITHOUT SKIN, roasted, 3.5 oz, 100 gm	161	30	4	0	0	21	1.31	60	304	68
1 c, 140 gm	226	42	5	0	0	29	1.83	84	425	95
½ turkey, 748 gm	1204	224	28	0	0	157	9.80	449	2274	509
DARK FLESH WITHOUT SKIN, roasted, 3.5 oz, 100 gm	192	28	8	0	0	30	2.33	75	292	80
1 c, 140 gm	268	40	11	0	0	42	3.26	105	409	111
½ turkey, 580 gm	1114	165	45	0	0	174	13.51	435	1694	464
BACK, FLESH WITH SKIN, roasted, 3.5 oz, 100 gm	254	26	16	0	0	31	2.22	69	263	85
½ back, 217 gm	551	57	34	0	0	67	4.81	149	571	185

FOOD & DESCRIPTION MEASURE OR QUANTITY	CALORIES	PROTEIN (GM)	FAT (GM)	CARBO-HYDRATE (GM)	FIBER (GM)	CALCIUM (MG)	IRON (MG)	SODIUM (MG)	POTASSIUM (MG)	CHOLES-TEROL (MG)
BREAST, FLESH WITH SKIN,										
roasted, 3.5 oz, 100 gm	194	29	8	0	0	22	1.36	58	289	72
½ breast, 686 gm	1330	198	54	0	0	152	9.33	401	1980	492
LEG, FLESH WITH SKIN,										
roasted, 3.5 oz, 100 gm	213	28	11	0	0	30	2.29	73	282	82
1 leg, 448 gm	955	124	47	0	0	136	10.25	326	1264	365
WING, FLESH WITH SKIN,										
roasted, 3.5 oz, 100 gm	238	27	13	0	0	24	1.43	56	268	77
1 leg, 174 gm	414	48	23	0	0	41	2.49	98	467	134
TURKEY, YOUNG TOM										
[Figures are for a										
23-pound turkey,										
approximately.]										
FLESH WITH SKIN, roasted,										
3.5 oz, 100 gm	202	28	9	0	0	27	1.78	72	282	82
½ turkey, 2750 gm	5545	773	249	0	0	735	48.87	1993	7761	2265
FLESH WITHOUT SKIN,										
roasted, 3.5 oz, 100 gm	168	29	5	0	0	25	1.78	74	301	77
1 c, 140 gm	235	41	7	0	0	35	2.49	104	422	108
½ turkey, 2376 gm	3992	698	111	0	0	594	42.29	1758	7152	1830
LIGHT FLESH WITH SKIN,										
roasted, 3.5 oz, 100 gm	191	28	8	0	0	21	1.41	67	287	75
½ turkey, 1566 gm	2992	446	121	0	0	323	22.13	1051	4495	1182
DARK FLESH WITH SKIN,										
roasted, 3.5 oz, 100 gm	216	28	11	0	0	35	2.26	80	276	91
½ turkey, 1184 gm	2553	327	128	0	0	413	26.73	942	3268	1081
LIGHT FLESH WITHOUT										
SKIN, roasted, 3.5 oz,										
100 gm	154	30	3	0	0	18	1.36	68	308	69
1 c, 140 gm	215	42	4	0	0	25	1.90	95	431	97
½ turkey, 1344 gm	2070	402	39	0	0	242	18.28	914	4140	927
DARK FLESH WITHOUT SKIN,										
roasted, 3.5 oz, 100 gm	185	29	7	0	0	35	2.33	82	293	88
1 c, 140 gm	260	40	10	0	0	48	3.26	115	410	123
½ turkey, 1033 gm	1911	296	72	0	0	362	24.07	847	3027	909
BACK, FLESH WITH SKIN,										
roasted, 3.5 oz, 100 gm	238	27	14	0	0	35	2.21	77	264	94
½ back, 380 gm	903	102	52	0	0	133	8.38	294	1002	358
BREAST, FLESH WITH SKIN,										
roasted, 3.5 oz, 100 gm	189	29	7	0	0	21	1.41	67	289	75
½ breast, 1329 gm	2510	380	98	0	0	273	18.74	892	3839	1002
LEG, FLESH WITH SKIN,										
roasted, 3.5 oz, 100 gm	206	28	10	0	0	35	2.28	80	281	90
1 leg, 805 gm	1660	225	78	0	0	280	18.36	648	2264	727
WING, FLESH WITH SKIN,										
roasted, 3.5 oz, 100 gm	221	27	12	0	0	23	1.46	66	271	81
1 wing, 237 gm	524	65	27	0	0	54	3.46	157	643	192

Processed Poultry

Banquet

BREADED CHICKEN NUGGETS,										
3 oz, 85 gm	233	14	14	14	—	9	.90	169	44	—
BREADED CHICKEN PATTIES,										
3 oz, 85 gm	225	13	14	13	—	8	.90	151	44	—
BREADED CHICKEN STICKS, 3										
oz, 85 gm	228	14	13	15	—	8	.90	166	47	—
FRIED CHICKEN, 6.4 oz, 181										
gm	325	18	19	20	—	21	1.00	1201	144	—
FRIED CHICKEN, BREAST										
PORTION, 4.4 oz, 125										
gm	238	17	12	14	—	16	1.00	772	141	—
FRIED CHICKEN, THIGH &										

FOOD & DESCRIPTION MEASURE OR QUANTITY	CALORIES	PROTEIN (GM)	FAT (GM)	CARBO-HYDRATE (GM)	FIBER (GM)	CALCIUM (MG)	IRON (MG)	SODIUM (MG)	POTASSIUM (MG)	CHOLES-TEROL (MG)
DRUMSTICKS, 5 oz, 142 gm	277	16	16	16	—	16	1.00	892	136	—
FRIED CHICKEN, WING PORTION, 6.75 oz, 191 gm	346	16	22	21	—	22	1.00	1226	117	—

Featherweight

CHICKEN, cnd, 3 oz, 85 gm	186	20	11	0	—	—	—	38	129	—

Hormel

CHUNK BREAST OF CHICKEN, cnd, 6.75 oz, 191 gm	350	41	20	0	—	—	—	855	—	—
CHUNK DARK CHICKEN, cnd, 6.75 oz, 191 gm	327	42	18	0	—	—	—	933	—	—
CHUNK TURKEY, cnd, 6.75 oz, 191 gm	230	37	10	0	—	—	—	1278	—	—
CHUNK WHITE & DARK CHICKEN, cnd, 6.75 oz, 191 gm	340	39	20	0	—	—	—	857	—	—
SALT-FREE, 6.75 oz, 191 gm	330	42	18	0	—	—	—	75	—	—

Land O'Lakes

BUTTER BASTED YOUNG TURKEY, 3 oz, 85 gm	140	17	8	<1	—	*	.72	135	265	85
BUTTERMOIST TURKEY ROAST										
WHITE, WITH GRAVY, 3 oz, 85 gm	110	14	5	1	—	*	.72	510	170	20
WHITE/DARK, WITH GRAVY, 3 oz, 85 gm	120	13	7	1	—	*	1.08	490	155	20
DICED TURKEY, WHITE/DARK MIXED, 3 oz, 85 gm	120	15	6	<1	—	20	1.08	590	160	35
OVEN-COOKED TURKEY BREAST										
BRONZE LABEL, 3 oz, 85 gm	100	15	4	2	—	*	.72	510	220	50
GOLD LABEL										
BROWNED, 3 oz, 85 gm	120	19	5	0	—	*	.72	635	235	55
SKINLESS, 3 oz, 85 gm	90	21	1	0	—	*	.36	715	215	50
SKIN ON, 3 oz, 85 gm	120	20	4	0	—	*	.72	640	210	55
SILVER LABEL, 3 oz, 85 gm	100	19	2	0	—	*	.36	565	210	50
SELF-BASTING YOUNG TURKEY (with broth), 3 oz, 85 gm	120	18	5	<1	—	*	.72	145	265	77
TURKEY										
BREAST, 3 oz, 85 gm	100	20	1	0	—	*	1.08	55	260	50
BREAST FILLETS WITH CHEESE, 5 oz, 142 gm	300	25	16	16	—	150	1.44	835	315	35
DRUMSTICKS, 3 oz, 85 gm	120	17	5	0	—	*	1.08	85	245	—
HINDQUARTER ROAST, 3 oz, 85 gm	140	17	8	0	—	*	1.08	80	240	—
PATTIES, 2.25 oz, 64 gm	170	8	11	10	—	40	1.44	330	80	30
ROLLS										
BLUE LABEL										
MIXED, 3 oz, 85 gm	120	14	6	1	—	*	.72	550	175	50
WHITE, 3 oz, 85 gm	110	14	5	2	—	*	.36	560	185	50
RED LABEL										
MIXED, 3 oz, 85 gm	110	13	5	4	—	*	1.08	510	245	50
WHITE, 3 oz, 85 gm	110	14	5	3	—	*	1.08	530	225	50
STICKS, 2 oz, 57 gm	150	7	10	9	—	20	1.08	295	70	25
THIGHS, 3 oz, 85 gm	150	17	10	0	—	*	1.08	75	230	—
WINGS, 3 oz, 85 gm	120	18	5	0	—	*	.36	65	205	—

FOOD & DESCRIPTION MEASURE OR QUANTITY	CALORIES	PROTEIN (GM)	FAT (GM)	CARBO-HYDRATE (GM)	FIBER (GM)	CALCIUM (MG)	IRON (MG)	SODIUM (MG)	POTASSIUM (MG)	CHOLES-TEROL (MG)
Louis Rich										
BARBEQUED BREAST OF TURKEY, 1 oz, 28 gm	40	6	1	0	—	2	.12	156	57	16
HICKORY SMOKED BREAST OF TURKEY, 1 oz, 28 gm	35	6	1	<1	—	1	.20	208	59	13
OVEN ROASTED BREAST OF TURKEY, 1 oz, 28 gm	35	6	1	0	—	1	.16	149	54	15
OVEN ROASTED TURKEY BREAST, 1 sl, 28 gm	30	6	<1	<1	—	2	.13	214	63	10
SMOKED TURKEY, 1 oz, 28 gm	30	5	1	<1	—	2	.13	272	65	12
SMOKED TURKEY BREAST, 1 sl, 21 gm	20	4	<1	<1	—	1	.09	181	52	6
SMOKED TURKEY DRUMSTICKS, 1 oz, 28 gm	40	6	2	<1	—	6	.40	399	55	23
SMOKED TURKEY WING DRUMMETTES, 1 oz, 28 gm	45	7	2	<1	—	4	.18	285	53	22
TURKEY BREAST, ckd, 1 oz, 28 gm	45	9	2	0	—	2	.25	25	67	12
TURKEY BREAST SLICES, ckd, 1 oz, 28 gm	40	9	<1	0	—	1	.26	24	98	12
TURKEY BREAST TENDERLOINS, ckd, 1 oz, 28 gm	40	9	<1	0	—	1	.26	29	97	10
TURKEY DRUMSTICKS, ckd, 1 oz, 28 gm	60	8	3	0	—	3	.67	24	45	33
TURKEY, GROUND, ckd, 1 oz, 28 gm	65	7	4	0	—	8	.46	32	66	26
TURKEY WINGS, ckd, 1 oz, 28 gm	55	8	3	0	—	2	.29	21	36	26
Swanson–Campbell										
CHUNK PREMIUM WHITE CHICKEN IN WATER, cnd, 2.5 oz, 71 gm	90	17	2	0	—	*	.36	230	—	—
CHUNK STYLE MIXIN' CHICKEN, cnd, 2.5 oz, 71 gm	130	14	8	0	—	20	.72	225		
CHUNK WHITE AND DARK CHICKEN IN WATER, cnd, 2.5 oz, 71 gm	100	16	3	0	—	*	.72	240	—	—
CHICKEN CUTLETS, 3.5 oz, 100 gm	230	14	13	14	—	*	1.08	440	—	—
CHICKEN DIPSTERS, 3 oz, 85 gm	220	11	14	13	—	*	1.08	400	—	—
CHICKEN DRUMLETS, 3 oz, 85 gm	220	11	13	15	—	*	1.08	390	—	—
CHICKEN NIBBLES (wing sections), 3.25 oz, 92 gm	300	13	20	16	—	20	1.80	640	—	—
FRIED CHICKEN BREAST QUARTERS, 4.5 oz, 128 gm	350	22	21	19	—	20	2.70	830	—	—
FRIED CHICKEN, ASSORTED PIECES, 3.25 oz, 92 gm	270	15	17	13	—	20	1.44	600	—	—
TAKE-OUT FRIED CHICKEN, ASSORTED PIECES, 3.25 oz, 92 gm	270	17	17	13	—	20	1.80	660	—	—
THIGHS & DRUMSTICKS, 3.25 oz, 92 gm	280	16	19	11	—	20	1.44	550	—	—

FOOD & DESCRIPTION MEASURE OR QUANTITY	CALORIES	PROTEIN (GM)	FAT (GM)	CARBO-HYDRATE (GM)	FIBER (GM)	CALCIUM (MG)	IRON (MG)	SODIUM (MG)	POTASSIUM (MG)	CHOLES-TEROL (MG)
Tyson										
BREAST FILLETS, 3 oz, 85 gm	190	15	8	14	—	—	—	—	—	—
BREAST PATTIE, 3 oz, 85 gm	240	13	17	10	—	—	—	—	—	—
CHICKEN CHEDDAR, 3 oz, 85 gm	260	13	17	13	—	—	—	—	—	—
CHICKEN CHUNKS, 6 chunks, 3 oz, 85 gm	250	13	16	13	—	—	—	—	—	—
CHICKEN KIEV, 5 oz, 142 gm	430	20	31	18	—	—	—	—	—	—
CHICKEN STICKS, 3 sticks, 3 oz, 85 gm	240	13	15	14	—	—	—	—	—	—
CORDON BLEU, 5 oz, 142 gm	310	23	15	19	—	—	—	—	—	—
ITALIAN HOAGIE, 3 oz, 85 gm	250	12	17	12	—	—	—	—	—	—
SWISS 'N BACON, 3 oz, 85 gm	280	12	20	14	—	—	—	—	—	—
TURKEY PATTIE, 3 oz, 85 gm	220	13	14	12	—	—	—	—	—	—
USDA										
CHICKEN, cnd, boned, with broth, 5 oz, 142 gm	234	31	11	0	0	20	2.25	714	196	—
GRAVY & TURKEY, fz, 3.5 oz, 100 gm	67	6	3	5	.3	14	.93	554	—	—
1 c, 240 gm	160	14	6	11	.71	33	2.22	1328	—	—
TURKEY, cnd, boned, with broth, 5 oz, 142 gm	231	34	10	0	0	17	2.64	663	—	—
TURKEY PATTIES, breaded, fried										
3.33 oz, 94 gm	266	13	17	15	—	13	2.07	752	259	—
2.25 oz, 64 gm	181	9	12	10	—	9	1.41	512	176	—
TURKEY, prebasted BREAST, FLESH WITH SKIN, roasted, 3.5 oz, 100 gm	126	22	3	0	0	9	.66	397	248	42
½ breast, 864 gm	1087	191	30	0	0	75	5.71	3434	2141	359
THIGH, FLESH WITH SKIN, roasted, 3.5 oz, 100 gm	157	19	9	0	0	8	1.51	437	241	62
1 thigh, 314 gm	494	59	27	0	0	25	4.74	1371	758	194
TURKEY ROAST, LIGHT & DARK FLESH, boneless, seasoned, roasted, 3.5 oz, 100 gm	155	21	6	3	—	5	1.63	680	298	53
TURKEY STICKS, breaded, battered, fried, 3.5 oz, 100 gm	279	14	17	17	—	14	2.20	838	260	—
1 stick, 2.25 oz, 64 gm	178	9	11	11	—	9	1.41	536	166	—

18

SAUCES & GRAVIES

FOOD & DESCRIPTION MEASURE OR QUANTITY	CALORIES	PROTEIN (GM)	FAT (GM)	CARBO- HYDRATE (GM)	FIBER (GM)	CALCIUM (MG)	IRON (MG)	SODIUM (MG)	POTASSIUM (MG)	CHOLES- TEROL (MG)
Cantisano										
CANTISANO or FRANCESCO RINALDI SPAGHETTI SAUCE, all flavors, 4 oz	80	2	4	9	—	*	1.08	570	—	—
NO SALT, NO SUGAR, 4 oz	80	2	4	9	—	*	1.08	35	—	—
Catelli										
MARINARA SAUCE, 5.3 oz, 159 gm	61	1	1	11	.38	16	1.24	938	335	—
MEAT SAUCE, 5.3 oz, 161 gm	142	6	9	9	.56	27	2.40	1095	486	—
MUSHROOM SAUCE, 5.3 oz, 160 gm	92	2	4	13	.58	23	1.68	1216	475	—
OLD FASHIONED SPAGHETTI SAUCE										
GARLIC, 5.3 oz, 159 gm	107	3	5	12	.80	12	2.39	811	633	—
HOT & SPICY, 5.3 oz, 159 gm	103	3	5	11	.80	12	2.39	827	633	—
MILD, 5.3 oz, 159 gm	105	3	5	13	.80	12	2.39	827	636	—
PIZZA PRONTO, MILD, 2 tbsp, 30 gm	17	<1	<1	3	.11	4	.41	186	107	—
SPICY, 2 tbsp, 30 gm	16	<1	<1	3	.11	4	.41	182	107	—
TOMATO SAUCE, 5.3 oz, 160 gm	88	2	6	12	.56	25	1.68	1072	443	—
Del Monte										
BURRITO SALSA, ¼ c, 57 gm	20	0	0	4	—	0	*	355	75	—
ENCHILADA SAUCE, HOT, ½ c, 113.5 gm	45	1	0	11	—	20	.72	1090	250	—
MILD, ½ c, 113.5 gm	45	1	0	11	—	20	1.08	1150	310	—
GREEN CHILE SALSA, MILD, ¼ c, 57 gm	20	0	0	3	—	20	*	590	120	—
SALSA PICANTA, HOT, ¼ c, 57 gm	20	0	0	4	—	20	.36	385	125	—
HOT AND CHUNKY, ¼ c, 57 gm	15	0	0	3	—	20	.36	405	125	—
SALSA ROJA, MILD, ¼ c, 57 gm	20	0	0	4	—	0	.36	510	125	—
TACO SAUCE, HOT, ¼ c, 57 gm	15	0	0	4	—	0	.36	440	115	—
MILD, ¼ c, 57 gm	15	0	0	4	—	0	.36	480	105	—
TACO STARTER, 8 oz, 227 gm	140	3	1	28	—	60	2.70	2180	765	—
Dia-Mel										
SPAGHETTI SAUCE, 4 oz	70	2	2	13	—	—	—	30	—	0

FOOD & DESCRIPTION MEASURE OR QUANTITY	CALORIES	PROTEIN (GM)	FAT (GM)	CARBO-HYDRATE (GM)	FIBER (GM)	CALCIUM (MG)	IRON (MG)	SODIUM (MG)	POTASSIUM (MG)	CHOLES-TEROL (MG)
Durkee										
A LA KING SAUCE MIX, prep,										
1 c	133	1	8	14	—	—	—	1384	31	—
AU JUS										
MIX, prep, 2 c	62	4	<1	13	—	—	—	1826	1	—
ROASTIN' BAG, 28.3 gm	64	<1	1	14	—	—	—	2628	38	—
BEEF STEW MIX, 49.6 gm,	99	<1	<1	22	—	—	—	6953	9	—
prep with beef, shortening,										
vegetables, 8 c	3032	182	192	134	—	—	—	7800	3167	—
BROWN GRAVY MIX, prep, 1 c	59	3	<1	10	—	—	—	1037	19	—
WITH MUSHROOMS, prep, 1 c	59	<1	<1	11	—	—	—	1402	115	—
WITH ONIONS, prep, 1 c	66	2	<1	13	—	—	—	1356	56	—
CHEESE SAUCE MIX, 31.9 gm	157	7	8	13	—	—	—	796	42	—
with 1 c milk, 1 c	316	16	17	25	—	—	—	1098	393	—
CHICKEN										
CREAMY GRAVY MIX, prep,										
1 c	156	3	9	14	—	—	—	1528	24	—
CREAMY GRAVY ROASTIN'										
BAG, 56.7 gm	242	4	12	22	—	—	—	2528	19	—
GRAVY MIX, prep, 1 c	92	2	1	15	—	—	—	1537	56	—
GRAVY ROASTIN' BAG,										
42.53 gm	122	3	1	24	—	—	—	3597	121	—
ITALIAN STYLE ROASTIN'										
BAG, dry, 42.5 gm	144	15	1	31	—	—	—	3614	103	—
CHILI CON CARNE MIX, 49.6										
gm	148	2	2	33	—	—	—	3239	155	—
with ground beef, tomatoes &										
kidney beans, 4 c	1859	150	100	125	—	—	—	3915	3317	—
CHOP SUEY SEASONING, 42.5										
gm	128	2	2	19	—	—	—	828	77	—
with pork & vegetables,										
3.5 c	1113	108	65	42	—	—	—	1274	9379	—
CREAMY DILL SAUCE FOR										
FISH ROASTIN' BAG,										
31.89 gm	153	<1	14	4	—	—	—	741	—	—
ENCHILADA SAUCE MIX,										
31.9 gm	89	3	2	18	—	—	—	320	177	—
with tomato paste, 4 c	229	8	2	50	—	—	—	385	1688	—
FRIED RICE SEASONING MIX,										
28.4 gm	62	2	1	11	—	—	—	1931	85	—
with rice, 2 c	430	8	1	93	—	—	—	2698	180	—
GROUND BEEF MIX, 31.9 gm	91	3	<1	18	—	—	—	1314	162	—
with ground beef, 2 c	1307	84	97	18	—	—	—	1598	1461	—
GROUND BEEF WITH ONION,										
dry, 31.8 gm	102	3	—	13	—	—	—	1914	18	—
with ground beef, prep, 2 c	1318	84	96	13	—	—	—	2198	1317	—
HAMBURGER SEASONING										
MIX, 28.3 gm	110	2	5	15	—	—	—	1739	2	—
with ground beef, 2 c	1326	83	101	15	—	—	—	2023	1301	—
HOLLANDAISE SAUCE MIX,										
prep, ¾ c	173	9	14	11	—	—	—	548	23	—
HOMESTYLE GRAVY MIX,										
prep, 1 c	70	<1	2	11	—	—	—	830	40	—
ITALIAN MEATBALL MIX, 28.3										
gm	22	4	<1	9	—	—	—	1755	57	—
with ground beef, 2 c	1238	86	97	9	—	—	—	2039	1356	—
LEMON BUTTER SEASONING										
FOR FISH ROASTIN'										
BAG, 24.8 gm	75	<1	<1	17	—	—	—	1347	7	—
MEATLOAF ROASTIN' BAG,										
42.5 gm	129	21	1	18	—	—	—	3472	53	—
MEAT MARINADE MIX, prep,										
½ c	47	<1	<1	9	—	—	—	4104	74	—

FOOD & DESCRIPTION MEASURE OR QUANTITY	CALORIES	PROTEIN (GM)	FAT (GM)	CARBO-HYDRATE (GM)	FIBER (GM)	CALCIUM (MG)	IRON (MG)	SODIUM (MG)	POTASSIUM (MG)	CHOLES-TEROL (MG)
MUSHROOM GRAVY MIX,										
prep, 1 c	60	2	1	11	—	—	—	1170	46	—
ONION GRAVY MIX, prep, 1 c	84	3	<1	15	—	—	—	953	78	—
ONION POT ROAST ROASTIN'										
BAG, 42.5 gm	124	4	<1	24	—	—	—	2864	123	—
POT ROAST & STEW										
ROASTIN' BAG, 42.5 gm	125	3	1	25	—	—	—	2965	185	—
PORK GRAVY										
MIX, prep, 1 c	70	2	<1	14	—	—	—	2175	60	—
ROASTIN' BAG, 42.5 gm	130	3	1	26	—	—	—	2579	80	—
SLOPPY JOE MIX, 42.5 gm	118	1	<1	29	—	—	—	3512	247	—
with ground beef & tomato										
paste. 2½ c	1453	88	97	60	—	—	—	3577	2827	—
ITALIAN STYLE MIX,										
28.3 gm	99	<1	5	12	—	—	—	936	55	—
with ground beef and tomato										
sauce, 2½ c	1492	90	102	52	—	—	—	3030	3286	—
SPAGHETTI SAUCE MIX, 42.5										
gm	85	1	<1	20	—	—	—	3863	149	—
with tomato paste, 2½ c	224	7	1	52	—	—	—	3937	1660	—
SPAGHETTI SAUCE, EXTRA										
THICK & RICH MIX, 37.7										
gm	72	2	<1	24	—	—	—	1808	—	—
with tomato paste, 2¼ c	212	8	1	55	—	—	—	1873	—	—
SPAGHETTI SAUCE WITH										
MUSHROOMS MIX, 31.8										
gm	69	2	<1	16	—	—	—	3042	191	—
with tomato paste, 2.67 c	208	7	<1	48	—	—	—	3106	1702	—
SPARERIB SAUCE ROASTIN'										
BAG, 53 gm	162	<1	2	37	—	—	—	2185	57	—
STROGANOFF MIX, 35.4 gm	90	4	<1	18	—	—	—	3002	166	—
with beef, oil & sour cream,										
4 c	3280	125	285	26	—	—	—	3480	2219	—
SWEET & SOUR SAUCE, prep,										
1 c, 56.7 gm	230	1	6	45	—	—	—	1053	25	—
SWISS STEAK										
GRAVY MIX, prep, 1½ c	68	1	<1	16	—	—	—	2222	9	—
ROASTIN' BAG, 42.5 gm	115	2	<1	28	—	—	—	3008	19	—
TACO SEASONING MIX, prep,										
31.9 gm	67	2	1	15	—	—	—	2106	202	—
with ground beef, 2 c	1283	83	97	15	—	—	—	2390	1272	—
TEXAS CHILE SEASONING,										
dry, 49.6 gm	151	5	4	23	—	—	—	2603	5823	—
with ground beef & tomato										
paste, 2 c	1544	94	102	75	—	—	—	4697	7963	—
TURKEY GRAVY MIX, prep, 1 c	87	3	<1	14	—	—	—	1010	31	—
WHITE SAUCE MIX, 28.4 gm	155	2	11	11	—	—	—	617	70	—
with milk, 1 c	317	11	20	23	—	—	—	799	422	—
Franco American–Campbell										
AU JUS GRAVY, 2 oz	5	0	0	1	—	*	*	290	—	—
BEEF GRAVY, 2 oz	25	1	1	3	—	*	*	310	—	—
BROWN GRAVY WITH										
ONIONS, 2 oz	25	0	1	4	—	*	*	340	—	—
CHICKEN GRAVY, 2 oz	50	0	4	3	—	*	*	320	—	—
CHICKEN GIBLET GRAVY, 2 oz	30	1	2	3	—	*	*	320	—	—
MUSHROOM GRAVY, 2 oz	25	0	1	3	—	*	*	320	—	—
PORK GRAVY, 2 oz	40	0	3	3	—	*	*	350	—	—
TURKEY GRAVY, 2 oz	30	0	2	3	—	*	*	300	—	—

FOOD & DESCRIPTION MEASURE OR QUANTITY	CALORIES	PROTEIN (GM)	FAT (GM)	CARBO- HYDRATE (GM)	FIBER (GM)	CALCIUM (MG)	IRON (MG)	SODIUM (MG)	POTASSIUM (MG)	CHOLES- TEROL (MG)
Heinz										
BROWN GRAVY, 2 oz	30	1	1	4	—	—	—	180	—	—
CHICKEN GRAVY, 2 oz	40	2	3	3	—	—	—	275	—	—
MUSHROOM GRAVY, 2 oz	30	1	1	4	—	—	—	220	—	—
ONION GRAVY, 2 oz	35	1	1	5	—	—	—	220	—	—
PORK GRAVY, 2 oz	30	1	2	4	—	—	—	280	—	—
TURKEY GRAVY, 2 oz	40	2	3	3	—	—	—	280	—	—
Hormel										
GREAT BEGINNINGS										
WITH CHUNKY BEEF, 5 oz	136	12	7	7	—	—	—	904	—	—
WITH CHUNKY CHICKEN, 5 oz	147	14	8	5	—	—	—	567	—	—
WITH CHUNKY PORK, 5 oz	140	14	8	5	—	—	—	567	—	—
WITH CHUNKY TURKEY, 5 oz	138	11	8	7	—	—	—	585	—	—
Libby										
SLOPPY JOE BARBEQUE SAUCE										
WITH BEEF, ⅓ c	110	5	7	7	—	*	.72	190	100	—
WITH PORK, ⅓ c	120	7	8	6	—	*	.72	—	—	—
McCormick										
BROWN GRAVY MIX, ¼ pkg	22	<1	<1	3	—	20	.12	337	22	—
CHICKEN GRAVY MIX, ¼ pkg	20	<1	<1	3	—	10	.10	348	23	—
ONION GRAVY MIX, ¼ pkg	18	<1	<1	2	—	9	.19	320	20	—
SPAGHETTI SAUCE MIX, ⅕ pkg	26	<1	<1	5	—	20	.25	492	63	—
Pillsbury										
BROWN GRAVY, prep, ¼ c	15	<1	0	3	—	0	0	300	5	—
CHICKEN GRAVY, prep, ¼ c	25	<1	1	4	—	0	0	230	20	—
HOMESTYLE GRAVY, prep, ¼ c	15	<1	0	3	—	0	0	300	5	—
Prego–Campbell										
PREGO PLUS										
GROUND BEEF SIRLOIN WITH ONIONS, 4 oz	160	4	7	20	—	40	1.44	420	—	—
ITALIAN SAUSAGE & GREEN PEPPERS, 4 oz	170	3	9	19	—	40	1.08	480	—	—
SLICED MUSHROOMS & CHUNK TOMATOES, 4 oz	130	2	5	18	—	40	1.08	400	—	—
VEAL & SLICED MUSHROOMS, 4 oz	150	5	5	20	—	40	1.08	380	—	—
PREGO SPAGHETTI SAUCE, 4 oz	140	2	6	20	—	20	.72	670	—	—
MEAT FLAVORED, 4 oz	150	2	6	21	—	20	.72	680	—	—
WITH MUSHROOMS, 4 oz	140	2	5	21	—	20	1.08	640	—	—
NO-SALT-ADDED, 4 oz	100	2	6	10	—	40	1.08	25	—	—
Ragu										
EXTRA THICK AND ZESTY SPAGHETTI SAUCE, 4 oz	100	2	4	15	—	20	1.44	740	—	0
FLAVORED WITH MEAT, 4 oz	100	2	4	14	—	20	1.44	740	—	2
FLAVORED WITH MUSHROOMS, 4 oz	110	2	5	13	—	20	1.44	740	—	0
HOMESTYLE SPAGHETTI SAUCE										
FLAVORED WITH MEAT, 4 oz	80	3	2	12	—	20	1.8	400	—	2

FOOD & DESCRIPTION MEASURE OR QUANTITY	CALORIES	PROTEIN (GM)	FAT (GM)	CARBO-HYDRATE (GM)	FIBER (GM)	CALCIUM (MG)	IRON (MG)	SODIUM (MG)	POTASSIUM (MG)	CHOLES-TEROL (MG)
FLAVORED WITH MUSHROOMS, 4 oz	70	2	2	12	—	20	1.8	400	—	0
PLAIN, 4 oz	70	2	2	12	—	20	1.8	400	—	0
MARINARA SAUCE, 4 oz	90	2	4	12	—	20	1.08	740	—	0
PIZZA QUICK SAUCE, TRADITIONAL, SAUSAGE & MUSHROOM, 3 tbsp	40	1	2	4	—	*	.36	300	—	0
CHUNKY STYLE, 3 tbsp	45	1	2	6	—	*	.36	320	—	0
PEPPERONI, 3 tbsp	50	2	3	4	—	*	.36	330	—	0
SPAGHETTI SAUCE, PLAIN, 4 oz	80	2	3	11	—	20	1.08	740	—	0
FLAVORED WITH MEAT, 4 oz	80	2	2	11	—	20	1.08	740	—	2
FLAVORED WITH MUSHROOMS, 4 oz	90	2	4	9	—	20	1.08	740	—	0

R.T. French

FOOD & DESCRIPTION MEASURE OR QUANTITY	CALORIES	PROTEIN (GM)	FAT (GM)	CARBO-HYDRATE (GM)	FIBER (GM)	CALCIUM (MG)	IRON (MG)	SODIUM (MG)	POTASSIUM (MG)	CHOLES-TEROL (MG)
AU JUS, prep, ¼ c, 2 oz	8	0	0	2	—	*	*	280	—	—
BBQ DIP'UM, 2 tbsp	45	1	0	10	—	*	*	390	90	—
BROWN GRAVY, prep, ¼ c, 2 oz	20	1	1	3	—	*	*	290	—	—
CHEESE SAUCE, ¼ pkg	40	1	2	4	—	60	*	365	—	—
prep, ¼ c	80	3	4	7	—	100	*	395	—	—
CHICKEN GRAVY, prep, ¼ c, 2 oz	25	1	1	4	—	*	*	310	—	—
CREAMY MUSTARD DIP'UM, 2 tbsp	80	1	3	12	—	*	*	300	20	—
HOLLANDAISE SAUCE, prep, 3 tbsp	45	1	4	2	—	20	*	285	—	—
HOMESTYLE, prep, ¼ c, 2 oz	25	1	1	4	—	*	*	350	—	—
HOT MUSTARD DIP'UM, 2 tbsp	70	1	1	14	—	*	*	550	35	—
ITALIAN STYLE SPAGHETTI SAUCE, ¼ pkg	30	1	0	7	—	*	*	890	—	—
prep , 5 oz	100	2	4	15	—	20	1.44	905	—	—
MUSHROOM GRAVY, prep, ¼ c, 2 oz	20	1	1	3	—	*	*	350	—	—
ONION GRAVY, prep, ¼ c, 2 oz	25	1	1	4	—	*	*	390	—	—
PORK GRAVY, prep, ¼ c, 2 oz	20	1	1	3	—	*	*	310	—	—
SOUR CREAM SAUCE, ¼ pkg	40	1	4	4	—	20	*	110	—	—
prep, 2½ tbsp	60	2	5	5	—	60	*	125	—	—
SPAGHETTI SAUCE WITH MUSHROOMS, ¼ pkg	30	1	1	5	—	20	*	920	—	—
prep, 5 oz	100	2	4	13	—	40	1.44	935	—	—
STROGANOFF SAUCE, ¼ pkg	55	2	2	7	—	80	*	505	—	—
prep, ⅓ c	110	5	5	11	—	100	*	545	—	—
SWEET 'N SOUR MIX, prep, ½ c	55	0	0	14	—	*	*	145	—	—
DIP'UM, 2 tbsp	80	0	0	20	—	*	*	25	25	—
TERIYAKI SAUCE, prep, 2 tbsp	35	1	0	7	—	20	.72	1200	—	—
TURKEY GRAVY, prep, ¼ c, 2 oz	25	1	1	4	—	*	*	360	—	—

Snow—Borden

FOOD & DESCRIPTION MEASURE OR QUANTITY	CALORIES	PROTEIN (GM)	FAT (GM)	CARBO-HYDRATE (GM)	FIBER (GM)	CALCIUM (MG)	IRON (MG)	SODIUM (MG)	POTASSIUM (MG)	CHOLES-TEROL (MG)
WELSH RAREBIT CHEESE SAUCE, ½ c	170	9	11	10	—	250	.36	460	25	—

Spatini—Lipton

FOOD & DESCRIPTION MEASURE OR QUANTITY	CALORIES	PROTEIN (GM)	FAT (GM)	CARBO-HYDRATE (GM)	FIBER (GM)	CALCIUM (MG)	IRON (MG)	SODIUM (MG)	POTASSIUM (MG)	CHOLES-TEROL (MG)
FAMILY STYLE BROWN GRAVY MIX, prep, 1 oz	8	0	0	2	—	*	*	205	—	—
SPAGHETTI SAUCE MIX, prep, 1 oz	20	1	0	4	—	*	.72	130	—	—

FOOD & DESCRIPTION MEASURE OR QUANTITY	CALORIES	PROTEIN (GM)	FAT (GM)	CARBO- HYDRATE (GM)	FIBER (GM)	CALCIUM (MG)	IRON (MG)	SODIUM (MG)	POTASSIUM (MG)	CHOLES- TEROL (MG)
Sweet 'N Low										
CHEESE SAUCE MIX, ¼ pkt	25	1	<1	5	—	40	*	70	85	<5
with 2% fat milk, ¼ c	55	3	2	7	—	100	*	100	180	5
USDA										
AU JUS										
cnd, 1 c	39	3	<1	6	—	10	1.43	—	—	1
1 can, 298 gm	48	4	<1	7	—	12	1.79	—	—	1
mix, dry pkt, 23.8 gm	79	3	3	10	.05	45	—	2392	—	4
with water, 1 c	19	<1	<1	2	.01	11	—	579	—	1
BARBECUE SAUCE, rts, 1 c	188	5	5	32	1.50	48	2.25	2038	435	0
BEARNAISE SAUCE, dry pkt,										
24.8 gm	90	3	2	15	.05	—	—	841	—	tr
with milk and butter, 1 c	701	8	68	18	.03	—	—	1265	—	189
BEEF GRAVY,										
cnd, 1 c	124	9	5	11	—	14	1.63	117	189	7
can, 291 gm	155	11	7	14	—	17	2.04	146	236	9
BROWN GRAVY MIX, dry pkt,										
24.8 gm	85	3	2	15	.11	70	.24	1214	65	2
with water, 1 c	9	<1	<1	2	.01	7	.03	125	7	tr
CHEESE SAUCE, dry pkt, 35.2										
gm	158	8	9	12	.04	280	.15	1447	183	18
with milk, 1 c	307	16	17	23	.04	570	.27	1566	554	53
CHICKEN GRAVY										
cnd, 1 c	189	5	14	13	—	48	1.12	1375	260	5
1 can, 298 gm	236	6	17	16	—	60	1.40	1718	325	6
mix, 1 dry pkt, 23.1 gm, with										
water, 1 c	83	3	2	14	.06	39	—	1133	—	2
CURRY SAUCE, dry pkt, 35.4										
gm	151	3	8	18	.46	—	—	1444	—	tr
with milk, 1 c	270	11	15	26	.37	485	—	1276	—	35
HOLLANDAISE WITH										
BUTTERFAT, dry pkt,										
33.7 gm	187	4	16	11	.03	97	.71	1230	98	40
with water, 1 c	237	5	20	14	.04	124	.90	1565	124	51
HOLLANDAISE WITH										
VEGETABLE OIL, dry										
pkt, 24.8 gm	93	3	2	15	.05	—	—	645	—	tr
with milk & butter, 1 c	703	8	68	18	.03	—	—	1134	—	189
MUSHROOM GRAVY										
cnd, 1 c	120	3	6	13	—	17	1.57	1359	253	0
1 can, 298 gm	150	4	8	16	—	22	1.96	1699	316	0
mix, dry pkt, 21.3 gm, with										
water, 1 c	70	2	<1	14	—	49	—	1402	—	1
MUSHROOM SAUCE, dry pkt,										
28.35 gm	99	4	3	16	.28	—	—	1766	—	0
with milk, 1 c	228	11	10	24	.23	—	—	1533	—	34
ONION GRAVY MIX, dry pkt,										
24 gm	77	2	<1	16	—	67	—	1005	—	tr
with water, 1 c	80	2	<1	17	—	69	—	1036	—	1
PORK GRAVY MIX, dry pkt,										
21.3 gm, with water, 1 c	76	2	2	13	—	32	—	1235	—	2
SOUR CREAM SAUCE, dry pkt,										
35.2 gm	180	6	11	17	—	128	.25	444	181	28
with milk, 1 c	509	19	30	45	—	546	.61	1007	733	91
SPAGHETTI SAUCE, dry pkt,										
42 gm	118	3	<1	27	—	72	1.12	3562	353	0
WITH MUSHROOMS, dry pkt,										
39 gm	118	4	4	19	—	156	.71	3674	160	11
STROGANOFF SAUCE, dry pkt,										
46 gm	161	6	4	27	.60	307	1.33	1863	398	12
with milk & water, 1 c	271	12	11	34	.56	521	1.33	1829	672	38
SWEET & SOUR SAUCE, dry										

FOOD & DESCRIPTION MEASURE OR QUANTITY	CALORIES	PROTEIN (GM)	FAT (GM)	CARBO-HYDRATE (GM)	FIBER (GM)	CALCIUM (MG)	IRON (MG)	SODIUM (MG)	POTASSIUM (MG)	CHOLES-TEROL (MG)
pkt, 56.7 gm	220	<1	<1	55	—	30	1.21	584	49	0
with water & vinegar, 1 c	294	<1	<1	73	—	41	1.62	779	66	0
TERIYAKI SAUCE MIX, dry pkt,										
46 gm	130	4	<1	28	—	112	2.79	4784	215	0
with water, 1 c	131	4	<1	28	—	112	2.79	4791	216	0
TURKEY GRAVY										
cnd, 1 c	122	6	5	12	—	10	1.67	—	—	5
1 can, 298 gm	152	8	6	15	—	12	2.09	—	—	6
mix, dry pkt, 24.8 gm										
with water, 1 c	87	3	2	15	.10	50	—	1498	—	3
WHITE SAUCE										
homemade										
thin, 1 c	303	10	22	18	—	305	.30	878	365	—
medium, 1 c	405	10	31	22	—	288	.50	948	348	—
thick, 1 c	495	10	39	28	—	268	.80	998	333	—
mix, 49.6 gm	230	5	13	25	.10	334	—	1691	184	tr
with milk, 1 c	241	10	13	21	.04	424	.26	796	443	34

Weight Watchers

BROWN GRAVY MIX										
with water, prep, ¼ c	8	1	0	1	—	—	—	335	—	—
WITH MUSHROOMS, prep,										
¼ c	12	1	0	2	—	—	—	374	—	—
WITH ONIONS, prep, ¼ c	13	1	0	2	—	—	—	370	—	—
CHICKEN GRAVY MIX, prep,										
¼ c	10	1	0	2	—	—	—	522	—	—
LEMON BUTTER SAUCE, prep,										
1 tbsp	6	1	0	1	—	—	—	118	—	—

19

SNACKS

FOOD & DESCRIPTION MEASURE OR QUANTITY	CALORIES	PROTEIN (GM)	FAT (GM)	CARBO-HYDRATE (GM)	FIBER (GM)	CALCIUM (MG)	IRON (MG)	SODIUM (MG)	POTASSIUM (MG)	CHOLES-TEROL (MG)
Granola & Snack Bars										
Arrowhead Mills										
APPLE AMARANTH GRANOLA, 2 oz	225	7	6	39	—	—	—	3	—	—
ARROWHEAD CRUNCH, 1 oz	120	3	3	18	—	—	—	40	—	—
MAPLE NUT GRANOLA, 2 oz	260	8	11	34	—	—	—	25	—	—
Figurines—Pillsbury										
CARAMEL NUT, 2 bars	275	11	16	21	—	250	4.50	280	45	—
CHOCOLATE, 2 bars	275	11	16	21	—	250	4.50	230	55	—
CHOCOLATE CARAMEL, 2 bars	275	11	16	21	—	250	4.50	180	35	—
CHOCOLATE MINT, 2 bars	275	11	16	21	—	250	4.50	240	35	—
CHOCOLATE PEANUT BUTTER, 2 bars	275	13	16	18	—	250	4.50	240	75	—
DOUBLE CHOCOLATE, 2 bars	275	11	16	21	—	250	4.50	230	105	—
LEMON YOGURT, 2 bars	275	11	16	21	—	250	4.50	180	30	—
STRAWBERRY YOGURT, 2 bars	275	11	16	21	—	250	4.50	160	30	—
VANILLA, 2 bars	275	11	16	21	—	250	4.50	210	30	—
General Mills										
DANDY BARS										
CHOCOLATE ALMOND, 1 bar	170	2	8	22	—	40	.36	105	100	—
DARK CHOCOLATE, 1 bar	160	2	7	23	—	20	.72	110	115	—
MILK CHOCOLATE, 1 bar	160	2	7	23	—	20	.36	105	95	—
PEANUT BUTTER, 1 bar	160	3	7	22	—	40	.36	110	110	—
PEANUT BUTTER BOPPERS										
FUDGE CHIP, 1 bar	160	3	10	15	—	*	.36	100	100	—
HONEY CRISP, 1 bar	160	4	10	14	—	*	*	105	100	—
PEANUT CRUNCH, 1 bar	180	5	12	12	—	20	.36	100	120	—
Kellogg										
CHOCOLATE CHIP RICE KRISPIES BAR, 1 oz	120	2	4	20	.6d	6	1.80	110	50	—
PEANUT BUTTER RICE KRISPIES BAR, 1 oz	130	2	5	20	.7d	7	1.80	125	65	—
RAISIN RICE KRISPIES BAR, 1 oz	110	2	2	21	.5d	7	1.80	105	65	—

FOOD & DESCRIPTION MEASURE OR QUANTITY	CALORIES	PROTEIN (GM)	FAT (GM)	CARBO-HYDRATE (GM)	FIBER (GM)	CALCIUM (MG)	IRON (MG)	SODIUM (MG)	POTASSIUM (MG)	CHOLES-TEROL (MG)
Nature Valley–General Mills										
CHEWY GRANOLA BARS										
APPLE, 1 bar	130	2	5	20	—	*	.72	70	90	—
CARAMEL CHOCOLATE CHIP, 1 bar	140	2	6	19	—	20	.36	80	85	—
CHOCOLATE CHOCOLATE CHIP, 1 bar	150	2	6	21	—	20	.36	110	80	—
CHOCOLATE CHIP, 1 bar	150	2	7	19	—	*	.72	80	115	—
PEANUT BUTTER, 1 bar	150	3	7	18	—	*	.36	80	90	—
PEANUT BUTTER CHOCOLATE CHIP, 1 bar	150	2	7	19	—	*	.72	80	80	—
RAISIN, 1 bar	130	2	5	20	—	*	.72	70	80	—
GRANOLA										
CINNAMON & RAISIN, 1 oz, ⅓ c	130	3	5	19	—	*	1.08	35	100	—
COCONUT & HONEY, 1 oz, ⅓ c	150	3	7	18	—	20	1.08	35	110	—
FRUIT & NUT, 1 oz, ⅓ c	130	3	5	19	—	20	.72	35	105	—
TOASTED OAT MIXTURE, 1 oz, ⅓ c	130	3	5	19	—	*	1.08	35	95	—
GRANOLA BARS										
ALMOND, 1 bar	120	2	5	17	—	*	.72	90	70	—
CHOCOLATE CHIP, 1 bar	110	2	4	16	—	*	.72	75	60	—
CINNAMON, 1 bar	120	2	5	17	—	*	.72	70	60	—
COCONUT, 1 bar	130	2	7	15	—	*	.72	65	70	—
OATS 'N HONEY, 1 bar	120	2	5	17	—	*	.72	65	55	—
PEANUT, 1 bar	130	3	6	16	—	*	.72	80	75	—
PEANUT BUTTER, 1 bar	120	2	6	15	—	*	.72	70	70	—
GRANOLA CLUSTERS										
ALMOND, 1 roll	160	2	4	28	—	20	.72	110	80	—
APPLE CINNAMON, 1 roll	150	2	4	27	—	20	.36	100	70	—
CARAMEL, 1 roll	150	2	3	28	—	40	.72	120	80	—
CHOCOLATE, 1 roll	140	2	3	27	—	40	.72	110	100	—
CHOCOLATE CHIP, 1 roll	150	2	4	27	—	20	.72	100	85	—
RAISIN, 1 roll	150	2	3	28	—	20	.72	110	80	—
Pillsbury										
MILK BREAK BAR										
CHOCOLATE, 1 bar	230	5	13	22	—	150	.36	75	260	—
CHOCOLATE MINT, 1 bar	230	5	14	21	—	150	.72	80	280	—
NATURAL FLAVOR, 1 bar	230	5	14	21	—	150	.36	75	230	—
PEANUT BUTTER, 1 bar	220	6	13	21	—	150	.36	115	260	—
Quaker										
CHEWY GRANOLA BARS										
CHOCOLATE CHIP, 1 bar, 1 oz	129	2	5	19	.20	26	.74	79	99	—
CHOCOLATE, GRAHAM & MARSHMALLOW, 1 bar, 1 oz	126	2	4	20	.20	25	.79	93	79	—
CHUNKY NUT & RAISINS, 1 bar, 1 oz	133	2	6	17	.50	24	.64	81	118	—
HONEY & OATS, 1 bar, 1 oz	125	2	4	19	.30	28	.76	93	97	—
PEANUT BUTTER, 1 bar, 1 oz	130	3	5	18	.20	26	.62	106	109	—
PEANUT BUTTER & CHOCOLATE CHIPS, 1 bar, 1 oz	131	3	6	17	.30	23	.49	92	108	—
RAISINS & CINNAMON, 1 bar, 1 oz	130	2	5	19	.20	28	.71	83	104	—
DIPPS BARS										
CARAMEL NUT, 1 bar, 1.1 oz	148	2	6	21	.20	30	.56	63	87	—

FOOD & DESCRIPTION MEASURE OR QUANTITY	CALORIES	PROTEIN (GM)	FAT (GM)	CARBO- HYDRATE (GM)	FIBER (GM)	CALCIUM (MG)	IRON (MG)	SODIUM (MG)	POTASSIUM (MG)	CHOLES- TEROL (MG)
CHOCOLATE CHIP, 1 bar, 1 oz	138	2	6	18	.30	29	.77	65	90	—
HONEY & OATS, 1 bar, 1 oz	137	2	6	19	.20	30	.62	66	82	—
MINT CHOCOLATE CHIP, 1 bar, 1 oz	140	2	6	19	.20	30	.70	56	86	—
PEANUT BUTTER, 1 bar, 1 oz	141	3	7	17	.30	23	.62	89	87	—
RAISIN & ALMOND, 1 bar, 1 oz	139	2	6	19	.20	26	.75	84	81	—
ROCKY ROAD, 1 bar, 1 oz	140	2	7	18	.20	30	.57	60	87	—

Snack Foods

Arrowhead Mills

POPCORN, 2 oz, dry weight	210	7	3	41	—	—	—	2	—	—

Bachman Company

CORN CHIPS										
BAR-B-Q, 1 oz, 28 gm	150	2	9	15	—	80	.36	170	130	0
PLAIN, 1 oz, 28 gm	150	2	9	15	—	40	.36	190	85	0
JAX										
BAKED, 1 oz, 28 gm	150	2	8	17	—	20	.36	340	105	0
CRUNCHY, 1 oz, 28 gm	160	2	11	14	—	20	.36	280	60	0
POPCORN										
CHEESE, 1 oz, 28 gm	180	2	12	14	—	*	*	330	130	0
PLAIN, 1 oz, 28 gm	160	2	11	13	—	*	.72	310	95	0
POTATO CHIPS										
BAR-B-QUE, 1 oz, 28 gm	150	2	9	14	—	*	.72	280	380	0
HOT, 1 oz, 28 gm	150	2	9	14	—	*	.36	200	360	0
PLAIN, FLAT, 1 oz, 28 gm	160	2	10	14	—	*	.72	270	510	0
PLAIN, RIDGES, 1 oz, 28 gm	160	2	10	14	—	*	.72	260	500	0
SOUR CREAM—ONION, 1 oz, 28 gm	150	2	9	14	—	*	.36	200	360	0
UNSALTED, 1 oz, 28 gm	160	2	10	14	—	*	.72	5	520	0
VINEGAR, 1 oz, 28 gm	150	2	9	15	—	*	.36	610	370	0
PRETZELS										
BUTTER TWIST, 1 oz, 28 gm	110	3	2	21	—	*	1.80	410	35	0
CHEESE STICKS, 1 oz, 28 gm	110	4	2	21	—	20	1.44	760	65	0
HARD, 1 oz, 28 gm	102	3	0	23	—	*	.36	550	—	0
LOGS, 1 oz, 28 gm	110	3	2	21	—	*	1.80	470	40	0
NUTZELS, 1 oz, 28 gm	110	3	2	21	—	*	1.80	470	40	0
PETITES, 1 oz, 28 gm	110	3	2	21	—	*	1.80	410	35	0
RINGS, 1 oz, 28 gm	110	3	2	21	—	*	1.80	410	35	0
RODS, 1 oz, 28 gm	110	3	2	21	—	*	1.80	240	40	0
STIX, 1 oz, 28 gm	110	3	2	21	—	*	1.80	610	55	0
TREATS, 1 oz, 28 gm	110	3	2	21	—	*	1.80	410	35	0
TWIST, 1 oz, 28 gm	110	3	2	21	—	*	1.80	410	35	0
UNSALTED PETITES, 1 oz, 28 gm	110	3	2	21	—	*	1.80	0	35	0
TORTILLA CHIPS										
NACHO, 1 oz, 28 gm	140	3	6	17	—	60	.36	180	85	0
PLAIN, 1 oz, 28 gm	140	2	8	16	—	*	*	105	70	0

Borden

BRAVOS NACHO CHEESE FLAVOR CRISPY ROUND TORTILLA CHIPS, 1 oz, 28 gm	150	2	8	17	—	60	.36	—	—	—
BUCKEYE KETCHUP and FRENCH FRY FLAVOR POTATO CHIPS, 1 oz, 28 gm	160	2	11	14	—	*	.36	230	370	—

264

FOOD & DESCRIPTION MEASURE OR QUANTITY	CALORIES	PROTEIN (GM)	FAT (GM)	CARBO-HYDRATE (GM)	FIBER (GM)	CALCIUM (MG)	IRON (MG)	SODIUM (MG)	POTASSIUM (MG)	CHOLES-TEROL (MG)
CHEEZ DOODLES										
CRUNCHY CHEESE FLAVORED FRIED CORN PUFFS, 1 oz, 28 gm	160	2	10	16	—	20	.72	—	—	—
PUFFED CHEESE FLAVORED BAKED CORN PUFFS, 1 oz, 28 gm	160	2	10	16	—	20	.72	—	—	—
CRACKER JACK CARAMEL COATED POPCORN AND PEANUTS, 1 oz, 28 gm	120	2	3	22	—	*	.72	85	100	—
GUY'S BAKED CHEESE BALLS, 1 oz, 28 gm	160	2	11	14	—	20	*	320	40	—
LITE-LINE										
NACHO CHEESE FLAVORED TORTILLA CHIPS, 1 oz, 28 gm	130	2	5	19	—	40	.36	165	50	—
PUFFED CHEESE CURLS, 1 oz, 28 gm	130	2	5	19	—	20	.72	—	—	—
MORTON'S RIDGIES BARBEQUE FLAVOR RIPPLED POTATO CHIPS, 1 oz, 28 gm	150	2	10	14	—	*	.36	—	—	—
OLD LONDON										
CHEEZ WAFFIES, 1 oz, 28 gm	140	3	8	14	—	60	*	—	—	—
CRUNCHY CHEESE FLAVORED FRIED CORN PUFFS, 1 oz, 28 gm	160	2	10	16	—	20	.72	—	—	—
PRETZ-L NUGGETS BITE-SIZE PRETZELS, 1 oz, 28 gm	110	2	2	22	—	*	*	365	35	—
PUFFED CHEESE FLAVORED BAKED CORN PUFFS, 1 oz, 28 gm	160	2	10	16	—	20	.72	—	—	—
SEYFERT'S BUTTER PRETZELS, 1 oz, 28 gm	110	3	1	21	—	*	.36	530	40	—
WISE										
BUTTER FLAVOR POPCORN, .5 oz, 14 gm	70	1	4	8	—	*	*	—	—	—
CHEEZ POPCORN, .5 oz, 14 gm	90	1	6	7	—	*	*	—	—	—
CHEEZ WAFFIES, 1 oz, 28 gm	140	3	8	14	—	60	*	—	—	—
CORN CRUNCHIES, 1 oz, 28 gm	160	2	10	16	—	20	.36	—	—	—
CRUNCHY CHEESE FLAVORED FRIED CORN PUFFS, 1 oz, 28 gm	160	2	10	16	—	20	.72	—	—	—
NATURAL FLAVOR POTATO CHIPS, 1 oz, 28 gm	160	2	11	14	—	*	.36	240	340	—
POTATO CHIPS, NO SALT ADDED, 1 oz, 28 gm	150	2	10	14	—	*	*	20	340	—
PRETZ-L NUGGETS BITE-SIZE PRETZELS, 1 oz, 28 gm	110	2	2	22	—	*	*	365	35	—
PUFFED CHEESE FLAVORED BAKED CORN PUFFS, 1 oz, 28 gm	160	2	10	16	—	20	.72	—	—	—
Estee										
UNSALTED PRETZELS, 5 pretzels	25	<1	<1	5	—	—	—	<5	—	0
Featherweight										
CHEESE CURLS, 1 oz, 28 gm	150	2	9	16	—	—	—	81	—	—

FOOD & DESCRIPTION MEASURE OR QUANTITY	CALORIES	PROTEIN (GM)	FAT (GM)	CARBO-HYDRATE (GM)	FIBER (GM)	CALCIUM (MG)	IRON (MG)	SODIUM (MG)	POTASSIUM (MG)	CHOLES-TEROL (MG)
CORN CHIPS, 1 oz, 28 gm	170	2	11	15	—	—	—	3	—	—
POTATO CHIPS, 1 oz, 28 gm	160	2	11	14	—	—	—	10	397	—
PRETZELS, 3 pretzels	20	1	0	4	—	—	—	5	40	—

Flavor Tree–Lipton

BUTTERED AND POPPED CORN STICKS, 1 oz, 28 gm	160	2	10	15	—	20	.36	220	—	—
CHEDDAR STICKS, 1 oz, 28 gm	160	3	11	12	—	60	.36	445	—	—
CORN CHIPS, 1 oz, 28 gm	150	2	8	17	—	40	.36	260	—	—
FRUIT ROLLS, APPLE, APRICOT, CHERRY, FRUIT PUNCH, GRAPE, RASPBERRY, STRAWBERRY, 1 roll, ¾ oz	80	0	<1	18	—	*	*	15	—	—
PARTY MIX, 1 oz, 28 gm	160	4	11	11	—	60	.36	400	—	—
NO SALT ADDED, 1 oz, 28 gm	160	4	11	11	—	40	.36	10	—	—
SESAME CHIPS, 1 oz, 28 gm	150	3	10	13	—	60	.36	410	—	—
SESAME CRUNCH, 1 oz, 28 gm	150	5	10	10	—	*	1.44	70	—	0
SESAME STICKS, 1 oz, 28 gm	150	3	10	13	—	60	.36	405	—	—
NO SALT ADDED, 1 oz, 28 gm	160	3	11	12	—	60	.36	10	—	—
WITH BRAN, 1 oz, 28 gm	160	4	11	11	—	60	.72	370	—	—
SOUR CREAM and ONION STICKS, 1 oz, 28 gm	150	3	10	13	—	60	.36	415	—	—
WHEAT NUTS, 1 oz, 28 gm	200	4	18	5	—	*	.72	185	—	0

Frito-Lay

CHEETOS										
CHEDDAR VALLEY SHARP CRUNCHY CHEESE FLAVORED SNACK, 1 oz, 28 gm	150	3	9	15	—	*	.36	260	55	0
CRUNCHY CHEESE FLAVORED SNACKS, 1 oz, 28 gm	160	2	10	15	—	*	.36	300	40	0
MELLOW CHEDDAR CHEESE FLAVORED SNACK, puffed balls, 1 oz, 28 gm	160	2	10	15	—	*	.36	350	45	0
MELLOW CHEDDAR CRUNCHY CHEESE FLAVORED SNACK, 1 oz, 28 gm	160	3	10	15	—	*	.36	270	45	0
MELLOW CHEESE FLAVORED SNACK, puffed rods, 1 oz, 28 gm	160	2	10	15	—	*	.36	370	45	0
DORITOS										
TORTILLA CHIPS, 1 oz, 28 gm	140	2	7	19	—	20	.36	190	50	0
TACO FLAVOR TORTILLA CHIPS, 1 oz, 28 gm	140	2	7	18	—	40	.36	260	70	0
FRITOS										
BARBQ FLAVORED CORN CHIPS, 1 oz, 28 gm	150	2	9	16	—	20	.36	310	55	0
CORN CHIPS, 1 oz, 28 gm	150	2	10	16	—	20	.36	220	45	0
CORN CHIPS, KING SIZE DIP CHIPS, 1 oz, 28 gm	150	2	9	16	—	40	*	190	55	0
LIGHTS CORN CHIPS, 1 oz, 28 gm	150	2	10	16	—	20	*	210	55	0

FOOD & DESCRIPTION MEASURE OR QUANTITY	CALORIES	PROTEIN (GM)	FAT (GM)	CARBO-HYDRATE (GM)	FIBER (GM)	CALCIUM (MG)	IRON (MG)	SODIUM (MG)	POTASSIUM (MG)	CHOLES-TEROL (MG)
LAY'S POTATO CHIPS										
BAR-B-Q FLAVORED, 1 oz, 28 gm	150	2	10	14	—	*	.36	360	380	0
REGULAR, 1.13 oz, 32 gm	170	2	11	17	—	*	.72	230	450	0
SALT & VINEGAR ARTIFICIALLY FLAVORED, 1 oz, 28 gm	150	2	9	15	—	*	.36	390	390	0
SOUR CREAM & ONION ARTIFICIALLY FLAVORED, 1.13 oz, 32 gm	170	3	11	16	—	20	.36	360	450	0
UNSALTED, 1 oz, 28 gm	160	2	11	14	—	*	.36	10	380	0
O'GRADY'S POTATO CHIPS										
EXTRA THICK AND CRUNCHY, 1 oz, 28 gm	150	2	9	16	—	*	.36	160	400	0
EXTRA THICK AND CRUNCHY AU GRATIN CHEESE FLAVORED, 1.13 oz, 28 gm	170	3	10	17	—	*	*	330	450	0
EXTRA THICK AND CRUNCHY HEARTY SEASONING, 1 oz, 28 gm	140	2	8	17	—	*	.36	390	380	0
RUFFLES POTATO CHIPS										
BACON AND SOUR CREAM ARTIFICIALLY FLAVORED, 1 oz, 28 gm	160	3	10	14	—	20	.36	325	—	—
BAR-B-Q FLAVORED, 1 oz, 28 gm	150	2	10	15	—	*	.36	260	—	—
REGULAR, 1 oz, 28 gm	150	2	10	15	—	*	.36	200	350	0
SOUR CREAM & ONION ARTIFICIALLY FLAVORED, 1 oz, 28 gm	150	2	9	15	—	20	.36	260	400	0
TOSTITOS										
CRISPY ROUND TORTILLA CHIPS, 1 oz, 28 gm	140	2	8	18	—	20	.36	180	70	0
NACHO CHEESE FLAVORED ROUND TORTILLA CHIPS, 1 oz, 28 gm	150	2	8	17	—	40	.36	220	90	0

General Mills

FOOD & DESCRIPTION MEASURE OR QUANTITY	CALORIES	PROTEIN (GM)	FAT (GM)	CARBO-HYDRATE (GM)	FIBER (GM)	CALCIUM (MG)	IRON (MG)	SODIUM (MG)	POTASSIUM (MG)	CHOLES-TEROL (MG)
BUGLES, 1 oz, 28 gm	150	2	8	18	—	*	.72	290	20	—
NACHO CHEESE BUGLES, 1 oz, 28 gm	160	2	9	17	—	*	.36	270	35	—
POP SECRET										
BUTTER FLAVOR, 4 c	230	4	14	27	—	*	.72	450	95	—
NATURAL FLAVOR, 4 c	230	4	13	27	—	*	.72	480	95	—

Mother's

FOOD & DESCRIPTION MEASURE OR QUANTITY	CALORIES	PROTEIN (GM)	FAT (GM)	CARBO-HYDRATE (GM)	FIBER (GM)	CALCIUM (MG)	IRON (MG)	SODIUM (MG)	POTASSIUM (MG)	CHOLES-TEROL (MG)
CRISPY CHINESE TV SNACKS, 1 oz, 28 gm	140	3	7	17	—	*	.36	—	—	—

Nabisco

FOOD & DESCRIPTION MEASURE OR QUANTITY	CALORIES	PROTEIN (GM)	FAT (GM)	CARBO-HYDRATE (GM)	FIBER (GM)	CALCIUM (MG)	IRON (MG)	SODIUM (MG)	POTASSIUM (MG)	CHOLES-TEROL (MG)
CHEESE 'N CRUNCH CHEESE FLAVORED SNACKS, 1 oz, 28 gm	160	2	11	15	—	20	.72	190	55	—
CHIPSTERS LIGHT 'N CRISPY POTATO SNACKS, 1 oz, 28 gm	120	1	5	19	—	*	.36	580	180	—
CORN DIGGERS CORN SNACK, 1 oz, 28 gm	150	2	8	17	—	*	*	260	25	—
DOO DADS										
CHEDDAR 'N BACON, ½ c, 1 oz	140	3	6	18	—	20	.72	350	90	—

FOOD & DESCRIPTION MEASURE OR QUANTITY	CALORIES	PROTEIN (GM)	FAT (GM)	CARBO-HYDRATE (GM)	FIBER (GM)	CALCIUM (MG)	IRON (MG)	SODIUM (MG)	POTASSIUM (MG)	CHOLES-TEROL (MG)
CHEDDAR 'N HERB, ½ c, 1 oz	140	3	6	18	—	20	.72	400	75	—
ORIGINAL, ½ c, 1 oz	140	3	6	18	—	20	.72	400	75	—
ZESTY CHEESE, ½ c, 1 oz	140	3	6	18	—	20	.72	420	80	—
MISTER SALTY										
DUTCH PRETZELS, 2 pretzels, 1 oz, 28 gm	110	3	1	22	—	*	1.08	440	35	—
JUNIORS, 1 oz, 28 gm	110	3	1	21	—	*	1.08	510	40	—
JUNIORS, BUTTER FLAVORED, 1 oz, 28 gm	110	3	1	21	—	*	1.08	510	40	—
PRETZELS, BUTTER FLAVORED RINGS, 1 oz, 28 gm	110	3	2	21	—	*	1.08	570	35	—
PRETZELS, BUTTER FLAVORED STICKS, 1 oz, 28 gm	110	3	1	22	—	*	1.08	620	35	—
PRETZELS, BUTTER FLAVORED TWISTS, 1 oz, 28 gm	110	3	1	22	—	*	1.08	510	35	—
PRETZEL LOGS, 1 oz, 28 gm	110	3	1	21	—	*	1.08	510	40	—
PRETZEL NUGGETS, 1 oz, 28 gm	110	3	1	21	—	*	1.08	550	45	—
PRETZEL MINI, 1 oz, 28 gm	110	3	1	21	—	*	1.08	450	40	—
PRETZEL MINI MIX, 1 oz, 28 gm	110	3	1	23	—	*	1.08	480	40	—
PRETZEL RINGS, 1 oz, 28 gm	110	3	2	21	—	*	1.08	510	40	—
PRETZEL RODS, 1 oz, 28 gm	110	3	1	21	—	*	1.08	500	40	—
PRETZEL STICKS, 1 oz, 28 gm	110	3	1	22	—	*	1.08	620	40	—
PRETZEL TWISTS, 1 oz, 28 gm	110	3	2	21	—	*	1.08	590	40	—
VERI-THIN PRETZEL STICKS, 1 oz, 28 gm	110	3	1	22	—	*	1.08	770	35	—

Ovaltine

FIDDLE FADDLE, 1.25 oz, 35.4 gm	160	2	5	27	.4	—	—	—	—	—
POPPYCOCK ORIGINAL, 1.5 oz, 42.5 gm	225	2	13	24	1.2	—	—	—	—	—
POPPYCOCK MAPLE-WALNUT, 1.5 oz, 42.5 gm	220	3	12	26	.6	—	—	—	—	—
SCREAMING YELLOW ZONKERS, .88 oz, 24 gm	110	<1	3	18	.5	—	—	—	—	—

Pillsbury

MICROWAVE POPCORN BUTTER FLAVORED, 4 c popped	260	4	14	29	—	0	1.08	410	100	—
ORIGINAL FLAVORED, 4 c popped	260	4	15	28	—	0	1.08	400	110	—
SALT FREE, 4 c popped	190	4	8	26	—	0	1.08	5	95	—

Planters—Nabisco

CHEESE CURLS, 1 oz, 28 gm	160	2	11	14	—	*	*	290	35	—
CHEEZ BALLS, 1 oz, 28 gm	160	2	11	14	—	*	*	270	45	—
CORN CHIPS, 1 oz, 28 gm	160	2	10	15	—	40	.36	160	40	—
NATURALLY NUT 'N FRUIT BARS										
ALMOND APRICOT, 1 oz, 28 gm	140	3	7	17	—	20	.72	75	140	—

FOOD & DESCRIPTION MEASURE OR QUANTITY	CALORIES	PROTEIN (GM)	FAT (GM)	CARBO-HYDRATE (GM)	FIBER (GM)	CALCIUM (MG)	IRON (MG)	SODIUM (MG)	POTASSIUM (MG)	CHOLES-TEROL (MG)
ALMOND PINEAPPLE, 1 oz, 28 gm	140	2	6	18	—	20	.72	80	80	—
PEANUT RAISIN, 1 oz, 28 gm	140	3	7	17	—	*	.36	70	105	—
WALNUT APPLE, 1 oz, 28 gm	150	2	8	16	—	*	.36	90	75	—
PIZZA CRUNCHIES, 1 oz, 28 gm	160	2	10	15	—	*	*	160	45	—
PRETZELS, 1 oz, 28 gm	110	3	1	22	—	*	1.44	700	40	—
SOUR CREAM & ONION PUFFS, 1 oz, 28 gm	160	1	10	16	—	*	*	300	45	—
TORTILLA CHIPS										
NACHO FLAVOR, 1 oz, 28 gm	150	2	8	18	—	40	.36	160	65	—
TRADITIONAL, 1 oz, 28 gm	150	2	8	18	—	40	.36	150	60	—

Procter & Gamble

PRINGLE'S POTATO CHIPS										
CHEEZ-UMS, 1 oz, 28 gm	170	2	12	13	—	40	.36	220	—	—
LIGHT, 1 oz, 28 gm	150	2	8	17	—	*	.36	145	—	—
REGULAR, 1 oz, 28 gm	170	2	13	12	—	*	.36	215	—	—
RIPPLED, 1 oz, 28 gm	170	2	12	13	—	*	.36	250	—	—
SOUR CREAM'N ONION, 1 oz, 28 gm	170	2	12	13	—	*	.36	136	—	—

Rokeach

PRETZELS										
BALDIES or NO SALT DUTCH, 1 oz, 28 gm	110	2	0	20	—	*	*	30	—	—
DUTCH STYLE, 1 oz, 28 gm	110	3	0	24	—	*	*	—	—	—
PARTY CANISTER, 1 oz, 28 gm	110	2	1	23	—	*	*	—	—	—

Sahadi–Lipton

PEANUT CRUNCH BAR, .75 oz, 21 gm	110	4	6	9	—	*	.36	10	—	0
SESAME CRUNCH BAR, .75 oz, 21 gm	110	4	7	7	—	*	1.08	55	—	0

Sunkist–Lipton

SUNKIST FRUIT ROLLS, CHERRY, GRAPE, ORANGE, RASPBERRY, STRAWBERRY, 1 roll, .5 oz	50	0	<1	12	—	*	*	10	—	—

Tastykake

COATED PRETZEL, 1 triple ring	108	2	5	14	—	—	—	69	—	—
COATED MINI-PRETZEL, 1 triple ring	24	<1	1	3	—	—	—	22	—	—

USDA

POPCORN										
unpopped, 1 c, 205 gm	742	24	10	148	—	21	5.1	6	—	—
popped, commercial, plain, large kernel, 1 c, 6 gm	23	<1	<1	5	—	1	.2	tr	—	—
popped, commercial, oil & salt added, large kernel, 1 c, 9 gm	41	<1	2	5	—	1	.2	175	—	—
popped, commerical, sugar-coated, 1 c, 35 gm	134	2	1	30	—	2	.5	tr	—	—
PRETZELS										
EXTRUDED LOGS, 3 × ½" diam, 10 pretzels, 50 gm	195	5	2	38	—	11	.8	840	65	—

FOOD & DESCRIPTION MEASURE OR QUANTITY	CALORIES	PROTEIN (GM)	FAT (GM)	CARBO-HYDRATE (GM)	FIBER (GM)	CALCIUM (MG)	IRON (MG)	SODIUM (MG)	POTASSIUM (MG)	CHOLES-TEROL (MG)
EXTRUDED RODS, 7½ × ½" diam, 1 pretzel, 14 gm	55	1	<1	11	—	3	.2	235	18	—
EXTRUDED STICKS, 3⅛ × ⅛" diam, 10 pretzels, 6 gm	23	<1	<1	5	—	1	.1	101	8	—
REGULAR, 1 oz, 28 gm	111	3	1	22	—	6	.4	476	37	—
TWISTED, ONE-RING, 1½ × ¼" diam, 10 pretzels, 20 gm	78	2	<1	15	—	4	.3	336	26	—
TWISTED, THREE-RING, 1⅞ × 1¾ × ¼", 10 pretzels, 30 gm	117	3	1	23	—	7	.5	504	39	—
TWISTED THINS, 3¼ × 2¼ × ¼", 10 pretzels, 60 gm	234	6	3	46	—	13	.9	1008	78	—

20

SOUPS

Note: For Condensed soups, 4 oz condensed = 8 oz prepared with water.

FOOD & DESCRIPTION MEASURE OR QUANTITY	CALORIES	PROTEIN (GM)	FAT (GM)	CARBO-HYDRATE (GM)	FIBER (GM)	CALCIUM (MG)	IRON (MG)	SODIUM (MG)	POTASSIUM (MG)	CHOLES-TEROL (MG)
Campbell Soup Company										
ASPARAGUS, CREAM OF, 4 oz cond	90	2	4	11	—	20	.36	900	—	5
BEAN WITH BACON, 4 oz cond	150	6	5	21	6d	60	1.8	860	—	5
BEEF, 4 oz cond	80	6	2	10	—	*	.72	850	—	10
BEEF BROTH or BOUILLON, 4 oz cond	16	3	0	1	—	*	*	860	—	0
BEEF NOODLE, 4 oz cond	70	4	3	7	—	*	.72	870	—	15
BEEF NOODLE, HOMESTYLE, 4 oz cond	80	6	3	8	—	*	.72	810	—	20
BEEFY MUSHROOM, 4 oz cond	60	4	3	5	—	*	.36	960	—	10
BLACK BEAN, 4 oz cond	110	5	2	17	4d	20	1.8	980	—	0
BURLY VEGETABLE BEEF & BACON, SOUP FOR ONE, 7¾ oz can, 11 oz prep	160	8	5	20	—	60	1.8	1480	—	—
CELERY, CREAM OF, 4 oz cond	10	1	7	8	—	20	*	860	—	5
CHEDDAR CHEESE, 4 oz cond	130	3	8	10	—	80	.36	800	—	10
DRY MIX, 8 oz prep	150	7	9	10	—	200	0	970	—	—
CHICKEN ALPHABET, 4 oz cond	80	3	3	10	—	*	.72	870	—	10
CHICKEN BROTH, 4 oz cond	35	1	2	3	—	*	*	790	—	0
CHICKEN BROTH, LOW SODIUM, rts, 10½ oz	40	3	2	2	—	*	1.08	70	—	—
CHICKEN BROTH AND NOODLES, 4 oz cond	60	2	2	8	—	*	.72	870	—	10
CHICKEN BROTH AND RICE, 4 oz cond	50	1	1	8	—	*	*	880	—	0
CHICKEN, CREAM OF, 4 oz cond	110	3	7	9	—	20	.36	850	—	10
CHICKEN 'N DUMPLINGS, 4 oz cond	80	4	3	9	—	*	.36	980	—	25
CHICKEN GUMBO, 4 oz cond	60	2	2	8	—	20	.36	910	—	5
CHICKEN NOODLE, 4 oz cond	70	3	2	8	—	*	.72	920	—	15
CHICKEN NOODLE, HOMESTYLE, 4 oz	70	3	3	8	—	*	.36	920	—	15
CHICKEN NOODLEO'S, 4 oz cond	70	3	2	9	—	*	.72	840	—	20
CHICKEN NOODLE WITH MEAT, dry 8 oz prep	100	5	2	15	—	0	.72	890	—	—
CHICKEN RICE, dry, 8 oz prep	90	4	2	16	—	0	0	820	—	—
CHICKEN WITH RICE, 4 oz cond	60	2	2	7	—	*	*	840	—	10
CHICKEN & STARS, 4 oz cond	60	3	2	7	—	*	.36	920	—	10

FOOD & DESCRIPTION MEASURE OR QUANTITY	CALORIES	PROTEIN (GM)	FAT (GM)	CARBO-HYDRATE (GM)	FIBER (GM)	CALCIUM (MG)	IRON (MG)	SODIUM (MG)	POTASSIUM (MG)	CHOLES-TEROL (MG)
CHICKEN VEGETABLE, 4 oz cond	70	3	3	8	—	*	.72	870	—	10
CHICKEN WITH NOODLES, ls, rts, 10¾ oz	160	14	5	15	—	20	1.80	85	—	—
CHILI BEEF, 4 oz cond	130	5	5	17	—	20	1.08	900	—	10
CHUNKY SOUPS, rts										
BEEF, 10¾ oz	190	14	5	23	—	20	1.80	1110	—	—
9½ oz	170	13	4	20	—	20	1.80	970	—	—
BEEF & MUSHROOM, ls, 10¾ oz	210	13	7	23	—	40	1.80	65	—	—
BEEF STROGANOFF, 10¾ oz	300	15	15	28	—	60	2.70	1290	—	—
CHICKEN NOODLE & MUSHROOMS, 10¾ oz	200	14	7	20	—	20	1.80	1190	—	—
9½ oz	180	12	6	18	—	20	1.80	1050	—	—
CHICKEN RICE, 9½ oz	140	10	4	15	—	20	.72	1080	—	—
CHICKEN VEGETABLE, 9½ oz	170	10	6	19	—	20	1.08	1100	—	—
ls, 10¾ oz	240	15	11	20	—	40	1.44	95	—	—
CHILI BEEF, 11 oz	290	21	7	37	—	60	4.50	1150	—	—
9¾ oz	260	19	6	33	—	60	3.60	1020	—	—
CLAM CHOWDER, MANHATTAN, 10¾ oz	160	7	5	24	—	60	1.80	1230	—	—
9½ oz	150	6	4	22	—	40	1.80	1080	—	—
CLAM CHOWDER, NEW ENGLAND, 10¾ oz	290	9	17	25	—	40	1.80	1180	—	—
9½ oz	250	8	15	22	—	40	1.80	1040	—	—
FISHERMAN CHOWDER, 10¾ oz	260	11	14	26	—	80	1.80	1320	—	—
9½ oz	230	10	13	23	—	60	1.44	1160	—	—
HAM 'N BUTTER BEAN, 10¾ oz	280	12	10	34	—	40	1.80	1180	—	—
MEDITERRANEAN VEGETABLE, 9½ oz	160	4	5	24	—	60	1.44	1020	—	—
MINESTRONE, 9½ oz	140	4	5	21	—	60	1.44	940	—	—
OLD FASHIONED BEAN 'N HAM, 11 oz	290	14	9	37	—	100	2.70	1150	—	—
9⅝ oz	260	12	8	33	—	80	2.70	1010	—	—
OLD FASHIONED CHICKEN, 10¾ oz	170	12	5	21	—	40	1.44	1340	—	—
9½ oz	150	10	4	18	—	20	1.44	1180	—	—
OLD FASHIONED VEGETABLE BEEF, 10¾ oz	180	12	5	20	—	40	1.80	1210	—	—
9½ oz	160	11	4	18	—	40	1.80	1070	—	—
SIRLOIN BURGER, 10¾ oz	220	12	9	23	—	20	1.80	1280	—	—
9½ oz	200	11	8	20	—	20	1.80	1130	—	—
SPLIT PEA 'N HAM, 10¾ oz	230	12	6	33	—	20	1.80	1070	—	—
9½ oz	200	11	5	29	—	20	1.80	950	—	—
STEAK 'N POTATO, 10¾ oz	200	14	5	24	—	*	1.80	1250	—	—
9½ oz	170	12	4	21	—	*	1.80	1110	—	—
TURKEY VEGETABLE, 9⅜ oz	150	9	6	16	—	40	1.08	1080	—	—
VEGETABLE, 10¾ oz	140	4	4	23	—	60	1.44	1100	—	—
9½ oz	130	3	4	21	—	40	1.44	970	—	—
VEGETABLE BEEF, ls, 10¾ oz	170	13	5	19	—	40	1.80	60	—	—
CLAM CHOWDER, MANHATTAN, 4 oz cond	70	2	2	11	—	20	.72	860	—	0
CLAM CHOWDER, NEW ENGLAND, 4 oz cond	80	3	3	11	—	20	.72	880	—	5
prep with milk, 8 oz prep	150	7	7	17	—	150	.72	930	—	—
SOUP FOR ONE, 7¾ oz										
prep with milk, 11 oz prep	190	9	7	23	—	150	1.44	1410	—	—
prep with water, 11 oz prep	130	6	4	19	—	60	1.44	1360	—	—
CONSOMME, BEEF, GELATIN ADDED, 4 oz cond	25	4	0	2	—	*	*	780	—	0
CREAMY CHICKEN MUSHROOM, 4 oz cond	120	3	8	9	—	20	.36	940	—	15

FOOD & DESCRIPTION MEASURE OR QUANTITY	CALORIES	PROTEIN (GM)	FAT (GM)	CARBO-HYDRATE (GM)	FIBER (GM)	CALCIUM (MG)	IRON (MG)	SODIUM (MG)	POTASSIUM (MG)	CHOLES-TEROL (MG)
CREAMY NATURAL SOUPS										
ASPARAGUS, 4 oz cond	130	1	10	8	—	*	.72	800	—	—
prep with milk, 8 oz	200	5	14	13	—	100	.72	855	—	—
BROCCOLI, 4 oz cond	70	1	4	8	—	20	.72	820	—	—
prep with milk, 8 oz	140	5	8	13	—	100	.72	875	—	—
CAULIFLOWER, 4 oz cond	130	1	9	13	—	*	.36	800	—	—
prep with milk, 8 oz	200	5	13	18	—	150	.36	850	—	—
POTATO, 4 oz cond	150	1	11	11	—	*	.36	810	—	—
prep with milk, 8 oz	220	5	15	16	—	100	.36	865	—	—
CURLY NOODLE WITH CHICKEN, 4 oz cond	70	3	3	9	—	*	.72	960	—	15
FRENCH ONION, 4 oz cond	60	2	2	9	—	20	.36	950	—	5
ls, rts, 10½ oz	80	2	4	8	—	20	1.08	50	—	—
dry mix, 8 oz prep	150	1	3	8	—	20	0	710	—	—
FULL FLAVORED CHICKEN VEGETABLE, SOUP FOR ONE, 7¾ oz, 11 oz prep	120	4	6	13	—	20	.72	1500	—	—
GAZPACHO, 4 oz cond	40	0	0	10	—	20	.36	590	—	0
GOLDEN CHICKEN & NOODLES, SOUP FOR ONE, 7¾ oz, 11 oz prep	120	6	4	14	—	20	1.08	1450	—	—
GREEN PEA, 4 oz cond	160	8	3	25	4d	*	1.44	840	—	5
MEATBALL ALPHABET, 4 oz cond	100	5	4	11	—	*	.72	970	—	10
MINESTRONE, 4 oz cond	80	4	2	12	2d	20	1.08	930	—	0
MUSHROOM, CREAM OF, 4 oz cond	100	1	7	9	—	20	*	820	—	0
ls, rts, 10½ oz	200	3	14	17	—	60	.72	55	—	—
MUSHROOM, GOLDEN, 4 oz cond	80	2	3	10	—	*	.36	900	—	5
NOODLE & GROUND BEEF, 4 oz cond	90	4	4	10	—	*	1.08	840	—	25
NOODLE SOUP WITH BROTH MIX, 8 oz prep	110	4	2	18	—	0	1.44	890	—	—
OLD FASHIONED BEAN WITH HAM, SOUP FOR ONE, 7¾ oz, 11 oz prep	220	8	7	30	—	80	1.80	1400	—	—
ONION, CREAM OF, 4 oz cond	100	2	5	12	—	20	*	830	—	15
prep with water & milk, 8 oz	140	4	7	15	—	80	.36	860	—	—
ONION MUSHROOM MIX, 8 oz prep	60	1	1	10	—	0	0	890	—	—
OYSTER STEW, 4 oz cond	80	3	5	5	—	*	1.44	850	—	25
prep with milk, 8 oz	150	6	9	10	—	100	1.44	900	—	—
PEPPER POT, 4 oz cond	90	5	4	9	—	*	.72	960	—	40
POTATO, CREAM OF, 4 oz cond	70	1	3	11	—	*	*	930	—	5
prep with milk & water, 8 oz	110	3	4	14	—	80	.36	960	—	—
SAVORY CREAM OF MUSHROOM, SOUP FOR ONE, 7½ oz, 11 oz prep	180	3	13	14	—	20	.36	1500	—	—
SCOTCH BROTH, 4 oz cond	80	4	3	9	—	*	.72	890	—	10
SHRIMP, CREAM OF, 4 oz cond	90	2	6	8	—	*	*	790	—	20
prep with milk, 8 oz	160	5	10	13	—	150	.36	850	—	—
SPLIT PEA, ls, 10¾ oz	240	11	5	38	—	40	2.70	25	—	—
SPLIT PEA WITH HAM & BACON, 4 oz cond	160	8	4	24	4d	*	1.80	800	—	5
TOMATO, 4 oz cond	90	1	2	17	—	*	.36	720	—	0
prep with milk, 8 oz	160	5	6	22	—	100	.72	770	—	—
TOMATO BISQUE, 4 oz cond	120	1	3	23	—	40	.36	830	—	5
TOMATO, CREAM OF, HOMESTYLE, 4 oz cond	110	1	3	20	—	*	.72	830	—	—
prep with milk, 8 oz cond	180	5	7	25	—	100	.72	880	—	—
TOMATO RICE, OLD										

FOOD & DESCRIPTION MEASURE OR QUANTITY	CALORIES	PROTEIN (GM)	FAT (GM)	CARBO-HYDRATE (GM)	FIBER (GM)	CALCIUM (MG)	IRON (MG)	SODIUM (MG)	POTASSIUM (MG)	CHOLES-TEROL (MG)
FASHIONED, 4 oz cond	110	1	2	22	—	*	.36	760	—	0
TOMATO ROYALE, SOUP FOR ONE, 7¾ oz, 11 oz prep	180	3	3	35	—	20	.72	1080	—	—
TOMATO WITH TOMATO PIECES, ls, rts, 10½ oz	180	3	5	29	—	40	1.08	40	—	—
TURKEY NOODLE, 4 oz cond	60	3	2	8	—	*	.72	910	—	15
TURKEY VEGETABLE, 4 oz cond	70	2	3	8	—	*	.36	820	—	10
VEGETABLE, 4 oz cond	80	3	2	13	2d	20	.72	770	—	0
VEGETABLE BEEF, 4 oz cond	70	4	2	8	1d	*	1.08	820	—	10
VEGETABLE, HOMESTYLE, 4 oz cond	60	2	2	10	—	20	.72	880	—	0
VEGETABLE, OLD FASHIONED, 4 oz cond	60	2	2	9	—	*	.36	910	—	0
VEGETABLE, OLD WORLD, SOUP FOR ONE, 7¾ oz, 11 oz prep	130	4	4	18	—	60	1.44	1470	—	—
VEGETARIAN VEGETABLE, 4 oz cond	80	2	2	13	2d	20	.72	770	—	0
WON TON, 4 oz cond	40	3	1	5	—	*	.36	870	—	10
Dia-Mel										
CHICKEN NOODLE, 8 oz	50	3	1	7	—	—	—	20	—	—
MUSHROOM, CREAM OF, 8 oz	85	2	5	9	—	—	—	30	—	—
TOMATO, 8 oz	50	1	<1	11	—	—	—	15	—	—
VEGETABLE BEEF, 8 oz	70	3	2	12	—	—	—	20	—	—
Estee										
BEEF VEGETABLE MIX, 6 oz prep	30	2	<1	3	—	—	—	115	—	<1
CHICKEN NOODLE MIX, 6 oz prep	35	2	1	2	—	—	—	140	—	4
CLAM CHOWDER, MANHATTAN, MIX, 6 oz prep	30	2	0	3	—	—	—	130	—	3
MUSHROOM MIX, 6 oz prep	30	2	1	2	—	—	—	140	—	<1
TOMATO MIX, 6 oz prep	40	1	<1	5	—	—	—	55	—	0
Featherweight										
BEEF BOUILLON, INSTANT, LOW SODIUM, 1 tsp	18	0	1	2	—	—	—	10	545	—
CHICKEN BOUILLON, INSTANT, LOW SODIUM, 1 tsp	18	0	1	2	—	—	—	5	510	—
CHICKEN NOODLE, LOW SODIUM, 1 c	60	4	2	8	—	—	—	40	6	—
MUSHROOM, LOW SODIUM, 1 c	50	1	2	9	—	—	—	15	474	—
TOMATO, LOW SODIUM, 1 c	60	2	0	15	—	—	—	10	670	—
VEGETABLE BEEF, LOW SODIUM, 1 c	80	4	3	12	—	—	—	20	420	—
Grandma Brown's										
BEAN SOUP, 8 oz, 227 gm	182	9	3	29	—	80	2.70	—	—	—
SPLIT PEA SOUP, 8 oz, 227 gm	184	11	3	28	—	20	2.16	—	—	—
Habitant—Catelli										
CABBAGE, 1 c	39	<1	2	6	.50	34	.25	881	147	—
CHICKEN, CREAM OF, 1 c	157	3	12	10	tr	42	.13	717	69	—
CHICKEN NOODLE, 1 c	85	5	3	8	.08	14	.48	901	95	—

FOOD & DESCRIPTION MEASURE OR QUANTITY	CALORIES	PROTEIN (GM)	FAT (GM)	CARBO-HYDRATE (GM)	FIBER (GM)	CALCIUM (MG)	IRON (MG)	SODIUM (MG)	POTASSIUM (MG)	CHOLES-TEROL (MG)
CHICKEN RICE, 1 c	83	5	3	8	.10	14	.46	807	91	—
MINESTRONE, 1 c	85	3	2	15	.41	24	.85	1105	208	—
MUSHROOM, CREAM OF, 1 c	113	1	8	9	tr	41	.13	508	51	—
PEA, 1 c	176	10	5	24	1.94	31	2.05	907	404	—
PEA WITH HAM, 1 c	194	12	6	25	1.97	33	2.26	926	439	—
TOMATO, CREAM OF, 1 c	112	3	2	21	.34	61	1.45	750	396	—
TOMATO VERMICELLI, 1 c	57	2	1	10	.15	12	.73	935	150	—
VEGETABLE, 1 c	74	2	2	13	.43	21	.84	1118	193	—

Hain

FOOD & DESCRIPTION MEASURE OR QUANTITY	CALORIES	PROTEIN (GM)	FAT (GM)	CARBO-HYDRATE (GM)	FIBER (GM)	CALCIUM (MG)	IRON (MG)	SODIUM (MG)	POTASSIUM (MG)	CHOLES-TEROL (MG)
CHICKEN VEGETABLE, 9½ oz prep	130	9	3	15	—	20	.72	—	—	—
UNSALTED, 9½ oz prep	130	9	3	15	—	40	1.08	100	—	—
LENTIL, 9½ oz prep	190	6	5	30	—	20	2.70	—	—	—
UNSALTED, 9½ oz prep	190	6	5	30	—	20	2.70	55	—	—
MINESTRONE, 9½ oz prep	190	5	4	33	—	40	1.80	—	—	—
UNSALTED, 9½ oz prep	190	6	5	33	—	40	2.16	35	—	—
SPLIT PEA, 9½ oz prep	210	9	2	37	—	20	3.34	—	—	—
UNSALTED, 9½ oz prep	220	10	1	40	—	20	1.80	40	—	—
VEGETARIAN VEGETABLE, 9½ oz prep	180	4	6	25	—	40	1.80	—	—	—
UNSALTED, 9½ oz prep	160	3	5	25	—	20	1.44	45	—	—

Herb-Ox

FOOD & DESCRIPTION MEASURE OR QUANTITY	CALORIES	PROTEIN (GM)	FAT (GM)	CARBO-HYDRATE (GM)	FIBER (GM)	CALCIUM (MG)	IRON (MG)	SODIUM (MG)	POTASSIUM (MG)	CHOLES-TEROL (MG)
BEEF BOUILLON CUBES, 1 cube, 3.7 gm	6	<1	<1	<1	—	—	—	840	—	—
BEEF BROTH & SEASONING, 1 pkt	8	<1	<1	<1	—	—	—	1040	—	—
BEEF BROTH, ls, 1 pkt	11	1	<1	2	—	—	—	10	550	—
CHICKEN BOUILLON CUBES, 1 cube, 3.8 gm	6	<1	<1	<1	—	—	—	960	—	—
CHICKEN BROTH & SEASONING, 1 pkt	12	<1	<1	2	—	—	—	960	—	—
CHICKEN BROTH, ls, 1 pkt	12	<1	<1	2	—	—	—	5	600	—
ONION BOUILLON CUBES, 1 cube, 3.8 gm	10	<1	<1	<1	—	—	—	560	—	—
ONION BROTH & SEASONING, 1 pkt	14	<1	<1	2	—	—	—	800	—	—
VEGETABLE BOUILLON CUBES, 1 cube, 3.6 gm	6	<1	<1	<1	—	—	—	920	—	—
VEGETABLE BROTH & SEASONING, 1 pkt	12	<1	<1	2	—	—	—	880	—	—

Lipton

FOOD & DESCRIPTION MEASURE OR QUANTITY	CALORIES	PROTEIN (GM)	FAT (GM)	CARBO-HYDRATE (GM)	FIBER (GM)	CALCIUM (MG)	IRON (MG)	SODIUM (MG)	POTASSIUM (MG)	CHOLES-TEROL (MG)
ASPARAGUS PARISIENNE, CREAM OF, ½ env	70	3	2	9	—	20	*	900	—	—
prep, 9 oz	150	7	7	15	—	150	*	960	—	—
BEEF FLAVORED MUSHROOM, 8 oz prep	40	2	<1	7	—	*	*	995	—	—
BEEF FLAVOR CUP-A-SOUP TRIM, 6 oz prep	10	1	0	1	—	*	*	695	—	—
LOTS-A-NOODLES, 7 oz prep	120	5	2	21	—	20	.72	780	—	—
NOODLE CUP-A-SOUP, 6 oz prep	45	2	<1	8	—	*	.36	830	—	—
BEEF VEGETABLE CUP-A-SOUP, 6 oz prep	80	3	<1	14	—	*	.36	905	—	—
BEEFY ONION, 8 oz prep	35	1	1	5	—	*	*	950	—	—
BEEFY TOMATO CUP-A-SOUP TRIM, 6 oz prep	10	<1	0	2	—	*	*	440	—	—
BEEF VEGETABLE NOODLE, HEARTY, 8 oz prep	80	3	<1	14	—	*	.36	905	—	—
CALIFORNIA CREAM OF										

FOOD & DESCRIPTION MEASURE OR QUANTITY	CALORIES	PROTEIN (GM)	FAT (GM)	CARBO- HYDRATE (GM)	FIBER (GM)	CALCIUM (MG)	IRON (MG)	SODIUM (MG)	POTASSIUM (MG)	CHOLES- TEROL (MG)
BROCCOLI, ½ env	90	3	3	11	—	40	.36	850	—	—
prep, 9 oz	160	7	8	16	—	150	.36	910	—	—
CHICKEN CUP-A-BROTH, 6 oz prep	25	1	<1	4	—	*	*	780	—	—
CHICKEN, CREAM OF CUP-A-SOUP, 6 oz prep	80	2	4	9	—	*	*	840	—	—
LOTS-A-NOODLES, 7 oz prep	150	5	5	22	—	*	.72	755	—	—
CHICKEN FLAVOR CUP-A-SOUP TRIM, 6 oz prep	10	<1	0	1	—	*	*	560	—	—
LOTS-A-NOODLES, 7 oz prep	120	5	1	23	—	*	.72	855	—	—
CHICKEN NOODLE, 8 oz prep	70	3	2	9	—	*	.36	900	—	—
HEARTY, 8 oz prep	90	4	2	14	—	*	.36	695	—	—
WITH MEAT, CUP-A-SOUP, 6 oz prep	45	3	1	6	—	*	.36	770	—	—
CHICKEN RICE CUP-A-SOUP, 6 oz prep	45	2	<1	7	—	*	.36	750	—	—
CHICKEN SUPREME CUP-A-SOUP, 6 oz prep	100	3	5	11	—	20	.36	870	—	—
CHICKEN VEGETABLES CUP-A-SOUP, 6 oz prep	40	2	<1	7	—	*	.36	800	—	—
COUNTRY VEGETABLE, 8 oz prep	80	3	1	14	—	*	.36	995	—	—
GARDEN VEGETABLE LOTS-A-NOODLES, 7 oz prep	130	5	2	23	—	*	1.08	745	—	—
GIGGLE NOODLE, 8 oz prep	80	3	2	12	—	*	.36	925	—	—
GOLDEN MUSHROOM, CHICKEN BROTH, 8 oz prep	60	2	2	8	—	*	*	900	—	—
GOLDEN ONION, CHICKEN BROTH, 8 oz prep	60	1	1	10	—	*	*	995	—	—
GREEN PEA CUP-A-SOUP, 6 oz prep	120	4	4	16	—	20	*	710	—	—
HARVEST VEGETABLE CUP-A-SOUP, 6 oz prep	90	2	<1	20	—	20	.72	625	—	—
HEARTY CHICKEN CUP-A-SOUP, 6 oz prep	70	4	1	10	—	*	.36	970	—	—
HERB VEGETABLE CUP-A-SOUP TRIM, 6 oz prep	10	1	0	1	—	*	*	560	—	—
LOBSTER BISQUE, ½ env	80	4	2	10	—	20	*	1030	—	—
prep, 9 oz	160	8	7	16	—	150	*	1090	—	—
MUSHROOM A LA REINE, CREAM OF, ½ env	100	4	3	13	—	20	.72	930	—	—
prep, 9 oz	180	8	8	19	—	150	.72	990	—	—
MUSHROOM, CREAM OF, CUP-A-SOUP, 6 oz prep	80	2	4	9	—	*	*	830	—	—
NEW ENGLAND CLAM CHOWDER, ½ env	120	5	2	19	—	40	.36	920	—	—
prep, 9 oz	190	9	7	24	—	200	.36	980	—	—
NOODLE WITH CHICKEN BROTH, 8 oz prep	70	2	2	10	—	*	.36	785	—	—
NOODLE WITH VEGETABLES, CHICKEN BROTH, HEARTY, 8 oz prep	80	3	2	12	—	*	.36	925	—	—
ONION, 8 oz prep	35	1	<1	6	—	*	*	640	—	—
ONION, CUP-A-SOUP, 6 oz prep	30	1	1	5	—	*	*	870	—	—
ONION, MUSHROOM, 8 oz prep	45	2	1	7	—	*	*	995	—	—
ORIENTAL STYLE LOTS-A-NOODLES, 7 oz prep	120	5	2	20	—	20	1.08	940	—	—
RING NOODLE CUP-A-SOUP, 6 oz prep	50	2	1	9	—	*	.36	745	—	—
RING-O-NOODLE, 8 oz prep	60	3	1	9	—	*	.36	855	—	—

FOOD & DESCRIPTION MEASURE OR QUANTITY	CALORIES	PROTEIN (GM)	FAT (GM)	CARBO-HYDRATE (GM)	FIBER (GM)	CALCIUM (MG)	IRON (MG)	SODIUM (MG)	POTASSIUM (MG)	CHOLES-TEROL (MG)
SPRING VEGETABLE CUP-A-SOUP, 6 oz prep	40	2	1	7	—	*	.36	865	—	—
TOMATO CUP-A-SOUP, 6 oz prep	80	1	1	17	—	20	.36	650	—	—
TOMATO ONION, 8 oz prep	80	1	<1	17	—	20	.36	900	—	—
TOMATO VEGETABLE LOTS-A-NOODLES, 7 oz prep	110	4	1	21	—	*	.72	885	—	—
TOMATO VEGETABLE NOODLE, HEARTY, 8 oz prep	80	3	1	15	—	*	.36	930	—	—
VEGETABLE BEEF CUP-A-SOUP, 6 oz prep	50	2	<1	8	—	*	.36	820	—	—
VEGETABLE SOUP FOR DIP, 8 oz prep	45	2	<1	8	—	20	.36	995	—	—
VEGETABLE WITH BEEF STOCK, 8 oz prep	50	2	<1	9	—	*	.36	995	—	—
VIRGINIA PEA CUP-A-SOUP, 6 oz prep	140	5	5	18	—	20	*	870	—	—

Lite-line—Borden

BEEF FLAVOR LOW SODIUM INSTANT BROTH, 1 tsp dry	12	<1	<1	2	—	*	*	10	600	—
CHICKEN FLAVOR LOW SODIUM INSTANT BROTH, 1 tsp dry	12	<1	<1	2	—	*	*	5	585	—

Manischewitz

BORSCHT, LOW CALORIE, 8 oz	20	—	0	—	—	—	—	640	—	0
MINESTRONE SOUP MIX, 6 oz prep	50	—	<1	—	—	—	—	160	—	—
PEA SOUP MIX, 6 oz prep	45	—	<1	—	—	—	—	320	—	0
VEGETABLE SOUP MIX, 6 oz prep	50	—	<1	—	—	—	—	25	—	—

Progresso

BEAN & HAM, 9½ oz	170	11	1	30	—	100	2.70	1170	—	—
BEEF, 9½ oz	150	9	4	19	—	40	2.70	1390	—	—
BEEF MINESTRONE, 9½ oz	150	11	4	19	—	40	2.70	1040	—	—
BEEF VEGETABLE, 9½ oz	150	12	2	19	—	40	1.80	1140	—	—
10½ oz	160	13	3	21	—	40	2.70	1310	—	—
CHICKARINA WITH TINY MEATBALLS, 9½ oz	90	8	6	8	—	20	1.44	1060	—	—
CHICKEN, HOMESTYLE, 9½ oz	90	9	2	8	—	*	1.08	1190	—	—
10½ oz	100	10	2	9	—	*	1.08	1320	—	—
CHICKEN MINESTRONE, 9½ oz	150	10	6	15	—	20	1.80	1210	—	—
CHICKEN NOODLE, 9½ oz	120	12	4	10	—	*	1.44	980	—	—
10½ oz	130	13	4	11	—	*	1.44	1080	—	—
CHICKEN RICE WITH VEGETABLES, 9½ oz	140	8	3	22	—	20	1.08	880	—	—
CLAM CHOWDER, MANHATTAN, 9½ oz	130	6	3	21	—	60	.72	1240	—	—
ESCAROLE IN CHICKEN BROTH, 9½ oz	35	2	3	3	—	60	1.44	1020	—	—
FRENCH ONION, 9½ oz	120	4	9	9	—	40	1.80	1270	—	—
LENTIL, 9½ oz	170	11	2	26	—	40	4.50	1000	—	—
10½ oz	180	12	2	28	—	40	4.50	1110	—	—
MACARONI & BEAN, 9½ oz	180	6	3	30	—	80	2.70	1290	—	—
MINESTRONE, 9½ oz	150	7	3	24	—	60	1.44	820	—	—
10½ oz	160	7	4	27	—	60	1.80	900	—	—

FOOD & DESCRIPTION MEASURE OR QUANTITY	CALORIES	PROTEIN (GM)	FAT (GM)	CARBO-HYDRATE (GM)	FIBER (GM)	CALCIUM (MG)	IRON (MG)	SODIUM (MG)	POTASSIUM (MG)	CHOLES-TEROL (MG)
PEA, 9½ oz	190	10	2	31	—	20	2.70	1050	—	—
SPLIT PEA WITH HAM, 9½ oz	170	10	3	26	—	20	1.44	1030	—	—
TOMATO WITH MACARONI SHELLS, 10½ oz	130	4	2	24	—	40	1.08	1270	—	—
TOMATO WITH VEGETABLES & MACARONI, 9½ oz	120	4	2	22	—	40	1.08	1150	—	—
TORTELLINI, 9½ oz	80	3	2	13	—	40	1.08	1080	—	—

Rokeach

BORSCHT										
DIET, 8 oz	29	<1	<1	6	.36	13	.46	897	—	—
REGULAR, 8 oz	96	<1	<1	23	.49	11	.37	985	—	—
UNSALTED, 8 oz	103	<1	<1	25	.45	12	.38	50	—	—
CELERY, CREAM OF, cond, 5 oz	90	2	4	12	—	60	.36	950	—	—
prep with milk, 10 oz	190	7	9	19	—	250	.36	1020	—	—
MUSHROOM, CREAM OF, cond, 5 oz	150	2	10	13	—	60	.36	1050	—	—
prep with milk, 10 oz	240	7	15	20	—	250	.36	1170	—	—
TOMATO, cond, 5 oz	90	2	1	20	—	20	.36	980	—	—
prep with milk, 10 oz	190	7	6	27	—	200	.36	1059	—	—
TOMATO RICE, cond, 5 oz	160	3	5	25	—	40	.72	815	—	—
VEGETARIAN VEGETABLE, cond, 5 oz	90	2	3	15	—	20	.36	1055	—	—

R.T. French

BEEF FLAVOR STOCK BASE, 1 tsp, 3.7 gm	8	<1	<1	2	—	*	*	470	—	—
CHICKEN FLAVOR STOCK BASE, 1 tsp, 3.2 gm	8	<1	<1	1	—	*	*	480	—	—

Snow's

CLAM CHOWDER, MANHATTAN, prep with water, 7½ oz	70	3	2	9	—	40	.72	635	215	—
CLAM CHOWDER, NEW ENGLAND, cond, 3¾ oz	70	5	2	8	—	*	.36	620	120	—
prep with milk, 7½ oz	140	8	6	13	—	150	.72	665	285	—
CORN CHOWDER, NEW ENGLAND, cond, 3¾ oz	80	2	2	13	—	*	.36	595	115	—
prep with milk, 7½ oz	150	5	6	18	—	150	.36	640	280	—
FISH CHOWDER, NEW ENGLAND, cond, 3¾ oz	60	5	2	6	—	*	.36	565	125	—
prep with milk, 7½ oz	130	9	6	11	—	150	.36	620	290	—
SEAFOOD CHOWDER, NEW ENGLAND, cond 3¾ oz	60	4	2	6	—	*	.36	640	115	—
prep with milk, 7½ oz	130	8	6	11	—	150	.36	690	280	—

Stouffer's

CLAM CHOWDER, NEW ENGLAND, 8 oz	200	8	11	16	—	80	1.44	790	370	—
SPINACH, CREAM OF, 8 oz	220	7	14	16	—	200	.72	1020	420	—
SPLIT PEA WITH HAM, 8¼ oz	200	12	3	30	—	20	1.44	1130	430	—

Swanson–Campbell

BEEF BROTH, rts, 7¼ oz	20	2	1	1	—	*	.36	750	—	—
CHICKEN BROTH, rts, 7¼ oz	30	2	2	2	—	*	.36	910	—	—
CHICKEN BROTH NATURAL GOODNESS, rts, 7¼ oz	18	2	1	1	—	*	.36	630	—	—

FOOD & DESCRIPTION MEASURE OR QUANTITY	CALORIES	PROTEIN (GM)	FAT (GM)	CARBO-HYDRATE (GM)	FIBER (GM)	CALCIUM (MG)	IRON (MG)	SODIUM (MG)	POTASSIUM (MG)	CHOLES-TEROL (MG)
USDA										
ASPARAGUS, CREAM OF,										
cond, 10.75 oz, 305 gm	210	6	10	26	1.83	70	1.95	2385	421	12
prep with milk, 1 c, 248 gm	161	6	8	16	.74	175	.87	1041	359	22
prep with water, 1 c, 244 gm	87	2	4	11	.73	29	.8	981	173	5
ASPARAGUS, CREAM OF, dry,										
1 pkt, 63.8 gm	234	9	7	36	.51	—	—	3177	—	1
prep with water, 1 c, 251 gm	59	2	2	9	.13	—	—	801	—	tr
BEAN, BLACK, cond, 11 oz,										
312 gm	285	15	4	48	—	110	4.68	3026	780	0
prep with water, 1 c, 247 gm	116	6	2	20	1.31	45	2.16	1198	273	0
BEAN WITH BACON, cond,										
11½ oz, 326 gm	420	19	14	55	4.24	196	4.97	2311	978	6
prep with water, 1 c, 253 gm	173	8	6	23	1.52	81	2.05	952	403	3
BEAN WITH BACON, dry, 1 pkt, prep with water, 1										
c, 265 gm	105	5	2	16	1.53	—	—	928	326	3
BEAN WITH FRANKFURTER,										
cond, 11¼ oz, 319 gm	454	24	17	53	4.15	210	5.68	2651	1158	29
prep with water, 1 c, 250 gm	187	10	7	22	1.5	86	2.34	1092	477	12
BEAN WITH HAM, CHUNKY,										
rts, 19¼ oz, 546 gm	519	28	19	61	—	177	7.26	2184	—	49
1 c, 243 gm	231	13	9	27	—	79	3.23	972	—	22
BEEF BROTH CUBE, 1 cube,										
3.6 gm, 6 oz prep	6	<1	<1	<1	—	—	.08	864	15	tr
BEEF BROTH or BOUILLON,										
dry, 1 pkt, 6 gm	14	<1	<1	1	.01	4	—	1019	27	1
prep with water, 1 c, 244 gm	19	1	<1	2	.01	5	—	1358	36	1
BEEF BROTH or BOUILLON,										
rts, 14 oz, 397 gm	27	5	<1	<1	tr	25	.67	1294	214	1
1 c, 240 gm	16	3	<1	<1	tr	15	.41	782	130	tr
BEEF, CHUNKY, rts, 19 oz,										
539 gm	383	26	12	44	1.62	69	5.2	1947	755	32
1 c, 240 gm	171	12	5	20	.72	31	2.32	867	336	14
BEEF NOODLE, cond, 10¾ oz,										
305 gm	204	12	7	22	.31	36	2.67	2313	241	12
prep with water, 1 c, 244 gm	84	5	3	9	tr	15	1.10	952	99	5
BEEF NOODLE, dry, 1 pkt, 9.2										
gm, 6 oz prep	30	2	<1	4	.04	4	.25	774	60	1
prep with water, 1 c, 251 gm	41	2	<1	6	.06	5	.33	1041	81	2
CAULIFLOWER, dry, 1 pkt, prep with water, 1 c,										
256 gm	68	3	2	11	.19	—	—	843	—	tr
CELERY, CREAM OF, cond,										
10¾ oz, 305 gm	219	4	14	21	.92	98	1.52	2308	299	34
prep with milk, 1 c, 248 gm	165	6	10	15	.38	186	.69	1010	309	32
1 can cond & 1 can milk, 602 gm	400	14	24	35	.92	451	1.67	2451	751	78
prep with water, 1 c, 244 gm	90	2	6	9	.38	40	.62	949	123	15
CELERY, CREAM OF, dry, prep										
with water, 1 c, 254 gm	63	3	2	10	.19	—	—	839	—	1
CHEESE, cond, 11 oz, 312 gm	377	13	25	26	—	345	1.81	2331	374	72
prep with milk, 1 c, 251 gm	230	9	15	16	—	288	.81	1020	340	48
1 can cond & 1 can milk, 609 gm	558	23	35	39	—	698	1.95	2474	826	116
prep with water, 1 c, 247 gm	155	5	10	11	—	142	.75	959	154	30
CHICKEN & DUMPLINGS,										
cond, 10½ oz, 298 gm	236	14	13	15	—	35	1.52	2093	283	80
prep with water, 1 c, 241 gm	97	6	6	6	—	15	.62	861	116	34
CHICKEN BROTH, cond, 10¾										
oz, 305 gm	94	13	3	2	tr	17	1.25	1909	519	3
prep with water, 1 c, 244 gm	39	5	1	<1	tr	9	.51	776	210	1

FOOD & DESCRIPTION MEASURE OR QUANTITY	CALORIES	PROTEIN (GM)	FAT (GM)	CARBO-HYDRATE (GM)	FIBER (GM)	CALCIUM (MG)	IRON (MG)	SODIUM (MG)	POTASSIUM (MG)	CHOLES-TEROL (MG)
CHICKEN BROTH/BOUILLON CUBE, 1 cube, 4.8 gm, 6 oz prep	9	<1	<1	1	—	—	.09	1152	18	1
CHICKEN BROTH or BOUILLON, 1 pkt, 6 gm	16	1	<1	1	.01	11	.06	1115	19	1
prep with water, 1 c, 244 gm	21	1	1	1	.01	15	.08	1484	25	1
CHICKEN, CHUNKY, rts, 10¾ oz, 305 gm	216	15	8	21	.31	29	2.1	1078	214	37
1 c, 251 gm	178	13	7	17	.25	24	1.73	887	176	30
CHICKEN, CREAM OF, dry, 1 pkt, 18.3 gm	80	1	4	10	.87	57	—	882	160	2
prep with water, 1 c, 261 gm	107	2	5	13	1.16	76	—	1184	215	3
CHICKEN, CREAM OF, cond, 10¾ oz, 305 gm	283	8	18	23	.31	83	1.47	2397	212	24
prep with milk, 1 c, 248 gm	191	7	11	15	.13	180	.67	1046	273	27
1 can cond & 1 can milk, 602 gm	464	18	28	36	.31	437	1.62	2540	664	66
prep with water, 1 c, 244 gm	116	3	7	9	.12	34	.61	986	87	10
CHICKEN GUMBO, cond, 10¾ oz, 305 gm	137	6	3	20	.61	59	2.17	2321	183	9
prep with water, 1 c, 244 gm	56	3	1	8	.24	24	.89	955	75	5
CHICKEN NOODLE, dry, 1 pkt, 11.1 gm	38	2	<1	5	.05	23	.36	931	23	2
1 pkt, 74.4 gm	257	14	6	36	.30	154	2.42	6243	153	10
prep with water, 1 c, 252 gm	53	3	1	7	.06	32	.50	1284	31	3
CHICKEN NOODLE, cond, 10½ oz, 298 gm	182	10	6	23	.30	32	1.84	2257	134	15
prep with water, 1 c, 241 gm	75	4	2	9	.24	17	.78	1107	55	7
CHICKEN NOODLE WITH MEATBALLS, rts, 20 oz, 567 gm	227	19	8	19	1.25	69	3.97	2376	—	23
1 c, 248 gm	99	8	4	8	.55	30	1.74	1039	—	10
CHICKEN RICE, CHUNKY, rts, 19 oz, 539 gm	286	28	7	29	—	78	4.20	1994	—	27
1 c, 240 gm	127	12	3	13	—	35	1.87	888	—	12
CHICKEN RICE, cond, 10½ oz, 298 gm	146	9	5	17	.30	42	1.82	1980	244	15
prep with water, 1 c, 241 gm	60	4	2	7	tr	17	.75	814	100	7
CHICKEN RICE, dry, prep with water, 1 c, 253 gm	60	2	1	9	—	8	—	980	10	3
CHICKEN VEGETABLE, CHUNKY, rts, 19 oz, 539 gm	374	28	11	42	—	57	3.31	2399	—	38
1 c, 240 gm	167	12	5	19	—	25	1.47	1068	—	17
CHICKEN VEGETABLE, cond, 10½ oz, 298 gm	181	9	7	21	.30	43	2.13	2297	374	21
prep with water, 1 c, 241 gm	74	4	3	9	.12	18	.87	944	154	10
CHICKEN VEGETABLE, dry, 1 pkt, 10.6 gm	37	2	<1	6	—	—	.44	604	51	2
prep with water, 1 c, 251 gm	49	3	<1	8	—	—	.59	808	68	3
CHILI BEEF, cond, 11¼ oz, 319 gm	411	16	16	52	3.51	105	5.18	2513	1275	32
prep with water, 1 c, 250 gm	169	7	7	21	1.45	43	2.13	1035	525	12
CLAM CHOWDER, MANHATTAN, CHUNKY, rts, 19 oz, 539 gm	299	16	8	42	1.08	151	5.93	2245	862	32
1 c, 240 gm	133	7	3	19	.48	67	2.64	1000	384	14
CLAM CHOWDER, MANHATTAN, cond, 10¾ oz, 305 gm	187	5	5	30	.92	56	3.97	2446	458	6
prep with water, 1 c, 244 gm	78	4	2	12	.49	34	1.89	1808	262	2
CLAM CHOWDER, MANHATTAN, dry, prep with water, 1 c, 18.9 gm	65	2	2	11	.57	—	—	1336	—	0

CLAM CHOWDER, NEW ENGLAND, cond, 10¾ oz, 305 gm	214	13	6	27	—	99	3.45	2266	278	12
prep with milk, 1 c, 248 gm	163	9	7	17	—	187	1.48	992	300	22
1 can cond & 1 can milk, 602 gm	396	23	16	40	—	453	3.59	2409	729	54
prep with water, 1 c, 244 gm	95	5	3	12	.27	43	1.48	914	146	5
CLAM CHOWDER, NEW ENGLAND, dry, 22.7 gm pkt, prep with water, 1 c	95	3	4	13	.20	76	—	745	205	1
CONSOMME WITH GELATIN, cond, 10½ oz, 298 gm	71	13	0	4	—	21	1.28	1550	373	0
prep with water, 1 c, 241 gm	29	5	0	2	—	8	.53	637	153	0
CONSOMME WITH GELATIN, dry, 1 pkt, 56.7 gm	77	10	<1	9	.06	—	—	14855	—	0
prep with water, 1 c, 249 gm	17	2	<1	2	.01	—	—	3299	—	0
CRAB, rts, 13 oz, 369 gm	114	8	2	16	.81	99	1.85	1866	493	10
1 c, 244 gm	76	5	2	10	.54	65	1.22	1234	326	10
ESCAROLE, rts, 19½ oz, 553 gm	61	3	4	4	1.66	72	1.66	8618	—	6
1 c, 248 gm	27	2	2	2	.74	32	.74	3865	—	2
GAZPACHO, rts, 13 oz, 369 gm	87	13	3	1	1.18	37	1.48	1790	338	0
1 c, 244 gm	57	9	2	<1	.78	24	.98	1183	224	0
LEEK, dry, 1 pkt, 78 gm	294	9	9	47	1.09	—	—	4009	—	9
prep with water, 1 c, 254 gm	71	2	2	11	.26	—	—	966	—	3
LENTIL WITH HAM, rts, 20 oz, 567 gm	320	21	6	46	3.20	96	6.04	3014	815	17
1 c, 248 gm	140	9	3	20	1.40	42	2.64	1318	356	7
MINESTRONE, CHUNKY, rts, 19 oz, 539 gm	285	11	6	47	—	136	3.97	1940	—	11
1 c, 240 gm	127	5	3	21	—	61	1.77	864	—	5
MINESTRONE, cond, 10½ oz, 298 gm	202	10	6	27	1.79	83	2.24	2217	760	3
prep with water, 1 c, 241 gm	83	4	3	11	.72	34	.92	911	312	2
MINESTRONE, dry, 1 pkt, 78 gm	279	16	6	42	1.48	—	—	3604	—	6
prep with water, 1 c, 254 gm	79	4	2	12	.42	—	—	1026	—	3
MUSHROOM, CREAM OF, cond, 10¾ oz, 305 gm	313	5	23	23	.61	78	1.28	2469	203	3
prep with milk, 1 c, 248 gm	203	6	14	15	.25	178	.59	1076	270	20
1 can cond & 1 can milk, 602 gm	494	15	33	36	.61	432	1.43	2612	655	48
prep with water, 1 c, 244 gm	129	2	9	9	.46	46	.51	1031	101	2
UNSALTED, 1 c, 244 gm	129	2	9	9	.46	46	.51	27	101	2
MUSHROOM, dry, 1 pkt, 74.4 gm	328	8	17	38	.25	228	—	3482	681	2
1 inst pkt, 16.7 gm	74	2	4	9	.06	51	—	782	153	0
prep with water, 1 c, 253 gm	96	2	5	11	.07	67	—	1019	199	1
MUSHROOM WITH BEEF STOCK, cond, 10¾ oz, 305 gm	208	8	10	23	—	25	2.04	2358	384	18
prep with water, 1 c, 244 gm	85	3	4	9	—	10	.84	970	158	7
ONION, cond, 10½ oz, 298 gm	138	9	4	20	1.19	64	1.64	2563	167	0
prep with water, 1 c, 241 gm	57	4	2	8	.48	26	.67	1053	69	0
ONION, dry, 1 pkt, 39 gm	115	5	2	21	.94	55	.58	3493	260	2
1 pkt, 7.1 gm	21	<1	<1	4	.17	10	.11	636	47	0
prep with water, 1 c, 246 gm	28	1	<1	5	.23	13	.14	848	63	0
OXTAIL, dry, 1 pkt, 74.4 gm	280	11	10	36	.52	—	—	4806	—	11
prep with water, 1 c, 253 gm	71	3	3	9	.13	—	—	1210	—	3
OYSTER STEW, cond, 10½ oz, 298 gm	144	5	9	10	—	52	2.38	2384	119	33
prep with milk, 1 c, 245 gm	134	6	8	10	—	167	1.04	1040	235	32
1 can cond & 1 can milk, 595										

FOOD & DESCRIPTION MEASURE OR QUANTITY	CALORIES	PROTEIN (GM)	FAT (GM)	CARBO- HYDRATE (GM)	FIBER (GM)	CALCIUM (MG)	IRON (MG)	SODIUM (MG)	POTASSIUM (MG)	CHOLES- TEROL (MG)
gm	325	15	19	24	—	406	2.53	2526	571	77
prep with water, 1 c, 241 gm	59	2	4	4	—	22	.98	980	49	14
PEA, GREEN, cond, 11¼ oz,										
319 gm	398	21	7	64	1.60	66	4.73	2397	463	0
prep with milk, 1 c, 254 gm	239	13	7	32	.66	173	2.01	1048	377	18
1 can cond & 1 can milk, 616										
gm	579	31	17	78	1.60	420	4.88	2541	914	43
prep with water, 1 c, 250 gm	164	9	3	27	.66	27	1.95	987	190	0
UNSALTED, 1 c, 250 gm	164	9	3	27	.66	27	1.95	33	190	0
PEA, GREEN, or SPLIT, dry, 1										
pkt, 113 gm	402	23	5	69	2.08	68	3.04	3687	718	1
1 pkt, 28 gm	100	6	1	17	.52	17	.75	914	178	0
prep with water, 1 c, 271 gm	133	8	2	23	.69	22	1.01	1220	238	3
PEA, SPLIT WITH HAM, CHUNKY, rts, 19 oz, 539										
gm	413	25	9	60	—	74	4.80	2167	—	16
1 c, 240 gm	184	11	4	27	—	33	2.14	965	—	7
PEA, SPLIT WITH HAM, cond,										
11½ oz, 326 gm	459	25	11	68	1.63	53	5.53	2446	969	20
prep with water, 1 c, 253 gm	189	10	4	28	.67	22	2.28	1008	339	8
PEPPER POT, cond, 10½ oz,										
298 gm	251	15	11	23	1.19	57	2.18	2360	370	24
prep with water, 1 c, 241 gm	103	6	5	9	.48	23	.89	970	152	10
POTATO, CREAM OF, cond,										
10¾ oz, 305 gm	178	4	6	28	—	48	1.16	2431	332	15
prep with milk, 1 c, 248 gm	148	6	6	17	—	166	.54	1060	323	22
1 can cond & 1 can milk, 602										
gm	360	14	16	42	—	402	1.31	2574	784	54
prep with water, 1 c, 244 gm	73	2	2	11	—	20	.48	1000	137	5
SCOTCH BROTH, cond, 10½										
oz, 298 gm	195	12	6	23	—	37	2.03	2461	387	12
prep with water, 1 c, 241 gm	80	5	3	9	—	15	.83	1012	159	5
SHRIMP, CREAM OF, cond,										
10¾ oz, 305 gm	219	7	13	20	—	43	1.28	2373	—	40
prep with milk, 1 c, 248 gm	165	7	9	14	—	164	.59	1036	—	35
1 can cond & 1 can milk, 602										
gm	400	17	23	34	—	397	1.43	2516	—	84
prep with water, 1 c, 244 gm	90	3	5	8	—	18	.53	976	—	17
STOCKPOT, cond, 11 oz, 312										
gm	242	12	9	28	1.25	53	2.11	2546	577	9
prep with water, 1 c, 247 gm	100	5	4	12	.49	22	.87	1048	238	5
TOMATO, cond, 10¾ oz, 305										
gm	208	5	5	40	1.22	32	4.27	2120	641	0
prep with milk, 1 c, 248 gm	160	6	6	22	.50	159	1.82	932	450	17
1 can cond & 1 can milk, 602										
gm	389	15	15	54	1.20	386	4.41	2263	1092	42
prep with water, 1 c, 244	86	2	2	17	.49	13	1.76	872	263	0
TOMATO, dry, 1 pkt, 21.3 gm	77	2	2	15	.32	40	.32	707	221	1
prep with water, 1 c, 265 gm	102	2	2	19	.43	54	.42	943	295	1
TOMATO BEEF WITH NOODLE,										
cond, 10¾ oz, 305 gm	341	11	10	51	—	43	2.71	2230	537	9
prep with water, 1 c, 244 gm	140	4	4	21	—	18	1.12	917	221	5
TOMATO BISQUE, cond, 11										
oz, 312 gm	300	5	6	58	—	98	1.99	2546	1014	11
prep with milk, 1 c, 251 gm	198	6	7	29	—	186	.88	1108	604	22
1 can cond & 1 can milk, 609										
gm	481	15	16	71	—	452	2.13	2689	1465	53
prep with water, 1 c, 247 gm	123	2	3	24	—	40	.82	1048	417	4
UNSALTED, 1 c, 247 gm	123	2	3	24	—	40	.82	30	417	4
TOMATO RICE, cond, 11 oz,										
312 gm	291	5	7	53	1.56	56	1.93	1981	803	3
prep with water, 1 c, 247 gm	120	2	3	22	.64	23	.79	815	330	2
TOMATO VEGETABLE, 1 pkt,										
38.5 gm	125	5	2	23	1.19	18	1.43	2588	233	1

FOOD & DESCRIPTION MEASURE OR QUANTITY	CALORIES	PROTEIN (GM)	FAT (GM)	CARBO-HYDRATE (GM)	FIBER (GM)	CALCIUM (MG)	IRON (MG)	SODIUM (MG)	POTASSIUM (MG)	CHOLES-TEROL (MG)
prep with water, 1 c, 253 gm	55	2	<1	10	.53	8	.63	1146	103	tr
TURKEY, CHUNKY, rts, 18¾ oz, 532 gm	306	23	10	32	2.13	112	4.31	2082	814	21
1 c, 236 gm	136	10	4	14	.94	50	1.91	923	361	9
TURKEY NOODLE, cond, 10¾ oz, 305 gm	168	9	5	21	.31	28	2.29	1983	183	12
prep with water, 1 c, 244 gm	69	4	2	9	.24	12	.94	815	75	5
UNSALTED, 1 c, 244 gm	69	4	2	9	.24	12	.94	41	75	5
TURKEY VEGETABLE, cond, 10½ oz, 298 gm	179	8	7	21	—	40	1.85	2202	426	3
prep with water, 1 c, 241 gm	74	3	3	9	—	17	.76	905	175	2
VEGETABLE BEEF, dry, 1 pkt, 74.4 gm	256	14	5	38	.74	—	4.10	4806	—	6
prep with water, 1 c, 253 gm	53	3	1	8	.15	—	.85	1000	—	1
VEGETABLE, CHUNKY, rts, 19 oz, 539 gm	274	8	8	43	2.7	126	3.67	2269	889	0
1 c, 240 gm	122	4	4	19	1.2	56	1.63	1010	396	0
VEGETABLE, CREAM OF, 1 pkt, 17.7 gm	79	1	4	9	.11	—	—	877	72	0
prep with water, 1 c, 260 gm	105	2	6	12	.14	—	—	1171	96	0
VEGETABLE WITH BEEF, cond, 10¾ oz, 305 gm	192	14	5	25	.76	41	2.70	2326	420	12
prep with water, 1 c, 244 gm	79	6	2	10	.31	17	1.11	957	173	5
UNSALTED, 1 c, 244 gm	79	6	2	10	.31	17	1.11	51	173	5
VEGETABLE WITH BEEF BROTH, cond, 10½ oz, 298 gm	197	7	5	32	1.49	43	2.35	1969	467	6
prep with water, 1 c, 241 gm	81	3	2	13	.72	18	.97	810	192	2
UNSALTED, 1 c, 241 gm	81	3	2	13	.72	18	.97	34	192	2
VEGETARIAN VEGETABLE, cond, 10½ oz, 298 gm	176	5	5	29	1.19	52	2.62	2001	509	0
prep with water, 1 c, 241 gm	72	2	2	12	.49	21	1.08	823	209	0

Weight Watchers

FOOD & DESCRIPTION MEASURE OR QUANTITY	CALORIES	PROTEIN (GM)	FAT (GM)	CARBO-HYDRATE (GM)	FIBER (GM)	CALCIUM (MG)	IRON (MG)	SODIUM (MG)	POTASSIUM (MG)	CHOLES-TEROL (MG)
BEEF BROTH & SEASONING MIX, 1 pkt, 4.5 gm	10	1	0	2	—	—	—	870	—	—
CHICKEN BROTH & SEASONING MIX, 1 pkt, 4.5 gm	8	1	0	2	—	—	—	940	—	—
ONION BROTH & SEASONING MIX, 1 pkt, 4.5 gm	10	1	0	2	—	—	—	699	—	—

Wyler's

FOOD & DESCRIPTION MEASURE OR QUANTITY	CALORIES	PROTEIN (GM)	FAT (GM)	CARBO-HYDRATE (GM)	FIBER (GM)	CALCIUM (MG)	IRON (MG)	SODIUM (MG)	POTASSIUM (MG)	CHOLES-TEROL (MG)
BEEF FLAVORED INSTANT BOUILLON, 1 tsp	6	<1	<1	1	—	*	*	930	5	—
CHICKEN FLAVORED INSTANT BOUILLON, 1 cube	8	<1	<1	1	—	*	*	850	5	—
ONION FLAVORED INSTANT BOUILLON, 1 tsp	10	<1	<1	1	—	*	*	—	—	—

21

STARCHES & SIDE DISHES

FOOD & DESCRIPTION MEASURE OR QUANTITY	CALORIES	PROTEIN (GM)	FAT (GM)	CARBO-HYDRATE (GM)	FIBER (GM)	CALCIUM (MG)	IRON (MG)	SODIUM (MG)	POTASSIUM (MG)	CHOLES-TEROL (MG)
Grains										
Arrowhead Mills										
BROWN RICE, LONG, 2 oz	200	4	1	44	—	—	—	5	—	—
BROWN RICE, LONG BASMATI, 2 oz	200	4	1	44	—	—	—	5	—	—
BROWN RICE, MEDIUM, 2 oz	200	4	1	44	—	—	—	5	—	—
BROWN RICE, SHORT, 2 oz	200	4	1	44	—	—	—	5	—	—
Golden Grain										
BEEF RICE-A-RONI, dry, ⅙ pkg, 1.3 oz	130	4	1	26	—	40	1.08	780	—	—
CHICKEN RICE-A-RONI, dry, ⅙ pkg, 1.3 oz	130	4	1	27	—	*	1.08	800	—	—
MACARONI AND CHEDDAR, dry, ¼ pkg, 1.8 oz	190	7	2	35	—	60	1.80	430	—	—
NOODLE RONI PARMESANO, dry, ⅕ pkg, 1.02 oz	130	5	3	21	—	40	1.08	270	—	—
SPANISH RICE-A-RONI, dry, ⅐ pkg, 1.07 oz	110	3	1	22	—	*	.72	720	—	—
Green Giant										
RICE ORIGINALS										
ITALIAN BLEND WHITE RICE & SPINACH IN A CHEESE SAUSE, ½ c	160	4	7	21	—	60	1.08	460	80	—
LONG GRAIN WHITE AND WILD RICE, ½ c	120	3	2	23	—	0	1.44	550	40	—
RICE 'N BROCCOLI IN FLAVORED CHEESE SAUCE, ½ c	120	3	4	18	—	40	1.44	510	70	—
RICE WITH HERB BUTTER SAUCE, ½ c	150	3	6	21	—	0	1.08	420	55	—
RICE MEDLEY, ½ c	120	3	3	21	—	0	1.80	260	55	—
RICE PILAF, ½ c	100	3	2	23	—	0	1.44	520	45	—
Hain										
SIDE DISHES										
CHICKEN, ½ c prep	100	4	1	17	—	—	—	390	85	—
ITALIAN, ½ c prep	130	6	2	22	—	—	—	445	265	—
SPANISH, ½ c prep	90	4	2	14	—	—	—	415	185	—
TERIYAKI, ½ c prep	130	3	4	20	—	—	—	510	170	—

FOOD & DESCRIPTION MEASURE OR QUANTITY	CALORIES	PROTEIN (GM)	FAT (GM)	CARBO-HYDRATE (GM)	FIBER (GM)	CALCIUM (MG)	IRON (MG)	SODIUM (MG)	POTASSIUM (MG)	CHOLES-TEROL (MG)
Lipton										
RICE AND SAUCE										
BEEF FLAVOR, ½ c prep	160	3	4	27	—	*	.72	665	—	—
CHICKEN FLAVOR, ½ c prep	150	3	4	26	—	*	.72	525	—	—
HERB AND BUTTER, ½ c prep	160	3	5	25	—	*	.72	500	—	—
MUSHROOM, ½ c prep	140	3	3	26	—	*	.72	560	—	—
SPANISH, ½ c prep	140	3	3	26	—	*	.72	520	—	—
RICE AND SAUCE COMBINATONS										
RICE AND PEAS, ½ c prep	150	4	3	26	—	*	.72	400	—	—
RICE MEDLEY, ½ c prep	150	4	3	26	—	*	.72	400	—	—
Minute—General Foods										
MINUTE RICE, prep without salt and butter, .67 c	120	3	0	27	tr	*	1.08	0	0	—
MINUTE RICE MIX DRUMSTICK RICE MIX, 1 serving	120	3	0	25	tr	*	1.08	650	20	—
prep with butter (salted), ½ c	150	3	4	25	tr	*	1.08	690	20	—
FRIED RICE MIX, 1 serving	120	3	0	25	tr	*	1.08	550	45	—
prep with oil, ½ c	160	3	5	25	tr	*	1.08	550	45	—
LONG GRAIN & WILD RICE MIX, 1 serving	120	3	0	25	tr	*	1.08	530	40	—
prep with butter (salted), ½ c	150	3	4	25	tr	*	1.08	570	40	—
RIB ROAST MIX, 1 serving	120	3	0	25	tr	*	1.08	680	25	—
prep with butter (salted), ½ c	150	3	4	25	tr	*	1.08	720	25	—
Ogilvie—Catelli										
BARLEY, PEARL, 1 c ckd	212	6	<1	45	.48	10	1.20	2	96	—
POT, 1 c ckd	211	6	<1	45	.60	20	1.62	—	178	—
WHEAT GERM, 1 tbsp	32	3	<1	5	.18	6	.99	<1	85	—
Quaker										
HOMINY GRITS, INSTANT										
WHITE, 1 pkt	79	2	<1	18	.10	7	.81	385	28	—
WITH HAM BITS, 1 pkt	99	3	<1	21	.10	7	.81	665	56	—
WITH IMITATION BACON BITS, 1 pkt	101	3	<1	22	.10	7	.81	544	62	—
WITH REAL CHEESE, 1 pkt	104	2	1	22	.10	14	.81	497	40	—
REGULAR or QUICK										
WHITE, 3 tbsp dry	101	2	<1	22	.10	1	.81	1	39	—
YELLOW, 3 tbsp dry	101	2	<1	22	.10	1	.81	1	45	—
Riviana										
CAROLINA										
ENRICHED RICE, 1 oz, ½ c ckd	100	2	0	22	—	*	.72	<10	—	—
ENRICHED LONG GRAIN PRE-COOKED INSTANT RICE, 1 oz, ½ c ckd	110	2	0	23	—	*	.72	—	—	—
MAHATMA										
INSTANT RICE, 1 oz, ½ c ckd	110	2	0	23	—	*	.72	—	—	—
LONG GRAIN ENRICHED RICE, 1 oz, ½ c ckd	100	2	0	22	—	*	.72	<10	—	—
NATURAL LONG GRAIN BROWN RICE, 1 oz, ½ c ckd	110	2	0	23	—	*	.36	<10	—	—
MAKE-IT-EASY										

FOOD & DESCRIPTION MEASURE OR QUANTITY	CALORIES	PROTEIN (GM)	FAT (GM)	CARBO-HYDRATE (GM)	FIBER (GM)	CALCIUM (MG)	IRON (MG)	SODIUM (MG)	POTASSIUM (MG)	CHOLES-TEROL (MG)
BEEF FLAVORED RICE AND VERMICELLI MIX, 1.3 oz, ½ c	130	3	1	28	—	*	1.08	—	—	—
CHICKEN FLAVORED RICE AND VERMICELLI MIX, 1.3 oz, ½ c	130	3	1	28	—	*	1.08	—	—	—
RIVER										
ENRICHED RICE, 1 oz, ½ c ckd	100	2	0	22	—	*	.72	<10	—	—
NATURAL LONG GRAIN BROWN RICE, 1 oz, ½ c ckd	110	2	0	23	—	*	.36	—	—	—
SUCCESS RICE, BOIL IN BAGS, .9 oz, ½ c ckd	100	2	0	21	—	*	.72	<10	—	—
WATER MAID ENRICHED RICE, 1 oz, ½ c ckd	100	2	0	22	—	*	.72	<10	—	—

R.T. French

SPICE YOUR RICE										
BEEF FLAVOR 'N ONION, ⅙ pkg	10	0	0	2	—	*	*	510	30	—
½ c prep	160	2	4	27	—	*	.72	560	60	—
BUTTERY HERB, ⅙ pkg	18	1	1	2	—	*	*	380	60	—
½ c prep	170	3	5	27	—	*	.72	430	80	—
CHEESE 'N CHIVES, ⅙ pkg	14	1	0	2	—	*	*	350	50	—
½ c prep	200	3	8	27	—	*	.72	440	80	—
CHICKEN FLAVOR 'N HERB, ⅙ pkg	12	1	1	1	—	*	*	390	35	—
½ c prep	160	3	4	26	—	*	.72	440	60	—
CHICKEN FLAVOR 'N PARMESAN, ⅙ pkg	14	1	1	2	—	*	*	400	50	—
½ c prep	200	3	8	27	—	*	.72	490	80	—

Uncle Ben's

RICE, WHITE, ENRICHED, LONG GRAIN, ckd, parboiled										
prep with butter and salt, .67 c, 133 gm	148	3	2	29	.1	43	1.07	463	56	—
prep with salt without butter, .67 c, 129 gm	129	3	<1	29	.1	42	1.07	437	55	—
prep without butter or salt, .67 c, 129 gm	129	3	<1	29	.1	41	1.07	2	55	—

USDA

BARLEY, PEARLED,										
LIGHT, 1 c, 200 gm	698	16	2	158	—	32	4.00	6	320	—
POT or SCOTCH, 1 c, 200 gm	696	19	2	154	—	68	5.40	—	592	—
BULGUR, COMMERCIAL cnd (from hard red winter wheat)										
seasoned, 1 c, 135 gm	246	8	5	44	—	27	1.90	621	151	—
unseasoned, 1 c, 135 gm	227	8	1	47	—	27	1.80	809	117	—
dry										
CLUB WHEAT, 1 c, 175 gm	628	15	3	139	—	53	8.20	—	459	—
HARD RED WINTER WHEAT, 1 c, 170 gm	602	19	3	129	—	49	6.30	—	389	—
WHITE WHEAT, 1 c, 155 gm	553	16	2	121	—	56	7.30	—	481	—
RICE, BROWN										
LONG GRAIN, 1 c, 185 gm	666	14	4	143	—	59	3.00	17	396	—
ckd, cold, 1 c, 145 gm	173	4	<1	37	—	17	.70	—	102	—
hot, 1 c, 195 gm	232	5	1	50	—	23	1.00	—	137	—

FOOD & DESCRIPTION MEASURE OR QUANTITY	CALORIES	PROTEIN (GM)	FAT (GM)	CARBO- HYDRATE (GM)	FIBER (GM)	CALCIUM (MG)	IRON (MG)	SODIUM (MG)	POTASSIUM (MG)	CHOLES- TEROL (MG)
SHORT GRAIN, 1 c, 200 gm	720	15	4	155	—	64	3.20	18	428	—
RICE, INSTANT LONG GRAIN										
dry, 1 c, 95 gm	355	7	<1	78	—	5	2.80	1	—	—
ckd cold, 1 c, 130 gm	142	3	tr	32	—	4	1.00	—	—	—
hot, 1 c, 165 gm	180	4	tr	40	—	5	1.30	—	—	—
RICE, WHITE ENRICHED										
LONG, 1 c, 185 gm	672	12	<1	149	—	44	5.40	9	170	—
ckd, cold, 1 c, 145 gm	158	3	<1	35	—	15	1.30	—	41	—
hot, 1 c, 205 gm	223	4	<1	50	—	21	1.80	—	57	—
MEDIUM, 1 c, 195 gm	708	13	<1	157	—	47	5.70	10	179	—
SHORT, 1 c, 200 gm	726	13	<1	161	—	48	5.80	10	184	—
RICE, PARBOILED LONG GRAIN										
dry, 1 c, 185 gm	683	14	<1	150	—	111	5.40	17	278	—
ckd, cold, 1 c, 145 gm	154	3	<1	34	—	28	1.20	—	62	—
hot, 1 c, 175 gm	186	4	<1	41	—	33	1.40	—	75	—
RICE, WILD, raw, 1 c, 160 gm	565	23	1	121	—	30	6.70	11	352	—

Van Camp

SPANISH RICE, 8 oz, 227 gm	150	3	3	28	.6	35	2.92	1358	260	—

Pasta

Buitoni

EGG NOODLE, 2 oz dry	220	8	3	40	—	20	1.80	—	—	—
HIGH PROTEIN, 2 oz dry	210	12	1	37	—	*	1.80	—	—	—
PASTA ROMANA 2 oz dry	210	7	1	41	—	*	1.80	—	—	—
SPINACH, 2 oz dry	210	12	1	37	—	*	1.80	—	—	—

Catelli

CATELLI PASTA, 3 oz, 85 gm	306	11	1	64	.26	14	1.40	2	167	—
CATELLI PLUS, 3 oz, 85 gm	306	14	1	60	—	36	—	54	255	—
EGG NOODLES, 3 oz, 85 gm	316	11	3	61	.3	28	1.70	5	167	—
SPINACH LASAGNA, 3 oz, 85 gm	304	11	1	63	.35	35	1.90	14	247	—
SPLENDER PASTA, 3 oz, 85 gm	306	11	1	64	.26	14	1.40	2	167	—

General Mills

INTERNATIONAL NOODLE MIXES										
FETTUCINE ALFREDO, prep, ¼ pkg	230	8	11	25	—	150	1.08	590	130	—
PARISIENNE, prep, ¼ pkg	190	5	9	22	—	20	.72	620	120	—
ROMANOFF, prep, ¼ pkg	220	7	11	24	—	40	.72	680	140	—
STROGANOFF, prep, ¼ pkg	230	6	11	25	—	80	.72	730	180	—

Lipton

DELUXE NOODLES AND SAUCE										
ALFREDO, ½ c prep	220	7	11	22	—	100	1.08	560	—	—
CHICKEN BOMBAY, ½ c prep	190	6	9	22	—	40	1.08	515	—	—
PARMESANO, ½ c prep	210	6	11	22	—	60	.72	445	—	—
STROGANOFF, ½ c prep	200	6	10	22	—	40	1.44	510	—	—
NOODLES AND SAUCE										
BEEF FLAVOR, ½ c prep	190	5	7	26	—	*	.72	595	—	—
BUTTER, ½ c prep	190	5	9	24	—	*	.72	565	—	—
BUTTER AND HERB, ½ c prep	180	5	9	23	—	*	.72	525	—	—
CHICKEN FLAVOR, ½ c prep	190	5	9	25	—	*	.72	465	—	—
CHEESE, ½ c prep	200	5	9	24	—	40	.72	540	—	—
SOUR CREAM AND CHIVE,										

FOOD & DESCRIPTION MEASURE OR QUANTITY	CALORIES	PROTEIN (GM)	FAT (GM)	CARBO- HYDRATE (GM)	FIBER (GM)	CALCIUM (MG)	IRON (MG)	SODIUM (MG)	POTASSIUM (MG)	CHOLES- TEROL (MG)
½ c prep	190	5	9	23	—	*	.72	455	—	—
SHELLS AND SAUCE										
CREAMY GARLIC, ½ c	200	5	9	27	—	40	1.08	535	—	—
HERB TOMATO, ½ c	170	5	6	25	—	*	1.08	435	—	—

Muellers—Best Foods

EGG NOODLES, 2 oz dry	220	8	2	41	.2	15	2.10	15	—	55
GOLDEN RICH EGG NOODLES, 2 oz dry	220	8	2	41	.2	15	2.10	15	—	70
LASAGNE, 2 oz dry	210	8	1	42	.1	8	1.80	2	—	0
MACARONI, SPAGHETTI, 2 oz dry	210	7	<1	44	.1	8	1.80	2	—	0

Prince

EGG NOODLE, ENRICHED, 2 oz dry, 1 c ckd	220	8	3	40	—	*	1.80	20	—	—
MACARONI, SPAGHETTI PRODUCTS, ENRICHED, 2 oz dry	210	8	1	42	—	*	1.80	5	—	—

USDA

MACARONI, ENRICHED, ckd firm stage										
1 c, 130 gm	192	7	<1	39	—	14	1.40	1	103	—
yield from 1 lb dry, 8⅕ c	1674	57	5	341	—	122	13.00	9	894	—
tender stage										
yield from 1 lb dry, 10⅔ c										
hot, 14 c cold	1674	57	5	341	—	122	13.00	9	894	—
cold, 1 c, 105 gm	117	4	<1	24	—	8	.90	1	64	—
hot, 1 c, 140 gm	155	5	<1	32	—	11	1.30	1	85	—
NOODLES										
CHOW MEIN, cnd, 5 oz can, 142 gm	694	19	33	82	—	—	—	—	—	—
1 c, 45 gm	220	6	11	26	—	—	—	—	—	—
EGG, ckd										
yield from 1 lb dry, 8⅕ c	1760	58	21	327	—	141	13.00	23	617	—
1 c, 160 gm	200	7	2	37	—	16	1.40	3	70	—
PASTINA, EGG ENRICHED, DRY FORM, 1 c, 170 gm	651	22	7	122	—	60	4.90	9	—	—
SPAGHETTI, ENRICHED, ckd firm stage										
yield from 1 lb, 8⅕ c	1674	57	5	341	—	122	13.00	9	894	—
1 c, 130 gm	192	7	<1	39	—	14	1.40	1	103	—
tender stage										
yield from 1 lb, 10⅗ c	1674	57	5	341	—	122	13.00	9	894	—
1 c, 140 gm	155	5	<1	32	—	11	1.30	1	85	—
DRY FORM, 1 lb	1674	57	5	341	—	122	13.00	9	894	—

Potatoes

Betty Crocker— General Mills

AU GRATIN, ½ c prep	150	3	6	21	—	80	.36	630	350	—
CHICKEN 'N HERB, ½ c prep	120	3	4	19	—	20	.36	600	240	—
HASH BROWNS WITH ONIONS, ½ c prep	160	2	6	24	—	*	.36	460	430	—
HICKORY SMOKE CHEESE, ½ c prep	150	3	6	22	—	80	.36	700	320	—
JULIENNE, ½ c prep	140	3	6	19	—	80	.36	600	240	—
PARSLEY, CREAMED, ½ c prep	180	4	8	22	—	60	.36	420	330	—

FOOD & DESCRIPTION MEASURE OR QUANTITY	CALORIES	PROTEIN (GM)	FAT (GM)	CARBO-HYDRATE (GM)	FIBER (GM)	CALCIUM (MG)	IRON (MG)	SODIUM (MG)	POTASSIUM (MG)	CHOLES-TEROL (MG)
POTATO BUDS										
dry, .33 c	70	2	0	16	—	*	*	20	180	—
prep, ½ c	130	3	6	17	—	20	*	360	210	—
SCALLOPED, ½ c prep	140	3	6	19	—	20	.36	570	280	—
SOUR CREAM 'N CHIVE, ½ c prep	160	3	7	21	—	20	.36	530	280	—
TWICE BAKED POTATOES MILD CHEDDAR WITH ONION, prep, ⅙ total	200	5	12	19	—	60	.72	630	390	—
SOUR CREAM 'N CHIVE, prep, ⅙ total	200	5	11	19	—	60	.72	520	360	—
Del Monte										
POTATOES, SLICED or WHOLE, ½ c, 113.5 gm	45	1	0	10	—	20	.36	355	290	—
Durkee										
O&C POTATO STICKS, 1.5 oz	231	3	15	22	—	—	—	383	481	—
Green Giant–Pillsbury										
POTATO ORIGINALS STUFFED BAKED POTATO WITH CHEESE FLAVORED TOPPING, 5 oz	200	4	6	33	—	40	.72	520	620	—
STUFFED BAKED POTATO WITH SOUR CREAM AND CHIVES, 5 oz	230	5	10	31	—	40	.72	580	570	—
Hormel										
AU GRATIN POTATOES AND BACON, 7.5 oz	240	9	14	20	—	—	—	942	—	—
Hungry Jack–Pillsbury										
MASHED POTATOES MIX only, 1 serving	70	1	0	16	—	0	0	25	280	—
prep, .5 c	140	3	7	17	—	40	0	380	320	—
Libby										
POTATO, cnd, ½ c	45	2	0	11	—	20	.36	310	—	—
POTATO CLASSICS AU GRATIN STYLE, ¾ c prep	130	3	3	22	—	20	.72	—	—	—
SCALLOPED STYLE, ¾ c prep	130	3	2	24	—	40	.72	—	—	—
Mother's										
POTATO LATKES (pancakes), fz, precooked MINI, 2.8 oz 10 pc	148	2	6	20	—	—	—	240	366	—
LARGE, 2.8 oz 2 pc	120	2	6	20	—	—	—	240	366	—
Ore-Ida–Heinz										
CHEDDAR BROWNS, 3 oz	80	2	2	14	—	0	1.08	315	315	10
COTTAGE FRIES, 3 oz	140	2	6	21	—	*	.36	40	220	0
COUNTRY STYLE DINNER FRIES, 3 oz	120	2	4	20	—	*	.36	50	180	0
CRISPERS, 3 oz	240	3	15	25	—	*	.72	560	180	0
CRISPY CROWNS, 3 oz	150	2	8	18	—	*	.36	370	200	0
WITH ONIONS, 3 oz	170	2	10	19	—	*	.36	480	200	0
GOLDEN CRINKLES, 3 oz	120	2	5	20	—	*	.36	40	220	0
GOLDEN FRIES, 3 oz	130	2	5	21	—	*	.36	40	200	0
GOLDEN PATTIES, 2.5 oz	130	2	10	17	—	*	.72	340	200	0

FOOD & DESCRIPTION MEASURE OR QUANTITY	CALORIES	PROTEIN (GM)	FAT (GM)	CARBO-HYDRATE (GM)	FIBER (GM)	CALCIUM (MG)	IRON (MG)	SODIUM (MG)	POTASSIUM (MG)	CHOLES-TEROL (MG)
HOME STYLE POTATOES										
PLANKS, 3 oz	110	2	5	18	—	*	.36	30	350	0
SLICES, 3 oz	110	2	4	17	—	*	.36	40	350	0
THINS, 3 oz	130	2	6	18	—	*	.36	40	260	0
WEDGES, 3 oz	100	2	4	17	—	*	.36	20	300	0
PIXIE CRINKLES, 3 oz	160	2	10	22	—	*	.36	40	170	0
POTATOES O'BRIEN, 3 oz	80	2	0	17	—	*	.36	50	160	0
SHOESTRINGS, 3 oz	160	2	7	24	—	*	.36	40	170	0
SHREDDED HASHBROWNS, 6 oz	130	3	0	29	—	*	.72	50	100	0
SOUTHERN STYLE HASHBROWNS, 3 oz	70	1	0	17	—	*	.36	60	130	0
TATER TOTS										
BACON FLAVORED, 3 oz	160	3	7	21	—	*	.36	720	200	0
ONION, 3 oz	160	2	8	21	—	*	.36	600	200	0
PLAIN, 3 oz	160	2	8	21	—	*	.36	550	200	0
USDA										
POTATO STICKS, .75 × 2.75 × .13″, 1 c, 35 gm	190	2	13	18	—	15	.60	—	46	—
POTATO STICKS, 1 oz	154	2	10	14	—	12	.50	—	320	—

Stuffing

General Mills

CHICKEN STUFFING MIX, ⅙ pkg prep	180	4	9	21	—	20	1.44	620	75	—
CORN BREAD STUFFING MIX, ⅙ pkg prep	180	3	9	23	—	20	1.08	710	75	—
PORK STUFFING MIX, ⅙ pkg prep	190	4	9	22	—	20	1.44	640	70	—
TRADITIONAL HERB STUFFING MIX, ⅙ pkg prep	190	4	9	22	—	20	1.44	640	70	—

Green Giant–Pillsbury

STUFFING ORIGINALS										
CHICKEN, ½ c	170	4	7	21	—	20	1.08	670	90	—
CORNBREAD, ½ c	170	3	6	25	—	0	1.08	660	100	—
MUSHROOM, ½ c	150	4	7	19	—	20	1.08	780	105	—

Pepperidge Farm–Campbell

CORN BREAD, 1 oz	110	3	1	22	—	20	1.08	320	—	—
CUBE, 1 oz	110	3	1	22	—	20	1.08	430	—	—
HERB SEASONED, 1 oz	110	3	1	22	—	40	1.08	410	—	—

Stove Top–General Foods

AMERICANA NEW ENGLAND, dry, ⅙ pkg	110	4	1	21	tr	40	1.08	560	100	—
prep, ½ c	180	4	9	21	tr	40	1.08	630	105	—
AMERICANA SAN FRANCISCO, dry, ⅙ pkg	110	4	1	20	tr	20	.72	560	75	—
prep, ½ c	170	4	9	20	tr	20	.72	640	80	—
BEEF, dry, ⅙ pkg	110	4	1	21	tr	20	1.08	500	75	—
prep, ½ c	180	4	9	21	tr	20	1.08	580	80	—
CHICKEN FLAVOR, dry, ⅙ pkg	110	4	1	20	tr	20	.72	560	80	—
prep, ½ c	180	4	9	20	tr	20	.72	640	80	—
CORNBREAD, dry, ⅙ pkg	110	3	1	21	tr	20	1.08	590	80	—
prep, ½ c	170	3	9	21	tr	20	1.08	660	80	—

FOOD & DESCRIPTION MEASURE OR QUANTITY	CALORIES	PROTEIN (GM)	FAT (GM)	CARBO-HYDRATE (GM)	FIBER (GM)	CALCIUM (MG)	IRON (MG)	SODIUM (MG)	POTASSIUM (MG)	CHOLES-TEROL (MG)
PORK, dry, ⅙ pkg	110	4	1	20	tr	40	1.08	540	85	—
prep, ½ c	170	4	9	20	tr	40	1.08	620	90	—
TURKEY, dry, ⅙ pkg	110	4	1	20	tr	20	.72	550	80	—
prep, ½ pkg	170	4	9	20	tr	20	.72	630	80	—
WILD RICE, dry, ⅙ pkg	110	3	1	23	tr	20	1.08	430	65	—
prep, ½ c	180	3	8	23	tr	20	1.08	500	70	—

USDA

BREAD STUFFING MIX										
coarse crumbs, 1 c, 70 gm	260	9	3	51	—	87	2.20	932	120	—
cubes, 1 c, 30 gm	111	4	1	22	—	37	1.00	399	52	—
dry, 8 oz, 1 pkg, 227 gm	842	29	9	164	—	281	7.30	3021	390	—
prep, dry & crumbly, with water & table fat										
1 c, 140 gm	501	9	31	50	—	92	2.20	1254	126	—
1 lb, 454 gm	1624	30	99	162	—	299	7.30	4064	408	—
prep, moist, with water, egg & table fat										
1 c, 200 gm	416	9	26	39	—	80	2.00	1008	116	—
1 lb, 454 gm	943	20	58	89	—	181	4.50	2286	263	—

22

VEGETABLES

FOOD & DESCRIPTION MEASURE OR QUANTITY	CALORIES	PROTEIN (GM)	FAT (GM)	CARBO-HYDRATE (GM)	FIBER (GM)	CALCIUM (MG)	IRON (MG)	SODIUM (MG)	POTASSIUM (MG)	CHOLES-TEROL (MG)
Arrowhead Mills										
ALFALFA SEED SPROUTS, 1 c	40	5	1	4	—	—	—	2	—	—
Birds Eye– **General Foods**										
ARTICHOKE HEARTS, 3 oz	30	2	0	7	.8	*	.72	40	210	—
ASPARAGUS CUTS, 3.3 oz	25	3	0	4	.8	20	.72	0	240	—
SPEARS, 3.3 oz	25	3	0	4	.7	20	.72	0	260	—
BAVARIAN STYLE RECIPE BEANS AND SPAETZLE, 3.3 oz	110	2	6	11	.5	40	.72	420	80	—
BEANS, GREEN CORN, CARROTS AND PEARL ONIONS, 3.2 oz	45	2	0	10	.8	20	.36	15	150	—
CUT, 3 oz	25	1	0	6	.9	40	.72	0	130	—
FRENCH CUT, 3 oz	25	1	0	6	1.0	40	.72	0	150	—
CAULIFLOWER AND CARROTS, 3.2 oz	25	1	0	6	1.0	20	.72	20	160	—
WITH TOASTED ALMONDS, 3 oz	50	3	2	8	1.0	40	.36	340	170	—
ITALIAN, 3 oz	30	2	0	7	.9	40	.72	0	180	—
WHOLE, 3 oz	25	1	0	5	.8	40	.72	0	150	—
BEANS, LIMA										
BABY, 3.3 oz	130	7	0	24	1.9	40	1.8	115	470	—
FORDHOOK, 3.3 oz	100	6	0	19	1.8	20	1.44	100	480	—
BROCCOLI										
CHOPPED, 3.3 oz	25	3	0	5	1.0	60	.72	20	200	—
CUTS, 3.3 oz	25	3	0	4	1.0	60	.72	25	200	—
FLORETS, 3.3 oz	25	3	0	5	.9	40	.72	20	230	
SPEARS, 3.3 oz	25	3	0	5	.9	40	.72	20	230	
BABY, 3.3 oz	30	3	0	5	1.1	40	.72	15	250	—
AND CAULIFLOWER WITH CREAMY ITALIAN CHEESE SAUCE, 4.5 oz	110	5	7	8	.8	100	.72	280	230	—
AND WATER CHESTNUTS, 3.3 oz	30	3	0	6	.9	40	.72	220	180	—
BEANS, GREEN, PEARL ONIONS AND RED PEPPERS, 3.2 oz	25	2	0	5	.9	40	.72	15	170	—
CARROTS AND PASTA TWISTS, 3.3 oz	90	2	4	11	.8	20	.36	270	160	—
CARROTS, BABY, AND WATER CHESTNUTS, 3.2 oz	30	2	0	6	.9	20	.72	25	190	—
CAULIFLOWER AND										

FOOD & DESCRIPTION MEASURE OR QUANTITY	CALORIES	PROTEIN (GM)	FAT (GM)	CARBO-HYDRATE (GM)	FIBER (GM)	CALCIUM (MG)	IRON (MG)	SODIUM (MG)	POTASSIUM (MG)	CHOLES-TEROL (MG)
CARROTS, 3.2 oz	25	2	0	5	.9	40	.72	25	190	—
CAULIFLOWER AND CARROTS WITH CHEESE SAUCE, 5 oz	110	4	5	12	.9	100	.72	390	280	—
CORN AND RED PEPPERS, 3.2 oz	50	3	0	11	.7	*	.36	10	200	—
WITH ALMONDS, 3.3 oz	50	4	3	6	1.0	60	1.08	220	210	—
WITH CHEESE SAUCE, 5 oz	120	5	7	13	.7	150	.72	510	300	—
WITH CREAMY ITALIAN CHEESE SAUCE, 4.5 oz	110	5	7	8	.9	100	1.08	280	230	—
BRUSSELS SPROUTS, 3.3 oz	35	3	0	7	1.2	20	.72	15	330	—
BABY, WITH CHEESE SAUCE, 4.5 oz	120	5	6	13	1.0	100	.72	440	380	—
CAULIFLOWER AND CARROTS, 3.2 oz	30	2	0	7	1.0	20	.72	20	240	—
CARROTS, BABY, 3.3 oz	40	1	0	9	1.2	20	.72	45	150	—
SWEET PEAS AND PEARL ONIONS, 3.3 oz	50	2	0	10	1.2	20	.72	60	150	—
CAULIFLOWER, 3.3 oz	25	2	0	5	.8	20	.36	20	190	—
GREEN BEANS AND CORN, 3.2 oz	35	2	0	8	.7	20	.36	10	170	—
WITH ALMONDS, 3.3 oz	40	3	2	5	.8	20	.72	270	200	—
WITH CHEESE SAUCE, 5 oz	120	4	7	12	.6	100	.36	500	260	—
CHINESE STYLE, 3.3 oz	80	2	5	8	.2	20	.72	360	135	—
STIR FRY, 3.3 oz	30	2	0	7	.8	40	1.08	480	170	—
CORN BIG EARS ON THE COB, 1 ear	160	5	1	37	1.5	*	1.08	0	490	—
GREEN BEANS & PASTA CURLS, 3.3 oz	110	3	5	15	.5	60	.36	280	140	—
LITTLE EARS ON THE COB, 2 ears	130	4	1	30	1.2	*	.72	0	400	—
ON THE COB, 1 ear	120	4	1	29	1.2	*	.72	0	380	—
SWEET, 3.3 oz	80	3	1	20	.5	*	.36	0	200	—
TENDERTREAT SWEET, 3.3 oz	80	3	1	20	.5	*	.36	0	200	—
FAR EASTERN STYLE, 3.3 oz	80	2	5	8	.8	20	.36	390	180	—
ITALIAN STYLE, 3.3 oz	110	2	7	11	.6	40	.72	570	140	—
JAPANESE STYLE, 3.3 oz	100	2	6	10	.6	20	.36	500	135	—
STIR FRY, 3.3 oz	30	2	0	6	.7	20	.72	570	115	—
MEXICANA STYLE, 3.3 oz	120	3	6	16	1.0	*	1.08	470	190	—
MIXED VEGETABLES, 3.3 oz	60	3	0	13	1.1	20	.72	45	200	—
WITH ONION SAUCE, 2.6 oz	100	2	5	11	.7	60	.36	350	170	—
NEW ENGLAND STYLE, 3.3 oz	130	3	7	14	.7	20	.36	410	160	—
OKRA CUT, 3.3 oz	25	1	0	6	.7	80	.36	0	180	—
WHOLE, 3.3 oz	30	2	0	7	.7	80	.36	0	220	—
ONIONS, SMALL, WITH CREAM SAUCE, 3 oz	110	1	6	11	.4	60	*	330	170	—
ONIONS, SMALL WHOLE, 4 oz	40	1	0	10	.7	40	.36	10	160	—
PEAS, GREEN, 3.3 oz	80	5	0	13	1.8	20	1.44	130	160	—
TENDER TINY, 3.3 oz	60	4	0	11	1.9	*	1.08	120	135	—
& PEARL ONIONS, 3.3 oz	70	5	0	13	1.7	*	.72	310	170	—
WITH CHEESE SAUCE, 5 oz	140	6	5	18	1.4	100	1.08	460	230	—
& POTATOES WITH CREAM SAUCE, 2.6 oz	140	4	7	15	.9	40	.36	480	230	—
WITH CREAM SAUCE, 2.6 oz	130	4	7	14	1.1	40	.36	440	200	—
RICE AND PEAS WITH MUSHROOMS, 2.3 oz	110	4	0	23	.6	*	.72	320	70	—
SAN FRANCISCO STYLE, 3.3 oz	100	2	5	11	.5	20	.36	400	160	—
SPINACH CHOPPED, 3.3 oz	20	3	0	3	.8	100	1.8	80	280	—
WHOLE LEAF, 3.3 oz	20	3	0	4	.8	100	1.8	90	300	—
AND WATER CHESTNUTS,										

FOOD & DESCRIPTION MEASURE OR QUANTITY	CALORIES	PROTEIN (GM)	FAT (GM)	CARBO-HYDRATE (GM)	FIBER (GM)	CALCIUM (MG)	IRON (MG)	SODIUM (MG)	POTASSIUM (MG)	CHOLES-TEROL (MG)
3.3 oz	25	2	0	5	.7	80	1.8	270	270	—
CREAMED, 3 oz	60	3	3	5	.7	60	.36	280	290	—
SQUASH, COOKED WINTER, 4 oz	45	1	0	11	1.4	20	.72	0	260	—

Campbell

TOMATO JUICE, 6 oz	35	1	0	8	—	*	.36	570	—	—
"V-8" VEGETABLE JUICE, 6 oz	35	1	0	8	—	20	.72	625	—	—
"V-8" VEGETABLE JUICE, NO-SALT-ADDED, 6 oz	40	1	0	9	—	20	.72	50	—	—
"V-8" SPICY HOT VEGETABLE JUICE, 6 oz	35	1	0	8	—	20	.72	625	—	—

Catelli

TOMATO PASTE, 1 tbsp	15	<1	<1	3	.16	5	.63	7	160	—

Del Monte

ASPARAGUS, ALL GREEN, ½ c, 114 gm	20	2	0	3	—	*	.36	355	205	—
BEANS, GREEN										
CUT, ½ c, 114 gm	20	1	0	4	—	20	.72	355	130	—
SALT FREE, ½ c, 114 gm	20	1	0	4	—	20	.72	<10	130	—
FRENCH STYLE, ½ c, 114 gm	20	1	0	4	—	20	.72	355	105	—
SALT FREE, ½ c, 114 gm	20	1	0	4	—	20	.72	<10	105	—
SEASONED, ½ c, 114 gm	20	1	0	4	—	20	.36	355	105	—
ITALIAN CUT, ½ c, 114 gm	25	1	0	6	—	20	.72	355	160	—
WHOLE, ½ c, 114 gm	20	1	0	4	—	*	.36	355	120	—
BEANS, LIMA, GREEN, ½ c, 114 gm	70	4	0	14	—	20	1.44	355	300	—
BEANS, WAX CUT, GOLDEN, ½ c, 114 gm	20	0	0	4	—	20	.36	355	130	—
BEETS, SLICED or WHOLE, ½ c, 114 gm	35	1	0	8	—	*	.36	290	150	—
SALT FREE, ½ c sliced, 114 gm	35	1	0	8	—	*	.36	100	150	—
PICKLED, CRINKLE SLICED, ½ c, 114 gm	80	1	0	19	—	*	.36	375	170	—
CARROTS, SLICED or CUT, ½ c, 114 gm	30	0	0	7	—	20	.36	265	235	—
CHILES, GREEN, WHOLE or DICED, ½ c, 113 gm	20	0	0	5	—	60	.72	690	160	—
CHILES, JALAPENO, WHOLE or SLICED, ½ c, 113 gm	30	1	1	6	—	20	2.70	1690	170	—
CORN, GOLDEN										
CREAM STYLE, ½ c, 114 gm	80	2	1	18	—	0	.36	355	145	—
SALT FREE, ½ c, 121 gm	80	2	1	20	—	0	.36	<10	145	—
WHOLE KERNEL, ½ c, 114 gm	70	2	1	17	—	0	.36	355	170	—
SALT FREE, ½ c, 121 gm	80	2	1	18	—	0	.36	<10	170	—
VACUUM PACK, ½ c, 114 gm	90	3	1	22	—	0	.36	355	210	—
SALT FREE, ½ c, 114 gm	90	3	1	22	—	0	.36	<10	210	—
CORN, WHITE										
CREAM STYLE, ½ c, 114 gm	90	2	0	21	—	0	.36	355	160	—
WHOLE KERNEL, ½ c, 114 gm	70	2	0	16	—	0	.36	355	185	—
MIXED VEGETABLES, ½ c, 114 gm	40	2	0	7	—	20	.72	355	171	—
PEAS										
SEASONED, ½ c, 114 gm	60	3	0	11	—	*	1.08	355	140	—
SWEET, ½ c, 114 gm	60	3	0	10	—	20	1.08	355	115	—
UNSALTED, ½ c, 121 gm	60	3	0	11	—	20	1.08	<10	115	—

FOOD & DESCRIPTION MEASURE OR QUANTITY	CALORIES	PROTEIN (GM)	FAT (GM)	CARBO-HYDRATE (GM)	FIBER (GM)	CALCIUM (MG)	IRON (MG)	SODIUM (MG)	POTASSIUM (MG)	CHOLES-TEROL (MG)
SMALL, ½ c, 114 gm	50	3	0	9	—	*	1.44	355	100	—
PEAS AND CARROTS, ½ c, 114 gm	50	2	0	10	—	20	.72	355	125	—
PUMPKIN, ½ c, 114 gm	35	1	0	9	—	20	.72	<10	240	—
SAUERKRAUT, ½ c, 114 gm	25	1	0	6	—	20	.36	775	185	—
SPINACH										
CHOPPED or WHOLE LEAF, ½ c, 114 gm	25	2	0	4	—	100	1.44	355	290	—
UNSALTED, WHOLE LEAF, ½ c, 114 gm	25	2	0	4	—	100	1.44	35	290	—
TOMATO AND CHILI COCKTAIL, SNAPPY TOM, 6 oz, 183 gm	40	2	0	7	—	20	1.08	980	520	—
TOMATO PASTE, ¾ c, 170 gm	150	6	1	34	—	60	2.70	110	1770	—
SALT FREE, 6 oz, 170 gm	150	6	1	34	—	60	2.70	110	1170	—
TOMATO SAUCE, 1 c, 227 gm	70	3	1	16	—	20	1.80	1330	870	—
SALT FREE, 1 c, 227 gm	70	3	1	16	—	20	1.80	50	890	—
WITH ONIONS, 1 c, 227 gm	100	3	1	23	—	20	1.80	1150	955	—
TOMATOES										
STEWED, ½ c, 114 gm	35	1	0	8	—	20	.36	355	285	—
SALT FREE, ½ c, 113 gm	35	1	0	8	—	20	.36	45	285	—
WEDGES, ½ c, 114 gm	30	1	0	8	—	20	.36	355	280	—
WHOLE, PEELED, ½ c, 114 gm	25	1	0	5	—	20	.36	220	285	—
ZUCCHINI IN TOMATO SAUCE, ½ c, 114 gm	30	1	0	8	—	20	.72	485	291	—
Duffy—Mott										
BEEFAMATO, 4 oz	42	0	0	9	—	—	—	—	—	—
CLAMATO, 6 oz	81	1	0	19	—	—	—	—	—	—
Durkee										
FRENCH FRIED ONIONS, 1 oz, 28 gm	175	2	15	9	—	—	—	178	83	—
SOUP GREENS, 1 jar, 2.5 oz	216	6	3	43	—	—	—	408	940	—
Featherweight										
BEANS, GREEN, SALT FREE, ½ c	25	1	0	5	—	—	—	<10	114	—
BEETS, SALT FREE, ½ c	45	1	0	10	—	—	—	55	206	—
CARROTS, SALT FREE, ½ c	30	1	0	6	—	—	—	30	148	—
CORN, SALT FREE, ½ c	80	2	1	16	—	—	—	40	345	—
LIMA BEANS, SALT FREE, ½ c	80	5	0	16	—	—	—	25	276	—
PEAS, SALT FREE, ½ c	70	5	0	12	—	—	—	<10	120	—
SPINACH, SALT FREE, ½ c	35	2	1	4	—	—	—	35	—	—
TOMATO										
cnd, SALT FREE, ½ c	20	1	0	4	—	—	—	<10	252	—
JUICE, SALT FREE, 6 oz	35	1	0	8	—	—	—	20	325	—
PASTE, SALT FREE, 1 oz	25	1	0	6	—	—	—	12	252	—
PUREE, 1 c	90	3	0	20	—	—	—	<10	960	—
VEGETABLE JUICE COCKTAIL, 6 oz	35	1	0	8	—	—	—	25	42	—
VEGETABLES, MIXED, SALT FREE, ½ c	40	2	0	8	—	—	—	25	175	—
Green Giant [All items are frozen unless otherwise indicated]										
ASPARAGUS, cnd CUTS, ½ c	20	3	0	2	—	0	.72	450	150	—

FOOD & DESCRIPTION MEASURE OR QUANTITY	CALORIES	PROTEIN (GM)	FAT (GM)	CARBO-HYDRATE (GM)	FIBER (GM)	CALCIUM (MG)	IRON (MG)	SODIUM (MG)	POTASSIUM (MG)	CHOLES-TEROL (MG)
drained, ½ c,	—	—	—	—	—	0	—	310	—	—
SPEARS, LE SUEUR, ½	30	3	0	4	—	0	.72	390	150	—
dr, ½ c	—	—	—	—	—	—	—	300	—	—
BEANS, GREEN										
cnd										
CUT, 1–1½" pieces, ½ c	20	1	1	3	—	20	.72	310	110	—
dr, ½ c	—	—	—	—	—	—	—	190	—	—
CUT, KTICHEN, ½ c	20	2	0	3	—	20	.72	260	110	—
dr, ½ c	—	—	—	—	—	—	—	150	—	—
FRENCH STYLE, CUT, ½ c	18	1	0	3	—	20	.72	270	110	—
dr, ½ c	—	—	—	—	—	—	—	140	—	—
fz, ½ c	30	1	0	6	—	20	.36	270	150	—
POLYBAG, ½ c	20	1	0	4	—	20	.36	10	110	—
CUT, IN BUTTER SAUCE, ½ c	35	1	1	5	—	20	.36	300	100	—
FRENCH STYLE, IN BUTTER SAUCE, ½ c	40	1	1	6	—	20	.36	360	125	—
BEANS, LIMA										
BABY, IN BUTTER SAUCE, ½ c	120	6	2	20	—	20	1.44	450	380	—
fz, ½ c	100	6	0	19	—	20	1.8	310	370	—
POLYBAG, ½ c	100	6	0	19	—	20	1.44	30	340	—
BROCCOLI										
fz										
CUT ½ c	30	2	0	5	—	20	.36	240	115	—
POLYBAG, ½ c	16	2	0	2	—	20	0	10	130	—
MINISPEARS, POLYBAG, ½ c	16	1	0	3	—	0	0	10	140	—
SPEARS, ½ c	30	3	0	4	—	20	.36	200	160	—
CARROT FANFARE, ½ c	25	1	0	5	—	20	.36	20	170	—
CAULIFLOWER AND CARROTS IN BUTTER SAUCE, ½ c	35	1	1	5	—	20	.36	380	150	—
CAULIFLOWER AND CARROTS IN CHEESE FLAVORED SAUCE, ½ c	70	3	2	9	—	60	.36	490	240	—
CAULIFLOWER MEDLEY, ½ c	60	2	1	10	—	20	.36	470	250	—
CAULIFLOWER SUPREME, ½ c	20	2	0	4	—	20	.36	30	190	—
FANFARE, ½ c	70	3	1	12	—	20	.36	470	150	—
IN CHEESE FLAVORED SAUCE, ½ c	70	3	2	9	—	60	.36	530	260	—
IN WHITE CHEDDAR CHEESE FLAVORED SAUCE, ½ c	60	3	3	6	—	60	0	450	160	—
SPEARS IN BUTTER SAUCE, ½ c	45	2	2	5	—	20	0	340	150	—
BRUSSELS SPROUTS										
BABY, IN CHEESE FLAVORED SAUCE, ½ c	80	3	2	13	—	60	.36	470	310	—
fz, POLYBAG, ½ c	30	2	0	6	—	20	.36	10	270	—
IN BUTTER SAUCE, ½ c	60	3	1	9	—	20	.36	270	280	—
CAULIFLOWER										
CARROT BONANZA, ½ c	60	2	3	7	—	0	.72	290	160	—
fz, CUTS, POLYBAG, ½ c	16	1	0	3	—	0	0	30	130	—
IN BUTTER SAUCE, ½ c	30	1	1	4	—	0	.36	320	150	—
IN CHEESE FLAVORED SAUCE, ½ c	60	2	2	10	—	60	.36	450	245	—
IN WHITE CHEDDAR CHEESE FLAVORED SAUCE, ½ c	70	3	3	7	—	60	.72	420	230	—
CORN										
BROCCOLI BOUNTY, ½ c	60	2	1	11	—	0	.36	10	150	—
cnd										
WHOLE KERNEL, LE SUEUR, ½ c	80	2	0	18	—	0	.36	290	170	—
dr, ½ c	—	—	—	—	—	—	—	230	—	—

FOOD & DESCRIPTION MEASURE OR QUANTITY	CALORIES	PROTEIN (GM)	FAT (GM)	CARBO-HYDRATE (GM)	FIBER (GM)	CALCIUM (MG)	IRON (MG)	SODIUM (MG)	POTASSIUM (MG)	CHOLES-TEROL (MG)
VACUUM PACKED, ½ c	90	2	0	20	—	0	.36	230	170	—
dr, ½ c	—	—	—	—	—	—	—	180	—	—
CREAM STYLE, ½ c	120	3	1	25	—	0	0	370	180	—
cnd, ½ c	100	2	1	21	—	0	0	320	120	—
GOLDEN SHOEPEG, ½ c	90	2	1	18	—	0	.36	270	190	—
dr, ½ c	—	—	—	—	—	—	—	160	—	—
MEXICORN WITH PEPPERS, ½ c	80	2	0	18	—	0	.36	330	160	—
dr, ½ c	—	—	—	—	—	—	—	280	—	—
NIBLETS, ½ c	100	3	1	24	—	0	0	200	200	—
IN BUTTER SAUCE, ½ c	100	2	2	18	—	0	.36	280	180	—
POLYBAG, ½ c	80	2	1	17	—	0	0	5	150	—
4 EAR CORN-ON-THE-COB, POLYBAG, 1 5½" piece	140	4	1	30	—	0	.36	20	340	—
6 EAR CORN-ON-THE-COB, POLYBAG, 1 piece	80	2	1	16	—	0	0	10	180	—
WHITE SHOEPEG, ½ c	80	2	1	16	—	0	0	160	—	—
cnd, VACUUM PACK, ½ c	90	2	0	20	—	0	0	270	210	—
dr, ½ c	—	—	—	—	—	—	—	220	—	—
IN BUTTER SAUCE, ½ c	110	3	2	21	—	0	0	310	210	—
JAPANESE VEGETABLES, ½ c	40	2	1	6	—	20	.36	370	160	—
MUSHROOM										
cnd, pieces, stems & buttons, 2 oz	14	1	0	2	—	0	.36	260	70	—
dr, solids from a 2 oz can	—	—	—	—	—	—	—	150	—	—
IN BUTTER SAUCE, ½ c	25	2	<1	3	—	0	.36	530	150	—
dr, ½ c	—	—	—	—	—	—	—	290	—	—
PEAS										
BABY EARLY AND SWEET PEAS IN BUTTER SAUCE, LE SUEUR, ½ c	90	4	1	14	—	20	.72	490	125	—
EARLY JUNE, cnd,	60	3	<1	11	—	20	1.08	380	100	—
dr, ½ c	—	—	—	—	—	—	—	230	—	—
fz, POLYBAG, ½ c	60	5	0	10	—	20	1.08	170	115	—
IN CREAM SAUCE, ½ c	100	4	4	12	—	40	1.08	320	150	—
MINI PEAS, PEA PODS & WATER CHESTNUTS BUTTER SAUCE, LE SUEUR, ½ c	80	4	2	10	—	20	1.08	410	120	—
MINI SWEET, cnd, ½ c	60	4	0	11	—	20	1.44	420	115	—
dr, ½ c	—	—	—	—	—	—	—	290	—	—
SWEET										
CAULIFLOWER MEDLEY, POLYBAG, ½ c	40	3	0	7	—	20	.72	35	160	—
cnd, ½ c	60	4	0	11	—	20	1.08	370	105	—
dr, ½ c	—	—	—	—	—	—	—	260	—	—
fz , ½ c	80	4	0	16	—	20	1.44	300	110	—
POLYBAG, ½ c	60	4	0	11	—	0	.72	110	110	—
SWEET, AND ONIONS, ½ c	60	3	<1	11	—	20	1.08	550	115	—
dr, ½ c	—	—	—	—	—	—	—	400	—	—
SPINACH										
CREAMED, ½ c	80	3	3	10	—	100	.72	480	390	—
CUT LEAF IN BUTTER SAUCE, ½ c	60	4	2	6	—	200	1.80	550	500	—
fz, ½ c	40	4	<1	5	—	100	1.44	440	510	—
THREE BEAN SALAD, ½ c	80	2	<1	18	—	20	3.60	540	120	—
VEGETABLES, MIXED, fz, ½ c	60	3	0	13	—	20	1.08	220	210	—
POLYBAG, ½ c	50	2	0	11	—	0	.36	30	180	—
IN BUTTER SAUCE, ½ c	80	3	2	13	—	20	.72	370	190	—

Heinz

ONIONS
SPICED, 1 oz	2	0	0	0	—	*	*	600	—	—

FOOD & DESCRIPTION MEASURE OR QUANTITY	CALORIES	PROTEIN (GM)	FAT (GM)	CARBO-HYDRATE (GM)	FIBER (GM)	CALCIUM (MG)	IRON (MG)	SODIUM (MG)	POTASSIUM (MG)	CHOLES-TEROL (MG)
SWEET, 1 oz	40	0	0	9	—	*	*	165	—	—
PEPPERS										
HOT BANANA, 1 oz	6	0	0	1	—	20	*	305	—	—
HOT CHERRY, 1 oz	8	0	0	2	—	20	*	310	—	—
HOT RINGS/SLICES, 1 oz	4	0	0	1	—	20	*	300	—	—
SWEET MEMENTOS, 1 oz	6	0	0	1	—	20	*	320	—	—
SWEET MILD CHERRY, 1 oz	8	0	0	2	—	20	*	315	—	—
SWEET MILD RINGS/SLICES, 1 oz	4	0	0	1	—	20	*	305	—	—

Hollywood

CARROT JUICE, 6 oz	70	1	0	16	—	40	1.08	200	—	—

Libby

PUMPKIN, SOLID PACK, 1 c	80	2	1	20	—	60	3.6	10	470	—
PUMPKIN PIE MIX, PLAIN, 1 c	210	2	0	58	—	40	1.44	420	345	—
TOMATO JUICE, cnd, 6 oz	35	1	0	8	—	*	.72	455	430	—

Libby & Seneca

BEANS, GREEN										
CUTS, ½ c	20	1	0	4	—	20	.72	340	110	—
NATURAL PACK, UNSALTED, ½ c	20	1	0	4	—	20	.72	10	110	—
FRENCH, ½ c	20	1	0	4	—	20	.72	340	100	—
NATURAL PACK, UNSALTED, ½ c	20	1	0	4	—	20	.72	10	100	—
WHOLE, ½ c	20	1	0	4	—	20	.72	340	110	—
BEANS, LIMA, ½ c	80	5	0	15	—	40	1.44	230	320	—
BEANS, WAX, ½ c	20	1	0	5	—	20	.36	340	125	—
BEETS										
CUTS, DICED, SLICED or WHOLE, cnd, ½ c	35	1	0	8	—	*	.72	270	160	—
SLICED or WHOLE, jar, ½ c	35	1	0	8	—	*	.36	270	160	—
HARVARD, ½ c	80	1	0	20	—	*	.36	270	200	—
PICKLED, jar, ½ c	80	0	0	18	—	*	.36	270	155	—
WITH ONION, ½ c	80	0	0	18	—	*	.36	270	155	—
CARROTS, SLICED or DICED, ½ c	20	0	0	5	—	20	*	250	135	—
CORN, CREAM STYLE, ½ c	80	2	0	16	—	*	.36	260	145	—
CORN, WHOLE KERNEL, ½ c	80	2	1	18	—	*	.36	300	175	—
NATURAL PACK, UNSALTED, ½ c	80	2	1	18	—	*	.36	10	175	—
MUSHROOMS, ¼ c	35	4	0	4	—	*	.36	240	115	—
PEAS, ½ c	60	4	0	12	—	*	1.08	320	120	—
NATURAL PACK, UNSALTED, ½ c	60	4	0	12	—	*	1.08	10	120	—
PEAS & CARROTS, ½ c	50	3	0	10	—	20	.72	300	125	—
SAUERKRAUT, cnd, ½ c	20	1	0	5	—	20	1.08	780	175	—
jar, ½ c	20	1	0	5	—	20	.36	780	170	—
SPINACH, ½ c	25	3	0	4	—	100	1.8	540	275	—
SUCCOTASH, ½ c	80	3	1	22	—	*	.72	270	245	—
VEGETABLES, MIXED, ½ c	40	1	0	9	—	20	.36	320	235	—

Mrs. Pauls—Campbell

CORN FRITTERS, 2 fritters	250	5	12	30	—	20	1.08	725	—	—
EGGPLANT PARMIGIANA, 11 oz	540	16	34	40	—	200	2.16	1810	—	—
EGGPLANT STICKS, FRIED, 3½ oz	240	4	12	29	—	20	1.44	610	—	—
ONION RINGS, FRENCH FRIED, 2¼ oz	150	3	6	20	—	20	.36	275	—	—
POTATO AND CHEESE										

FOOD & DESCRIPTION MEASURE OR QUANTITY	CALORIES	PROTEIN (GM)	FAT (GM)	CARBO- HYDRATE (GM)	FIBER (GM)	CALCIUM (MG)	IRON (MG)	SODIUM (MG)	POTASSIUM (MG)	CHOLES- TEROL (MG)
PIEROGIES, 3	280	10	7	44	—	20	4.50	720	—	—
YAMS, CANDIED, 4 oz	181	1	0	44	—	*	.72	105	—	—
'N APPLES, 4 oz	150	1	1	36	—	40	.72	50	—	—
ZUCCHINI STICKS, LIGHT BATTER, 3 oz	180	3	9	23	—	20	.72	630	—	—

Nabisco

DROMEDARY PIMIENTOS, all types, dr, 1 oz	10	0	0	2	—	*	.72	5	45	—

Pepperidge Farm–
Campbell

ASPARAGUS WITH MORNAY SAUCE, 1 pastry	240	5	16	19	—	40	1.44	250	—	—
BEANS, GREEN, WITH MUSHROOM SAUCE, 1 pastry	250	4	17	20	—	40	1.44	270	—	—
BROCCOLI WITH CHEESE, 1 pastry	230	5	16	18	—	60	1.44	380	—	—
CAULIFLOWER AND CHEESE SAUCE, 1 pastry	210	5	13	19	—	60	1.44	450	—	—
MUSHROOMS DIJON, 1 pastry	220	4	15	19	—	20	2.70	340	—	—

Progresso

BLACK-EYED PEAS, 8 oz	165	11	1	29	—	20	2.70	—	—	—

Stouffer's

BEAN, GREEN, MUSHROOM CASSEROLE, 4.75 oz	170	3	12	12	—	20	1.44	640	200	—
BROCCOLI IN CHEDDAR CHEESE SAUCE, 4.5 oz	150	8	10	7	—	150	.72	480	270	—
CORN SOUFFLE, 4 oz	150	5	7	16	—	40	.36	540	200	—
POTATOES										
AU GRATIN, 3.83 oz	120	3	6	13	—	80	*	480	290	—
SCALLOPED, 4 oz	110	3	6	11	—	80	.36	410	240	—
RATATOUILLE, 5 oz	80	2	4	8	—	20	1.08	800	150	—
SPINACH										
CREAMED, 4.5 oz	190	4	15	9	—	100	1.08	440	250	—
SOUFFLE, 4 oz	140	5	9	10	—	80	1.08	560	220	—
YAMS AND APPLES, 5 oz	160	1	3	33	—	20	.72	200	240	—

USDA

ALFALFA SPROUTS, raw, 1 tbsp, 3 gm	1	<1	<1	<1	.07d	1	.03	0	2	0
1 c, 33 gm	10	1	<1	1	.73d	10	.32	2	26	0
AMARANTH, raw, 1 leaf, 14 gm	4	<1	<1	<1	.14	30	.32	3	85	0
1 c, 28 gm	7	<1	<1	1	.27	60	.65	5	171	0
AMARANTH, ckd, dr, ½ c, 66 gm	14	1	<1	3	.86	138	1.49	14	423	0
ARROWHEAD, raw, 1 medium, 12 gm	12	<1	<1	2	.1	1	.31	3	111	0
1 large, 25 gm	26	1	<1	5	.21	3	.64	6	231	0
ARROWHEAD, ckd, dr, 1 medium, 12 gm	9	<1	<1	2	.18	1	.15	2	106	0
ARTICHOKE, raw, 1 medium, 128 gm	65	3	<1	15	1.36	61	2.1	102	434	0
1 large, 162 gm	83	4	<1	19	1.72	78	2.66	130	549	0
ARTICHOKE, ckd, dr, 1 medium, 120 gm	53	3	<1	12	1.1	47	1.62	79	316	0
½ c hearts, 84 gm	37	2	<1	9	.77	33	1.13	55	221	0

FOOD & DESCRIPTION MEASURE OR QUANTITY	CALORIES	PROTEIN (GM)	FAT (GM)	CARBO-HYDRATE (GM)	FIBER (GM)	CALCIUM (MG)	IRON (MG)	SODIUM (MG)	POTASSIUM (MG)	CHOLES-TEROL (MG)
ARTICHOKE HEARTS, fz, 9 oz										
pkg, 255 gm	96	7	1	20	1.98	48	1.27	120	632	0
1/3 9 oz pkg, 85 gm	32	2	<1	7	.66	16	.42	40	211	0
ARTICHOKE HEARTS, fz, ckd,										
dr, 9 oz pkg, 240 gm	108	7	1	22	2.21	50	1.34	127	634	0
1/3 pkg, 80 gm	36	2	<1	7	.74	17	.45	42	211	0
ASPARAGUS										
ckd, dr, 1/2 c, 90 gm	22	2	<1	4	.75	22	.59	4	279	0
4 spears, 60 gm	15	2	<1	3	.5	15	.4	3	186	0
cnd, dr, 1/2 c, 121 gm	24	3	<1	3	—	—	2.22	—	—	0
1 can, 248 gm	48	5	2	6	—	—	4.55	—	—	0
s & l, 1/2 c, 122 gm	17	2	<1	3	.64	17	.71	425	186	0
salt-free, 1/2 c, 122 gm	17	2	<1	3	.64	17	.71	5	186	0
1 can, 411 gm	58	7	<1	9	2.17	58	2.38	1432	628	0
salt-free, 1 can, 411 gm	58	7	<1	9	2.17	58	2.38	16	628	0
raw, 1/2 c, 67 gm	15	2	<1	2	.55	14	.45	1	202	0
4 spears, 58 gm	13	2	<1	2	.48	12	.39	1	175	0
fz, 10 oz pkg, 284 gm	69	9	<1	12	2.48	72	2.07	24	718	0
4 spears, 58 gm	14	2	<1	2	.51	15	.42	5	147	0
fz, ckd, dr, 10 oz pkg, 293 gm	82	9	1	14	2.45	68	1.87	12	640	0
4 spears, 60 gm	17	2	<1	3	.5	14	.38	2	131	0
BALSAM-PEAR LEAFY TIPS										
ckd, dr, 1/2 c, 29 gm	10	1	<1	2	.54	12	.3	4	174	0
raw, 1 leaf, 4 gm	1	<1	<1	<1	.09	3	.08	0	24	0
1/2 c, 24 gm	7	1	<1	<1	.55	20	.49	3	146	0
BALSAM-PEAR PODS										
ckd, dr, 1/2 c pieces, 62 gm	12	<1	<1	3	.65	6	.24	4	198	0
raw, 1 c pieces, 93 gm	16	<1	<1	3	1.3	18	.4	5	275	0
1 pear, 124 gm	21	1	<1	5	1.74	24	.53	6	367	0
BAMBOO SHOOTS										
ckd, dr, 1 shoot, 144 gm	18	2	<1	3	.94	17	.35	6	768	0
1/2 c sl, 120 gm	8	<1	<1	1	.39	7	.15	3	320	0
cnd, dr, 1 c, 1/8" sl, 131 gm	25	2	<1	4	.87	10	.42	9	104	0
1 can, 262 gm	50	5	<1	8	1.76	21	.84	18	210	0
raw, 1/2 c sl, 76 gm	21	2	<1	4	.53	10	.38	3	405	0
BEAN SPROUTS										
KIDNEY										
ckd, dr, 100 gm	33	5	<1	5	—	19	.89	—	194	0
raw, 1/2 c, 92 gm	27	4	<1	4	—	16	.75	—	172	0
MUNG										
ckd, dr, 1/2 c, 62 gm	13	1	<1	3	.32	7	.4	6	63	0
cnd, s, 1/2 c, 62 gm	8	<1	<1	1	.16	9	.27	—	17	0
raw, 1/2 c, 52 gm	16	2	<1	3	.57d	7	.47	3	77	0
12 oz pkg, 340 gm	102	10	<1	20	3.74d	43	3.08	19	505	0
stir-fried, 1/2 c, 62 gm	31	3	<1	7	.43	8	1.18	—	—	0
NAVY										
ckd, dr, 100 gm	78	7	<1	15	2.88	16	2.11	—	317	0
raw, 1/2 c, 52 gm	35	3	<1	7	1.3	8	1.00	—	159	0
PINTO										
ckd, dr, 100 gm	22	2	<1	4	.95	15	.66	51	98	0
raw, 100 gm	62	5	<1	12	2.7	43	1.97	153	307	0
BEANS, LIMA										
ckd, dr, 1/2 c, 85 gm	104	6	<1	20	3.57d	27	2.08	14	485	0
cnd, s & l, 1/2 c, 124 gm	93	6	<1	17	5.21d	35	1.97	309	334	0
salt-free, 1/2 c, 124 gm	93	6	<1	17	5.21d	35	1.97	5	334	0
1 can, 454 gm	339	21	1	63	19.07d	128	7.20	1131	1222	0
salt-free, 1 can, 454 gm	339	21	1	63	19.07d	128	7.20	18	1222	0
raw, 1/2 c, 78 gm	88	5	<1	16	2.89d	27	2.45	6	365	0
BEANS, LIMA, BABY, fz										
10 oz pkg, 284 gm	376	22	1	71	6.18	98	6.28	147	1283	0
1/2 c, 82 gm	108	6	<1	21	1.79	29	1.81	43	371	0
ckd, dr, 10 oz pkg, 311 gm	326	21	<1	60	—	89	6.1	90	1277	0
1/2 c, 90 gm	94	6	<1	18	—	25	1.76	26	370	0

FOOD & DESCRIPTION MEASURE OR QUANTITY	CALORIES	PROTEIN (GM)	FAT (GM)	CARBO-HYDRATE (GM)	FIBER (GM)	CALCIUM (MG)	IRON (MG)	SODIUM (MG)	POTASSIUM (MG)	CHOLES-TEROL (MG)
BEANS, LIMA, FORDHOOK, fz										
10 oz pkg, 284 gm	301	18	1	56	5.61	68	4.29	166	1357	0
½ c, 80 gm	85	5	<1	16	1.58	19	1.21	46	382	0
ckd, dr, 10 oz pkg, 311 gm	312	19	1	58	5.82	67	4.23	164	1268	0
½ c, 85 gm	85	5	<1	16	1.59	19	1.16	45	347	0
BEANS, PINTO, fz										
10 oz pkg, 284 gm	484	28	1	92	—	165	8.52	—	—	0
⅓ 10 oz pkg, 94 gm	160	9	<1	31	—	55	2.82	—	—	0
ckd, dr, 10 oz pkg, 284 gm	460	26	1	88	—	149	7.70	—	—	0
⅓ pkg, 94 gm	152	9	<1	29	—	49	2.55	—	—	0
BEANS, SHELLIE, cnd, s & l,										
½ c, 122 gm	37	2	<1	8	.73	36	1.21	408	133	0
BEANS, SNAP [includes ITALIAN, GREEN & YELLOW VARIETIES]										
ckd, dr, ½ c, 62 gm	22	1	<1	5	1.12d	29	.79	2	185	0
cnd, s & l, ½ c, 120 gm	18	1	<1	4	.72d	29	1.05	442	117	0
salt-free, ½ c, 120 gm	18	1	<1	4	.72d	29	1.05	2	117	0
1 can, 439 gm	68	4	<1	15	2.63d	104	3.85	1615	428	0
salt-free, 1 can, 439 gm	68	4	<1	15	2.63d	104	3.85	9	428	0
cnd, dr, ½ c, 68 gm	13	<1	<1	3	.88d	18	.61	170	74	0
salt-free, ½ c, 68 gm	13	<1	<1	3	.88d	18	.61	1	74	0
1 can, 262 gm	52	3	<1	12	3.41d	69	2.36	657	286	0
salt-free, 1 can, 262 gm	52	3	<1	12	3.41d	69	2.36	5	286	0
cnd, season, s & l, ½ c, 114 gm	18	<1	<1	4	.97	25	.54	425	106	0
1 can, 439 gm	71	4	<1	15	3.73	98	2.08	1637	407	0
fz, ½ c, 62 gm	21	1	<1	5	1.12d	26	.53	2	115	0
10 oz pkg, 284 gm	94	5	<1	22	5.11d	118	2.45	8	529	0
fz, ckd, dr, ½ c, 68 gm	18	<1	<1	4	1.09d	31	.56	9	76	0
raw, ½ c, 55 gm	17	1	<1	4	1.16d	21	.57	3	115	0
BEET GREENS										
ckd, dr, ½ c, 72 gm	20	2	<1	4	.76	82	1.37	173	654	0
raw, pieces, ½ c, 19 gm	4	<1	<1	<1	.25	23	.63	38	104	0
1 leaf, 32 gm	6	<1	<1	1	.42	38	1.06	64	175	0
BEETS										
ckd, dr, ½ c sl, 85 gm	26	<1	<1	6	.72	9	.53	42	266	0
2 beets, 100 gm	31	1	<1	7	.85	11	.62	49	312	0
cnd, dr, ½ c sl, 85 gm	27	<1	<1	6	—	—	1.55	—	—	0
1 can, 294 gm	92	3	<1	21	—	—	5.36	—	—	0
cnd, s & l, 123 gm	36	1	<1	8	.75	17	.82	324	175	0
salt-free, ½ c, 123 gm	36	1	<1	8	.75	17	.82	57	175	0
raw, ½ c sl, 68 gm	30	1	<1	7	.68d	11	.62	49	220	0
2 beets, 163 gm	71	2	<1	16	1.63d	25	1.49	118	528	0
BEETS, HARVARD, cnd, s & l,										
½ c, 123 gm	89	1	<1	22	—	13	.44	199	201	0
BEETS, PICKLED, cnd, s & l,										
½ c, 114 gm	75	<1	<1	19	.71	13	.47	301	169	0
BORAGE										
ckd, dr, 100 gm	25	2	<1	4	1.07	102	3.64	88	491	0
raw, pieces, ½ c, 44 gm	9	<1	<1	1	.4	41	1.45	35	207	0
BROAD BEANS,										
ckd, dr, 100 gm	56	5	<1	10	1.9	18	1.5	41	193	0
raw, 1 bean, 8 gm	6	<1	<1	<1	.18	2	.15	4	20	0
1 c, 109 gm	79	6	<1	13	2.4	24	2.07	55	273	0
BROCCOLI										
ckd, dr, ½ c, chopped, 78 gm	23	2	<1	4	.94	89	.89	8	127	0
1 spear, 180 gm	53	5	<1	10	2.16	205	2.06	19	293	0
fz										
chopped										
⅓ pkg, 95 gm	25	3	<1	5	1.61d	53	.77	23	201	0
10 oz pkg, 284 gm	75	8	<1	14	4.83d	159	2.3	68	602	0
ckd, dr, ½ c, 92 gm	25	3	<1	5	2.02d	47	.56	22	166	0

FOOD & DESCRIPTION MEASURE OR QUANTITY	CALORIES	PROTEIN (GM)	FAT (GM)	CARBO-HYDRATE (GM)	FIBER (GM)	CALCIUM (MG)	IRON (MG)	SODIUM (MG)	POTASSIUM (MG)	CHOLES-TEROL (MG)
spears										
⅓ pkg, 95 gm	28	3	<1	5	1.99d	38	.68	16	237	0
10 oz pkg, 284 gm	84	9	<1	15	5.96d	115	2.03	49	710	0
ckd, dr,										
½ c, 92 gm	25	3	<1	5	2.02d	47	.56	22	166	0
10 oz pkg, 250 gm	69	8	<1	13	5.50d	127	1.53	60	451	0
raw, ½ c, chopped, 44 gm	12	1	<1	2	.62d	21	.39	12	143	0
1 spear, 151 gm	42	5	<1	8	2.11d	73	1.33	40	490	0
BRUSSELS SPROUTS										
ckd, dr, 1 sprout, 21 gm	8	<1	<1	2	.29d	7	.25	4	67	0
½ c, 78 gm	30	2	<1	7	1.09d	28	.94	17	247	0
fz, ⅓ pkg, 95 gm	39	4	<1	7	2.08d	25	.88	9	351	0
10 oz pkg, 284 gm	116	11	1	22	6.25d	75	2.65	28	1052	0
ckd, dr, ½ c, 78 gm	33	3	<1	6	1.40d	19	.58	18	254	0
raw, 1 sprout, 19 gm	8	<1	<1	2	.29	8	.27	5	74	0
½ c, 44 gm	19	1	<1	4	.66	18	.62	11	171	0
BURDOCK ROOT										
ckd, dr, ½ c, 63 gm	55	1	<1	13	1.15	31	.48	3	225	0
1 root, 166 gm	146	3	<1	35	3.04	82	1.28	7	597	0
raw, ½ c pieces, 59 gm	43	<1	<1	10	1.15	24	.47	3	182	0
1 root, 156 gm	112	2	<1	27	3.03	64	1.25	8	480	0
BUTTERBUR [FUKI]										
ckd, dr, 100 gm	8	<1	<1	2	.78	59	.1	4	354	0
cnd, 3 stalks, 45 gm	1	<1	<1	<1	.39	15	.28	2	5	0
1 c chopped, 124 gm	3	<1	<1	<1	1.08	42	.78	5	15	0
raw, 1 petiole, 5 gm	1	<1	0	<1	.07	5	.01	0	33	0
½ c, 47 gm	7	<1	<1	2	.61	49	.05	4	308	0
CABBAGE										
ckd, shredded, dr, ½ c, 75 gm	16	<1	<1	4	.45	25	.29	14	154	0
1 head, 1262 gm	270	12	3	60	7.57	413	4.96	239	2593	0
raw, shredded, ½ c, 35 gm	8	<1	<1	2	.39d	16	.2	6	86	0
1 head, 908 gm	215	11	2	49	9.99d	424	5.09	164	2231	0
CABBAGE, CHINESE [PAK-CHOI], shredded, ckd,										
dr, ½ c, 85 gm	10	1	<1	2	.51	79	.88	29	315	0
raw, ½ c, 35 gm	5	<1	<1	<1	.21	37	.28	23	88	0
CABBAGE, CHINESE [PE-TSAI], shredded, ckd,										
dr, ½ c, 60 gm	8	<1	<1	1	.3	19	.18	6	134	0
raw, ½ c, 38 gm	6	<1	<1	1	.23	29	.12	3	90	0
CABBAGE, RED, shredded,										
ckd, dr, 1 leaf, 22 gm	5	<1	<1	1	.17	8	.08	2	31	0
½ c, 75 gm	16	<1	<1	3	.57	28	.27	6	105	0
raw, ½ c, 35 gm	10	<1	<1	2	.39d	18	.17	4	72	0
CABBAGE, SAVOY, shredded,										
ckd, dr, ½ c, 73 gm	18	1	<1	4	.51	22	.28	17	134	0
raw, ½ c, 35 gm	10	<1	<1	2	.28	12	.14	10	81	0
CARDOON, ckd, dr, 100 gm	22	<1	<1	5	—	72	.73	176	392	0
raw, ½ c, 89 gm	18	<1	<1	4	—	62	.62	151	356	0
CARROTS										
ckd, dr, ½ c, 78 gm	35	<1	<1	8	1.48d	24	.48	52	177	0
1 carrot, 46 gm	21	<1	<1	5	.87d	14	.28	30	104	0
cnd, dr, sl, ½ c, 73 gm	17	<1	<1	4	.88d	19	.47	176	131	0
salt-free, ½ c, 73 gm	17	<1	<1	4	.88d	19	.47	31	131	0
1 can, 284 gm	65	2	<1	16	3.41d	71	1.82	684	508	0
salt-free, 1 can, 284 gm	65	2	<1	16	3.41d	71	1.82	119	508	0
cnd, s & l, ½ c, 123 gm	28	<1	<1	6	1.35d	31	.75	297	213	0
salt-free, ½ c, 123 gm	28	<1	<1	6	1.35d	31	.75	48	213	0
1 can, 454 gm	102	3	<1	23	4.99d	114	2.76	1095	784	0
salt-free, 1 can 454 gm	102	3	<1	23	4.99d	114	2.76	177	784	0
fz, sl, ½ c, 64 gm	25	<1	<1	6	.90d	21	.39	38	116	0
10 oz pkg, 284 gm	112	3	<1	26	3.98d	92	1.72	167	515	0
ckd, dr, ½ c, 73 gm	26	<1	<1	6	1.31d	21	.35	43	115	0

FOOD & DESCRIPTION MEASURE OR QUANTITY	CALORIES	PROTEIN (GM)	FAT (GM)	CARBO-HYDRATE (GM)	FIBER (GM)	CALCIUM (MG)	IRON (MG)	SODIUM (MG)	POTASSIUM (MG)	CHOLES-TEROL (MG)
raw, shredded, ½ c, 55 gm	24	<1	<1	6	.83d	15	.27	19	178	0
1 carrot, 72 gm	31	<1	<1	7	1.08d	19	.36	25	233	0
CARROT JUICE, cnd, ½ c, 123										
gm	49	1	<1	11	1.17	29	.57	36	360	0
6 oz, 184 gm	73	2	<1	17	1.75	44	.85	54	538	0
CASSAVA, raw, 100 gm	120	3	<1	27	2.49	91	3.6	8	764	0
CAULIFLOWER										
ckd, dr, pieces, ½ c, 62 gm	15	1	<1	3	.99d	17	.26	4	200	0
3 florets, 54 gm	13	1	<1	3	.86d	14	.23	3	174	0
fz, ½ c, 66 gm	16	1	<1	3	.66	15	.36	16	127	0
10 oz pkg, 284 gm	68	6	<1	13	2.84	63	1.54	68	548	0
ckd, dr, ½ c, 90 gm	17	1	<1	3	.72	15	.37	16	125	0
raw, pieces, ½ c, 50 gm	12	<1	<1	2	.42	14	.29	7	178	0
3 florets, 56 gm	13	1	<1	3	.47	16	.32	8	199	0
CELERIAC										
ckd, dr, 100 gm	25	<1	<1	6	.83	26	.43	61	173	0
raw, ½ c, 78 gm	31	1	<1	7	1.01	34	.55	78	234	0
CELERY										
ckd, dr, diced, ½ c, 75 gm	11	<1	<1	3	.49	27	.1	48	266	0
raw, 1 stalk, 40 gm	6	<1	<1	1	.36d	14	.19	35	114	0
diced, ½ c, 60 gm	9	<1	<1	2	.54d	22	.29	53	170	0
CELTUCE, raw, 1 leaf, 8 gm	2	<1	<1	<1	.03	3	.04	1	26	0
CHARD, SWISS										
ckd, dr, ½ c, 88 gm	18	2	<1	4	.83	51	1.99	158	483	0
raw, chopped, ½ c, 18 gm	3	<1	<1	<1	.14	9	.32	38	68	0
1 leaf, 48 gm	9	<1	<1	2	.38	24	.86	102	182	0
CHAYOTE FRUIT										
ckd, dr, ½ c pieces, 80 gm	19	<1	<1	4	.46	10	.18	1	138	0
raw, pieces, ½ c, 66 gm	16	<1	<1	4	.46	13	.27	3	99	0
1 fruit, 203 gm	49	2	<1	11	1.42	39	.81	8	305	0
CHICORY GREENS, raw, ½ c, 90 gm	21	2	<1	4	.72	90	.81	41	378	0
CHICORY ROOTS, raw, pieces, ½ c, 45 gm	33	<1	<1	8	.88	18	.36	23	131	0
1 root, 60 gm	44	<1	<1	11	1.17	25	.48	30	174	0
CHICORY, WITLOOF, raw, ½ c, 45 gm	7	<1	<1	1	—	—	.23	3	82	0
1 head, 53 gm	8	<1	<1	2	—	—	.26	4	96	0
CHIVES, raw,										
1 tsp chopped, 1 gm	<1	<1	<1	<1	.01	1	.02	0	3	0
1 tbsp, 3 gm	1	<1	<1	<1	.03	2	.05	0	8	0
CHIVES, freeze-dried, 1 tbsp, .2 gm	1	<1	<1	<1	.02	2	.04	—	6	0
CHRYSANTHEMUM, GARLAND										
ckd, dr, ½ c, 50 gm	10	<1	<1	2	.58	34	1.87	27	284	0
raw, 1 stem, 14 gm	2	<1	<1	<1	.12	8	.44	7	80	0
½ c, 13 gm	2	<1	<1	<1	.11	7	.39	7	72	0
COLESLAW, ½ c, 60 gm	42	<1	2	7	.36	27	.35	14	109	0
COLLARDS										
ckd, dr, ½ c, 95 gm	13	1	<1	3	.38	74	.39	18	88	0
fz, ⅓ pkg, 95 gm	31	3	<1	6	.93	190	1.01	45	240	0
10 oz pkg, 284 gm	93	8	1	18	2.78	570	3.03	136	719	0
ckd, dr, ½ c, 85 gm	31	3	<1	6	.92	179	.95	42	214	0
raw, chopped, ½ c, 93 gm	18	1	<1	4	.53	109	.58	26	137	0
CORIANDER, raw										
¼ c, 4 gm	1	<1	<1	<1	.03	4	.08	1	22	0
9 plants, 20 gm	4	<1	<1	<1	.16	20	.39	6	108	0
CORN, SWEET										
ckd, dr, ½ c, 82 gm	89	3	1	21	.49	2	.5	14	204	0
kernels from 1 ear, 77 gm	83	3	<1	19	.46	2	.47	13	192	0
cnd, cream-style, ½ c, 128 gm	93	2	<1	23	.62	4	.49	365	172	0
salt-free, ½ c, 128 gm	93	2	<1	23	.62	4	.49	4	172	0
1 can, 482 gm	349	8	2	87	2.35	15	1.83	1376	646	0

FOOD & DESCRIPTION MEASURE OR QUANTITY	CALORIES	PROTEIN (GM)	FAT (GM)	CARBO-HYDRATE (GM)	FIBER (GM)	CALCIUM (MG)	IRON (MG)	SODIUM (MG)	POTASSIUM (MG)	CHOLES-TEROL (MG)
salt-free, 1 can, 482 gm	349	8	2	87	2.35	15	1.83	14	—	0
cnd, dr, ½ c, 82 gm	66	2	<1	15	1.07d	—	.70	—	—	0
1 can, 298 gm	242	8	3	55	3.87d	—	2.55	—	—	0
cnd, s & l, ½ c, 128 gm	79	2	<1	19	1.66d	5	.44	324	196	0
salt-free, ½ c, 128 gm	79	2	<1	19	1.66d	5	.44	4	196	0
1 can, 482 gm	294	9	2	71	6.27d	19	1.69	1220	738	0
salt-free, 1 can, 482 gm	294	9	2	71	6.27d	19	1.69	14	738	0
cnd, vacuum-packed, ½ c, 105 gm	83	3	<1	20	.82	5	.44	286	195	0
salt-free, ½ c, 105 gm	83	3	<1	20	.82	5	.44	3	195	0
1 can, 340 gm	270	8	2	66	2.66	16	1.44	925	632	0
salt-free, 1 can, 340 gm	270	8	2	66	2.66	16	1.44	10	632	0
fz, kernels, ½ c, 82 gm	72	2	<1	17	1.72d	4	.35	3	172	0
10 oz pkg, 284 gm	250	9	2	59	5.96d	12	1.2	9	596	0
ckd, dr, ½ c, 82 gm	67	2	<1	17	1.72d	2	.25	4	114	0
10 oz pkg, 284 gm	231	9	<1	58	5.96d	6	.86	14	394	0
on cob, fz, ½ c kernels, 82 gm	81	3	<1	19	.56	3	.56	4	241	0
1 ear, 125 gm	123	4	<1	29	.86	4	.85	6	367	0
ckd, dr, ½ c, kernels, 82 gm	77	3	<1	18	.53	3	.5	3	206	0
1 ear, 63 gm	59	2	<1	14	.41	2	.39	3	158	0
raw, ½ c, 77 gm	66	2	<1	15	1.23d	2	.40	12	208	0
kernels from 1 ear, 90 gm	77	3	1	17	1.44d	2	.46	14	243	0
CORN WITH PEPPERS [MEXICALI], cnd, s & l, ½ c, 114 gm	86	3	<1	21	.71	5	.9	396	174	0
CORN PUDDING, ½ c, 125 gm	136	5	7	16	.45	50	.7	69	201	0
CORN SALAD, raw, ½ c, 28 gm	6	<1	<1	1	.22	—	—	—	—	0
COWPEAS										
ckd, dr, ½ c, 82 gm	89	7	<1	15	1.46	23	1.17	4	344	0
fz, ½ c, 80 gm	111	7	<1	20	1.29	21	1.88	5	353	0
10 oz pkg, 284 gm	396	25	2	71	4.57	73	6.69	17	1252	0
ckd, dr, ½ c, 85 gm	112	7	<1	20	1.29	20	1.80	5	319	0
raw, ½ c, 72 gm	91	6	<1	16	1.3	19	.79	3	311	0
COWPEAS, LEAFY TIPS										
ckd, dr, chopped, ½ c, 26 gm	6	1	<1	<1	.68	18	.28	2	91	0
raw, 1 leaf, 3 gm	1	<1	<1	<1	.04	2	.06	0	14	0
1 c, chopped, 36 gm	10	1	<1	2	.47	23	.69	2	164	0
COWPEAS, PODS WITH SEEDS										
ckd, dr, ½ c, 47 gm	16	1	<1	3	.8	26	.33	1	92	0
raw, 1 pod, 12 gm	5	<1	<1	1	.2	8	.12	0	26	0
½ c, 47 gm	21	2	<1	4	.8	31	.47	2	101	0
CRESS, GARDEN										
ckd, dr, ½ c, 68 gm	16	1	<1	3	.61	41	.54	5	240	0
raw, 1 sprig, 1 gm	<1	<1	<1	<1	.01	1	.01	0	6	0
½ c, 25 gm	8	<1	<1	1	.28	20	.33	4	152	0
CUCUMBER, raw, ½ c sl, 52 gm	7	<1	<1	2	.26d	7	.14	1	78	0
1 cucumber, 301 gm	39	2	<1	9	1.51d	42	.84	6	448	0
DANDELION GREENS, chopped										
ckd, dr, ½ c, 52 gm	17	1	<1	3	.68	73	.94	23	121	0
raw, ½ c, 28 gm	13	<1	<1	3	.45	52	.87	21	111	0
DOCK, chopped										
ckd, dr, 100 gm	20	2	<1	3	.73	38	2.08	3	321	0
raw, ½ c, 67 gm	15	1	<1	2	.54	29	1.61	3	261	0
EGGPLANT										
ckd, dr, ½ c cubes, 48 gm	13	<1	<1	3	.47	3	.17	2	119	0
raw, ½ c pieces, 41 gm	11	<1	<1	3	.62d	15	.22	1	90	0
1 eggplant, Hawaiian, 103										

304

FOOD & DESCRIPTION MEASURE OR QUANTITY	CALORIES	PROTEIN (GM)	FAT (GM)	CARBO-HYDRATE (GM)	FIBER (GM)	CALCIUM (MG)	IRON (MG)	SODIUM (MG)	POTASSIUM (MG)	CHOLES-TEROL (MG)
gm	27	1	<1	6	1.55d	37	.56	4	225	0
ENDIVE, raw, chopped, ½ c,										
25 gm	4	<1	<1	<1	.23	13	.21	6	79	0
1 head, 513 gm	86	6	1	17	4.62	267	4.23	115	1611	0
EPPAW, raw, ½ c, 50 gm	75	2	<1	16	—	55	.58	6	170	0
GARLIC, raw, 1 clove, 3 gm	4	<1	<1	<1	.05	5	.05	1	12	0
GINGER ROOT, raw, 5 sl, 11										
gm	8	<1	<1	2	.11	2	.05	1	46	0
¼ c sl, 24 gm	17	<1	<1	4	.25	4	.12	3	100	0
GOURD, DISHCLOTH										
ckd, dr, ½ c, 89 gm	50	<1	<1	13	.36d	8	.32	18	403	0
raw, 1 c sl, 95 gm	19	1	<1	4	.48	19	.34	3	132	0
1 gourd, 178 gm	36	2	<1	8	.89	36	.64	6	247	0
GOURD, WHITE-FLOWERED										
ckd, dr, ½ c, 73 gm	11	<1	<1	3	.46	18	.18	1	124	0
raw, ½ c cubes, 89 gm	8	<1	<1	2	.64d	15	.12	1	87	0
1 gourd, 771 gm	106	5	<1	26	8.48d	200	1.54	19	1154	0
HORSERADISH-TREE, LEAFY TIPS,										
ckd, dr, ½ c, 21 gm	13	1	<1	2	.36	—	.49	2	72	0
raw, ½ c chopped, 10 gm	6	<1	<1	<1	.15	—	.4	1	34	0
HORSERADISH-TREE, PODS										
ckd, dr, ½ c, 59 gm	21	1	<1	5	1.09	12	.27	25	270	0
raw, 1 pod, 11 gm	4	<1	<1	<1	.14	3	.04	5	51	0
1 c, 100 gm	37	2	<1	9	1.30	30	.36	42	461	0
HYACINTH BEANS										
ckd, dr, ½ c, 44 gm	22	1	<1	4	.78	18	.33	1	115	0
raw, ½ c, 40 gm	19	<1	<1	4	.52	20	.30	1	101	0
JERUSALEM ARTICHOKES,										
raw, sliced, ½ c, 75 gm	57	2	<1	13	.6	10	2.55	—	—	0
JUTE, POTHERB										
ckd, dr, ½ c, 43 gm	16	2	<1	3	.84	91	1.35	5	237	0
raw, ½ c, 14 gm	5	1	<1	<1	.17	29	.67	1	78	0
KALE, chopped										
ckd, dr, ½ c, 65 gm	21	1	<1	4	.52	47	.59	15	148	0
fz, ⅓ pkg, 94 gm	26	3	<1	5	.81	127	.87	14	313	0
10 oz pkg, 284 gm	79	8	1	14	2.46	385	2.63	43	947	0
fz, ckd, dr, ½ c, 65 gm	20	2	<1	3	.6	90	.61	10	209	0
raw, ½ c, 34 gm	17	1	<1	3	.51	46	.58	15	152	0
KALE, SCOTCH, chopped										
ckd, dr, ½ c, 65 gm	18	1	<1	4	.55	86	1.25	29	178	0
raw, ½ c, 34 gm	14	<1	<1	3	.42	70	1.02	24	153	0
KANPYO, dried, 3 strips, 19										
gm	49	2	<1	12	1.73	53	.97	3	301	0
½ c, 27 gm	70	2	<1	18	2.47	76	1.38	4	427	0
KOHLRABI, sliced										
ckd, dr, ½ c, 82 gm	24	1	<1	5	.90	20	.33	17	279	0
raw, ½ c, 70 gm	19	1	<1	4	.77d	17	.28	14	245	0
LAMBSQUARTERS										
ckd, dr, ½ c chopped, 90 gm	29	3	<1	5	1.62	232	.63	—	—	0
raw, 100 gm	43	4	<1	7	2.10	309	1.20	—	—	0
LEEKS										
ckd, dr, ¼ c chopped, 236 gm	8	<1	<1	2	.21	8	.29	3	23	0
1 leek, 124 gm	38	1	<1	9	1.02	37	1.36	13	108	0
freeze-dried, 1 tbsp, .2 gm	1	<1	0	<1	.02	1	.02	0	5	0
¼ c, .8 gm	3	<1	<1	<1	.07	3	.06	0	19	0
raw, ¼ c, 26 gm	16	<1	<1	4	.31d	15	.55	5	47	0
1 leek, 124 gm	76	2	<1	18	1.49d	73	2.6	25	223	0
LENTIL SPROUTS										
ckd, stir-fried, no fat, 100 gm	101	9	<1	21	1.10	14	3.1	—	284	0
raw, ½ c, 38 gm	40	3	<1	8	1.16	9	1.22	4	122	0
LETTUCE, BUTTERHEAD, raw,										
2 leaves, 15 gm	2	<1	<1	<1	.11d	—	.04	1	39	0

305

FOOD & DESCRIPTION MEASURE OR QUANTITY	CALORIES	PROTEIN (GM)	FAT (GM)	CARBO-HYDRATE (GM)	FIBER (GM)	CALCIUM (MG)	IRON (MG)	SODIUM (MG)	POTASSIUM (MG)	CHOLES-TEROL (MG)
1 head, 163 gm	21	2	<1	4	1.14d	—	.49	8	416	0
LETTUCE, COS/ROMAINE,										
raw, inner leaf, 10 gm	2	<1	<1	<1	.07	4	.11	1	29	0
½ c shredded, 28 gm	4	<1	<1	<1	.2	10	.31	2	81	0
LETTUCE, ICEBERG, raw, 1										
leaf, 20 gm	3	<1	<1	<1	.18d	4	.1	2	32	0
1 head, 539 gm	70	5	1	11	4.85d	102	2.7	48	852	0
LETTUCE, LOOSELEAF, raw, 1										
leaf, 10 gm	2	<1	<1	<1	.07	7	.14	1	26	0
½ c shredded, 28 gm	5	<1	<1	<1	.20	19	.39	3	74	0
LOTUS ROOT										
ckd, dr, 10 sl, 89 gm	59	1	<1	14	.76	23	.8	40	323	0
raw, 10 sl, 81 gm	45	2	<1	14	.64	36	.94	33	450	0
1 root, 115 gm	64	3	<1	20	.91	52	1.33	47	639	0
MIXED VEGETABLES										
cnd, dr, ½ c, 82 gm	39	2	<1	8	1.97d	22	.86	122	239	0
cnd, s & l, ½ c, 122 gm	44	2	<1	9	1.46	26	.79	273	169	0
fz, 10 oz pkg, 284 gm	201	9	1	38	3.34	72	2.7	132	603	0
ckd, dr, ½ c, 91 gm	54	3	<1	12	2.09d	22	.75	32	154	0
10 oz pkg, 275 gm	163	8	<1	36	6.33d	67	2.26	96	464	0
MOUNTAIN YAM, HAWAII										
raw, ½ c cubed, 68 gm	46	<1	<1	11	.31	18	.3	9	284	0
1 yam, 420 gm	282	6	<1	68	1.89	108	1.85	55	1756	0
steamed, ½ c, cubed, 72 gm	59	1	<1	14	.4	5	.31	9	356	0
MUSHROOMS										
ckd, dr, 1 mushroom, 12 gm	3	<1	<1	<1	.1	1	.21	0	43	0
½ c, 78 gm	21	2	<1	4	.68	4	1.36	2	277	0
cnd, dr, 1 mushroom, 12 gm	3	<1	<1	<1	—	—	.1	—	—	0
½ c, 78 gm	19	1	<1	4	—	—	.62	—	—	0
raw, 1 mushroom, 18 gm	5	<1	<1	<1	.13	1	.22	1	67	0
½ c, 35 gm	9	<1	<1	2	.26	2	.43	1	130	0
MUSHROOMS, SHIITAKE										
ckd, 4 mushrooms, 72 gm	40	1	<1	10	1.41	2	.32	3	85	0
½ c, pieces, 73 gm	40	1	<1	10	1.42	2	.32	3	85	0
dried, 1 mushroom, 3.6 gm	11	<1	<1	3	.41	0	.06	0	55	0
MUSTARD GREENS, chopped										
ckd, dr, ½ c, 70 gm	11	2	<1	1	.48	52	.49	11	141	0
fz, ½ c, 73 gm	15	2	<1	2	.58	85	.94	21	124	0
10 oz, 284 gm	58	7	<1	10	2.27	329	3.67	83	481	0
fz, ckd, dr, ½ c, 75 gm	14	2	<1	2	.55	75	.84	19	104	0
10 oz pkg, 212 gm	40	5	<1	7	1.55	213	2.38	53	295	0
raw, ½ c, 28 gm	7	<1	<1	1	.17d	29	.41	7	99	0
MUSTARD SPINACH, chopped										
ckd, dr, ½ c, 90 gm	14	2	<1	3	.72	142	.72	—	—	0
raw, ½ c, 75 gm	17	2	<1	3	.75	158	1.13	—	—	0
NEW ZEALAND SPINACH, chopped										
ckd, dr, ½ c, 90 gm	11	1	<1	2	.55	43	.59	97	92	0
raw, ½ c, 28 gm	4	<1	<1	<1	.2	16	.22	36	36	0
OKRA, sliced										
ckd, dr, ½ c, 80 gm	25	1	<1	6	.72	50	.36	4	257	0
8 pods, 85 gm	27	2	<1	6	.77	54	.38	5	273	0
fz, 10 oz pkg, 284 gm	85	5	<1	19	2.35	231	1.62	7	600	0
ckd, dr, ½ c, 92 gm	34	2	<1	8	.94	88	.62	3	215	0
10 oz pkg, 255 gm	94	5	<1	21	2.6	245	1.71	8	597	0
raw, ½ c, 50 gm	19	1	<1	4	.47	41	.4	4	151	0
8 pods, 95 gm	36	2	<1	7	.89	77	.76	8	287	0
ONION RINGS, fz										
9 oz pkg, 255 gm	658	8	36	78	—	117	2.37	627	483	0
heated, 2 rings, 20 gm	81	1	5	8	.08	6	.34	75	26	0
ONIONS										
ckd, dr, chopped, 1 tbsp, 15 gm	4	<1	<1	<1	.06	4	.03	1	23	0
½ c, 105 gm	29	<1	<1	7	.44	29	.21	8	159	0

FOOD & DESCRIPTION MEASURE OR QUANTITY	CALORIES	PROTEIN (GM)	FAT (GM)	CARBO-HYDRATE (GM)	FIBER (GM)	CALCIUM (MG)	IRON (MG)	SODIUM (MG)	POTASSIUM (MG)	CHOLES-TEROL (MG)
cnd, s & l, 1 onion, 63 gm	12	<1	<1	3	.69d	29	.08	234	70	0
½ c, chopped, 112 gm	21	<1	<1	5	1.23d	51	.15	416	124	0
dehydrated, flakes, 1 tbsp, 5 gm	16	<1	<1	4	.23	13	.08	1	81	0
¼ c, 14 gm	45	1	<1	12	.64	36	.22	3	227	0
fz, chopped, 10 oz pkg, 284 gm	83	2	<1	19	2.27d	50	.93	35	353	0
ckd, dr, 1 tbsp, 15 gm	4	<1	<1	<1	.07	2	.05	2	16	0
½ c, 105 gm	30	<1	<1	7	.48	17	.32	13	114	0
fz, whole, ⅓ pkg, 94 gm	33	<1	<1	8	.65	34	.43	9	133	0
10 oz pkg, 284 gm	101	3	<1	24	1.96	102	1.29	27	402	0
ckd, dr, 100 gm	28	<1	<1	7	.55	27	.34	8	101	0
raw, chopped, 1 tbsp, 10 gm	3	<1	<1	<1	.08d	2	.04	0	16	0
½ c, 80 gm	27	<1	<1	6	.64d	20	.29	2	124	0
ONIONS, SPRING, raw, chopped, 1 tbsp, 6 gm	2	<1	<1	<1	.05	4	.11	0	15	0
½ c, 50 gm	13	<1	<1	3	.42	30	.94	2	128	0
ONIONS, WELSH, raw, 100 gm	34	2	<1	7	1	18	—	—	—	0
PARSLEY										
freeze-dried, 1 tbsp, .4 gm	1	<1	<1	<1	.04	1	.22	2	25	0
¼ c, 1.4 gm	4	<1	<1	<1	.14	2	.75	5	88	0
raw, 10 sprigs, 10 gm	3	<1	<1	<1	.12	13	.62	4	54	0
½ c, chopped, 30 gm	10	<1	<1	2	.36	39	1.86	12	161	0
PARSNIPS										
ckd, dr, sliced, ½ c, 78 gm	63	1	<1	15	2.11d	29	.45	8	287	0
1 parsnip, 160 gm	130	2	<1	31	4.32d	59	.92	17	588	0
raw, sliced, ½ c, 67 gm	50	<1	<1	12	1.34	24	.39	7	251	0
PEA PODS										
ckd, dr, ½ c, 80 gm	34	3	<1	6	1.28d	33	1.58	3	192	0
fz, ½ c, 72 gm	30	2	<1	5	1.73	36	1.44	3	139	0
10 oz pkg, 284 gm	118	8	<1	20	6.82	142	5.68	11	546	0
ckd, dr, ½ c, 80 gm	42	3	<1	7	2.4	48	1.92	4	173	0
10 oz pkg, 253 gm	132	9	<1	23	7.61	150	6.07	12	549	0
raw, ½ c, 72 gm	30	2	<1	5	1.37d	31	1.5	3	144	0
PEAS, GREEN										
ckd, ½ c, 80 gm	67	4	<1	13	2.96d	22	1.24	2	217	0
cnd, dr, ½ c, 85 gm	59	4	<1	11	3.49d	17	.81	186	147	0
salt-free, ½ c, 85 gm	59	4	<1	11	3.49d	17	.81	2	147	0
1 can, 313 gm	217	14	1	39	12.83d	62	2.97	685	541	0
salt-free, 1 can, 313 gm	217	14	1	39	12.83d	62	2.97	6	541	0
cnd, s & l, ½ c, 124 gm	61	4	<1	11	2.23d	22	1.37	.340	108	0
salt-free, ½ c, 124 gm	61	4	<1	11	2.23d	22	1.37	2	108	0
1 can, 482 gm	237	14	1	43	8.68d	86	5.33	1321	419	0
salt-free, 1 can, 482 gm	237	14	1	43	8.68d	86	5.33	10	419	0
cnd, seasoned, s & l, ½ c, 114 gm	57	4	<1	11	1.93	18	1.37	290	139	0
fz, ½ c, 72 gm	55	4	<1	10	2.74d	16	1.1	81	107	0
10 oz pkg, 284 gm	219	15	1	39	10.79d	61	4.33	319	424	0
ckd, dr, ½ c, 80 gm	63	4	<1	11	3.04d	19	1.26	70	134	0
10 oz pkg, 253 gm	198	13	<1	36	9.61d	61	3.98	221	424	0
raw, ½ c, 78 gm	63	4	<1	11	2.65d	19	1.15	4	190	0
PEA SPROUTS										
ckd, dr, 100 gm	118	7	<1	22	3.30d	26	1.67	3	268	0
raw, ½ c, 60 gm	77	5	<1	17	1.67	21	1.35	12	229	0
PEAS & CARROTS										
cnd, s & l, ½ c, 128 gm	48	3	<1	11	1.46	29	.97	332	128	0
salt-free, ½ c, 128 gm	48	3	<1	11	1.46	29	.97	5	128	0
fz, ½ c, 70 gm	37	2	<1	8	1.07	19	.76	55	136	0
10 oz pkg, 284 gm	150	10	1	32	4.34	75	3.1	225	551	0
fz, ckd, dr, ½ c, 80 gm	38	2	<1	8	1.11	18	.75	55	127	0
10 oz pkg, 278 gm	133	9	1	28	3.86	64	2.62	190	441	0
PEAS & ONIONS										
cnd, s & l, ½ c, 60 gm	30	2	<1	5	.74	10	.52	265	57	0

FOOD & DESCRIPTION MEASURE OR QUANTITY	CALORIES	PROTEIN (GM)	FAT (GM)	CARBO-HYDRATE (GM)	FIBER (GM)	CALCIUM (MG)	IRON (MG)	SODIUM (MG)	POTASSIUM (MG)	CHOLES-TEROL (MG)
fz, ½ c, 69 gm	48	3	<1	9	—	16	1.06	—	—	0
10 oz pkg, 284 gm	199	11	<1	38	—	65	4.37	—	—	0
fz, ckd, dr, ½ c, 90 gm	40	2	<1	8	—	13	.84	—	—	0
PEPEAO										
dried, ½ c, 12 gm	36	<1	<1	10	3.71	14	.74	8	85	0
raw, 1 piece, 6 gm	2	<1	0	<1	.13	1	.03	1	3	0
½ c, 50 gm	13	<1	<1	3	1.06	8	.28	5	21	0
PEPPER, HOT CHILI										
cnd, s & l, 1 pepper, 73 gm	18	<1	<1	4	.88	5	.37	—	—	0
½ c, 68 gm	17	<1	<1	4	.82	5	.34	—	—	0
raw, 1 pepper, 45 gm	18	<1	<1	4	.81	8	.54	3	153	0
½ c, chopped, 75 gm	30	2	<1	7	1.35	13	.9	5	255	0
PEPPERS, JALAPENO, cnd, s & l, chopped, ½ c, 68 gm	17	<1	<1	3	1.56	18	1.9	995	92	0
PEPPERS, SWEET										
ckd, dr, 1 pepper, 73 gm	13	<1	<1	3	.64	3	.64	2	94	0
½ c, 68 gm	12	<1	<1	3	.6	3	.6	1	88	0
cnd, s & l, ½ c, 70 gm	13	<1	<1	3	.56	28	.56	958	102	0
fz, ⅒ pkg, 28 gm	6	<1	<1	1	.28	3	.17	1	26	0
10 oz pkg, 284 gm	58	3	<1	13	2.84	26	1.76	15	259	0
fz, ckd, dr, 100 gm	18	<1	<1	4	.88	8	.52	4	72	0
freeze-dried, 1 tbsp, .4 gm	1	<1	<1	<1	.07	1	.04	1	13	0
¼ c, 1.6 gm	5	<1	<1	1	.26	2	.17	3	51	0
raw, 1 pepper, 74 gm	18	<1	<1	4	.81d	4	.94	2	144	0
½ c, chopped, 50 gm	12	<1	<1	3	.55d	3	.63	2	98	0
PIGEONPEAS										
ckd, dr, ½ c, 77 gm	86	5	1	15	2.23	27	1.02	3	351	0
raw, 10 seeds, 4 gm	5	<1	<1	<1	.11	2	.06	0	22	0
½ c, 77 gm	105	6	1	18	2.06	32	1.23	4	425	0
POI, ½ c, 120 gm	134	<1	<1	33	.65	19	1.06	14	220	0
POKEBERRY SHOOTS										
ckd, dr, ½ c, 82 gm	16	2	<1	3	—	43	.98	—	—	0
raw, ½ c, 80 gm	18	2	<1	3	—	42	1.36	—	—	0
POTATO										
baked										
flesh only, 1 potato, 156 gm	145	3	<1	34	.59	8	.55	8	610	0
½ c, 61 gm	57	1	<1	13	.23	3	.22	3	238	0
flesh & skin, 1 potato, 202 gm	220	5	<1	51	1.33	20	2.75	16	844	0
skin, from 1 potato, 58 gm	115	2	<1	27	1.32	20	4.08	12	332	0
boiled in skin										
flesh, ½ c, 78 gm	68	1	<1	16	.25	4	.24	3	295	0
1 potato, 136 gm	119	3	<1	27	.43	7	.42	6	515	0
skin, from 1 potato, 34 gm	27	1	<1	6	1.25	15	2.06	5	138	0
boiled without skin										
flesh, ½ c, 78 gm	67	1	<1	16	.29	6	.24	4	256	0
1 potato, 135 gm	116	2	<1	27	.51	10	.42	7	443	0
cnd										
dr, 1 potato, 35 gm	21	<1	<1	5	.09	2	.44	—	80	0
½ c, 90 gm	54	1	<1	12	.24	5	1.13	—	206	0
s & l, whole, 1 c, 300 gm	120	4	<1	26	.71	89	2.92	904	729	0
1 can, 454 gm	181	6	<1	39	1.07	134	4.41	1367	1103	0
fz										
french-fried										
cottage cut, heated										
10 strips, 50 gm	109	2	4	17	.36	5	.75	23	240	0
9 oz pkg, 198 gm	431	7	16	67	1.41	19	2.96	90	951	0
extruded, unheated										
10 strips, 65 gm	169	2	10	20	.37	6	.86	318	280	0
9 oz pkg, 255 gm	663	7	38	77	1.45	24	3.38	1248	1097	0
heated										
10 strips, 50 gm	163	2	9	19	.35	6	.83	307	270	0
9 oz pkg, 198 gm	645	7	37	75	1.39	24	3.29	1214	1067	0

FOOD & DESCRIPTION MEASURE OR QUANTITY	CALORIES	PROTEIN (GM)	FAT (GM)	CARBO- HYDRATE (GM)	FIBER (GM)	CALCIUM (MG)	IRON (MG)	SODIUM (MG)	POTASSIUM (MG)	CHOLES- TEROL (MG)
strips, unheated										
10 strips, 65 gm	107	2	4	16	.33	4	.64	15	219	0
9 oz pkg, 255 gm	419	7	16	64	1.29	17	2.5	58	861	0
heated in the oven										
10 strips, 50 gm	111	2	4	17	.34	4	.67	15	229	0
9 oz pkg, 198 gm	440	7	17	67	1.36	17	2.63	61	905	0
fried in vegetable oil										
10 strips, 50 gm	158	2	8	20	.37	10	.38	108	366	0
1 c, 57 gm	180	2	9	23	.42	11	.43	123	417	0
fried in vegetable & animal oils										
10 strips, 50 gm	158	2	8	20	.37	10	.38	108	366	6
1 c, 57 gm	180	2	9	23	.42	11	.43	123	417	7
hash browned										
½ c, 105 gm	86	2	<1	19	.37	11	1.03	23	299	0
12 oz pkg, 340 gm	280	7	2	60	1.19	34	3.34	76	968	0
prep										
½ c, 78 gm	170	2	9	22	.42	12	1.17	27	340	0
12 oz pkg, 205 gm	447	6	24	58	1.1	31	3.09	70	894	0
whole, ½ c, 91 gm	71	2	<1	16	.36	7	.91	22	314	0
ckd, dr, 100 gm	65	2	<1	15	.33	7	.84	20	287	0
mashed										
home prep, with whole milk & margarine, ½ c, 105 gm	111	2	4	18	.32	27	.28	309	303	2
with whole milk, ½ c, 105 gm	81	2	<1	18	.33	28	.29	318	314	2
dehyd, flakes, without milk, ½ c, 100 gm	361	8	1	83	3.1	35	1.06	137	662	0
prep with milk and butter, ½ c, 105 gm	118	2	6	16	.5	52	.23	349	245	15
dry granules without milk, ½ c, 22 gm	80	2	<1	18	.35	13	.4	24	199	0
prep with milk and butter, ½ c, 105 gm	137	2	7	18	—	57	4.27	358	223	18
dry granules with milk, ½ c, 100 gm	358	11	1	78	1.5	142	3.5	82	1848	0
prep, ½ c, 105 gm	83	2	2	14	.32	33	.63	246	352	0
microwaved in skin										
flesh, ½ c, 78 gm	78	2	<1	18	.32	4	.32	5	321	0
1 potato, 156 gm	156	3	<1	17	1.79	27	3.44	9	377	0
flesh & skin, 1 potato, 202 gm	212	5	<1	49	1.64	22	2.50	16	903	0
skin, from 1 potato, 58 gm	77	3	<1	17	1.79	27	3.44	9	377	0
raw, flesh, ½ c, 75 gm	59	2	<1	13	.33	5	.57	5	407	0
1 potato, 112 gm	88	2	<1	20	.49	8	.85	7	608	0
skin, from 1 potato, 38 gm	22	<1	<1	5	.68	11	1.23	4	157	0
POTATOES AU GRATIN										
dry mix										
⅙ pkg, 26 gm	82	2	<1	19	.24	81	.42	545	257	—
5½ oz pkg, 156 gm	490	14	6	116	1.45	485	2.54	3268	1544	—
dry mix, prep										
⅙ pkg, 137 gm	127	3	6	18	.23	114	.44	601	300	—
5½ oz pkg, 822 gm	764	19	34	106	1.4	682	2.63	3609	1800	—
home prep, ½ c, 122 gm	160	6	9	14	.33	146	.78	528	483	—
POTATO CHIPS										
10 chips, 20 gm	105	1	7	10	.28	5	.24	94	260	0
salt-free, 10 chips, 20 gm	105	1	7	10	.28	5	.24	2	260	0
1 oz, 28 gm	148	2	10	15	.40	7	.34	133	369	0
salt-free, 1 oz, 28 gm	148	2	10	15	.40	7	.34	2	369	0
from dried potatoes, 1 oz, 28 gm	164	2	13	12	.37	6	.43	216	312	0
POTATO FLOUR, ½ c, 90 gm	316	7	1	72	1.44	30	15.48	31	1429	0
POTATO PANCAKES, home										

FOOD & DESCRIPTION MEASURE OR QUANTITY	CALORIES	PROTEIN (GM)	FAT (GM)	CARBO-HYDRATE (GM)	FIBER (GM)	CALCIUM (MG)	IRON (MG)	SODIUM (MG)	POTASSIUM (MG)	CHOLES-TEROL (MG)
prep, 1 pancake, 76 gm	495	5	13	26	.50	21	1.21	388	538	0
POTATO PUFFS, fz, prep, 1 puff, 7 gm	16	<1	<1	2	.04	2	.11	52	27	0
½ c, 62 gm	138	2	7	19	.37	19	.97	462	236	0
POTATO SALAD, ½ c, 125 gm	179	3	10	14	.46	24	.81	661	317	86
POTATO STICKS, 1 oz, 28 gm	148	2	10	15	.34	5	.65	71	351	0
½ c, 18 gm	94	1	6	10	.22	3	.41	45	223	0
POTATOES O'BRIEN										
home prep, 1 c, 194 gm	157	5	2	30	.83	70	.91	421	516	7
fz										
unheated, 100 gm	76	2	<1	17	—	13	1.03	33	249	0
prep, 100 gm	204	2	13	22	—	20	.96	43	—	0
POTATOES, SCALLOPED										
home prep, ½ c, 122 gm	105	4	4	13	.36	70	.7	409	461	14
dry mix										
⅙ pkg, 26 gm	93	2	1	19	.37	16	.52	410	235	—
5½ oz pkg, 156 gm	558	12	7	115	2.23	97	3.14	2462	1412	—
prep										
⅙ pkg, 137 gm	127	3	6	18	.37	49	.52	467	278	—
5½ oz pkg, 822 gm	764	17	35	105	2.22	296	3.12	2803	1669	—
PUMPKIN										
ckd, dr, ½ c mashed, 122 gm	24	<1	<1	6	1.01	18	.7	2	281	0
cnd, ½ c, 122 gm	41	1	<1	10	1.97	32	1.7	6	251	0
raw, ½ c cubed, 58 gm	15	<1	<1	4	.64	12	.46	1	197	0
PUMPKIN FLOWERS										
ckd, dr, ½ c, 67 gm	10	<1	<1	2	.62	25	.59	4	71	0
raw										
1 flower, 2 gm	<1	<1	0	<1	.01	1	.01	0	3	0
1 c, 33 gm	5	<1	<1	1	.21	13	.23	2	57	0
PUMPKIN LEAVES										
ckd, dr, ½ c, 35 gm	7	<1	<1	1	.37	15	1.12	3	153	0
raw, ½ c, 20 gm	4	<1	<1	<1	.2	8	.44	2	87	0
PUMPKIN PIE MIX, cnd, ½ c, 135 gm	141	1	<1	36	1.61	49	1.43	280	186	0
PURSLANE										
ckd, dr, ½ c, 58 gm	10	<1	<1	2	.47	45	.45	26	283	0
raw										
1 plant, 3 gm	1	<1	0	<1	.02	2	.06	1	15	0
1 c, 43 gm	7	<1	<1	1	.34	28	.86	20	213	0
RADISH SPROUTS, raw, ½ c, 19 gm	8	<1	<1	<1	—	10	.16	1	16	0
RADISHES, raw, 10 radishes, 45 gm	7	<1	<1	2	.24	9	.13	11	104	0
½ c, sliced, 58 gm	10	<1	<1	2	.32	12	.17	14	134	0
RADISHES, ORIENTAL										
raw										
1 radish, 338 gm	62	2	<1	14	2.16	91	1.35	71	767	0
½ c, sliced, 44 gm	8	<1	<1	2	.28	12	.18	9	100	0
ckd, dr, ½ c, sliced, 74 gm	13	<1	<1	3	.36	12	.11	10	211	0
dried, ½ c, 58 gm	157	5	<1	37	4.85	365	3.9	161	2027	0
RADISHES, WHITE ICICLE, raw, ½ c, sliced, 50 gm	7	<1	<1	1	.35	14	.4	8	140	0
1 radish, 100 gm	14	1	<1	3	.70	27	.8	16	280	0
RUTABAGAS										
ckd, dr										
½ c cubed, 85 gm	29	<1	<1	7	.89	36	.4	15	244	0
½ c mashed, 120 gm	41	1	<1	9	1.25	50	.56	22	344	0
raw, ½ c cubed, 70 gm	25	<1	<1	6	.77	33	.36	14	236	0
SALSIFY										
ckd, dr, ½ c, sliced, 68 gm	46	2	<1	10	1.01	32	.37	11	192	0
raw, ½ c, sliced, 67 gm	55	2	<1	12	1.21	40	.47	13	255	0
SAUERKRAUT, cnd, s & l, ½ c, 118 gm	22	1	<1	5	1.26	36	1.73	780	201	0
SEAWEED										

FOOD & DESCRIPTION MEASURE OR QUANTITY	CALORIES	PROTEIN (GM)	FAT (GM)	CARBO-HYDRATE (GM)	FIBER (GM)	CALCIUM (MG)	IRON (MG)	SODIUM (MG)	POTASSIUM (MG)	CHOLES-TEROL (MG)
AGAR										
dried, 100 gm	306	6	<1	81	.71	625	21.4	102	1125	0
raw, 100 gm	26	<1	<1	7	.45	54	1.86	9	226	0
IRISHMOSS, raw, 100 gm	49	2	<1	12	—	72	8.9	67	63	0
KELP, raw, 100 gm	43	2	<1	10	1.33	168	2.85	233	89	0
LAVER, raw, 100 gm	35	6	<1	5	.27	70	1.8	48	356	0
SPIRULINA										
dried, 100 gm	290	57	8	24	3.64	—	28.5	1048	1363	0
raw, 100 gm	26	6	<1	2	.34	—	—	98	127	0
WAKAME, raw, 100 gm	45	3	<1	9	.54	150	2.18	872	50	0
SESBANIA FLOWERS										
steamed, ½ c, 52 gm	11	<1	<1	3	.81	11	.29	6	56	0
raw										
1 flower, 3 gm	1	<1	0	<1	.04	1	.02	0	5	0
½ c, 10 gm	3	<1	<1	<1	.15	2	.09	2	19	0
SHALLOTS										
freeze-dried										
1 tbsp, .9 gm	3	<1	0	<1	.04	2	.05	1	15	0
¼ c, 3.6 gm	13	<1	<1	3	.17	7	.22	2	59	0
raw, chopped, 1 tbsp, 10 gm	7	<1	<1	2	.07	4	.12	1	33	0
SOYBEANS, GREEN										
ckd, dr, ½ c, 90 gm	127	11	6	10	1.67	131	2.25	—	—	0
raw, ½ c, 128 gm	188	17	9	14	2.62	252	4.54	—	—	0
SOYBEAN SPROUTS										
raw										
10 sprouts, 10 gm	12	1	<1	1	.22	6	.2	1	46	0
½ c, 35 gm	45	5	2	4	.81	24	.74	5	169	0
steamed, ½ c, 47 gm	38	4	2	3	.92	28	.62	5	167	0
stir-fried, 100 gm	125	13	7	9	2.5	82	.4	—	567	0
SPINACH										
ckd, dr, ½ c, 90 gm	21	3	<1	3	1.71d	122	3.21	63	419	0
cnd, dr, salt-free, ½ c, 107 gm	25	3	<1	4	3.00d	135	2.46	29	370	0
cnd, s & l, ½ c, 117 gm	22	2	<1	3	1.05d	97	1.85	373	269	0
fz										
1 c, 156 gm	37	5	<1	6	3.28d	173	3.2	116	504	0
10 oz pkg, 284 gm	68	8	1	11	5.96d	314	5.83	211	918	0
ckd, dr										
½ c, 95 gm	27	3	<1	5	2.00d	139	1.44	82	283	0
10 oz pkg, 220 gm	63	7	<1	12	4.62d	321	3.34	190	656	0
raw, chopped										
½ c, 28 gm	6	<1	<1	<1	.90d	28	.76	22	156	0
10 oz pkg, 284 gm	46	6	<1	7	9.09d	202	5.52	160	1139	0
SQUASH, SUMMER										
ckd, dr, sliced, ½ c, 90 gm	18	<1	<1	4	.99d	24	.32	1	173	0
raw, sliced, ½ c, 65 gm	13	<1	<1	3	.72d	13	.3	1	126	0
CROOKNECK										
ckd, dr, sliced, ½ c, 90 gm	18	<1	<1	4	.99d	24	.32	1	173	0
cnd, dr, salt-free, sliced										
½ c, 108 gm	14	<1	<1	3	1.08d	13	.77	5	104	0
1 can, 241 gm	31	1	<1	7	2.41d	30	1.71	11	231	0
fz, sliced, ½ c, 65 gm	13	<1	<1	3	.78d	12	.31	3	136	0
ckd, dr, sliced, ½ c, 96 gm	24	1	<1	5	1.15d	19	.49	6	243	0
raw, sliced, ½ c, 65 gm	12	<1	<1	3	.72d	14	.31	1	138	0
SCALLOP										
ckd, dr										
½ c sliced, 90 gm	14	<1	<1	3	.43	14	.29	1	126	0
½ c mashed, 120 gm	19	1	<1	4	.57	19	.39	1	169	0
raw, sliced, ½ c, 65 gm	12	<1	<1	3	.36	12	.26	1	118	0
ZUCCHINI										
ckd, dr										
½ c sliced, 90 gm	14	<1	<1	4	.45	12	.32	2	228	0
½ c mashed, 120 gm	19	<1	<1	5	.6	16	.42	3	303	0
cnd, in tomato juice, ½ c,										

FOOD & DESCRIPTION MEASURE OR QUANTITY	CALORIES	PROTEIN (GM)	FAT (GM)	CARBO- HYDRATE (GM)	FIBER (GM)	CALCIUM (MG)	IRON (MG)	SODIUM (MG)	POTASSIUM (MG)	CHOLES- TEROL (MG)
114 gm	33	1	<1	8	.58	19	.78	427	312	0
fz, 10 oz pkg, 284 gm	48	3	<1	10	2.56d	52	1.46	7	619	0
ckd, dr ½ c, 112 gm	119	1	<1	4	.62	19	.54	2	218	0
raw, sliced, ½ c, 65 gm	9	<1	<1	2	.33d	10	.28	2	161	0
SQUASH, WINTER										
baked, ½ c cubed, 102 gm	39	<1	<1	9	1.22d	14	.33	1	445	0
raw, ½ c cubed, 58 gm	21	<1	<1	5	.81	18	.33	2	203	0
ACORN										
baked, ½ c cubed, 102 gm	57	1	<1	15	2	45	.95	4	446	0
ckd, mashed, ½ c, 122 gm	41	<1	<1	11	1.44	32	.68	3	321	0
raw										
½ c cubed, 70 gm	28	<1	<1	7	.98d	23	.49	3	243	0
1 squash, 431 gm	172	3	<1	45	6.03	142	3.02	14	1496	
BUTTERNUT										
bkd, ½ c cubed, 102 gm	41	<1	<1	11	1.28	42	.61	4	290	0
fz, 12 oz pkg, 340 gm	192	6	<1	49	4.22	97	2.99	8	722	0
boiled, mashed, ½ c, 120 gm	47	1	<1	12	1.04	23	.7	2	160	0
raw, ½ c cubed, 70 gm	32	<1	<1	8	.98	34	.49	3	246	0
HUBBARD										
baked, ½ c cubed, 102 gm	51	3	<1	11	1.77	17	.48	8	365	0
ckd, mashed, ½ c, 118 gm	35	2	<1	8	1.22	12	.33	6	252	0
raw, ½ c cubed, 5 gm	23	1	<1	5	.81	8	.23	4	186	0
SPAGHETTI										
ckd, dr, ½ c cubed, 78 gm	23	<1	<1	5	1.09	17	.26	14	91	0
raw, ½ c, cubed, 50 gm	17	<1	<1	3	.7	11	.16	9	54	0
SUCCOTASH										
ckd, dr, ½ c, 96 gm	111	5	<1	23	1.29	16	1.46	16	393	0
cnd, whole corn, s & l, ½ c, 128 gm	81	3	<1	18	.79	14	.68	283	209	0
cnd, with cream-style corn, ½ c, 133 gm	102	4	<1	23	1.71	15	.73	325	243	0
fz, ½ c, 78 gm	73	3	<1	16	.8	12	.73	35	230	0
10 oz pkg, 284 gm	265	12	3	57	2.92	45	2.66	128	836	0
ckd, dr, ½ c, 85 gm	79	4	<1	17	.87	13	.76	38	225	0
raw, 100 gm	99	5	1	20	2.60d	18	1.83	4	369	0
SWAMP CABBAGE										
ckd, dr, ½ c, 49 gm	10	1	<1	2	.42	26	.65	60	139	0
raw										
1 shoot, 13 gm	2	<1	<1	<1	.14	10	.22	15	41	0
½ c chopped, 28 gm	6	<1	<1	<1	.31	22	.47	32	87	0
SWEET POTATO LEAVES										
raw										
1 leaf, 16 gm	6	<1	<1	1	.19	6	.16	1	83	0
1 c chopped, 35 gm	12	<1	<1	2	.42	13	.35	3	181	0
steamed, ½ c, 32 gm	11	<1	<1	2	.42	8	.19	4	153	0
SWEET POTATOES										
baked in skin, flesh only										
½ c mashed, 100 gm	103	2	<1	24	1.80d	28	.45	10	348	0
1 potato, 114 gm	118	2	<1	28	2.05d	32	.52	12	397	0
boiled without skin										
½ c mashed, 164 gm	172	3	<1	40	1.39	35	.92	21	301	0
candied, 1 piece, 105 gm	144	<1	3	29	.41	27	1.19	73	198	0
cnd										
mashed, ½ c, 128 gm	129	3	<1	30	—	38	1.7	96	268	0
1 can, 496 gm	499	10	<1	115	—	151	6.61	372	1043	0
syrup pack										
dr, ½ c, 98 gm	106	1	<1	25	.55	16	.93	38	189	0
s & l, ½ c, 114 gm	101	1	<1	24	.53	18	.92	50	212	0
1 can, 638 gm	566	6	1	134	2.93	99	5.11	279	1183	0
vacuum-packed										
½ c mashed, 128 gm	117	2	<1	27	.90	28	1.13	68	398	0
½ c pieces, 100 gm	92	2	<1	21	.71	22	.89	54	313	0
fz, ½ c cubed, 88 gm	84	2	<1	20	1.50d	33	.47	6	321	0

FOOD & DESCRIPTION MEASURE OR QUANTITY	CALORIES	PROTEIN (GM)	FAT (GM)	CARBO-HYDRATE (GM)	FIBER (GM)	CALCIUM (MG)	IRON (MG)	SODIUM (MG)	POTASSIUM (MG)	CHOLES-TEROL (MG)
bkd, ½ c, 88 gm	88	2	<1	21	1.32d	31	.47	7	332	0
raw										
1 potato, 130 gm	136	2	<1	32	2.73d	29	.76	17	265	0
½ c cubed, 67 gm	72	1	<1	17	1.40d	16	.4	9	140	0
TARO, sliced										
ckd, ½ c, 66 gm	94	<1	<1	23	.57	12	.48	10	319	0
raw, ½ c, 52 gm	56	<1	<1	14	.42	22	.29	6	307	0
TARO CHIPS, 10 chips, 23 gm	110	<1	6	15	.27	10	.31	85	189	0
½ c, 12 gm	57	<1	3	8	.14	5	.16	44	99	0
TARO LEAVES										
raw, 1 leaf, 10 gm	4	<1	<1	<1	.2	11	.23	0	65	0
½ c, 14 gm	6	<1	<1	<1	.29	15	.32	<1	91	0
steamed, ½ c, 74 gm	18	2	<1	3	.4	63	.87	2	341	0
TARO SHOOTS, sliced										
ckd, ½ c, 70 gm	10	<1	<1	2	.38	9	.29	1	240	0
raw, ½ c, 43 gm	5	<1	<1	1	.25	5	.26	0	143	0
1 shoot, 83 gm	9	<1	<1	2	.48	10	.5	1	275	0
TARO, TAHITIAN, sliced										
ckd, ½ c, 68 gm	30	3	<1	5	1.55	101	1.06	37	423	0
raw, ½ c, 62 gm	25	2	<1	4	1.09	80	.81	31	376	0
TOMATO JUICE, cnd										
½ c, 120 gm	21	<1	<1	5	.48	10	.71	441	268	0
salt-free, ½ c, 120 gm	21	<1	<1	5	.48	10	.71	12	268	0
6 oz, 182 gm	32	1	<1	8	.72	16	1.06	658	400	0
salt-free, 6 oz, 182 gm	32	1	<1	8	.72	16	1.06	18	400	0
TOMATO PASTE, cnd										
½ c, 131 gm	110	5	1	25	1.25	46	3.91	1035	1221	0
salt-free, ½ c, 131 gm	110	5	1	25	1.25	46	3.91	86	1221	0
1 can, 170 gm	143	6	2	32	1.62	60	5.08	1343	1585	0
salt-free, 1 can, 170 gm	143	6	2	32	1.62	60	5.08	111	1585	0
TOMATO POWDER, 100 gm	302	13	<1	75	6.65	166	4.56	134	1927	0
TOMATO PUREE, cnd										
½ c, 125 gm	51	2	<1	13	1.03	19	1.16	499	526	0
salt-free, ½ c, 125 gm	51	2	<1	13	1.03	19	1.16	25	526	0
1 can, 822 gm	335	14	<1	82	6.74	122	7.61	3280	3454	0
salt-free, 1 can, 822 gm	335	14	<1	82	6.74	122	7.61	161	3454	0
TOMATO SAUCE, cnd										
salt added, ½ c, 122 gm	37	2	<1	9	.87	17	.94	738	452	0
Spanish-style										
½ c, 122 gm	40	2	<1	9	—	20	4.25	576	—	0
1 can, 425 gm	139	6	1	31	—	70	14.8	2006	—	0
with herbs & cheese										
½ c, 122 gm	72	3	2	13	—	45	1.06	—	—	0
1 can, 425 gm	252	9	8	44	—	156	3.68	—	—	0
with mushrooms, ½ c, 122 gm	42	2	<1	10	1.03	16	1.08	552	464	0
with onions, ½ c, 122 gm	52	2	<1	12	.98	20	1.13	672	504	0
with onions, green peppers, & celery										
½ c, 122 gm	50	1	<1	11	—	16	.92	—	—	0
1 can, 411 gm	168	4	3	36	—	55	3.10	—	—	0
with tomato tidbits										
½ c, 122 gm	39	2	<1	9	1.34	13	.83	18	455	0
1 can, 425 gm	135	6	2	30	4.68	44	2.91	64	1585	0
spaghetti sauce, cnd										
½ c, 125 gm	136	2	6	20	1.17	35	.81	618	479	0
15.5 oz jar, 439 gm	479	8	21	70	4.1	124	2.85	2179	1687	0
TOMATOES, GREEN, raw, 1 tomato, 123 gm	30	1	<1	6	.62	16	.63	16	251	0
TOMATOES, RED										
boiled, ½ c, 120 gm	30	1	<1	7	.92	10	.72	13	312	0
cnd										
in tomato juice, ½ c, 131 gm	34	<1	<1	8	.58	34	.61	285	329	0

FOOD & DESCRIPTION MEASURE OR QUANTITY	CALORIES	PROTEIN (GM)	FAT (GM)	CARBO- HYDRATE (GM)	FIBER (GM)	CALCIUM (MG)	IRON (MG)	SODIUM (MG)	POTASSIUM (MG)	CHOLES- TEROL (MG)
stewed, ½ c, 128 gm	34	1	<1	8	.54	42	.93	325	307	0
whole, ½ c, 120 gm	24	1	<1	5	.84d	32	.73	195	265	0
with green chilies, ½ c, 120 gm	18	<1	<1	4	.42	24	.31	481	129	0
raw, 1 tomato, 123 gm	24	1	<1	5	.98d	8	.59	10	254	0
½ c chopped, 90 gm	18	<1	<1	4	.72d	6	.43	8	186	0
stewed, ½ c, 51 gm	30	<1	1	5	.24	10	.39	187	85	0
TREE FERN, ckd										
1 frond, 31 gm	12	<1	<1	3	.19	2	.05	2	1	0
½ c chopped, 71 gm	28	<1	<1	8	.43	6	.11	3	3	0
TURNIPS										
ckd, dr										
½ c cubed, 78 gm	14	<1	<1	4	.55	18	.17	39	106	0
½ c mashed, 115 gm	21	<1	<1	6	.82	26	.26	58	156	0
fz, mashed										
⅓ 10 oz pkg, 94 gm	15	<1	<1	3	.43	21	.66	23	128	0
10 oz pkg, 284 gm	44	3	<1	8	1.3	64	1.99	71	388	0
fz, ckd, dr, 100 gm	23	2	<1	4	.68	32	.98	36	182	0
raw, ½ c cubed, 65 gm	18	<1	<1	4	.59	20	.2	44	124	0
TURNIP GREENS										
ckd, dr, ½ c chopped, 72 gm	15	<1	<1	3	.44	99	.57	21	146	0
cnd, s & l										
½ c, 117 gm	17	2	<1	3	.71	138	1.77	325	165	0
1 can, 425 gm	62	6	1	10	2.59	502	6.42	1179	600	0
fz, chopped										
½ c, 82 gm	18	2	<1	3	.62	97	1.23	9	151	0
10 oz pkg, 284 gm	62	7	<1	10	2.16	335	4.27	33	522	0
ckd, dr										
½ c, 82 gm	24	3	<1	4	.85	125	1.59	12	184	0
10 oz pkg, 220 gm	65	7	<1	11	2.27	335	4.27	33	494	0
raw, ½ c chopped, 28 gm	7	<1	<1	2	.22	53	.31	11	83	0
TURNIP GREENS & TURNIPS,										
fz, 10 oz pkg, 284 gm	59	7	<1	10	1.73	322	4.62	52	233	0
ckd, dr, 100 gm	17	2	<1	3	.52	91	1.33	15	62	0
VEGETABLE JUICE COCKTAIL,										
cnd										
½ c, 121 gm	22	<1	<1	6	.28	13	.51	442	234	0
6 oz, 182 gm	34	1	<1	8	.42	20	.77	664	351	0
VINESPINACH, raw, 100 gm	19	2	<1	3	.7	109	1.2	—	—	0
WATER CHESTNUTS, CHINESE										
cnd, s & l, 4 chestnuts, 28 gm	14	<1	<1	3	.16	1	.24	2	33	0
½ c sliced, 70 gm	35	<1	<1	9	.41	3	.61	6	82	0
raw										
4 chestnuts, 36 gm	38	<1	<1	9	.29	4	.22	5	210	0
½ c sliced, 62 gm	66	<1	<1	15	.50	7	.37	9	362	0
WATERCRESS, raw										
1 sprig, 2.5 gm	<1	<1	0	<1	.02	3	.01	1	8	0
½ c chopped, 17 gm	2	<1	<1	<1	.12	20	.03	7	56	0
WAXGOURD, cubed										
ckd, dr, ½ c, 87 gm	11	<1	<1	3	.44	16	.33	93	5	0
raw, ½ c, 66 gm	9	<1	<1	2	.40d	13	.27	74	4	0
WINGED BEAN LEAVES, raw, 100 gm	74	6	1	14	2.5	224	4	—	176	0
WINGED BEAN TUBER, raw, 100 gm	159	12	<1	28	7.4	30	2	—	—	0
WINGED BEANS										
ckd, dr, ½ c, 31 gm	12	2	<1	1	.43	19	.34	1	85	0
raw, 1 pod, 16 gm	8	1	<1	<1	.41	13	.24	1	36	0
½ c, 22 gm	11	2	<1	<1	.57	19	.33	1	49	0
YAM, cubed										
ckd, dr, bkd, ½ c, 68 gm	79	1	<1	19	—	9	.35	6	455	0
raw, ½ c, 75 gm	89	1	<1	21	—	12	.41	7	612	0
YAMBEAN [JICAMA]										

FOOD & DESCRIPTION MEASURE OR QUANTITY	CALORIES	PROTEIN (GM)	FAT (GM)	CARBO-HYDRATE (GM)	FIBER (GM)	CALCIUM (MG)	IRON (MG)	SODIUM (MG)	POTASSIUM (MG)	CHOLES-TEROL (MG)
ckd, dr, 100 gm	46	1	<1	10	1.12	16	.29	6	181	0
raw, 1 sliced, 6 gm	2	<1	<1	<1	.04	1	.04	0	11	0
1 c, sliced, 120 gm	49	2	<1	11	.84	18	.72	8	210	0
YARDLONG BEAN										
ckd, dr, 1 pod, 14 gm	7	<1	<1	1	.21	6	.14	1	41	0
½ c sliced, 52 gm	25	1	<1	5	.79	23	.51	2	151	0
raw, 1 pod, 12 gm	6	<1	<1	1	—	6	.06	0	29	0
½ c sliced, 46 gm	22	1	<1	4	—	23	.21	2	109	0

Van Camp

HOMINY										
GOLDEN, 8 oz	128	3	<1	28	.8	9	2.27	701	33	—
WITH RED & GREEN										
PEPPERS, 8 oz	129	3	<1	29	.7	10	1.46	685	46	—
WHITE, 8 oz	138	3	<1	30	.8	10	1.44	708	37	—

Welch

TOMATO JUICE, 6 oz	35	1	0	7	—	*	.36	550	400	—